DYP Survival Guide

For Post Graduate Dermatology Examinations

PART-1

DYP Survival Guide
For Post Graduate Dermatology Examinations
PART-1

Editors

Nitin Nadkarni MD DVD DDV
Professor, Department of Dermatology
Dr DY Patil Medical College and Research Centre
Nerul, Navi Mumbai, Maharashtra, India

Sharmila Patil MD DDV
Professor and Head, Department of Dermatology
Dr DY Patil Medical College and Research Centre
Nerul, Navi Mumbai, Maharashtra, India

Kiran Godse MD PhD FRCP (Glasgow)
Professor, Department of Dermatology
Dr DY Patil Medical College and Research Centre
Nerul, Navi Mumbai, Maharashtra, India

Assistant Editor

Aishwarya Rai MBBS
Senior Resident, Department of Dermatology
Dr DY Patil Medical College and Research Centre
Nerul, Navi Mumbai, Maharashtra, India

Foreword

Satish L Wadhwa MD DVD DDV FCPS

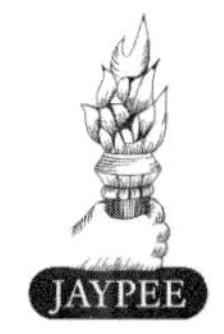

JAYPEE BROTHERS MEDICAL PUBLISHERS
The Health Sciences Publisher
New Delhi | London

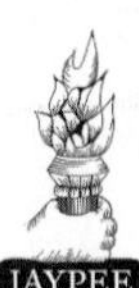

JAYPEE **Jaypee Brothers Medical Publishers (P) Ltd**

Headquarters

EMCA House, 23/23-B
Ansari Road, Daryaganj
New Delhi 110 002, India
Landline: +91-11-23272143, +91-11-23272703
+91-11-23282021, +91-11-23245672
e-mail: jaypee@jaypeebrothers.com

Corporate Office

4838/24, Ansari Road, Daryaganj
New Delhi 110 002, India
Phone: +91-11-43574357
Fax: +91-11-43574314
e-mail: jaypee@jaypeebrothers.com

Overseas Office

JP Medical Ltd.
83, Victoria Street, London
SW1H 0HW (UK)
Phone: +44-20 3170 8910
e-mail: info@jpmedpub.com

EU GPSR Authorised Representative

Logos Europe, 9 rue Nicolas Poussin
17000, La Rochelle, France
Phone: +33 (0) 6 67 93 73 78
e-mail: contact@logoseurope.eu

Website: www.jaypeebrothers.com
Website: www.jaypeedigital.com

Inquiries for bulk sales may be solicited at: jaypee@jaypeebrothers.com

DYP Survival Guide for Post Graduate Dermatology Examinations Part-1 / Nitin Nadkarni, Sharmila Patil, Kiran Godse

First Edition: 2014

Second Edition: **2023**

Reprint : 2024, 2025, **2026**

ISBN: 978-93-5465-981-2

Printed at: Sterling Graphics Pvt. Ltd.

Contributors

Manjyot Gautam MD (Dermatology)
Professor, Department of Dermatology
Dr DY Patil Medical College and Research Centre
Nerul, Navi Mumbai, Maharashtra, India

Parag Chaudhari MD (Dermatology)
Assistant Professor, Department of Dermatology
Dr DY Patil Medical College and Research Centre
Nerul, Navi Mumbai, Maharashtra, India

Swagat Waghmare MD (Dermatology)
Assistant Professor, Department of Dermatology
Dr DY Patil Medical College and Research Centre
Nerul, Navi Mumbai, Maharashtra, India

Vedant Ghuse MD (Dermatology)
Assistant Professor, Department of Dermatology
Dr DY Patil Medical College and Research Centre
Nerul, Navi Mumbai, Maharashtra, India

Aswathy Radhakrishnan MD (Dermatology)
Assistant Professor, Department of Dermatology
Dr DY Patil Medical College and Research Centre
Nerul, Navi Mumbai, Maharashtra, India

Notice

Foreword

It gives me great pleasure to introduce the second edition of *DYP Survival Guide for Post Graduate Dermatology Examinations*.

Success in exams is a matter of knowledge, hard work, presence of mind, and a proper attitude.

Ultimately, this requires not only hours and days of intense theoretical preparation but also practical presentation and rehearsals just as one would practice for a drama or a play.

I have the pleasure of knowing all the authors of this book personally. I have worked with Dr Nitin Nadkarni way back in 1984, when he was a lecturer in BYL Nair Hospital. Dr Kiran Godse has been my student in Nair for 3 years has proved to be hardworking and diligent. Dr Sharmila Patil has a very good name in Dermatology as Professor and Head of Dr DY Patil Hospital.

All these experienced teachers have come together and produced a book which gives a comprehensive approved to the practical examination at various levels in dermatology.

I am very sure this book will help in the understanding of the students of the various tips and tricks to succeed in the examination.

My best wishes to the authors and also to the readers of this book for a stress free and enjoyable exam experience.

Dr Satish L Wadhwa MD DVD DDV FCPS
Formerly Professor and Head
Department of Dermatology
Topiwala National Medical College and
BYL Nair Charitable Hospital
Professor of Dermatology
KJ Somaiya Medical College
Mumbai, Maharashtra, India

Preface to the Second Edition

Examinations are nothing but an ordeal, both for the students and (nowadays) for the examiners. It is a test of knowledge, competency, but above all, technique and temperament.

All of us have been candidates for examinations as well as examiners in our greater days. We have got (hopefully useful) experience which may help the unwary students to escape unscathed through the swampy fields of the viva and the practicals.

The aim of this book is to give advise on questions asked by examiners in tricky situations. We have divided the book into various sections including Long Cases, Short Cases, Spots and Viva. We have got feedback from various candidates who have emerged unscathed from the Post Graduate Examination in Dermatology.

In this book, we have tried to include recent information but omitted references for the sake of brevity. Some of these questions we have asked ourselves to the helpless candidates but we won't reveal which are our personal questions.

We gratefully acknowledge the help and cooperation by the Chancellor of the DY Patil Deemed-to-be-University Dr Vijay D Patil, as well as former Vice Chancellor of DY Patil University, Dr Shirish Patil, and our Dean Dr Rajiv Rao.

We would like to thank all the residents of our department who went through the proofs and also contributed to a few sections. We especially thank Bandhavi Muppalla, Aastha Menon, Edavally Sainath Reddy, Kazomi Shingala, Pooja Patel, Sahil Sethi, Jaisingh Solanki, Meghna Singh, Isheeta Manchandana and Sejal Kumar.

We would be remiss if we don't thank our own teachers, like Dr Satish L Wadhwa who wrote the Foreword, Dr Rui Fernandes and the doyens of Dermatology that are no more with us like Dr RG Valia and Dr VR Mehta. We are eternally grateful to all the teachers for have made us what we are today.

गुरु देवो भव!

We would also like to thank Torrent Pharmaceuticals and Jaypee Publishers for their help in distributing this book.

Nitin Nadkarni
Sharmila Patil
Kiran Godse

Preface to the First Edition

Examinations are a test, not only of knowledge and competence, but also of technique and temperament. Having (collectively) appeared for more than a dozen examinations, and having been examiners for a lot more, we are too aware of the foibles of examiners (including ourselves) and the follies of examinees. This book is a humble attempt to guide the unwary candidate through the pitfalls of dermatology postgraduate examinations at various levels (MD, DNB, DVD, FCPS, etc).

This book is intended for the examination-going candidate who is appearing (hopefully for the first and last time) for an important PG examination. We aim to give reliable advice on both simple and tricky questions asked by examiners in different clinical situations. We have divided the book into various sections, including long cases, short cases (and spots) as well as viva. We have collected common questions asked in the examinations, through "chatting up" our examiner friends, as well as quizzing candidates who have recently appeared for examinations (when their traumatic experiences are still fresh!). We have included lots of questions but have purposely omitted any references for the sake of brevity. Some of the questions (and the answers) reflect our own personal preferences and idiosyncrasies, but we think that is to be expected in a book of this nature.

We are extremely thankful to our teacher Dr Rui Fernandez, who went through the entire draft of this book and gave valuable suggestions, besides consenting to write the foreword. We gratefully acknowledge the help and cooperation given by the director of the Dr DY Patil Group of Hospitals, Mr Vijay D Patil as well as Dr Shirish Patil, dean of our hospital.

Lastly, we would like to thank the residents of our department, who helped with the nitty-gritty of preparing this book. Special mention must be made of Dr Aditya Mahajan and Dr Zubin Mandlewala, whose contribution to proofreading was invaluable. Many thanks to both of them.

Nitin Nadkarni
Sharmila Patil
Kiran Godse

Contents

1 Hints for Appearing in Examination

In our opinion, spots are the "make or break" section of the practicals. First impression is the last impression. Since the examiner encounters the candidate for the first time during the spots, what impression he gets will have a bearing on the final result. Hence it is imperative that a candidate does reasonably well in this section. If you get through the spots comfortably, for all practical purposes, you have passed!

IMPORTANT TIPS

1. The candidate should be well equipped. He should be wearing a clean (not tattered) apron with multiple pockets without any name on it. The pockets should contain: Pen, Magnifying lens (illuminated), Small Pen torch, Measuring tape, Glass slide, Pin, Cotton piece and a blotting paper (to demonstrate Auspitz sign). However, there is absolutely NO need to carry a mobile (actually, it is banned!).
2. Since most of the candidates are females, it is advisable (please accept our apologies if we sound sexist) that they should avoid the following items: Heavy makeup, streaked hair, painted and untrimmed nails, *mehendi*, jewellery, dangling earrings and prominent nose rings, pencil heels (they make a distracting noise). Both males and females should wear modest clothes. You should fit in the crowd and not stand out (for the wrong reasons!).
3. Greet the examiners respectfully during the first interaction. The following instructions are targeted towards the spots.
4. Make the patient comfortable and take his permission before examining
5. Keep both your hands free. All the accessories should be kept in the pocket s of your apron.
6. Look at the lesion through a magnifying glass (which you should carry and not borrow from the examiner!).
7. Touch the lesion. You cannot make out whether the lesion is flat or raised by just looking. If you suspect erythema or purpura, do a diascopy. If you suspect psoriasis, or pityriasis versicolor, do grattage. Remove the scale to see the "carpet tacking" if you suspect lupus erythematosus. Spots do not mean you take a cursory glance at the patient and give your diagnosis. Please do not put your hands

in your pockets or fold them. This implies you have already become a consultant (which you have not become yet).

8. If you want to look at other sites besides the one you are asked to see, ask the permission of the examiner before doing so.
9. If you want to ask questions of the patient, seek the permission of the examiner (some examiners do not allow it, but no harm in asking!).
10. If you suspect any infectious or neoplastic process, palpate the regional nodes (after taking permission).
11. As far as possible, give a single diagnosis, which is SIMPLE and COMMON. DON'T use short forms like LP, LE, PLE, (though they are used in this book for sake of brevity). Spots test your ability to come out with a single diagnosis. Try not to impress the examiner with "rare" diagnosis. We know of a candidate who came into trouble by giving a diagnosis of "porokeratosis palmaris et plantaris" when it was a case of palmoplantar warts. Remember, sounds of hoofs imply approaching horses and not zebras.
12. Usually the question asked is "How will you treat"? The examiner wants ONE treatment for the "SPECIFIC" patient sitting before you. Do not impress the examiner with a long list of possible treatments. First say the most common treatment you would give, with the dose (or concentration and frequency, in case of a topical medication) and duration. Also mention the general measures you would advice the patient (after talking about the specific treatment). If there is no satisfactory or specific treatment for a condition, say it, BUT immediately come out with SOME treatment or at least some general measures you would advice in case of an absolutely untreatable condition. Don't say, there is no satisfactory treatment and stop. In a series of cases of viral infections (warts, molluscum, etc.), a candidate said, there is no specific treatment at least 3 consecutive times, without saying anything more. The examiner asked him why he was trying to become a dermatologist when he didn't want to treat patients. Such embarrassing encounters should be avoided.

We will try to discuss the common "spots" which are kept in the examination. The list is NOT inclusive, since potentially any lesion on the skin (including a tattoo) is worthy of being kept as a spot!

In Case of Short and Long Cases, Following Hints will be Helpful

1. Write down all the history and examination findings as you would write in the ward notes. Many examiners look at them and criticize them.
2. Take a targeted history in short cases but a detailed history in long cases.
3. When time is limited, try to do the history taking and examination at the same time. This is especially true of leprosy cases, where you will be really pressed for time.
4. Give a specific yet detailed diagnosis. For example, in psoriasis, tell about the type of psoriasis, extent of involvement, stable or unstable, etc.
5. When examiner asks "how will you manage", start with investigations; when he asks how you will treat, start with the treatment.
6. Always talk about counseling and advice to the patient in the beginning of your treatment.
7. DON'T use trade names of medications. Always mention the dose or concentration of the medications even without being asked.
8. Do not forget to look at special sites—genitals, palms, soles, mouth, perianal areas, scalp, nails.
9. In case a patient refuses to allow you to examine a particular site, do not forcibly make him/her strip, but just inform the supervisor about it.
10. Ask for a tongue retractor, vaginal speculum but do not insist that the patient allows you to use it. In case of any controversy, inform the supervisor.

In general, please remember, DO NOT ARGUE WITH THE EXAMINERS. They are INFALLIBLE during the course of the examinations. As one of my respected teachers said, if the examiner says that the sun rises in the west, nod respectfully and say that it has been reported. Do not however, quote textbooks at the examiners to quote your point. Remember, there is such a thing as winning the battle and losing the war!

2 Signs in Dermatology

PAPULOSQUAMOUS DISORDERS

1. Auspitz Sign

- Seen in psoriasis vulgaris, actinic keratosis, Darier's disease.
- On scraping the scales of psoriasis with the pin head, the scales come off in layers and leave behind a moist membrane (membrane of Bulkeley). On removing this membrane, pin point bleeding is seen.
- NOT seen in palmoplantar psoriasis, scalp psoriasis, nail psoriasis or pustular psoriasis.

This sign is due to:

a. Parakeratosis—which helps in easy removal of scales
b. Suprapapillary thinned epidermis—represents Bulkeley's membrane
c. Dialatation and tortuosity of the capillaries in the dermal papillae

2. Antenna Sign

- Seen in keratosis pilaris
- Individual follicles showing glistening shine of keratin

3. Besnier's Sign or Scratch Sign also Called as Nail's Sign (Do not Use Your Own Nail to Do This)

- Seen in pityriasis versicolor. On scraping the lesion of pityriasis versicolor with a blunt end of pin head or edge of a slide, a previously non scaly lesion becomes scaly.
- Will NOT be see if the patient is partially treated or had a recent bath.

4. Grattage Sign

- Seen in lichen planus
- When lesions of active lichen planus are scratched with the head of the pin, a scale comes off and is followed by diffuse bleeding and pain.

5. Hanging Curtain Sign

- Seen in pityriasis rosea.
- When a lesion of pityriasis rosea is stretched, you can see a ring of scales at the periphery, attached on the outer surface and free on the inner surface.

6. Lake of Pus Sign

- Initially pustules are discrete, coalesce to form lake of pus
- Seen in acute pustular psoriasis

7. Nappes Claires Sign

- Seen in pityriasis rubra pilaris
- Islands of sparing in an area of diffuse erythema. The erythema is often described as salmon colored.

8. Pup-tent Sign

- Seen in nail lichen planus
- The nail splits in the center and then elevates. There is sloping on either side of this elevation.

9. Trailing Sign

- Seen in erythema annulare centrifugum.
- The scale is being the active border of the lesion

CONNECTIVE TISSUE DISORDERS

10. Barnette Sign

- Seen in scleroderma.
- On extending the neck, tightening and ridging of the neck with a visible and palpable platysma.

11. Carpet Tack Sign also Called Tin Tack Sign, Cat's Tongue Sign

- Seen in plaque type of discoid lupus erythematosus (DLE), seborrheic dermatitis, pemphigus foliaceus.
- When the scales of DLE is scraped off, the under surface of the scale shows small tacks and plugs.
- It is due to patulous hair follicles which contain parakeratotic cells protruding from the undersurface of the scale of DLE.
- It is NOT seen in systemic LE, or subacute LE.

12. Gottron's Papule

- Seen in dematomyositis
- Flat topped slightly erythematous papule seen on the knuckles

13. Gottron's Sign

- Scaly erythematous eruptions seen on the dorsum of the hands, metacarpophalangeal joints, and the proximal interphalangeal joints
  [*Note*: Erythema and scaling are seen on the knuckles are seen in dermatomyositis, but in between the knuckles in systemic lupus erythematosus (SLE)]

14. Holster Sign

- Seen in dermatomyositis.
- Confluent macular erythema seen on the lateral side of hip and the thighs.

15. Ingram's Sign

- Seen in systemic sclerosis
- Inability to retract the lower eyelid

16. Round Finger Pad Sign or Mizutani Sign

- Seen in systemic sclerosis
- The pink contour of the finger pads disappears and is replaced by a rounded fingerpad, especially on ring finger

17. Samitz Sign

- Seen in dermatomyositis
- Ragged cuticles seen at the base of the finger nails

18. Schuster's Sign

- Erythema and follicular plugging in the concha of ears seen in cutaneous lupus erythematosus (CLE)

19. Shawl Sign

- Seen in dermatomyositis.
- Confluent macular erythema seen on the neck and the shoulder

BLISTERING DISORDERS

20. Nikolsky Sign

- Giving tangential pressure on an apparently normal skin in a blistering disease causes separation of the epidermis.
- This can be elicited close to the active lesion (moderate disease) or away from the active lesions (severe disease). The former is sometimes called marginal Nikolsky sign while later is called direct Nikolsky sign.
- This sign is classically positive in all variants of pemphigus and staphylococcal scalded skin syndrome (SSSS).

21. Pseudo Nikolsky Sign

- Seen on erythematous areas, which on tangential pressure, peel off.
- Seen in erythema multiforme (EM), toxic epidermal necrosis (TEN), and pemphigoid group of disease.

22. Microscopic Nikolsky Sign

- The skin adjacent to the blister is given rotatory pressure with the head of the pencil and a biopsy is taken where acanthosis can be demonstrated.

23. Blister Spread Sign or Loot's Sign or Asboe-Hansen Sign

- It is the ability to enlarge a blister into the normal skin by applying mechanical pressure on the edge of the blister.
- Preferably outline the blister with a ball pen before doing this test.
- It is classically seen with pemphigus (mild) where the blister extension occurs at the sharp angle.
- Also seen in pemphigoid of various types, dermatitis herpetiformis, epidermolysis bullosa acquisita (EBA), porphyria, bullous SLE where the Nikolsky sign is negative but Asboe-Hansen is positive and the blister extension has a rounded border.

24. Hypopyon Sign

- Classically seen in bullous impetigo, or secondarily infected autoimmune vesicular conditions
- Pus accumulated in the lower half of the lesion, upper surface shows a fluid layer.

25. Pavithran's Nose Sign

- Seen in exfoliative dermatitis
- Complete absence to erythema and scaling of nose and perinatal areas

26. Pear's Sign

- Old blisters become flaccid and acquire a pear like shape
- Seen in pemphigus group of disease.

27. Sheklakov Sign

- It is the ability to extend the edge of a ruptured blister producing small limited erosions.
- Seen in pemphigoid group of disease, EM syndromes and TEN.

MISCELLANEOUS

28. Dermographism or Dermatographism

- It is an exaggerated triple response on scratching the skin with one's finger or with a special instrument (Frick's test).
- This is seen in chronic inducible urticaria (CIndU) (physical urticaria) and sometimes in spontaneous urticaria too.

29. Buschke–Ollendorff Sign (Deep Dermal Tenderness)

Classically described in secondary syphilis and also in cutaneous vasculitis. However, other conditions which show positive deep dermal tenderness are (a)neoplastic (b) inflammatory:

a. Neoplastic (mnemonic-**BLEND TAN EGG**)
    - **B:** Blue rubber bleb nevi
    - **L:** Leiomyoma
    - **E:** Eccrine spiradenoma
    - **N:** Neuroma
    - **D:** Dermatofibroma
    - **T:** Tufted angioma
    - **A:** Angiolipoma
    - **N:** Neurilemmoma
    - **E:** Endometrioma
    - **G:** Granular cell tumor
    - **G:** Glomus tumors

b. *Inflammatory*: Folliculitis, furunculosis, erythema nodosum, panniculitis—
  - The cause is perineurial and periappendegeal inflammation
  - Can be elicited by head of the pin pressing on the lesion

30. Button Hole Sign

- Seen in neurofibromatosis type I (NF-1)
- Due to a defect in the fascia, cutaneous neurofibromas can be pushed back into the subcutaneous tissue. On releasing the pressure, they reappear.
- It can also be found in dermatofibroma and anetoderma.

31. Breakfast, Lunch, Dinner Sign

- Seen in bed bugs (Cimex lectularius)
- Linear papules in groups 3–5 are seen on the skin.

32. Coudability Sign

- Seen in alopecia areata
- Hair that taper at the proximal end and when pushed inwards, kink or bend at the center

33. Darier's sign

- Seen in cutaneous mastocytosis.
- On rubbing or scratching a lesion of suspected mastocytosis, the lesion will show wheal formation with surrounding erythema.
- Should be distinguished from pseudo-Darier's sign—where contraction of underlying smooth muscle in response to rubbing causes a wheal like area seen in Becker's nevus or smooth muscle hamartoma.
- Darier's sign is NOT seen in telangiectasia macularis eruptiva perstans (TMEP)
- Multiple lesions should not be rubbed simultaneously as the patient can get flushing and hypotension.
- After eliciting Darier's sign in a lesion, the lesion becomes refractory for a few hours.
- Other causes of Darier's—leukemia cutis, lymphoma, hystiocytosis and juvenile xanthogranuloma.

34. Dory Flop Sign

- Seen in primary syphilis (syphilitic chancre)
- On retraction of the prepuce the ulcer flips out as the ulcer has an underlying button like induration

35. Frank's Sign

- Diagonal crease in the ear lobe
- Seen in atherosclerotic heart disease

36. Friar Tuck Sign

- Seen in trichotillomania.
- Hair in the center of the scalp are plucked out in the center while periphery is spared

37. Gorlin's Sign

- Seen in Ehlers-Danlos
- Ability of a patient to touch the tip of the nose with the tongue

38. Hair Collar Sign

- Seen in meningocele, encephalocele, ectopic neural tissue
- The lesion is surrounded by a collar of coarse hair

39. Hertoghe's Sign (also Called Queen Anne's Sign)

- Classically seen in atopic dermatitis
- Loss of lateral 1/3rd of eyebrows
- However, such loss is also seen in hypothyroidism, lepromatous leprosy, alopecia areata, trichotillomania, ulerythema ophryogenes

40. Hutchinson Sign

- Seen in herpes zoster
- Vesicles on the tip of the nose due to involvement of nasociliary branch of ophthalmic division of trigeminal nerve

41. Leser Treat Sign

- Sudden appearance of multiple (some pruritic) seborrheic keratosis due to an internal malignancy

42. Love's Sign

- Exact localization of a deep glomus tumor by presence of tenderness on pressing with a pin head

43. Matchbox Sign

- Seen in delusions of parasitosis
- Patient brings skin debris to the doctor in a box in the mistaken belief that it contains parasites

44. Patrick Yesudian Sign

- Palmar melanotic macules varying 2–4 mm in neurofibromatosis

45. Pastia's Sign

- Seen in streptococcal scarlet fever
- Linear petechial eruption in skin folds, especially in the antecubital fossa and axillary fold.

46. Prayers Sign

- Seen in diabetic microangiopathy and diabetic cheiroarthropathy
- Patient is unable to bring together his fingers completely. It indicates limited joint mobility due to glycosylation of collagen.

47. Reverse Prayers Sign

- Ability of the patient to oppose the back of hands together without any gap.
- Seen in Ehlers-Danlos syndrome

48. Thumb (Steinberg) Sign

- Extension of the thumb past the medical border of hand
- Seen in Ehlers-Danlos syndrome

49. Wrist Sign

- Overlapping of the thumb and little finger when encircling the opposite wrist
- Seen in Ehlers-Danlos syndrome

HISTOPATHOLOGICAL SIGNS

50. Hamberger Sign

- Histopathology of trichotillomania
- There is vertically oriented split of hair shafts and proteinaceous material and erythrocytes are present in the split resembling a hamburger within a bun.

51. Checkerboard Sign

- Seen in histopathology of pityriasis rubra pilaris (PRP)
- Alternating parakeratosis and orthokeratosis in both vertical and horizontal direction

LONG CASES

1 Anogenital Warts

Q. What are anogenital warts?

A. Anogenital warts are hyperplastic lesions of the genital and anorectal areas. They are one of the common sexually transmitted infections (STIs) and are caused by human papillomavirus (HPV) which has various strains.

Q. What are the genital lesion associated with HPV infections?

A. 1. Condyloma acuminata—HPV6, 11
2. Non-condylomatous lesions and/or intraepithelial neoplasia (mucocutaneous warts of various types)—mainly HPV6, 11, 16, 18, 31, 33, 40, 42, 43, etc.
3. Buschke-Löwenstein tumor—HPV6, 11

Genital HPV are divided into:

1. Low oncogenic risk: HPV types 6, 11, 42, 43 and 44
2. Intermediate risk: HPV types-31, 33 and 35
3. High risk: HPV types16, 18, 45 and 46

Q. What are the types clinical types of genital warts?

A. 1. Condyloma acuminata
2. Keratotic warts
3. Macular warts
4. Papular warts
5. Bowenoid papulosis
6. Giant condyloma acuminata

Q. How anogenital warts are transmitted?

A. ADULTS:

- Mostly sexual transmission.
- Autoinoculation: From cutaneous warts. Though transmission from genital to cutaneous is very rare.

B. CHILDREN—warts can be acquired from the mother's genital tract at delivery

- These are most common in the larynx
- Infection in older children may be indicator of sexual abuse.
- Rarely nonsexual transmission due to sharing of articles or sleeping in the same bed can occur

Q. Describe the clinical appearance of condyloma acuminata (acuminate warts).

A.
- (condyloma = knuckle, acuminatum = pointed; plural condylomata acuminata).
- The lesions are found on frenulum, glans, urethral meatus, prepuce (in males) labia minora, introitus, vagina, cervix (in females).
- Anal and perianal area (both)
- They are soft, pink, pedunculated papilliferous masses (cauliflower like) with finger-like peduncles and an irregular surface. It does not bleed on touch.
- A paper can be slid under the condylomata acuminate unlike condyloma lata (Paper test).

Q. What is giant condyloma acuminata?

A.
- Giant condyloma acuminata, also known as Buschke–Löwenstein tumor is a rare, aggressive wart-like growth
- It is a large cauliflower-like growth which is locally aggressive in spreading
- Most commonly occurs in uncircumcised male
- May spread deeply into the underlying benign tissue but rarely metastasises.
- It is classified as a verrucous carcinoma.

Q. Describe the clinical appearance of flat warts.

A. Flat warts are slightly raised, with an undulating wavy surface. Located anywhere on genital epithelium.

Q. Describe about papular warts.

A. Pedunculated, dome-shaped, or hemispherical masses are located in fully keratinized epithelium.

Q. Describe about macular variants.

A. Macular lesions are usually found on mucosal surfaces, a grayish-white color being most common manifestation. There may be slight vascularity seen.

Q. Describe the histopathology of warts.

A. Most characteristic feature is presence of koilocytes which are epithelial cells with perinuclear vacuolization. There is peripheral rim of condensed cytoplasm with hyperchromatic and large nucleus.

Q. Is there a simple test to diagnose warts?

A. Yes. Acetoacetic white test.

A gauze is soaked in glacial acetic acid test is applied, the affected areas becomes white. This is often used for inconspicuous macular lesions.

Q. What is the treatment of external genital warts?

A. There are multiple options of treatment for genital warts.

Divided into: (A) Patient applied treatment and (B) Physician applied treatment.

A. Patient applied treatment are:

1. Imiquimod 5% cream applied to affected areas thrice weekly at night for a maximum period of 16 weeks. It gives a clearance of 40–50% but a recurrence rate of 15%.
   Imiquimod upregulates toll-like receptors and topically activates immune enhancers that stimulate production of interferon and other cytokines.
2. Podophyllotoxin 0.5%: It is applied twice daily to the affected areas, for 3 days in a week with a 4-day gap in between therapies. The clearance rate is higher 50–70%. Recurrence rate is lower 4–10%.
3. Sinecatechins (extract of green tea leaves) to make a 15% ointment: 0.5 cm is applied on each wart thrice daily. Maximum period of 16 weeks. Clearance rate is about 15%. Recurrence rate is 5%

B. Physician applied:

1. Cryotherapy: Liquid nitrogen on an applicator or cryoprobe is applied on affected lesions until a halo appears around each lesions. About 2–3 cycles can be given at a time. Treatment is done weekly. Clearance rate is high 75%. Recurrence is high 50%.
2. Electrosurgery: The lesion is excised at the base and an electric current on coagulation mode is applied. Clearance is 95%. Recurrence is 20%.
3. Podophylline resin 25% in a compound tincture of benzoin: Apply < 0.5 mL to about 10 cm^2 of the wart. Wash off after 1–4 hours. Weekly applications for 6 weeks is needed. Clearance is 60%. Recurrence is 25%.
4. Trichloroacetic acid (TCA) or bichloroacetic acid (BCA) 1–3 times a week application. Repeat as many times. Clearance is 75%. Recurrence is 35%
5. Surgical excision—under local anesthesia. Clearance is 90%. Recurrence is 25%

Q. Discuss podophylline.

A.
- Podophyllotoxin is a purified extract of *Podophyllum peltatum* plant or *Podophyllum indicum*. The toxin, podophyllotoxin is a cellular toxin which binds to cellular microtubules, inhibits mitotic division at metaphase, and induces necrosis of warts that is 3–5 days after administration.
- Podofilox solution (0.5%) or 0.15% cream should be applied carefully after covering surrounding areas with petroleum jelly. It should be washed off after 1–4 hours.
- It cannot be used in pregnancy as it is a abortifacient.
- Excessive application can cause irritation.
- Podophylline can also cause renal toxicity
- If applied to plantar warts it can cause peripheral neuropathy and gangrene (called podophylline foot). It is always better in suspicious cases to take a biopsy before applying podophylline because it can cause dyskeratosis and normal mitotic figures (podophylline cells).

To avoid the possibility of complications associated with systemic absorption and toxicity, two guidelines should be followed:

1. Application should be limited to <0.5 mL of podophylline or an area of <10 cm^2 of warts per session, and
2. The area to which treatment is administered should not contain any open lesions or wounds. The preparation should be thoroughly washed off 1–4 hours after application to reduce local irritation.

Q. What is the choice of treatment of condylomata acuminate in pregnancy?

A.
- The best treatment of choice in pregnancy is TCA (trichloroacetic acid) which in not abortifacient or teratogenic.
- Electrodessication can also be done but pregnancy tissues are vascular and a lot of bleeding can occur.
- Cesarean section can be considered if the condylomas are very large and like to obstruct labour.

Q. How do you treat urethral condylomas?

A.
- Can be treated with imiquimod OR Surgery OR Lasers maybe used.
- Chemical cauterization is not recommended due to risk of stricture.

Q. Discuss the prevention of warts.

A. 1. One feasible option is male circumcision. It reduces the prevalence of HPV by at least 35%. It also decreases transmission of HIV and herpes simplex

2. Vaccination

Two HPV vaccines are available, both of which offer protection against the HPV types that cause 70% of cervical cancers (i.e., types 16 and 18):

1. Nonavalent vaccine (Gardasil 9) protects against types 6, 11, 16, 18, 31, 33, 45, 52, 58. It contains HPV L1 specific DNA fragments. It should be administered intramuscular over the deltoid or anterolateral area of thigh. A 2-dose schedule can be given 6–12 months apart for individuals from 9 to 14 years of age. A 3-dose schedule can be given at 0, 2 and 6 months for females between 15 to 45 years of age.
2. The quadrivalent vaccine (Gardasil) protects against the types 6, 11, 16 and 18 of HPV. Contains recombinant virus-like particles from the L1 proteins of HPV6, 11, 16, and 18. Recommended to be given to females between 9 and 26 years. Given in arm muscle in three doses. Dose 1, Dose 2: 1 month after dose 1, Dose 3: 6 months after dose 1.
3. The bivalent vaccine (Cervarix) protects against HPV16, 18 types. Contains L1 protein of viral capsid. Vaccine has no live virus so do not infect the patient. Given to females between 10–45 years of age.

2 Chancroid

Q. What is chancroid also known as?

A. Soft chancre, soft sore, ulcus molle.

Q. What is causative organism for chancroid?

A. *Haemophilus ducreyi* [Ducrey bacillus].

Q. Describe the biology of organism.

A. Gram-negative, coccobacillus which grows best in low concentration of oxygen. May be arranged in small groups or whorls or in parallel chains giving a 'school of fish', 'rail-road track' appearance.

Q. What is the incidence of acquiring infection after a single sexual exposure?

A. 60%.

Q. What is the incubation period of chancroid?

A. 3–10 days.

Q. Does carrier state exists for the disease?

A. Asymptomatic carrier seems to be rare.

Q. Classical lesions of chancroid (bubo).

A. *Site*:

- In males—glans, coronal sulcus, around the urethra
- In females—fourchette and labia minor
- Number of ulcers—multiple
- Evolution—lesion starts as a papule, which ulcerates to form small (usually <5 mm) superficial ulcer with necrotic floor that bleeds on touch. The edge of ulcer is undermined, it has a soft base, tender, usually heals without scarring.
- Within about 10 days patient develops lymphadenopathy which is mostly unilateral, involves only a single lymph node, it is soft, unilocular
- Overlying skin is stretched and erythematous.
- The center become suppurative, ruptures with a single sinus which discharge and often at site of rupture a giant chancroid can develop.

Q. Differential of bubo.

A. A bubo is an inflammatory suppurative lymphadenitis. It can mostly occur in the groins but can also occur in the axilla and neck. The causes can be sexually transmitted and nonsexually transmitted:

The sexually transmitted causes are:

1. Chancroid
2. Lymphogranuloma venereum (LGV)
3. Donovanosis—pseudobubo, i.e., it involves only the subcutaneous tissues and not lymph nodes

The nonsexual causes are:

1. Septic (pyogenic) bubo
2. Filariasis
3. Plague
4. Tularemia
5. Cat scratch disease

Note: The enlargement of lymph node in syphilis is not a bubo since there is no suppuration. In tuberculosis, malignancy and lymphomas as well it is not a bubo. However, these four can be considered as a differential of bubo.

Q. What are the types of chancroid?

A.
1. Classical chancroid
2. Dwarf chancroid
3. Giant chancroid
4. Herpetiform chancroid
5. Follicular chancroid
6. Transient chancroid
7. Phagedenic chancroid
8. Pseudogranuloma inguinale
9. Serpiginous chancroid
10. Mixed chancroid (chancroid with syphilis)

Q. What is chancroidal ulcer?

A.
- They are lesions resembling chancroid but caused by anaerobic organisms (Vincent's bacilli) are called chancroidal ulcers.
- Tender, non indurated single or multiple large ulcers with no lymphadenopathy

Q. Why is chancroid more common in males?

A. Occlusive environment provided by the prepuce makes men more susceptible to the infection. Also there is underreporting in women because of asymptomatic and hidden nature of lesions in women.

Q. What are the risk factors for chancroid?

A.
- Lack of circumcision
- Poor hygiene
- Unprotected sexual activity
- Males having sex with male
- Migratory population
- Alcoholism
- Drug abuse
- Human immunodeficiency virus (HIV)

Chancroid predisposes to HIV and vice versa

Q. Diagnostic methods of chancroid.

A.
1. Smear from edge of ulcer. It has 50% sensitivity.
2. Culture—with chocolate agar admixed with metal calf serum
3. PCR—highly sensitive
4. Histopathology—shows three zones:
   a. Upper zone: Necrotic debris, fibrin and neutrophils.
   b. Middle zone: Area of granulation tissue.
   c. Deepest zone: Lymphocytes and plasma cells.

Q. What are the differential diagnosis of chancroid?

A.
- Herpes genitalis
- Syphilis
- Donovanosis
- Early lesions of LGV

Non sexual lesions of the genitals—mnemonic is **FAINT PB**
- **F :** Fixed drug eruption
- **A :** Allergic irritant contact dermatitis
- **I :** Infections with pyogenic or tuberculous organisms
- **N :** Neoplasms
- **T :** Trauma
- **P :** Psoriasis/Pseudoepitheliomatous keratotic and micaceous balanitis
- **B :** Other causes of balanitis—candidiasis and Zoon's balanitis

Q. What are the complications of chancroid?

A.
1. Balanoposthitis
2. Phagedena—anaerobic mutilating necrosis of genital and perigenital area due to superinfection with anaerobic bacilli
3. Phimosis
4. Paraphimosis
5. Bubo with giant chancroid
6. Rarely, autoinoculation to other areas.

Q. What is the work up of chancroid?

A.
- REMEMBER in every case of genital ulcer, swab needs to be subjected to Dark-ground illumination for *Treponema pallidum* for 3 consecutive days before being declared negative.
- Venereal Disease Research Laboratories (VDRL) and enzyme-linked immunosorbent assay (ELISA) test should be done in all cases.

Q. What is the treatment of chancroid?

A. Recommended regimens:

Tablet Azithromycin 1 g orally in a single dose

OR

Injection Ceftriaxone 500 mg intramuscularly (IM) in a single dose

OR

Tablet Ciprofloxacin 500 mg orally twice a day for 3 days*

OR

Tablet Erythromycin base 500 mg orally QID for 7 days

Q. When will you follow-up this patient?

A.
- Bubo starts showing improvement in 3 days and heals substantially by the 7th day.
- If no suppuration, lymphadenopathy will subside in 2 weeks. If there is suppuration the bubo has to be aspirated with a wide bore needle from a non dependant area using Z technique
- Sometimes, incision and drainage has to be done

Q. Even after treatment, if patient doesn't improve. What can be the reasons?

A.
1. Incorrect diagnosis
2. Noncompliance
3. Coinfection with another sexually transmitted disease (STD)
4. HIV coinfection
5. *Haemophilus ducreyi* strain resistant to the prescribed antimicrobial

---

*Ciprofloxacin is contraindicated in pregnant and lactating women.

3 Dermatomyositis (Wegener's Disease)

Name/Age/Sex/Occupation/Marital status/Residing at/Hailing from ...

CHIEF COMPLAINTS

Cutaneous symptoms:

- Swelling around the eyes with discoloration since ...
- Rash over shoulders or thighs since ...
- Asymptomatic pink purple lesions on elbows or knuckles since ...
- Rash exacerbating on exposure to sunlight since ...

Muscular symptoms:

- H/O difficulty from standing to sitting position/getting up from the chair/climbing a staircase/combing hair
- H/O recurrent episodes of pain in shoulders and hips (bursitis often precedes myositis)
- H/O difficulty swallowing/burning pain in epigastrium/regurgitation
- H/O difficulty in speech

For overlap syndrome:

- H/O dry lips/mouth
- H/O tightness of skin, discoloration of fingers/difficulty opening of mouth
- H/O oral ulcerations
- H/O psychiatric symptoms

Systemic symptoms:

- H/O palpitations/chest pain/cough/difficulty breathing
- H/O unexplained weight loss (malignancy)
- H/O difficulty in breathing
- H/O respiratory and gastrointestinal (GI) infections in children

Past history:

- H/O tuberculosis/diabetes mellitus/hypertension (TB/DM/HTN)/cardiac problems/drug allergies
- H/O medical/surgical illnesses

Menstrual/Obstetric history in females:

- Quality of life (QOL)—interference of disease in professional/social/personal/sexual life

General examination:

- General condition
- Patient is conscious, cooperative well oriented to time space and person
- Pulse/blood pressure (BP)/respiratory rate (RR)
- Body mass index (BMI)
- Pallor/cyanosis/icterus/lymphadeopathy/edema feet

Cutaneous features:

- Face—periorbital edema with violaceous hue (heliotrope bloating; heliotrope = sun)
- Facial telangiectasia
- Sunburn and suntan sign—the former refers to erythema on convexities of face in active stage of DM, while the latter refers to pigmentation and scaling on same area when DM is inactive
- Poikiloderma on nails
- Shawl sign—poikiloderma over the upper back and shoulders
- Holster sign (belt used for carrying guns)—poikiloderma, erythema and pigmentation over hips and thighs

Hands:

- Mechanic's sign: Hyperkeratotic fissured plaques of the fingers
- Hiker's feet: Hyperkeratotic plaques over the soles
- Gottron's papules: Violaceous papules and plaques on knuckles/ elbow/knee/ankle
- Gottron's sign: Violaceous erythema on the dorm of the hands the interdigital spaces of dorsa of hands.
- Keining sign: Periungual telangiectasia, small hemorrhagic infarcts
- Inverse Gottron's sign: Hyperkeratotic papules on interphalangeal creases (palmar aspect)
- Flagellate erythema—parallel lines of erythema on trunk as if the patient is beaten
- Nails—ragged cuticles (Samitz's sign)
- Calcinosis cutis—firm yellow/flesh colored nodules-plaques on bony prominences

For muscles:

- Examine power of large group of muscles.
- Look for tenderness, nodules, and check for reflexes.

Systemic examination:

- Respiratory sounds (RS)—crepts/rhonchi
- Cardiovascular system (CVS)—S1, S2 normal

Q. What is your diagnosis?

A. Dermatomyositis (DMS)—Adult/Juvenile—Muscle group involved—Respiratory involvement—Any overlap features.

Q. Why do you diagnose it as dermatomyositis?

A. This is dermatomyositis because of the characteristic rash, Gottron's papules, and the proximal muscle weakness.

Q. Any radiological finding specific for dermatomyositis?

A. X-ray shows opacities in muscle as calcinosis but no terminal resorption of tips of digits (contrast with systemic sclerosis).

Q. How do you differentiate it from other myopathies?

A.
- Dermatomyositis is more rapid in onset and remissions are frequent.
- Erythrocyte sedimentation rate (ESR)—moderately increased
- Serum globulin may be elevated

Q. What are the potential markers of malignancy in DMS?

A.
- Elevated ESR
- Lack of Raynaud's phenomenon
- Lack of interstitial lung disease (ILD)
- Cutaneous necrosis.
- Fever malaise and weight loss

Q. What are markers for overlap syndrome?

A. Antinuclear antibody (ANA), anti-double-stranded deoxyribonucleic acid (anti-dsDNA), anti-ribonucleoprotein (anti-RNP) +ve.

Q. Heliotrope sign is seen in how many patients?

A.
- Seen in 30–60%
- The violaceous hue is because of mucin deposition and edema, the dermal vasculature goes deep. Deoxygenation of blood through abnormal dermal vasculature causes tyndall effect resulting in a violaceous hue.

Q. What are Mechanic's hands?

A. Hyperkeratotic, scaly, fissured hands, hyperpigmentation of radial and palmar aspect of fingers. Correlates with antisynthetase antibodies.

Q. How will you differentiate rash of systemic lupus erythematosus (SLE) from that of DMS?

A. Presence of pruritus and rash involves of nasolabial fold is suggestive of DMS. The rash is often associated with edema. The rash pieces muscle weakness in 50% cases.

Q. Nail changes of DM.

A. 1. Ragged cuticles (Samitz sign)
2. Diffuse redness and shininess of nails
3. On capillaroscopy—dilated, tortuous irregular capillary loops of nail folds
4. Raynaud's phenomenon

Q. Less common signs of DM.

A. 1. Spreading erythema and persisting edema of face and neck or limbs
2. Flagellate lesions
3. Urticarial lesions
4. Bullous lesions
5. Erythema nodosum
6. Erythema multiforme
7. Hypertrichosis
8. Pityriasis rubra pilaris (PRP) like follicular papule (Wong-type of DM)
9. Exfoliative dermatitis
10. Ichthyosis
11. Lived reticular
12. Anasarca (ominous sign)

Q. How is childhood DMS different from adult?

A.
- Calcinosis is very common in childhood and often universal
- Lipodystrophy is common in juvenile
- Malignancy common—in adults
- Hypertrichosis and vasculitis—children

Q. What are the variants of juvenile DMS?

A.
- Banker type—poor prognosis, widespread, vasculitis of various organs
- Brunsting type—better prognosis, slow course, no vasculitis, calcinosis, responsive to steroids

Q. What are the other causes of calcinosis?

A.
- Systemic sclerosis
- Mixed connective tissue disease (MCTD)
- SLE

Q. What is sclerodermatomyositis?

A. This is an overlap syndrome in which cutaneous changes of scleroderma and DMS are associated with myositis and homogenous nucleolar pattern of ANA but there is no visceral involvement and changes of DMS are transient.

Q. What is the effect of dermatomyositis on pregnancy and vice versa?

A.
- Half of pregnancies end prematurely
- Overall fetal loss is over 50%
- Fertility is impaired
- Pregnancy exacerbates disease in 50% and remission in 20%
- Pregnancy should be planned at time of remission and patient monitored atleast every month. If possible treatment to be confined to oral steroids.

Q. How many percentage of patients with dermatomyositis have Raynaud's phenomenon positive?

A. 10%.

Q. Which are the infections associated with DMS?

A.
- Staphylococcal osteomyelitis and arthritis
- Streptococcal infection (antigenic homology)
- Toxoplasmosis
- Parvovirus B19
- Coxsackie B virus

Q. Which are the autoantibodies found in DMS?

A.
- Jo-1 and PL-12 antibodies are directed against tRNA synthetase enzymes and are associated with interstitial pulmonary fibrosis.
- Anti-Mi-2—associated with acute onset and V neck sign
- Anti-SRP—associated with sever myositis
- Anti-MDA5—severe cutaneous involvement, myopathic type of DMS

Q. Which muscles are most affected?

A. Proximal striated muscles of lower limb and upper limb, especially extensors, limb girdle, pharynx and tongue.

Q. How will you investigate?

A.
- Diagnostic investigations are:
  1. Muscle enzymes like CPK-MB, aldolase, lactate dehydrogenase
  2. Positive ANA test
  3. Anti-Jo, anti-MI2, anti-tRNA synthetase, anti-SRP (signal recognition particle)
  4. Electromyography (EMG)
  5. MRI scan
  6. Muscle biopsy

- Prognostic investigations are:
    1. CBC—leukocytosis/anemia
    2. ESR and CRP may be increased
    3. LFT
    4. CT scan of lungs (HRCT)
    5. ECG, if indicated

Q. How will you investigate a patient suspected to have malignancy?

A.
- Look for weight loss, pallor, malaise, lymphadenopathy
- Palpate breast, abdomen
- Examine chest
- Do PR examination
- Hemoglobin, ESR, CRP, urine for hematuria, stool for occult blood, chest X-ray, USG of abdomen
- CT scan abdomen/pelvis/thorax
- Mammography
- Tumor specific markers [prostate-specific antigen (PSA), carcinoembryonic antigen (CEA)]

Q. What are the noninvasive tests for DMS?

A.
- MRI scan
- EMG
- Muscle enzymes

Q. How will you assess disease activity?

A.
1. Serial estimation of the 24 hours urinary creatine
2. MRI of the muscles

Q. Differential diagnosis of puffy heliotrope eyelids.

A.
1. Emotional stress
2. Dermatomyositis
3. Systemic sclerosis
4. Erysipelas
5. Aldosteronism
6. SLE
7. Angioedema
8. Erythema multiforme

Q. What are D/Ds of myositis?

A.
1. DMS
2. Systemic sclerosis

Q. What are the lung manifestations of DMS?

A. Interstitial lung disease, pulmonary hypertension, pneumonia, interstitial pneumonitis, pneumothorax, infections, malignancy, Bronchiolitis obliterans.

Q. What are the cardiac manifestations?

A. • Conduction abnormalities
- Pericarditis
- Pericardial effusion
- Arrhythmias
- Congestive cardiac failure (CCF)

Q. How is the eye involved in DMS?

A. • Conjunctival edema
- Nystagmus
- Iritis
- Retinitis
- Cotton wool spots
- Optic atrophy
- Extraocular muscle imbalance.

Q. What is the significance of arthritis in dermatomyositis?

A. Patients with arthritis frequently have pulmonary involvement.

Q. Which are the malignancies associated with dermatomyositis?

A. • Ovary, breast in females
- Lung and testes in males
- Stomach, rectum, kidney in both

Q. What are the factors associated with malignancy?

A. 1. Older age
2. Constitutional symptoms—fever weight loss malaise
3. Rapid onset of dermatomyositis
4. Lack of Raynaud's phenomenon
5. Grossly elevated ESR
6. Presence of leukocytoclastic vasculitis
7. Frequent relapse

Q. How many percentage of DMS have malignancy?

A. About 20% and in 40% it precedes neoplasm.

Q. What is Wong type DMS?

A. • DM associated with PRP like lesions where there are follicular hyperkeratotic papule in a liner fashion on the neck, back and bony prominences
- It may have a higher incidence of neoplasms

Q. Antisynthetase syndrome.

A. • It is the most common cause of overlap symptoms there are myositis specific antibodies directed against tRNA synthesize

- Multiple autoantibodies are described where anti-Jo1 is most common (histidine tRNA synthetases).
- It is often associated with ILD, mechanic hands

Q. What are the findings in skin biopsy?

A.
- Early: Interface dermatitis, dermal edema, there is usually some lymphocytic infiltrate, mucin deposits in the dermis is suggestive of dermatomyositis.
- Late: Thickening homogenization and sclerosis of the collagen, thickening of the walls of cutaneous blood vessels. Atrophic epidermis and increased basal layer pigmentation.

Q. How will you differentiate skin biopsy of lupus erythematosus (LE) and DMS?

A. Dermatomyositis shows less eccrine coil involvement and fewer vertical columns of lymphocytes in fibrous tract remnants.

Q. Why is MRI of muscle preferred to a muscle biopsy?

A.
- The muscle involvement in dermatomyositis is not uniform so histology may often be falsely negative so MRI is preferred.
- MRI changes are more uniform
- Also MRI is a non invasive procedure.

Q. From which muscle should a biopsy be taken?

A.
1. From a muscle that is tender, clinically weak.
2. Muscle identified as abnormal on EMG/MRI scan.
3. Nonatrophic usually deltoid, trapezius and quadriceps are chosen for biopsy

Q. What are the histopathological findings of a muscle biopsy in dermatomyositis?

A.
- Loss of transverse striations, hyalinization of the sarcoplasm, increase in sarcolemmal nuclei
- Later the fragmentation and vacuolar degeneration of fibers takes place.
- Intimal thickening of blood vessels may be seen.

Q. Why is ulceration and hemorrhage seen in skin/fat/GI tract?

A. Intimal proliferation and thrombosis of arteries and arterioles of skin, fat and alimentary tract causes ulceration.

Q. Which are the systems involved in dermatomyositis?

A. Lungs, GI tract, kidney, heart/vasculitis of cerebral vessels.

Q. Which are the drugs which can cause dermatomyositis?

A. Statins, tamoxifen (for breast cancer), oral progesterone, penicillamine.

Q. What are the diseases associated with DMS?

A.
- Thymoma
- Hyperthyroidism
- Aplastic anemia
- Hemolytic anemia
- Genaralized amyloidosis
- Multiple myeloma

Q. How do you treat DMS?

A.
1. General measures:
   - Avoidance of sunlight, alcohol, smoking, stress
   - Advice rest during acute phase
   - 1st line therapies—topical steroids and antimalarials
   - 2nd line therapies are—systemic corticosteroid with or without immunomodulators
   - 3rd line—IV immunoglobulins
   - 4th line—rituximab
2. Other drugs that have been used—oral tacrolimus, sirolimus, thalidomide, dapsone
3. Refractory DM has been treated with plasmapheresis, autologous stem cell transplantation and total body irradiation

Q. How do you treat a rash of DM?

A.
1. Topical steroids/topical calcineurin inhibitors
2. Antimalarials—HCQS 6.5 mg/kg/day

Q. How is the response?

A. The muscle weakness and response occurs in 1–2 weeks of high dose steroids.

Q. What are the causes of weakness in DM?

A.
- Myopathy because of DMS
- Steroid induced myopathy
- Electrolyte myopathy (hypokalemia)

Q. How to differentiate myopathy of DM and steroid induced?

A.
- Steroid myopathy—normal muscle enzymes but may have increased urinary creatine levels
- It takes about 4 months to recover after the stopping of steroids

Q. What are the adverse prognostic factors?

A.
- Acute pulmonary infiltration
- Dysphagia
- Cutaneous necrosis—increase in age

Q. What are the good prognostic factors?

A.
- Calcinosis
- Amyopathic DMS

Q. What is the cause of GI hemorrhagic in DM?

A. The disease itself and steroid intake.

Q. Cause of osteoporosis in DM.

A.
1. Immobility
2. Steroid

Q. Cause of death in DM.

A.
1. Respiratory involvement
2. Heart failure
3. Malnutrition due to difficulty in swallowing
4. Underlying malignancies
5. Side effects of steroids

Q. Treatment for DM.

A. Tablet prednisolone 1–2 mg/kg/day gradually reduced as a patient improves clinically and biochemically, maintenance dose 5–50 mg/day for months/years
- 1 g methylprednisolone IV for 3 days (if patient doesn't respond to the above therapy)
- Azathioprine 1.5–3 mg/kg/day in divided doses
- Oral methotrexate 7.5–15 mg weekly

Q. What if patient does not respond to above line of treatment?

A.
- Cyclosporine 5 mg/kg/day
- Cyclophosphamide 100 mg/day or as pulsed IV
- Intravenous immunoglobulin (IVIG) 1 mg/kg for 2 days every month for 4–6 months
- Infliximab (directed against tumor necrosis factor)
- Rituximab (directed against CD20 molecule on B lymphocyte precursors)
- Plasmapheresis
- Dapsone, pentoxifylline and aspirin (for digital ischemia) have also been tried with some success
- Octreotide (for constipation)
- Bisphosphonates and calcium supplements (for osteoporosis)
- Aluminium oxide and diltiazem (for calcinosis)
- Physiotherapy

4 Erythroderma

Name/Age/Sex/Occupation/Residing at ... /Hailing from ... /Marital status

Chief complaints:

- Redness and scaling all over body since ...
- How did the rash start?
- Sudden or gradual onset?
- Diffuse from beginning or initially discrete?
- Itching since ...
- Initially non itchy and later itchy points to lymphoma
- Fever since ...
- Edema feet since ...
- Any H/O a previous skin disease
- Patient could have psoriasis—lesions common on extensor aspect, could have PRP—lesions common on knuckles, could have eczema—initially more common on legs
- H/O recently starting drugs—herbal medication?
- Has patient had any allergic reaction to drugs in the past?
- Has the patient got H/O photosensitivity?
- Has patient got systemic symptoms—shivering, thirst, symptoms of underlying, malignancy (weight loss, cough, hemoptysis)?
- Patient was apparently alright ... back when he developed generalized redness and scaling on ... scalp/limbs/trunk
- Started from ... Spread to ... involve ... (was it cephalocaudal)
- Gradual/sudden onset, rapidly increased/slow spread
- Starting from ... cephalocaudal spread? Any areas which were spared. (On enquiry)

How are the scales?

- Type/color/amount (whether handful scales or bed is full of scales)
- Any associated pruritus/burning/dryness/irritation
- Any preexisting red raised scaly lesions on the body/scalp?
- (psoriasis/PRP/atopic eczema) H/O joint pains (psoriasis)
- Personal/familial H/O bronchial asthma/allergic rhinitis/allergic conjunctivitis

- H/O preceding itchy raised red lesions in the flexural areas (atopic dermatitis)
- H/O any areas that are spared (pityriasis rubra pilaris) H/O photosensitivity (photodermatitis)
- H/O any exposure to airborne allergens (congress grass)
- H/O weight loss (malignancy)
- H/O sexual exposure (HIV erythroderma/secondary syphilis/ Reiter's disease)
- H/O discharge per urethral/diarrhea (Reiter's syndrome)
- H/O any preceding drug taken for any other condition
- H/O fluid filled lesions in the past (pemphigus foliaceus)
- H/O proximal muscle weakness/rash around the eyes or photo-exposed areas/malar rash with photosensitivity [dermatomyositis (DM) and systemic lupus erythematosus (SLE)]
- H/O varicose veins/oozing itchy lesions on the legs H/O edema feet (stasis dermatitis)
- H/O fever/illness before episode
- H/O acute stress
- Winter exacerbation/Summer remission
- H/O overtreatment with any topical medication application/ withdrawal of any medicines or drugs (steroids)
- H/O any systemic medications prior to scaling/phototherapy
- H/O response to previous treatment
- H/O shivering/feeling of extremes of temperature (cold)/malaise and bodyache
- H/O shortness of breath or easy fatiguability (cardiac failure)
- H/O increased thirst (dehydration)
- H/O oliguria, edema feet (renal)
- H/O diarrhea (dermatopathic enteropathy)
- H/O cramps in hands and feet (electrolyte imbalance–hypokalemia)
- H/O pigmentation, itching/watering (ectropion) if longstanding

Past history:

- Past history similar episode
- Past history of illness in detail
- H/O TB/DM/HTN/IHD/Drug allergy/medical/surgical illness

Family history of similar complaints:

- Especially in neonatal and infantile erythroderma
- In adults if family members have got tinea or scabies

Personal history:
- H/O addictions/sleep/bowel/bladder/appetite
- Menstrual history
- Sexual exposure/HIV

Quality of life (work/personal)—general examination:
- Patients general condition fair
- Conscious, cooperative, well oriented in time place and person
- Pallor/clubbing/icterus/edema (feet/face)/lymphadenopathy
- TPR/BP (tachycardia/poikilothermic/hypotension/tachypnea)
- Signs of dehydration (dry tongue)
- Respiratory rate

Local examination:
- Distribution: Face/Trunk/Neck/Upper limb/Lower limb

Arrangement:
- Morphology
- Face/Trunk/Neck/Upper limb/Lower limb
- Diffuse erythema and scaling
- Amount-minimal/copious
- Color (White/Brown)
- Types of scale (adherent)
- Shedding/Adherent
- More in flexures?
- Any oozing?
- Any raw areas?
- Look for tenderness (TEN, secondary syphilis) and Nikolsky's sign for pemphigus foliaceus.
- Sparing of nose (Pavithran's sign)
- Eyes-normal/ectropion/entropion
- Oral mucosa
- Hair loss (axillary/inguinal)/Palms and soles involvement
- Nails
- Genital mucosa
- Lymph nodes (to rule out secondary syphilis/malignancy)
- Bones and joints (psoriatic arthritis)
- Testicular sensation
- Gynecomastia—liver failure

Systemic examination:

- RS—air entry is bilaterally equal (AEBE), no added sounds
- CVS-S1, S2 normal/increased JVP/tachycardia/high output cardiac failure
- CNS:
  - P/A—soft/no T/G/R, hepatosplenomegaly
  - P/R
  - P/V

Impression:

- Erythroderma secondary to ... with ... metabolic complications.

Systemic complications of erythroderma:

1. Hypercatabolic—daily protein loss is increased by 30% in psoriatic erythroderma and 10–15% in others
   This can cause loss of muscle mass and peripheral edema
2. Thermoregulation—since 25–30% of the blood supply is diverted to the skin (normal is 1%), the heart has to pump to supply blood to essential organs. Patient can develop high output cardiac failure
3. Adult respiratory distress syndrome
4. Capillary leak syndrome
5. Widespread endothelial activation results to increase level of adhesion molecules leading to immunosuppression.
6. Due to compromized barrier function, the bacteria can enter the skin and can cause a cytokine reaction which will aggravate the erythroderma
7. Patients of erythroderma often develop dermatopathic lymphadenopathy that can resemble malignancy
8. Patient can develop renal insufficiency
9. Endocrine effects–due to testicular atrophy can leave to hair loss from axilla and groins and also gynecomastia
10. Patients may develop subclinical enteropathy (diagnosed only by intestinal biopsy) or clinical enteropathy presenting with frothy stools and diagnosed by stool analysis
11. Lack of blood supply to brain can precipitate psychosis which can also be caused by steroids or strokes.

Q. What is the definition of erythroderma?

A. It is defined as generalized scaling and erythema of skin that involves more than 90% of the body surface. By 70–90% body involvement is called suberythroderma.

Q. Is erythroderma is the same as exfoliative dermatitis?

A. Yes. Not commonly used.

Q. What are the various causes of erythroderma?

A.

Preexisting skin disease	***Infections***	***Systemic diseases***	***Hematologic diseases***	***Malignancy***
Plaque and other types of psoriasis	Chronic or steroid treated dermato-phytosis	Lupus erythe-matosus	Cutaneous T-cell lymphoma and Sézary syndrome	Genitourinary tract malignancy in females
Pityriasis rubra pilaris	Crusted and hyperkera-totic scabies	Dermato-myositis	B-cell lymphoma	Prostate cancer in males
Contact dermatitis with dissemination	Toxoplas-mosis	Sarcoidosis	Anaplastic large cell lymphoma	Thyroid, lung, rectum, stomach malignancy
Seborrheic dermatitis with dissemination	HIV	Leiner's disease	Leukemia of various types	
Neuroderma-titis with dis-semination		Severe com-bined immu-nodeficiency (SCID)	Pseudolym-phoma	
Actinic dermatitis with dissemination		Graft-versus-host disease	Myelodys-plasia	
Pemphigus foliaceus				
Hailey–Hailey disease				
Drug reaction				

Q. Classify neonatal and infantile erythroderma.

A. [I] On the basis of duration—acute and chronic

[II] On basis of age of onset:

1. Congenital—ichthyosis, primary immunodeficiency syndrome (PIDS)
2. Neonatal (<28 days)—ichthyosis, PIDS, nutritional disorders, dermatophytosis
3. Infantile erythroderma (28 days to 1 year)— PIDS, seborrheic dermatitis, psoriasis, PRP, atopic dermatitis, ichthyosis, drug induced, nutritional, cutaneous T-cell lymphoma, DM, Pemphigus foliaceus, sarcoidosis

[III] On the basis of cause:

Infections	*Ichthyosis*	*Immuno-deficiency*	*Drug induced*	*Nutritional/ Metabolic*	*Eczematous*	*Papulo-squamous disorders*	*Malignan-cies*	*Autoimmune*
SSSS	Non bullous erythroderma	Omenn's syndrome	Boric acid toxicity	Acrodermatitis enteropathica	Infantile seborrhoeic dermatitis	Psoriasis	Mastocy-tosis	Dermato-myositis
TSS	Bullous ichthyosis erythroderma	SCID	Ceftrixone	Biotin metabolism disorder	Atopic dermatitis	PRP	Cutaneous T-cell lymphoma	Sarcoidosis
Candidiasis	Harlequin ichthyosis	GVHD	Vancomycin	Essential fatty acid deficiency				Pemphigus foliaceus
Congenital herpes simplex	Netherton syndrome	DiGeorge syndrome	Ampicillin/ Amoxicillin	Cystic fibrosis				
Dermato-phytosis	Sjögren–Larsson syndrome		Antiepileptics	Leiner's disease				
Norwegian scabies	KID syndrome		Sulfonamides					
Scarlet fever	Lipid storage disorder		Cimetidine					

(GVHD: graft-versus-host disease; KID: Keratitis–ichthyosis–deafness; PRP: pityriasis rubra pilaris; SCID: severe combined immunodeficiency; SSSS: Staphylococcal scalded skin syndrome; TSS: toxic shock syndrome)

Q. Clues to specific diagnosis of erythroderma.

A. 1. Psoriasis—typical psoriasiform plaques maybe seen, pustular lesions, nail changes and arthritis may be present
2. PRP—initially there is a seborrheic like rash which become generalized after sun exposure, patient has a salmon (bright pink) color erythema and islands of sparing (nappes claires)
3. Palmoplantar keratoderma and nail changes are seen
4. Pemphigus foliaceus—superficial erosions resembling impetigo as well as collarettes of scales.
5. Pemphigoid—tense blisters with erythroderma
6. Dermatomyositis—typical signs of DM as described in previous chapter
7. Sézary syndrome—may show erythema and thickening of the skin (leonine facies)
8. Sarcoidosis—ichthyosis like lesions, apple jelly lesions and keratotic follicular
9. Drug rash—acute onset, H/O drug ingestion in past 6 weeks. Patient appears toxic and may develop fever, hepato-splenomegaly, lymphadenopathy, edema. Sterile pustules may be present.

   Phenytoin can cause erythroderma resembling Sézary syndrome called pseudolymphoma.

   Sometimes, initially the disease is thought to be due to phenytoin and turns out to be an actual lymphoma. This is called pseudopseudolymphoma.

Q. What is Leiner's disease (erythroderma desquativum/red scaly syndrome)?

A.
- It is an erythroderma in infants due to C5 deficiency
- Patient has failure to thrive, low birth weight, diarrhea, seborrheic dermatitis like lesions, erythroderma, painful lesions and joint pain.

Q. What suggests diagnosis of phytophotodermatitis?

A. Involvement of retroauricular area, upper eyelids, submental area suggests phytodermatits.

Q. What suggests involvement of photodermatitis?

A.
- Sparing of area behind auricle the Wilkinson's triangle
- Sparing of upper eyelid and submental area—suggest photo-dermatitis
- If all are involved—suggests airborne contact dermatitis

Q. What is Alibert–Bazin disease?

A. Classical mycosis fungoides (MF) characterized by typical evolution of patches, plaques and tumors or a clinicopathologic variants showing a similar clinical course.

Q. What is Woringer–Kolopp?

A. It is the localized involvement of in MF, also called Woringer-Kolopp disease or Pagetoid reticulosis.

Q. What is erythrodermic cutaneous T-cell lymphoma (E-CTCL)?

A. A variant of CTCL characterized by chronic erythroderma and three types:

1. Sézary syndrome (SS): Presence of erythroderma, lymphadenopathy, and abnormal Sézary cells—large lymphocytes with convoluted cerebriform nucleus

   May include lymphadenopathy, hepatosplenomegaly, palmoplantar keratoderma, ectropion, and alopecia, may develop de novo (classic SS), but may be preceded by a prodrome of pruritus alone or nonspecific dermatitis.
2. E-MF: E-CTCL lacking the blood findings of SS that develops during the course of disease in patients with otherwise clinically typical MF.
3. E-CTCL, not otherwise specified (NOS): Cases of E-CTCL that fail to fulfill the diagnostic criteria for either E-MF or SS as defined above.

Q. What is Pseudo-CTCL erythroderma?

A. Benign non-malignant inflammatory conditions characterized by erythroderma and other findings that suggest the diagnosis of CTCL. Typically this refers to compatible skin histology, but occasionally cases of actinic reticuloid and certain drug eruptions may have increased numbers of Sézary cells in the blood that are suspected to be SS.

Q. What are the types of SS?

A. Small cell variant of SS when more than 80% of the Sézary cells are small (<12 μm in diameter) and large-cell variant of SS when 20% or more of the Sézary cells are very large (>14 μm in diameter). mixed cell variant is the one with an intermediate picture.

Q. What is Russell–Jones and Whittaker criteria for SS?

A. Erythroderma, compatible skin histology, more than 5% circulating mononuclear cells (Sézary cells), and evidence of a peripheral blood T-cell clone by means of at least one of the following specific tests:

- Very large Sézary cells (>14 μm diameter)
- Cytogenetic evidence of an abnormal clone

- Loss of pan-T cell antigen by immunophenotyping
- T-cell clone shown by Southern blot or PCR analysis

Q. What is a Sézary cell?

A. An atypical lymphocyte with a moderately to highly in folded or grooved nucleus (e.g., a cerebriform lymphocyte with nuclear contour index of 6.5 or more). Sézary cells, mycosis cells, Lutzner cells, and cerebriform lymphocytes are synonymous terms.

Q. Where do you get Lutzner cells?

A. Lutzner cells are atypical lymphocytes which are confined to the epidermis. It is seen in:

- They are seen in localized variant of MF
- Can also be seen in:
    - Actinic reticuloid,
    - Pseudolymphomatous drug eruptions
    - Severe eczemas

Q. Types of Sézary cell.

A.
A. Small Sézary cell: <12 μm diameter
B. Large Sézary cell: >12 μm diameter
C. Very large Sézary cell with cell diameter >14 μm is clearly neoplastic

Q. What are the drugs commonly causing erythroderma?

A. The list is very long. We can learn it alphabetically:

- Allopurinol
- Barbiturates
- Carbamazepine
- Dapsone
- Ephedrine
- Fluorouracil
- Gentamicin
- Hypoglycemic agents like sulfonylureas
- Isoniazid
- Lithium
- Minocycline
- Muscle relaxants
- Nifedipine
- NSAIDs (nonsteroidal anti-inflammatory drugs)
- Omeprazole
- Phenytoin
- Quinidine
- Retinoids

- Sulfasalazine
- Terbinafine
- Vancomycin (red man syndrome)
- Zidovudine

Q. How do you differentiate acute from chronic erythroderma?

A.
- In acute stages scales: Duration of the disease, presence of systemic symptoms are more evident. Scales are large and moist.
- Scales are small and dry in chronic erythroderma

Q. An erythrodermic patient with lymphadenopathy and hepatosplenomegaly, What are the possibilities?

A.
- Particularly in association with liver dysfunction and fever, may suggest a drug hypersensitivity syndrome or malignancy.

Note: This can occur with drug hypersensitive syndrome, lymphomas, and even in nonmalignant erythroderma there can be lymphadenopathy (lipomelanotic reticulosis)

Q. Enumerate different types of scales seen in various disorders.

A.
1. Micaceous scales (silvery)—Psoriasis
2. Branny (furfuraceous) scales—Pityriasis versicolor
3. Collarette of scales—Pityriasis rosea
4. Wafer like scale (oblaten)—Pityriasis lichenoides chronica
5. Thick fish like scales—Ichthyosis
6. Double edged scale—Netherton syndrome (ichthyosis linearis circumflexa)
7. Carpet tack like scales—Discoid lupus erythematosus
8. Trailing sign—Erythema annulare centrifugum (EAC)
9. Meuserung scales—Ichthyosis bullosa
10. Greasy scales—Seborrheic dermatits
11. Ichthyosiform scale—Ichthyosis vulgaris
12. Cornflake scale—Pemphigus foliaceus

Q. Why does one lose hair in erythroderma?

A. In erythroderma:
1. Scales are lost which results in sulfur loss. (Sulfur is needed for hail and nail growth), hence it is attributed in half of the cases
2. Hypoproteinemia due to loss of scales
3. Hyperestrogenemia which causes loss axillary and pubic hair

Q. What are Shoreline nails?

A. Transverse line of discontinuity proceeded by transverse leukonychia seen in drug-induced erythroderma.

Q. What is ebonization?

A. Shiny nails because of constant rubbing.

Q. What are the other nail changes?

A. Nails become thickened, ridged and may be shed. Beau's lines may be seen.

Q. Why does one get edema in this condition?

A.
1. Vasodilatation resulting in fluid permeability seeping from intracellular compartment to the extracellular compartment
2. Proteins are lost in scales resulting in hypoalbuminemia (hypoproteinemia), decreased lymphatic drainage
3. High-output cardiac failure
4. Inflammation resulting from primary skin disease

Q. What is the normal requirement of proteins?

A. 1 g/kg/day.

Q. How many scales and proteins are lost in erythroderma?

A.
- 20–30 g of scales (9 $g/m^2/day$)
- 200 g protein per day.

Q. Why hypoalbuminemia?

A.
- Decreased synthesis of albumin
- Increased metabolism of albumin
- Proteins lost in scales
- Decreased liver function
- Increased catabolism of albumin

Q. Why does a patient get gynecomastia?

A. Decreased perfusion in liver results in increased estrogens which causes gynecomastia.

Q. What is the rule of 9? (Rule of Wallace)

A.
- Face: 9%
- Upper limbs: 9 + 9%
- Chest: 18%
- Back: 18%
- Lower limbs: 18 + 18%
- Genitals: 1%

Q. Most common cause of erythroderma in India.

A. Psoriasis and phytophotodermatitis.

Q. Which drugs can precipitate erythroderma in psoriasis?

A.
- Overtreatment with tar, salicylic acid, dithranol
- Phototherapy in unstable psoriasis

- Gold, lithium, cimetidine, carbamazepine, omeprazole, hydantoin
- Beta blockers

Q. In AIDS when does a patient get erythroderma?

A. Seroconversion phase and late stage.

Q. What are the characteristics of pemphigus foliaceus?

A. Cornflake like scale crusts in seborrheic distribution usually without mucosal involvement and mousy odor.

Q. What is Norwegian scabies?

A. Hyperkeratotic crusted lesions all over the body in immunocompromized and debilitated people. Subungual hyperkeratosis of the nails.

Q. What are the causes of collodion baby?

A.
1. Nonbullous ichthyosiform erythroderma
2. Lamellar icthyosis
3. Sjögren–Larsson syndrome
4. Conradi–Hünermann syndrome
5. Netherton syndrome

Q. What is postoperative erythroderma?

A. A type of graft-versus-host disease following surgery along with blood transfusion, is marked by erythroderma, fever, pancytopenia, hepatic insufficiency and diarrhea and may be fatal.

Q. What is pavithran sign?

A. Sparing of nose and paranasal areas in erythroderma.

Q. What is dermatopathic lymphadenopathy? (lipomelanotic reticulosis)

A. Reactive lymphadenopathy because of macrophages which collect melanin from dermis and take it to lymphnode.

Q. What is Parkland formula?

A.

$$\text{Input} = 4 \text{ mL/kg} \times \text{BSA involved for burns}$$

In TEN 3/4 of this is given (Ringer lactate)
One half in the first 8 hours
Other half over next 16 hours

Q. What are the complications of erythroderma?

A.

Cutaneous	***Systemic***
Hair changes	Hypothermia
Nail changes	Hypoproteinemia
Epiphora	Anemia
Ectropion	Renal failure
Pruritus	Dermatopathic enteropathy
TEWL	High-output cardiac failure
Dry and fissured palms and soles	Acute skin failure
	Precipitation of stroke

Q. What is the effect of erythroderma on quality of life?

A. Since it's a chronic disease, patient can get depression. Also because of decreased circulation to the brain, patients having borderline psychosis can manifest overt signs. If steroids are given, they can also cause psychosis.

Q. What should be the humidity of the room?

A. 70%, room temperature should be 35°C.

Q. What is the normal core body temperature?

A. The normal core body temperature of a healthy, resting adult human being is stated to be at 98.6°F or 37.0°C.

Q. What is the axillary, oral and rectal temperature?

A. Oral temperatures, which are the most convenient type of temperature measurement, is at 37.0°C. Axillary temperature is the longest and most inaccurate way of measuring body temperature, the normal temperature falls at 97.6°F or 36.4°C. Rectal temperature fall at 99.6°F or 37.6°C. It is the least time consuming and most accurate type of body temperature measurement, being an internal measurement but not comfortable.

Q. Is erythroderma infectious?

A.
- It is infectious in the sense that the scales harbor bacteria which thus serve as a source of infection to others. It can infect patients in the wards.
- It is more prone for infections because barrier function of skin is lost and immune responses are altered. (CD4 Tcells lymphocytopenia and increased gamma globulin), therefore patient can get infectious from the surrounding patients.

Q. What is acute skin failure?

A. Skin failure is defined as loss of normal temperature control with inability to maintain the core body temperature, and failure to prevent percutaneous loss of fluids, electrolytes and proteins, with resulting imbalance and failure of mechanical barrier to prevent penetration of foreign material.

Q. What is concealed pyrexia?

A. In erythroderma, body feels warm because of increased peripheral skin perfusion and so even if patient gets fever, its not noticed. This is concealed pyrexia. Therfore rectal temperature must be taken.

Q. Why is barrier nursing important in erythroderma?

A. Scales harbor bacteria which thus serve as a source of infection to others.

Q. What is the pathogenesis of erythroderma?

A. The number of germinative cells as well as their mitotic rates is increased, meanwhile their transit time through the epidermis is decreased.

Q. What are the investigations in erythroderma?

A.
1. CBC—anemia due to chronic disease leukocytosis with eosinophilia,
2. ESR—increased
3. Serum albumin—hypoalbuminemia
4. Serum electrolytes—electrolyte imbalance
5. Serum IgE—increased in atopic erythroderma,
6. increased uric acid, abnormal serum protein electrophoresis with elevation in the gamma globulin
7. Skin scrapings—to rule out scabies and dermatophyte infection
8. Histopathology—in acute stages there is spongiosis and parakeratosis.

There is non-specific infiltrate, vasodilatation and perivascular infiltrates.

In chronic cases there is acanthosis, elongation of rete ridges. Histopathology can help identify the cause in 50% of cases.

Q. What is the significance of eosinophilia?

A. It is generally a nonspecific finding, although a highly elevated count raises the possibility of a lymphoma or drug hypersensitivity syndrome.

Q. What is Sézary syndrome?

A. It is a lymphoma of skin homing T-cells characterized by erythroderma, lymphadenopathy and Sézary cells in blood.

Q. In which circumstances direct immunofluorescence (DIF) should be done?

A. Direct immunofluorescence studies may be of diagnostic utility in cases of erythroderma secondary to pemphigus foliaceus, bullous pemphigoid, graft-versus-host disease and connective tissue disorders.

Q. What is red man syndrome?

A. Usually related to vancomycin. It is characterized by dermatopathic lymphadenopathy, palmoplantar keratoderma and relapsing erythroderma.

Q. What is Omenn syndrome?

A. It is characterized by immunodeficiency, failure to thrive, hypogammaglobulinemia, increased IgE, erythroderma and diffuse alopecia.Treatment is by bone marrow transplantation It is fatal if untreated.

Q. How will you manage a case of erythroderma?

A. Hospitalize the patient. Initial management consists of correction of fluid and electrolyte imbalance and treatment of secondary infections. The environmental temperature must be regulated. Cooling and overheating must be avoided by use of extra blankets and fans respectively. The possibility that the erythroderma is due to drug reaction must be considered in every case and all non essential drugs must be withdrawn. Sedating oral antihistamines will help to ease the pruritus. The cutaneous inflammation should be treated with bland emollient creams or mild topical steroids. Systemic steroids may be necessary in idiopathic erythroderma and drug reactions. Prednisone can be given in a dose of 1–2 mg/kg/day and a maintenance dose of 0.5 mg/kg/day. Due to increased transcutaneous absorption topical salicylic acid or lactic acid should be avoided. In refractory cases cyclosporine (5 mg/kg/day), retinoids, vitamin A, methotrexate and azathioprine can be given.

Many dermatologists prefer to avoid systemic steroids due to chances of fluid retention secondary infection diabetes but in persistent cases it may become necessary.

The diagnosis of underlying cause may be very difficult. The history and multiple biopsies is often helpful.

Q. How will you manage a case of psoriatic erythroderma?

A. In psoriatic erythroderma low dose methotrexate, acitretin or cyclosporine can be given avoid topical tar and UV therapy.

Q. What is deckchair sign?

A. Papuloerythroderma of Ofuji presents in elderly men as flat-topped red pruritic papules that become generalized erythrodermic plaques. There is sparing of abdominal skin folds ("deck chair" sign).

Q. What is emulsifying ointment BP?

A.
- Emulsifying wax—20 g
- Liquid paraffin—30 g
- White soft paraffin—40 g

It is a good moisturizing agent. It can be used by making a soapy solution in warm water which can be used in place of soap for bathing.

Q. How will you treat sezary syndrome?

A.
- Retinoids
- Bexarotene
- Interferon
- Extracorporeal photopheresis
- Granulocyte-macrophage colony-stimulating factor (GM-CSF)

Q. Why should eyes be examined?

A.
- Drug induced
- AD (blepharitis)

5 Genital Ulcer

Name/Age/Sex/Occupation/Residing at ... /Hailing from ... /Marital status

Chief complaints:

History of presenting illness (HOPI):

Three cardinal symptoms:

1. Ulcerative lesions of the genital
2. Urethral or vaginal discharge
3. Pain and swelling in the groins

Other symptoms:

- Skin rash (syphilis)
- Joint complaints (Reiter's, disseminated gonococcal infections)
- Eye symptoms
- Constitutional symptoms
- Urinary complaints

Genital ulcer:

- Duration ...
- Number/Site/Size/Pain/Discharge/Color started initially as what?
- Initial lesions—Were they raised/fluid filled/ulcers?
- Any prodromal symptoms
- H/O preceding drug intake
- H/O mucosal membrane involvement—oral/rectal/conjunctival
- H/O application of medications
- H/O any other medicines taken
- Urethral/Vaginal discharge since ...
- Amount/color/odor/site/irritation/itching/relation with intercourse/bloodstained/pain in the testicles/pain in lower abdomen/difficulty in intecourse/pain during defecation

Groin swelling:

- Bilateral/Unilateral
- Number/Site/Size/Pain/Overlying skin/Associated ulcer
- Associated complaints
- Fever/arthralgia/myalgia/eye complaints/abdominal pain/headache

History of sexual exposure:

- When was the latest exposure?
- Whether marital/extramarital/whether paid/unpaid sex/use of contraception
- Frequency of exposure
- Homosexual or heterosexual exposure
- H/O peno-vaginal/peno-oral/peno-anal exposure
- H/O multiple sex partner
- H/O trauma
- H/O drug intake
- H/O fever, loss of weight/loss of appetite
- H/O joint pain
- H/O itching all over the body

History of complication:

- If discharge—abdominal pain/obstruction/stools
- If ulcer—extent/bleeding/non healing lesion
- If discharge—burning/fever/chills inability to retract the preputial skin
- Swelling of the penis/scrotum
- Foul smelling discharge with black color

History of etiology:

- Syphilis: Primary (painless ulcer)/shotty lymphadenopathy
- Secondary: Skin lesions/oral lesions/painless lymphadenopathy
- Tertiary: Tabes dorsalis/neurological/cardiovascular system (CVS) complications
- Chancroid: Painful/multiple/Extragenital/Lymphadenopathy
- Lymphogranuloma venereum (LGV): Swelling of scrotum/leg/vulva/groin
    - Ribbon like stools/fissures/ulcers
    - Ophthalmic complaints
    - Beefy red/chronic
    - Scabies—H/O itching in the groins with crawling sensation

Past history:

- Past H/O sexually transmitted disease (STD) or similar complaints
- What type?
- If treated or not
- Human immunodeficiency virus (HIV)—known serostatus
    - Weight loss/diarrhea/Recurrent upper respiratory tract infection (URTI)
    - Herpes zoster/Tuberculosis/Bedridden/Cachexia
    - H/O IV drug abuse

  - H/O blood transfusion/needle prick
  - Any H/O jaundice (HBV)
- TB/DM/HTN/IHD/Bronchial asthma/drug allergy
- H/O medical and surgical illnesses

Sexual history: As detailed earlier

Menstrual history:
- LMP
- 1st menstrual period (menarche)
- irregularity/flow/painful or painless/intermenstrual bleeding/dyspareunia /duration/excessive bleeding

Obstetric history:
- Gravida/para/live births/abortion
- Infertility (PID)
- Abortion/stillbirth/infertility

Personal history:
- Sleep/bowel-bladder/addiction

Family history:
- H/O any complaints in the spouse
- H/O any similar complaints in the past
- H/O blood transfusion in the spouse
- H/O itching (scabies/pediculosis)
- Obstetric history in the spouse or other family members
- Any children born defective

General examination:
- General condition/orientation
- Patient is conscious, cooperative, well oriented in time, place and person
- Vitals
  - Weight/height/TPR/BP
  - Pallor, cyanosis, clubbing, icterus, edema feet
  - All lymph nodes should be systematically palpated for—number/size/consistency/mobility
  - Oral cavity
  - Examine skin for any type of rash
  - Hair, nails, palms, soles
  - Eyes (conjuctival redness, watering of eyes)
  - Per vaginal and per rectal examination
  - Pubic hair/nits (*Pthirus pubis*)/folliculitis
  - Groin-lymphadenopathy

- Bilateral/unilateral, discrete/matted
- Which group of lymph nodes are involved?
- Shape/size/tenderness/fluctuation/warmth/consistency (firm/hard/shotty)
- Impulse on coughing
- Skin overlying the lymph node—normal/sinuses/bluish/erythematous/ruptured buboes

Ulcer:

- Location/number/size/shape/edge/floor/base/margin/surrounding skin/bleeding on touch/pain on touch/induration of the base/smell
- Look at the mouth, perianal area, nails, palms and soles
- Look for scars/skin tags/fissures in perianal area
- Look at inguinal LN— bilateral/unilateral/single/multiple/tender/nontender/mobile/fixed/firm/soft/fluctuant/non-fluctuant/opening/not opening on the skin
- Nature of discharge—Thin/thick/purulent/serous/serosanguinous/blood staining of undergarments
- Discharge-site (urethral/vaginal)
    - Retract prepuce
    - Color/amount/smell/adherent/meatal redness
    - Milk urethra
- Scrotum/testes/epididymis/spermatic cord/cervix/vagina/bartholin/fourchette
- Perianal area-patulous
    - Warts/skin tags/sphincter elasticity/fissures
    - Scars
    - Bimanual pelvic examination

P/A-soft:

- Liver/Spleen tenderness
- Respiratory system (RS)
- Cardiovascular system (CVS)
- Central nervous system (CNS)
- **Impression:** Sexually transmitted disease with complications with HIV status,VDRL status/HBV in a high-risk patient.
- **Syphilis:** Single painless rounded well defined indurated button like induration on the ulcer with dull red clean granulation tissue with serous discharge on ... site.
- **Lymph nodes:** Bilateral, multiple, firm, discrete, mobile, non tender, move freely under finger (shotty, rubbery).

- **Chancroid:** Soft tender papule breaks down to form an ulcer, multiple 1–2 mm ulcers with sharp ragged, undermined edge, non indurated, painful base with yellow gray necrotic exudate covering granulation tissue that bleeds easily.
- Edema of prepuce +/–
- Unilateral tender fluctuant warm mass in inguinal region of ... size with normal overlying skin.

SYPHILIS

Q. What is the other name of syphilis?

A. • Great pox, because of the high mortality rate in Europe when it was 1st introduced.
  • LUES—(Lues = pest in French)

Q. How was the name syphilis derived?

A. • From a poem by Fracastorius (physician and poet), who wrote the poem about a shepherd named Syphiulus who offended the Gods and got a disease.
  • Two stages have been quite well described in the poem.

Q. What is the chance of syphilis after single exposure with infected person?

A. 30%.

Q. When is a syphilis patient infectious?

A. During the first year of untreated infection.

Q. What is the risk of mother infecting fetus with subsequent pregnancies?

A. Patient is infectious for many years, although risk of infecting fetus declines gradually during untreated illness after 8 years there is little risk even in untreated mother.

Q. Why is the incubation period of syphilis so long? (9–90 days)

A. As the doubling time of *Treponema pallidum* for each cell division is 33 hours.

Q. How will we differentiate between syphilitic chancre and chancroid?

A.

Syphilitic chancre (Hunterian chancre)	*Chancroid*
Painless	Painful
Usually single	Multiple

Continued

Continued

Syphilitic chancre (Hunterian chancre)	*Chancroid*
Clear ham colored base	Necrotic base
No exudate	Yellow exudate
Rolled edges	Jagged edges
Bilateral inguinal	Unilateral inguinal
Overlying skin normal	Overlying skin thin and shiny

Q. What is Dory flop sign?

A. The induration of the ulcer on the inner side of the prepuce often gives rise to flip on retraction of the preputial skin. This is Dory flop sign (dory—a small flat bottomed boat).

Q. What are kissing ulcers?

A. Ulcers on the coronal sulcus and prepuce are called kissing ulcers.

Q. What is condom chancre?

A. An ulcer occurring at the hilt of shaft of penis is called condom chancre.

Q. What are the usual sites of chancre?

A.
- Males: Coronal sulcus, Glans, Shaft, Prepuce, frenulum, urinary meatus
- Females: Vulva, vagina or cervix
- Extra genital sites (12–14%): Anorectal (receptive anal sex), oral cavity, hands and arms, rarely as paronychia.

Q. What is syphilis d'emblée?

A. Syphilis without a chancre as a result of direct inoculation into the blood as a result of transfusion of infected blood or blood component or punctured with an infective needle.

Q. What are the types of chancre?

A.
- Mixed chancre
  - Erosive chancre
  - Papuloerosive chancre
  - Condom chancre
  - Kissing chancre
  - Chancre redux (recurrence of primary chancre at site of original chancre—it is infectious and shows treponemes)
  - Psudo-chancre redux—recurrence of gum at set of original lesion. Doesn't contain treponemes and is non infectious
  - Follmann balanitis (only inflammation without ulcer)

    - Phagedenic chancre—anaerobic infection (due to conifection with fusospirochaetes characterized by necrotizing perforation of prepuce or in some patients gangrene)
    - Penetrating chancre—penetrates through prepuce to glans
    - Intraurethral chancre
- Syphilis without chancre (syphilis d'emblée)—due to blood transfusions

Q. What are the complications of primary chancre?

A. Edema, phimosis, erosive balanitis, lymphangitis, phagedenic chancre.

Q. What are the non STD causes of genital ulcers?

A. Fixed drug eruption, squamous cell carcinoma, Behçet's disease, Crohn's disease.

Q. Which is an important diagnostic clue in patients presenting with rash of secondary syphilis?

A. A thin depressed scar seen in 10% patients on the site of pre-existing ulcer.

Q. In how many patients the chancre persists even after the appearance of secondary rash?

A. 10–40%.

Q. Which are the most common manifestations of secondary syphilis?

A. Rash (raw-ham or copper colored) and Lymphadenopathy.

Q. What is roseola syphilitica?

A. Macular eruptions consisting of 0.5–2 cm pink, discrete, round or oval over trunk, flexor aspect of upper extremities, palms and soles which are transient.

Q. What is Corona veneris?

A. Papules along the hairline on forehead arranged in a crown like pattern (other causes of corona are- psoriasis, seborrheic dermatitis, reactive arthritis).

Q. What is Buschke-Ollendorff sign? (remember other causes of DDT)

A. Deep dermal tenderness elicited by wincing on applying pressure with a blunt end of a pin over a papule. Also seen with furuncle, vasculitis, erythema nodosum etc. Or neoplastic-remember the BLEND AN EGG mnemonic.

Q. What is necklace/collar of venus?

A. Resolving rash of secondary syphilis which leaves depigmented patches on the back and sides of the neck referred as leukoderma syphiliticum.

Q. Which variants of syphilis are associated with itching?

A.
- Follicular syphilis
- Lichenoid syphilis

Q. Enumerate the morphological variant of syphilis.

A.
- Macular or roseolar/maculopapular rash
  - Papular (Nickel and Dime)
  - Papulosquamous-most common
  - Psoriasiform
  - Annular
  - Pustular
  - Follicular
  - Lenticular
  - Corymbose
  - Lichenoid
  - Rupioid
  - Nodular (seen in late syphilis more than secondary syphilis)
  - Ulcerative or necrotic (lues maligna)

Q. Describe rash of secondary syphilis.

A.
1. Generalized rash of skin and mucous membranes
2. Bilateral and symmetrical
3. More prominent on upper limbs > abdomen> lower extremities with special predilection for palms and soles
4. More discrete than confluent,
5. Sharply demarcated
6. Polymorphous-usually non itchy
7. Deep dermal tenderness positivity.
8. Heals without scarring but with pigmentation

Q. Can you get vesicular rash in syphilis?

A. Yes extremely rare, called varioliform syphilis.

Q. What is lichenoid syphilis?

A. Characterized by maculopapular lesions with lichenoid (violaceous) hue with increased incidence now being attributed to HIV.

Q. What is lenticular syphilis?

A. Pinhead to lentil bean sized papules on face and genitalia.

Q. Which are the most common sites of annular syphilis?
A. Face,anogenital area, axillae, palms and soles.

Q. What are bombshell like eruptions?
A. They are corymbose lesions characterized by a central plaque and surrounding smaller satellite papules which occurs months after infection.

Q. What is syphilis cornee?
A. Corn like lesions over soles.

Q. What is Clous Syphilitiques?
A. Diffuse hyperkeratosis of soles seen in syphilis.

Q. What is Biette's collarette?
A. A zone of scaling surrounding papules of syphilis on palms and soles.

Q. What is the initial finding in secondary syphilis?
A. A coppery evanescent macular rash often overlooked.

Q. Describe mucous patches.
A. Large grayish plaques or small superficial ulcerated areas.

Q. How do we differentiate condyloma lata with condyloma acuminata?
A.

Condyloma lata	*Condyloma acuminata*
Pale	Pinkish
Flat topped	Thrown into folds
Moist	Dry
Broad at the base so a paper cannot be passed under it	Narrower at the base so a paper can be passed under it (paper test)
Bilateral, firm, rubbery, shotty, painless discrete and non tender Lymph node	No lymphadenopathy
Dark-ground illumination (DGI) positive	Negative DGI
Caused by *Treponema pallidum*	Caused by human papillomavirus

Q. What is the most infectious lesion in syplihis?
A. Condyloma lata.

Q. What are split papules?

A. Split papules are lesions similar to condyloma lata which become fissured at the labial commissures, nasolabial folds,behind ears,axilla, inframammary area.

Q. Why are the mucosal lesions morphologically different from the rash on the body?

A. Local irritation, moisture and trauma modify the morphology of rash at mucosal sites.

Q. What are snail track ulcers?

A. They are serpiginous ulcers in the mucosa.

Q. Why are mucosal lesions more common in women?

A. They are due to moisture, friction and some irritation.

Q. What are the types of hair loss seen in secondary syphilis?

A.
1. Telogen effluvium
2. Irregular patchy nonscarring alopecia (moth eaten alopecia)
3. Alopecia areata like lesions
4. In gummatous syphilis—areas of scarring alopecia

Q. Where is moth eaten alopecia observed?

A. Margins of the scalp, beard, eyebrows, legs.

Q. Nail changes in secondary syphilis.

A. Pitting, onycholysis, onychodystrophy, beaus lines, paronychia, onychia.

Q. What are the CSF findings in secondary syphilis?

A. 1/4th of the patients with early syphilis regardless of HIV status show elevated wbc count and proteins in CSF with a reactive VDRL.

Q. Why does a patient get syphilitic periostitis?

A. It is due to vasculitis.

Q. Which lymph nodes are commonly involved?

A.
- Inguinal nodes: 75%
- Axillary: 38%
- Posterior cervical: 28%
- Femoral: 18%
- Epitrochlear: 17%

Q. In which bones will you see periosteal inflammation?

A. Skull, tibia, sternum, ribs.

Q. Why is liver function test to be done in secondary syphilis?

A. Subclinical hepatitis may occur and occasionally symptomatic hepatitis (increased alkaline phosphatase).

Q. Why does a patient get systemic symptoms like glomerulonephritis/nephrotic syndrome/iritis/anterior uveitis?

A. Circulating immune complexes get deposited on the respective sites.

Q. Differential diagnosis of fever with sore throat and adenopathy.

A. Infectious mononucleosis, HIV, secondary syphilis (diffuse pharyngitis in secondary syphilis).

Q. What do you mean by latent syphilis?

A. Serological or historical evidence syphilis but who has never received treatment for this disease and who have no clinical manifestations.

Q. What are the types of latent syphilis?

A.
- Early: Potentially infectious and defined by one of the following:
  1. Documented seroconversion
  2. Unequivocal symptoms of primary or secondary syphilis
  3. Sexual partner documented to have primary or secondary or early latent syphilis.
- Late: More than 1 year on the basis of time when untreated individuals likely to have spontaneous mucocutaneous relapses.

Q. What is interval from acute infection to clinical onset of late or tertiary stage of disease?

A. 1–20 years.

Q. What is Merritt classification of neurosyphilis?

A.
1. **Asymptomatic**
   - Early
   - Late
2. **Meningeal**
   - Acute syphilitic meningitis
   - Meningovascular
   - Cerebral
   - Spinal form
3. **Parenchymatous**
   - General paresis
   - Tabes dorsalis
   - Taboparesis (mixed)
   - Optic atrophy
4. **Gummatous**
   - Cerebral
   - Spinal

Q. When can a patient get meningovascular syphilis and tabes dorsalis?

A.
- 5–12 years after primary infection (meningovascular syphilis)
- 8–25 years after primary infection (tabes/paresis)

Q. Why is syphilis not diagnosed in women until the secondary stage?

A. Because the chancre is not visible in women and it is painless.

Q. How much time does it take for a primary chancre to heal if untreated?

A. 3–6 weeks.

Q. Can a single ulcer on the genitals be due to herpes simplex virus?

A. Yes, recurrent herpes simplex virus often present with a single ulcer.

Q. How many patients of syphilis have abnormal CSF findings in primary and secondary stage?

A.
- Primary syphilis: 13%
- Secondary syphilis: 25%

Q. After how many days of a primary chancre will a patient get secondary syphilis?

A. Few weeks or months (both may co-exist).

Q. What is lues maligna?

A. Malignant secondary syphilis is widespread form produced by prodrome of fever, myalgia and headache followed by papulopustular eruption that rapidly transforms into necrotic, sharply marginated ulcers with erythematous halo, clean looking floor hemorrhagic brown crusts that are organized in rupioid layers (layers of crusts resembling oyster shell). More common in HIV positive patients.

Q. What are the four clinical characteristics of lues maligna?

A.
1. Short incubation period
2. Prodrome
3. Pleomorphic lesions
4. Noduloulcerative lesions of skin and mucosa

Q. What is Fisher's criteria for lues maligna?

A.
1. Compatible gross and microscopic morphology
2. A high titer of positivity for serologic tests for syphilis
3. Jarisch–Herxheimer reaction following treatment
4. Dramatic response to antibiotic treatment

Q. What are the systemic manifestations of secondary syphilis?

A. 1. Malaise, low grade fever, headache mild hepatitis, hepatosplenomegaly, jaundice
2. Pulmonary changes
3. Glomerulonephritis
4. Asymptomatic neurosyphilis
5. Gastrointestinal involvement (anorexia, nausea, vomiting, antral ulcers)
6. Myocarditis rarely, periostitis
7. Iritis, uveitis, parotitis

Q. What is the natural course of secondary syphilis?

A. It can last for several weeks till 1 year but relapses can occur in 20–25% of patients.

Q. How do you differentiate relapse from reinfection?

A. Occurrence of a chancre at a different location from the previous one or detection of early syphilis in a current sexual partner indicates reinfection.

Q. What are the types of relapse?

A. 1. Clinical relapse
2. Serological relapse-reagin tests becomes positive after having been negative, or shows a progressive rise in titers after a decline (often precedes a clinical relapse—CSF examination is recommended).
3. Pregnancy relapse—patient who is apparently cured of syphilis gives birth to a child with secondary syphilis. Also called transplacental syphilis.

Q. How do you diagnose a case of secondary syphilis?

A.
- Positive serology for syphilis
- Demonstration of *Treponema pallidum*

Q. How many treponemes are required for syphilis?

A. 1,000 treponemes.

Q. Difference between initial episode and relapse?

A. Lesions are fewer in number and smaller in size in relapses and asymmetrical. It is less severe.

Q. From which sites should a Dark-ground illumination (DGI) be done?

A. Moist lesions on mucous membranes which are full of treponemes are the best sites.

Q. Are lesions on the mouth or genital area more better for DGI?
A. Nonpathogenic treponemes are part of their normal flora. And so lesions from mouth should not be selected as a site for DGI.

Q. Which diseases mimic the pustular rash of secondary syphilis?
A. Vons zumbusch type of pustular psoriasis.

Q. Does the duration of infection hold any significance in the treatment of syphilis?
A. Yes, as the duration of infection increases *T. pallidum* divides more slowly requiring a more prolonged duration of therapy.

Q. What is syphilis incognito?
A. It is a subtype of latent syphilis (early/late) which runs a subclinical course from the time of infection until its diagnosis by routine serological screening. Improved personal hygiene—soaps or antiseptics may cause the chancre to stop developing or to heal rapidly. Coincidental use of antibiotics for some other disease may minimize or abolish symptoms of early disease but the dose may be insufficient to cure syphilis.

Q. What is the risk of getting late syphilis in the above case?
A. Dark ground illumination of these patients develop late syphilis.

Q. How do you visualize treponemes in histopathology?
A. Levaditi or Warthin-Starry stains.

Q. What is the histopathology in secondary syphilis?
A. Lymphomononuclear infiltrate most intense in papillary dermis. Plasma cells are seen as focal corrections around the skin appendages and on the periphery of epithelioid cell granulomas.

Q. How does syphilis in HIV differ from the usual form?
A. Larger primary chancre, multiple ulcers, more frequent systemic symptoms in the secondary stage, simultaneous multiorgan involvement, accelerated course and development of uveitis and neurosyphilis (within 2 years) in the early stages of infection.

Q. What is the rate of transmission to the fetus in untreated women in various stages of syphilis?
A.
- 70–100% in primary and secondary syphilis
- 40% in early latent syphilis
- 10% in late latent syphilis

Q. Which trimester infection is associated with high fetal mortality?
A. First and second trimester infection.

Q. What is Kassowitz's law?

A. Longer the interval between infection and pregnancy, the more benign is the outcome in the infant.

Q. Infection of the fetus does not occur before 18 weeks—TRUE/FALSE.

A. False. It has been shown that *T. pallidum* gains access to the fetal compartment as early as 9–10 weeks.

Q. Which is the most specific test in early congenital syphilis and early acquired syphilis?

A. Dark-field miocroscopy.

Q. Why don't you use a light microscope?

A. Treponemes cant be detected with light microscope because of its narrow width.

Q. What is the principle of dark-field microscopy?

A. In dark-field microscopy, dark-field condenser allows the light rays to strike the object in the field at an oblique angle so that no direct light but only rays reflected from from the object enter the microscope objective. This gives the object a luminous appearance against a black background.

Q. How do you collect specimen for the above test?

A. The lesion is cleaned gently with a saline soaked gauze and then squeezed with the index finger and thumb to produce a serous exudate. It is then transferred directly on a glass slide by pressing it on the lesion. A drop of saline is added to make it homogenous.

Q. Why should the specimen be immediately be examined?

A. The specimen should be immediately examined because any delay reduces the motility of treponemes.

Q. From where all can treponemes be isolated?

A.
1. Mucocutaneous lesions
2. Lymph node puncture
3. Amniotic fluid

Q. How is the lymph node puncture done?

A. The area is cleaned and draped. overlying skin over enlarged LN is infiltrated with 1% lignocaine. The overlying skin is stretched and the lymph node is held firmly. The 0.2 mL of sterile normal saline is injected, the lymph node is massaged gently and with a 20G needle and syringe, fluid is aspirated and expressed on a glass slide.

This is also called as indirect burning and Hoffman technique.

Q. How is *T. Pallidum* differentiated from nonpathogenic treponemes?

A. It is distinguished from other treponemes by the: *T. palladium* has tight spirals, regular coils and characteristic cork screw movement unlike the non pathogenic treponemes that have loose spirals and random movements.

Q. What are the advantages of direct fluorescent antibody-*T. pallidum* (DFA-TP) over dark-field microscopy?

A.
1. It is more sensitive and specific.
2. Samples from oral mucosa can be examined by this method.
3. Slides need not be examined immediately and may be sent to a laboratory.

Recently a so-called "reverse algorithm" is done where the specific test is done first, followed by the venereal disease research laboratory (VDRL).

Q. Which is the screening and confirmatory test for syphilis?

A.
- Non treponemal serological test—like VDRL are inexpensive, high in sensitivity and have a high negative predictive value, therefore are suitable for screening.
- Treponemal test [fluorescent treponemal antibody absorption (FTA-ABS)] are more specific and have a high positive predictive value, therefore are used for confirmation.

Q. What is the antigen in VDRL?

A. The antigen comprises mixture of lecithin, cholesterol and purified cardiolipin (a component of mammalian cell membrane).

Q. How is the VDRL test done?

A. Serum is heated at 56°C for 30 minutes. Serum and antigen are mixed within a ring on a glass slide by rotating it mechanically and results are read in a microscope at 100× magnification. If anticardiolipin antibodies are present, the antigen rods aggregate to form clumps.

Q. How much is the sensitivity of the above test?

A.
- The sensitivity of VDRL test is 70–90% in primary syphilis, while it is 100% in secondary syphilis.
- VDRL becomes positive after 15 days of the ulcer.

Q. What is the advantage of RPR test over VDRL?

A. It can be read macroscopically because of addition of charcoal particles, the antigen used is stabilized and cards are used instead of slides.

Q. What are the causes of false positive VDRL tests?

A. As the antigen used in nontreponemal test is a component of all mammalian cell membranes, the damage to the host tissue by infection (leprosy, HIV tuberculosis, malaria), immunization, pregnancy, age related changes, or autoimmune diseases (connective tissue diseases) can result into false positive VDRL.

Q. What are the types of false positive reactions?

A.
1. Acute (<6 months duration)
2. Chronic (>6 months duration). It is recommended that serology should be repeated at 10 weeks as by that time most cases will return to VDRL nonreactive.

Q. What is prozone phenomenon?

A. This phenomenon occurs when there is excess of antibodies in the patient's serum that interferes with the binding to antigen in the flocculation test, so if syphilis is strongly suspected the test should be repeated in serial dilutions.

Q. What is the zone of equivalence?

A. The optimal ratio of antigen to antibody yields an insoluble precipitate that is visible in a positive test. The zone of equivalence defines this optimal ratio.

Q. What is the appropriate temperature for storage of blood samples?

A. 27°C since false negative treponemal tests can occur in patients with titers of <1: 4 dilutions. If the blood samples are stored at cold temperature (4°C) before testing.

Q. Can treponemal tests be used for monitoring purposes?

A.
- No, because these tests remain reactive for years or even lifetime inspite of adequate therapy.
- On the other hand, VDRL becomes negative within 1 year of treatment of early syphilis and 2–3 years in late syphilis.

Q. What are the causes of positive and negative treponemal tests?

A.
- False positive: Leprosy, malaria, infectious mononucleosis, SLE
- False negative: Advanced immunodeficiency associated with HIV and early congenital syphilis.

Q. Which is the test to come positive first in early syphilis?

A. The FTA-ABS IgM is the first to become positive in early syphilis and has a higher sensitivity than the VDRL test in late syphilis.

Q. How is FTA-ABS done?

A. In this test, *T. pallidum* subspecies *pallidum* (Nichol's strain are fixed on glass slides). The patient's serum is first diluted 1:5 in sorbent (an extract from cultures of the nonpathogenic reiter treponeme) to remove nonspecific treponeme antibodies. The serum is then added to the glass slide. If it contains antibodies, it coats the treponemes. Then FITC—labeled antihuman immunoglobulin is added to the slide that combines with the patient's antibody attached to the *T. pallidum*. The slide is examined under fluorescent microscope.

Q. Which is the only test for sexually transmitted diseases which can be used with CSF?

A. Venereal disease research laboratory test.

Q. When does the VDRL test becomes reactive?

A. Two weeks after ulcer appears infection which reverts to negative in 1/4th cases during late latency.

Q. What is titer?

A.
- Titer is the highest dilution of the serum which shows a positive reaction (in the VDRL test)
- The higher the titer, the more the probability of patient having syphilis.

Q. How are the reports read?

A. Reactive, nonreactive, weakly reactive or in titers 1:2, 1:4, 1:8.

Q. What is the treatment of syphilis?

A.
- Primary, secondary or early latent syphilis
- Recommended: Benzathine penicillin 2.4 million units in a single dose IM.
- Penicillin allergy—Doxycycline 100 mg oral twice daily for 14 days
- Inj Ceftrixone 1 g IM or IV daily for 10 days (there is controversy whether ceftriaxone can be given for penicillin allergic individuals)
- Late latent syphilis, syphilis of unknown duration, tertiary syphilis
- Recommended: Benzathine penicillin 2.4 million units weekly for 3 weeks IM
- Penicillin allergy—Doxycycline 100 mg twice daily for 28 days
- Neurosyphilis, syphilitic eye disease, syphilitic auditory disease
- Recommended: Aqueous crystalline penicillin G, 18–24 million units/day administered as 3–4 million units IV every 4 hours/ continuous infusion for 10–14 days.

- Alternate: Procaine penicillin 2.4 million units IM once daily with probenecid 500 mg orally 4 times a day, both for 10–14 days.

Q. How is penicillin administered?

A. Benzathine penicillin 2.4 mega-units, 1.2 in each buttocks deep IM with a wide bore 18 no. needle (after test dose).

Q. How will you treat a pregnant woman with syphilis who also has a penicillin allergy?

A.
- Desensitization and treatment with penicillin. Oral step-wise penicillin dose challenge or skin testing might be helpful in identifying women at risk.
- Erythromycin and azithromycin should not be used, because neither reliably cures maternal infection or treats an infected fetus. Data are insufficient to recommend ceftriaxone for treatment of maternal infection and prevention of congenital syphilis

Q. A woman in her second trimester diagnosed as syphilis. How will you manage?

A. When syphilis is diagnosed during the second half of pregnancy, management should include a sonographic fetal evaluation for congenital syphilis and usual treatment. Sonographic signs of fetal or placental syphilis (i.e., hepatomegaly, ascites, hydrops, fetal anemia, or a thickened placenta) indicate a greater risk for fetal treatment failure.

Q. What are the reactions which a patient can get with injection penicillin?

A.
1. Anaphylactic reaction
2. Vasovagal reaction
3. Hoigne phenomenon
4. Jarisch–Herxheimer reaction

Q. What is Jarisch–Herxheimer reaction? (Therapeutic paradox)

A. It is an all or none phenomenon which may occur within the first 24 hours (usually 2–8 hours) after initiation of penicillin.
- Primary syphilis:
  - Edema and phimosis
  - Chancre becomes more prominent
- Secondary syphilis:
  - Lesions become more obvious
  - Papule at the site of primary chancre
- Signs of meningeal irritation:
  - Arthralgia/myalgia

- Late syphilis:
  - CNS and CVS affected
- Occlusion of coronary arteries, headache, nausea/vomiting, tender adenopathy, pharyngitis or fever.The reaction is believed to be a result of the rapid killing of spirochetes and is seen most commonly among patients treated for primary or secondary syphilis (1/3 to 2/3 of cases).
- Treatment is supportive utilizing antipyretics and analgesics and symptoms usually resolve within 24 hours. During pregnancy, the Jarisch–Herxheimer reaction has been associated with fetal distress and preterm labor (the greatest risk occurring during the first 48 hours after treatment).

Q. How do you prevent Jarisch–Herxheimer reaction?
A. Oral steroids.

Q. What is Mazzotti reaction?
A. Sudden increase in fever after starting within a few hours after antifilarial medication.

Q. Why does a patient get CNS symptoms after treatment?
A. After treatment, organisms is killed resulting in liberation of toxins from organism—act as superantigens-meningism like symptoms but CSF is normal (Shwartzman phenomenon).

Q. What is Hoigne's phenomenon?
A. Microcrystals of procaine penicillin enter the cerebral circulation resulting in abnormal behavior/anxiety/angor animi (feeling of impending death).

Q. How do you desensitize?
A. Intravenous protocol for penicillin desensitization.

*Step**	*Solution (U/mL)†*	*Dose (mL)*	*Dose (U)*
1	100	0.1	10
2	100	0.2	20
3	100	0.4	40
4	100	0.8	80
5	1,000	0.15	150
6	1,000	0.30	300
7	1,000	0.60	600

Continued

Continued

*Step**	*Solution (U/mL)†*	*Dose (mL)*	*Dose (U)*
8	1,000	1.00	1,000
9	10,000	0.2	2,000
10	10,000	0.4	4,000
11	10,000	0.8	8,000
12	100,000	0.15	15,000
13	100,000	0.30	30,000
14	100,000	0.60	60,000
15	100,000	1.00	100,000
16	200,000	25	200,000
17	400,000	25	400,000
18	800,000	25	800,000
19	1,600,000	25	1,600,000
20	3,200,000	25	3,200,000
21	5,000,000	25	5,000,000

* Each step is administered at 15-minute intervals.

† Use penicillin G for dilutions in 0.9% sodium chloride.

Q. When should screening for syphilis be done in a pregnant woman?

A. Most states mandate screening at the first prenatal visit for all women. For communities and populations in which the prevalence of syphilis is high and for patients at high risk, serologic testing should be performed twice during the third trimester (ideally at 28–32 weeks' gestation) and at delivery. Any woman who delivers a stillborn infant after 20 weeks' gestation should be tested for syphilis.

Q. When will you repeat the titers?

A. Serologic titers should be repeated at 28–32 weeks' gestation and at delivery as recommended for the disease stage. Inadequate maternal treatment is likely if delivery occurs within 30 days of therapy, if clinical signs of infection are present at delivery, or if the maternal antibody titer at delivery is fourfold higher than the pretreatment titer. Serologic titers can be checked monthly in women at high risk for reinfection or in geographic areas in which the prevalence of syphilis is high.

Q. In which stage of syphilis does one get bullous lesions?

A. Congenital syphilis.

Q. What is Hutchinson's triad?

A. Sir Jonathan Hutchinson (1828–1913) from England described a triad in late congenital syphilis consisting of

1. notched incisors,
2. interstitial keratitis, and
3. eighth cranial nerve deafness

Q. What is Dattner Thomas concept?

A. If cellular count in CSF is high (>5 cells/mm^3) then it is suggestive of active neurosyphilis in which case retreatment is essential even if VDRL is negative. While if the protein count is high with the cell count being low then it is not significant.

Q. Stigmata of syphilis.

Syphilitic facies	Frontal bossing, saddle nose, short maxilla, protuberant mandible
Ophthalmologic	Interstitial keratitis, chorioretinitis, secondary glaucoma, corneal scarring, optic atrophy
Ears	Sensorineural hearing loss
Oropharynx	Hutchinson teeth, mulberry molars, perforation of hard palate
Cutaneous	Rhagades, gummas
Central nervous system	Intellectual disability, arrested hydrocephalus, seizures, optic atrophy, juvenile general paresis
Skeletal	Saber shins (anterior bowing of the tibia), Higoumenakis sign (enlargement of the sternoclavicular portion of the clavicle), Clutton's joints (painless arthritis), scaphoid scapula

Q. What are the differentiating features of various STD ulcers?

Features	***Syphilis***	***Herpes***	***Chancroid***	***LGV***	***Donovanosis***
Incubation period	9–90 days	2–7 days	1–14 days	3 days to 6 weeks	1–4 weeks (up to 6 months)
Primary lesion	Papule	Vesicle (erosion)	Papule/ pustule	Papule, pustule, or vesicle	Papule
Number of lesions	Usually one	Multiple, may coalesce	Multiple, may co-alesce	Usually one	Variable

Continued

Continued

Features	***Syphilis***	***Herpes***	***Chancroid***	***LGV***	***Donovanosis***
Edges	Sharp, well demarcated, round or oval	Erythematous, cratered	Ragged, undermined, irregular	Elevated, round, or oval	Elevated, irregular
Depth	Deep or superficial	Superficial	Excavated	Superficial or deep	Superficial or deep
Base	Smooth, nonpurulent, relatively nonvascular	Serous, erythematous, nonvascular	Purulent, vascular, friable	Variable, nonvascular	Red and velvety, bleeds readily
Induration	Indurated	None	Soft	Occasionally firm	Firm
Pain	Rare	Often tender	Very tender	Variable	Uncommon
Lymph nodes					
Fluctuance	Firm	None	May suppurate	May suppurate	None; pseudobuboes
Tenderness	None	Tender	Tender	Tender	None; pseudobuboes
Distribution	Bilateral	Bilateral with primary infection	Usually unilateral	Usually unilateral	None; pseudobuboes

"If you know syphilis and all its manifestations, you will know medicine."

—Osler

HERPES GENITALIS

Q. What does the word 'HERPES' means?

A. The word Herpes is derived from Greek word which means to creep.

Q. What is the causative organism for Herpes genitalis?

A. Human herpes virus-2 is the most common organism implicated in Herpes Genitalis. However HHV 1 can cause the same in case of oral intercourse.

Q. What is primary herpes infection, first episode infection and what is recurrent herpes infection?

A.
- Primary herpes infection—'Primary infection' denotes initial herpes simplex virus (HSV) infection in individuals without preexisting antibodies to HSV-1 or HSV-2.
- First episode infection denotes—initial clinical attack of HSV in individuals with preexisting antibodies to HSV-1 or HSV-2 due to previous subclinical infection with the virus
- Recurrent herpes infection—The reactivation of HSV after the establishment of latency.
- Nonprimary genital infection—Refers to an infection with one HSV type in an individual who already has preexisting antibodies to the other HSV type.

Q. What are the risk factor for transmission of genital herpes?

A. Risk factors associated with the transmission of genital herpes include:

1. An age of 15–30 years (period of greatest sexual activity)
2. An increased number of sexual partners
3. Black or Hispanic race
4. Lower income levels and education
5. Female gender
6. Homosexuality
7. HIV positivity

Q. Describe the pathogenesis of Herpes infection.

A. The causative organism of herpes genitalis, HSV-2 spreads primarily by sexual contact

Virus will replicate at the site of infection (i.e., the mucocutaneous surface)

PRIMARY HERPES INFECTION

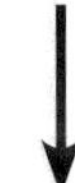

Virus then travel by retrograde axonal flow to the dorsal root ganglia and establish latency. Latency enables the virus to exist in a relatively noninfectious state for varying periods of time in its host.

LATENCY

Stress, UV light, fever, tissue damage, immunosuppression.

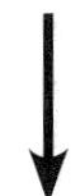

REACTIVATION OF VIRUS RECURRENT HERPES INFECTION

Q. How do you differentiate primary and recurrent herpes genitalis?

A.

	Primary (sometimes asymptomatic)	*Recurrent*
Prodromal symptoms	More severe	Less severe
Number of lesions	more	Limited
Severity (pain and extent)	more	less
Time taken for resolution	2–6 weeks	1 week
Complications	More common	Uncommon
Regional lymph nodes	Enlarged and tender	Not involved
Scarring	Sometimes	Never

Q. Why does nonprimary genital herpes lesion heal faster?

A. Patients with nonprimary first episode have neutralizing antibodies to HSV-1 which interrupts the spread of HSV infection. Thus they have lower frequencies of systemic symptoms, shorter duration of pain, fewer lesions and shorter healing time compared to true primary infections.

Q. What are the atypical presentations of genital herpes?

A.
1. Vaginal discharge (unrelated to candidiasis)
2. Genitourinary pain
3. Nonspecific vulvar erythema
4. Prostatitis and lower back pain
5. Itching, burning, soreness, pain over genital area (without obvious lesions)
6. Unexplained systemic symptoms—fever, malaise, myalgia
7. Vulvar, penile or perianal fissures
8. Folliculitis

Q. How does herpes in HIV present?

A.
1. Hyperkeratotic, verrucous lesions
2. Vegetating plaques
3. Chronic, persistent ulceration
4. Generalized papular eruptions

Q. How will you investigate the case of genital HSV?

A. 1. Collection of specimen—a large vesicle should be chosen and fluid should be aspirated with a tuberculin syringe. If large vesicle is not present, then exudates of a small vesicle or open lesion is collected by vigorously rubbing with a cotton-tipped swab on a wire shaft and sent for culture.

   To collect cervical specimens, swabs should be taken from ectocervix and the entry of the endocervical canal, as the HSV involves squamous rather than columnar epithelium.

   The specimen should be placed immediately into vials containing 1 mL of viral transport medium and should be kept at 4° until cultured.

2. Culture—gold standard for diagnosis of acute HSV infections.

   Human diploid fibroblast cell lines is used—HSV takes 12–18 hours for replication.

3. Confirmatory tests—neutralization with type specific antisera, immunological assays, nucleic acid hybridization.

Q. Describe the bedside test for herpes infection.

A. Tzanck test is the bedside investigation for herpes infection.

Specimen collected
Slide is air-dried

↓

Slide is covered with Giemsa-stain (which is diluted 1:10 with distilled water) for 15 minutes.

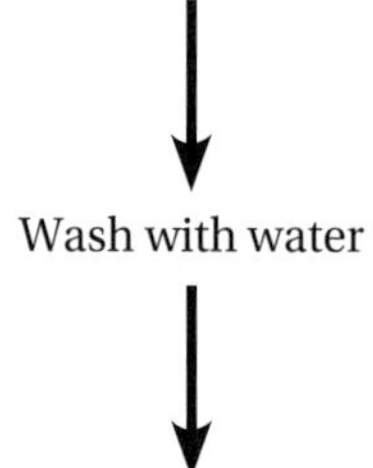

Wash with water

↓

Air dry the slide and examine under oil immersion

Q. What will you see in Tzanck smear?

A. Acantholytic cells (secondary acantholysis) with multinucleated gaint cell.

Q. What is the significance of HSV antibody titers?

A.
- HSV IgG: Past infection
- HSV IgM: Recent infection

Q. What are the sequelae of genital herpes?

A. 1. Psychological morbidity associated with recurrences.
2. Psychological morbidity related to transmission to partner or fetus or newborn.
3. Systemic complication.
4. Increased risk of acquiring or transmitting HIV infections.

Q. What are the systemic complications associated with herpes infections?

A. 1. Aseptic meningitis.
2. Radiculomyelopathy—urinary retention, numbness, paresthesias, neuralgic pain of buttocks, constipation, impotency.
3. HSV encephalitis.
4. Disseminated infections
5. Transmission to newborn
6. Secondary microbial infection
7. Pelvic inflammatory disease
8. Extragenital lesions

Q. What measures can be helpful for prevention of HSV infections?

A. 1. Abstinence
2. Limiting number of sexual partners
3. Avoiding partners who have a history of genital herpes
4. Consistent and correct condom use
5. Vaginal and rectal microbicides
6. Antiviral therapy
7. Vaccines

Q. How will you manage genital herpes infections?

A. General measures:

1. Counselling
2. Maintenance of local hygiene
3. Sitz bath

Topical treatment:

Topical antibiotics to avoid secondary infection.

Systemic treatment:

- Paracetamol- 500 mg, 4 hourly may relief pain.
- Antivirals (acyclovir, valacyclovir, and famciclovir) reduce viral shedding, itching, average healing time, and frequency of new lesion formation.

CDC GUIDELINES—2010

First episode	*Episodic therapy for recurrent genital herpes*	*Suppressive therapy for recurrent genital herpes (>6 attacks in a year)*	*Genital herpes in HIV infected individuals and other immunocompromized*
Acyclovir 400 mg orally three times a day for 7–10 days OR Acyclovir 200 mg orally five times a day for 7–10 days OR Famciclovir 250 mg orally three times a day for 7–10 days OR Valacyclovir 1 g orally twice a day for 7–10 days *Note*: Treatment can be extended if healing is incomplete after 10 days of therapy.	Acyclovir 400 mg orally three times a day for 5 days OR Acyclovir 800 mg orally twice a day for 5 days OR Famciclovir 125 mg orally twice daily for 5 days OR Valacyclovir 1 g orally once a day for 5 days	Acyclovir 400 mg orally twice a day OR Famciclovir 250 mg orally twice a day OR Valacyclovir 1 g orally once a day	**Episodic treatment**—Acyclovir 400 mg orally three times a day for 5–10 days OR Famciclovir 500 mg orally twice a day for 5 –10 days OR Valacyclovir 1 g orally twice a day for 5–10 days Suppressive T/T: Acyclovir 400–800 mg twice to thrice a day OR Famciclovir 500 mg orally BD OR Valacyclovir 500 mg oraly BD

Q. What are the indications of IV acyclovir?

A.
- Immunocompromized patient with disseminated herpes
- CNS complications (Herpetic meningoencephalitis)
- Pneumonitis, or hepatitis
- Severe initial clinical episodes in immunocompetent patient
- Neonatal Herpes simplex virus infections
- Varicella zoster infection in immunocompromized infections
- Patient is unable to swallow or tolerate oral acyclovir because of vomiting

Q. How is IV acyclovir administered?

A. About 5–10 mg/kg, 8 hourly infused at a constant rate over 1 hour for 3–7 days or until clinical improvement observed, followed by oral antiviral therapy to complete at least 10 days of total therapy. Acyclovir dose adjustment is required in renal failure.

Q. How is acyclovir injection available?

A. It is available as sterile solution containing acyclovir containing 25 mg/mL (as 20 mL and 40 mL vials).

Q. How will you manage asymptomatic sex partners of patients with genital herpes?

A. Asymptomatic sex partners of patients who have genital herpes should be questioned concerning histories of genital lesions and offered type-specific serologic testing for HSV infection.

Q. What is the risk of transmission of genital herpes from mother to neonate?

A. The risk for transmission to the neonate from an infected mother is high (30–50%) among women who acquire genital herpes near the time of delivery and low (<1%) among women with histories of recurrent herpes at term or who acquire genital HSV during the first half of pregnancy.

Q. What is the treatment of Genital herpes in pregnancy?

A. Oral or IV acyclovir in standard doses. Cesarean section should be considered for women developing genital herpes within 6 weeks of delivery.

Q. What is the treatment of neonatal herpes infection?

A. The recommended regimen for infants treated for known or suspected neonatal herpes is acyclovir 20 mg/kg IV every 8 hours for 21 days for disseminated and CNS disease or for 14 days for disease limited to the skin and mucous membranes.

Q. Name some vaccines available for HSV?

A. 1. Inactivated virion derived vaccines
2. Adjuvanted subunit vaccines

Q. Management of herpes simlex in pregnancy.

A.
- The number of women who acquire HSV-1 or 2 in pregnancy has been estimated to 0.5–2%.
- Female partners of men with genital herpes could not themselves have H/O genital herpres. Should be strongly advised not to have sexual intercouse at the time of recurrence and use condoms regularly throughout pregnancy
- The diagnosis can be confirmed by a Tzanck test or detecting HSV DNA by PCR.

Treatment:
- All primary episodes in pregnancy should be treated with Acyclovir orally which does not show teratogenic effects.
- Suppressive therapy with acyclovir from 36 weeks onwards reduces frequency of clinical disease and viral shedding at the time of delivery.

Prevention and therapy in neonates:
- If active herpetic lesions or if positive test for herpes is present at the time of delivery, it is better to do a Cesarean section.
- In case of recurrent herpes, vaginal delivery can be considered.
- All neonates with a confirmed or suspected HSV should be isolated.
- All visitors to take precautions to prevent direct contact with the skin.

Diagnosis:
PCR is the gold standard for detecting HSV from vesicular and conjunctival, oropharyngeal, stool, urine and CSF.

Therapy:
- IV Acyclovir significantly reduces mortality of disease.
- Dose: 10–20 mg/kg/day IV for 7 days.
- In case of cutaneous recurrences, 300 mg/m^2 is given orally 2–3 times a day for several months.

DONOVANOSIS [GRANULOMA INGUINALE]

Q. What is donovanosis?

A. Donovanosis is chronic, progressive ulcerative bacterial infection with *Calymmatobacterium (Klebsiella) granulomatis*, a gram-negative bacillus, as the causative microorganism.

Q. What is donovanosis also known as?

A. Granuloma venereum, granuloma inguinale tropicum, serpiginous ulcer.

Q. Is granuloma inguinale a misnomer?

A. Yes, this is because inguinal lesions occur only in up to 20% of patients.

Q. Name two important scientists involved in study of donovanosis.

A. Rajam and Rangaiah.

Q. Describe the bacillus *Calymmatobacterium granulomatis*.

A. *Calymmatobacterium granulomatis* is a small, pleomorphic, nonmotile, gram negative, fastidious bacillus showing bipolar staining (safety pin appearance).

Q. In which conditions safety pin appearance seen?

A.
- *Burkholderia pseudomallei (Pseudomonas pseudomallei)*
- *Francisella pestis (Yersinia pestis)*
- *Francisella tularensis*
- *Calymmatobacterium granulomatis*

Q. Who identified the causative organism?

A. The microorganism was first identified in 1905 by Donovan, who noted the characteristic Donovan bodies in macrophages and epithelial cells of the stratum malpighii.

Q. What are the predisposing factors for donovanosis?

A.
1. Sex: Male preponderance
2. Uncircumcised state.
3. Poor personal hygiene—who do not retract the prepuce and clean the area regularly.
4. Low socioeconomic status.
5. HLA-B57
6. Climate: High humidity and heavy rainfall.

Q. What is the primary lesion of donovanosis?

A. The primary lesion is a small cutaneous papule or nodule that contains mononuclear cells with cytoplasmic vacuoles filled with microorganisms. The cytoplasmic vacuoles can rupture and release bipolar Donovan bodies of coccoid, coccobacillary and bacillary morphology.

Q. What is the incubation period of donovanosis?

A. The exact incubation period is unclear—although the average period is about 17 days, may range from 1 day to 1 year.

Q. Describe the clinical features of donovanosis.

A.

Small papule or nodule

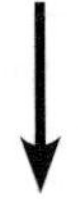

Breaks to form a nontender beefy red ulcer
Which bleeds on touch with sharply defined
edges and no adenitis. Inguinal abscesses (pseudobubo)
occur only in up to 20% of patients and are often
combined with genital involvement.

Q. What are the extragenital sites of donovanosis?

A. Often due to autoinoculation or secondary to dissemination, occurs in skin, bones (most common), intra-abdominal cavity and oral cavity.

Q. Describe the morphological variants of donovanosis.

A.
1. Ulcerative/Ulcerogranulomatous form (most common)
2. Hypertrophic/Verrucous form.
3. Necrotic type (Phagedena)
4. Sclerotic/Cicatricial type.

Q. What is the culture media for donovanosis?

A. Human peripheral blood mononuclear cells and HEp-2 cells.

Q. Which serological test available for diagnosis of donovanosis?

A. No serological test available for diagnosis of donovanosis.

Q. What is gold standard in diagnosis of donovanosis?

A. Demonstration of organism and identification of Donovan bodies in lesions is gold standard for diagnosis of donovanosis (Giemsa or Wright or Leishman's stain).

Q. Where and how crush smears are done?

A. For confirming the diagnosis of donovanosis, first the lesion is cleaned with gauze soaked in saline and then a dry gauze.

The infected tissue is usually friable and can be easily detached with a toothed forceps, a curette, scalpel blade, or a biopsy punch. The active edge of ulcer gives best yield.

Alternatively, lesion can be scraped with a scalpel or a cotton swab can be rolled over the lesion.

The pinched tissue is crushed in between two slides.

Slides are air-dried.

The smears are then stained with Giemsa, Leishmann or Wright's stain. In tissue scrapings stained by Wright's method.

Within large mononuclear cells, *C. granulomatis* organisms are found with bipolar staining at its two ends (Donovan bodies), giving them a 'safety pin' appearance.

Q. Describe the procedure of Leishman staining.

A.

Specimen collected
Slide is air-dried

Slide is covered with diluted Leishman stain for 10 minutes.

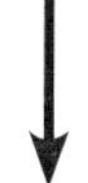

Rinse in steam of buffered water [ph 7.0–7.2]
Water is left on smear for 2–3 minutes.

Air dry the slide and examine under oil immersion

Q. What are the complications of donovanosis?

A.
1. Lymphedema [common in women] leading to pseudoelephantiasis or pseudoesthiomine/saxophone penis.
2. Autoamputation of penis in males, mutilation and destruction of labia in females in long standing cases.

3. Phimosis, paraphimosis and stenosis of urethral, vaginal, oral, or anal orifices in sclerotic variant of disease.
4. Local spread—involvement of fallopian tubes and ovaries leading to Pelvic Inflammatory disease.
5. Malignancy—development of SCC.

Q. How is pregnancy and donovanosis related?

A. Lesions of donovanosis tend to proliferate or reoccur during pregnancy. Cervical lesions may extend to pelvic structures and disseminate resulting in fatal hemorrhage at the time of delivery. These events are due to increased vascularity of tissues and immunosuppressive effects of pregnancy.

Q. What are the differential diagnosis of donovanosis?

A.
1. Squamous cell carcinoma
2. Amoebiasis
3. Tuberculosis
4. Dimorphic fungal infections
5. Pyoderma vegetans
6. Crohn's disease
7. Pyoderma gangrenosum
8. Atypical variant of secondary syphilis.

Q. What is pseudogranuloma inguinale?

A. The lesions of chancroid may closely resemble granuloma inguinale and is then known as pseudogranuloma inguinale.

Q. What is pseudobubo?

A. The bubo like swellings in the groins due to subcutaneous tissue involvement in the groins. The lymph nodes are NOT involved.

Q. Can donovanosis be eradicated?

A. For eradication of any disease the following criteria should be fulfilled:
1. Humans should be essential for the life cycle of the agent, which should not be able to amplify in the environment.
2. Diagnostic tests with sufficient sensitivity and specificity should be available to detect levels of infection that can lead to transmission.
3. Effective intervention should be available to interrupt the transmission of agent.

DONOVANOSIS FULFILLS ALL THE ABOVE CRITERIA FOR ERADICABILITY

Q. How will you treat donovanosis?

A. Recommended regimen:

- Doxycycline 100 mg orally twice a day for at least 3 weeks and until all lesions have completely healed.

Alternative regimen:

- Azithromycin 1 g orally once per week for at least 3 weeks and until all lesions have completely healed.

  OR

  Ciprofloxacin 750 mg orally twice a day for at least 3 weeks and until all lesions have completely healed.

  OR

  Erythromycin base 500 mg orally four times a day for at least 3 weeks and until all lesions have completely healed.

  OR

  Trimethoprim-sulfamethoxazole one double-strength (160 mg/800 mg) tablet orally twice a day for at least 3 weeks and until all lesions have completely healed.

Q. What is the treatment of donovanosis in pregnancy?

A. Erythromycin regimen or azithromycin should be given in pregnancy.

Q. How will you treat sex partners of donovanosis?

A. Persons who have had sexual contact with a patient who has granuloma inguinale within the 60 days before onset of the patient's symptoms should be examined and offered therapy.

Q. How does donovanosis in HIV differ from the usual pattern?

A.

Donovanosis and HIV infection:
Clinical features • Morphology: Longer ulcer duration, greater tissue destruction • Atypical sites: Extra genital sites (chin)
Course • Increased severity, slow healing and treatment failure
Investigation • Tissue smear and biopsy

Continued

Continued

Treatment

Recommended

1. Trimethoprim sulfamethoxazole double strength tablets 2 times a day or 3 weeks or until lesions heal
2. Doxycycline 100 mg 2 times a day in 3 weeks (or until lesions heal)

Alternative regimen

1. Ciprofloxacin 750 mg 2 times a day for 3 weeks (or until lesions heal)
2. Erythromycin 500 mg every 6 hours for 3 weeks (or until lesions heal)
3. Azithromycin 1 g orally once per week for atleast 3 weeks
4. Add Gentamicin 1 mg/kg body weight by slow IV infusion every 8 hours for 3 weeks (or until lesions heal) if slow healing

Donovanosis like any other STD can increase the chances of acquiring HIV infection.

6 Gonorrhea

Q. What is gonorrhea?

A. Gonorrhea is a sexually transmitted bacterial disease, caused by gram-negative, pear-shaped or reniform, fastidious, diplococcus, *Neisseria gonorrhoeae*. Derived from greek word 'gono' means seed; 'rrhoea'' means flow (the discharge was confused with semen).

Q. Which structures are more prone to get infected?

A. *N. gonorrhoeae* principally infects host mucous membranes lined by columnar, cuboidal epithelium and noncornified cells.

Q. What is the mode of transmission of gonorrhea?

A.
- Sexual contact—most common mode (vaginal, anal or oral intercourse).
- Vertical transmission—infected mother to the newborn during parturition, may lead to gonococcal conjunctivitis, pneumonia or even vulvovaginal infections.
- Fomites or nonsexual transmission—extremely rare (many patients claim to have been infected through toilet seats!).

Q. What is the risk of acquiring gonorrhea for a man following single vaginal intercourse with an infected female?

A.
- 20%, rising to an estimated 60–80% following 4 exposures.
- Whereas acquiring gonorrhea for a female following single intercourse with an infected male is 80%.

Q. What are the clinical features of gonorrhea?

A.
- Incubation period—1–14 days.
- Asymptomatic infections, local symptomatic mucosal infections (with or without local complications), and systemic dissemination.

Men	*Women*
10% asymptomatic infections	50% asymptomatic infections
• Acute anterior urethritis • Urethral discharge—purulent and profuse	• Endocervicitis • Increased vaginal discharge (prepubertal females) • Intermenstrual uterine bleeding • Menorrhagia • Deep dyspareunia

Continued

Continued

Men	**Women**
Dysuria	Dysuria
Without treatment, the clinical symptoms disappear in most patients after about 6 months	Swabbing of the endocervical canal results in a characteristic yellow swab, indicating gonococcal cervicitis
	Occasionally, inflammation of Bartholin's glands, with acute swelling of the labial folds and a discrete purulent discharge that appears when pressure is applied to the gland

Q. Why is gonorrhea not a cause of vaginal discharge in adult females?

A. This is because gonorrhea does not involves stratified squamous epithelium.

Q. What are the features of local complications of gonorrhea?

A.

Men	**Women**
Inflammation of the Cowper's and Tyson's glands	Inflammation of Bartholin's gland
Epididymitis	Salpingitis
Acute and chronic prostatitis	Oophoritis
Seminal vesiculitis	Pelvic inflammatory disease
Proctitis	Proctitis
Phimosis, paraphimosis, trigonitis, sterility	Parametritis
Watering can perineum (urine coming out through multiple openings on the perineum as a consequence of urethral stricture)	

Q. What are the complications of genital gonorrhea in pregnancy?

A.
- Spontaneous abortion
- Premature ruptures of membranes
- Premature delivery
- Acute chorioamnionitis
- Ophthalmia neonatorum (in newborn)
- Pharyngeal infections (in newborn)

Q. Enumerate extragenital gonorrhea.

A.
- Pharyngeal gonorrhea
- Rectal gonorrhea (asymptomatic in 50%)

- *Gonococcal ophthalmia*: Major cause of blindness in the developing world, primarily due to self-inoculation and unusual sexual practices. Characterized by purulent conjunctivitis progressing to a devastating keratitis followed by corneal opacification.

Q. What are the syndromes associated with disseminated gonococcal infections?

A. • Arthritis-dermatosis syndrome (gonococcemia)
- Acute perihepatitis (Fitz-Hugh–Curtis syndrome)

Q. Describe arthritis-dermatosis syndrome.

A. Occurs in 0.5–1% of patients with mucosal gonorrhea characterized by fever, gonococcal tenosynovitis affecting primarily larger joints, sometimes visible as erythema overlying the tendons and necrotic pustules due to embolic septic vasculitis seen on the distal portions of the extremities.

Q. What is Fitz-Hugh–Curtis syndrome?

A. • Occur with either gonorrhea, Chlamydia or mixed infections. It presents as fever and a complaint of right upper quadrant pain and tenderness that mimics acute cholecystitis.
- Fitz-Hugh–Curtis syndrome is inflammation of the liver capsule associated with genital tract infection.

Q. What are the risk factors of disseminated gonococcal infection?

A. Risk factors for disseminated gonococcal infection include:
- Menstruation (with the majority of cases in women developing during or immediately following menses).
- Deficiencies in the late complement components (C5–C9).
- Systemic lupus erythematosus.

Q. What is NGU?

A. Nongonococcal urethritis (NGU) that is not caused by *N. gonorrhoeae* but might be caused by *C. trachomatis.*

Q. What are the causes of nongonococcal urethritis?

A. • *Chlamydia trachomatis*
- *Ureaplasma urealyticum*
- *Mycoplasma genitalium/hominis*
- Trichomonas vaginalis
- *Gardnerella vaginalis*
- HSV
- Adenovirus
- Enteric bacteria

Q. What is the most common cause of gonococcal infections in children?

A. Sexual abuse is the most frequent cause of gonococcal infection in preadolescent children.

Q. How will you diagnose gonococcal infections?

A.
- Collection of specimen—in women, samples are obtained from the endocervical canal (after cleansing of any external exudate of vaginal secretions) and from the urethra.
- In men, specimen collection from the urethra is performed by using a small swab or bacteriologic loop.
- Anorectal specimens should be obtained under direct vision using anoscopy.
- Swabs of the posterior pharynx, including the tonsillar area, can be plated directly onto supplemented selective media.
- Staining—using grams stain or methylene blue stain.
- Culture—gold standard for the diagnosis of gonococcal infection.
- Culture media available—Thayer Martin media, New York City media.
- Nucleic acid amplification tests (NAATs)—polymerase chain reaction.

Q. What is the treatment of gonorrhea?

A. Uncomplicated gonococcal infections of the urethra, cervix, rectum: Recommended regimens:

- Ceftriaxone 500 mg IM in a single dose
  OR, IF NOT AN OPTION
  Cefixime 400 mg orally in a single dose
  OR
  Single-dose injectable cephalosporin regimen
  PLUS
  Azithromycin 1 g orally in a single dose
  OR
  Doxycycline 100 mg orally twice a day for 7 days
- Uncomplicated gonococcal infections of the pharynx:
  Ceftriaxone 500 mg IM in a single dose
  PLUS
  Azithromycin 1 g orally in a single dose
  OR
  Doxycycline 100 mg orally twice a day for 7 days
- Gonococcal conjunctivitis:
  Ceftriaxone 1 g IM in a single dose
- Gonococcal meningitis and endocarditis:
  Ceftriaxone 1–2 g IV every 12 hours

Therapy for meningitis should be continued for 10–14 days; therapy for endocarditis should be continued for at least 4 weeks.

- Disseminated gonococcal infections:
  Recommended regimen:
  Ceftriaxone 1 g IM or IV every 24 hours
  Alternative regimens:
- Cefotaxime 1 g IV every 8 hours OR
- Ceftizoxime 1 g IV every 8 hours
  All of the preceding regimens should be continued for 24–48 hours after improvement begins, at which time therapy can be switched to cefixime 400 mg orally twice daily to complete at least 1 week of antimicrobial therapy.
- Ophthalmia neonatorum:
  Ceftriaxone 25–50 mg/kg IV or IM in a single dose, not to exceed 125 mg
- Prophylactic treatment for infants whose mothers have gonococcal infection:
  - Recommended regimen in the absence of signs of gonococcal infection
  - Ceftriaxone 25–50 mg/kg IV or IM, not to exceed 125 mg, in a single dose.
  - Gonococcal infections in pregnancy:
  - Pregnancy/Breastfeeding:
    - Ceftriaxone, 500 mg IM as single dose OR
    - Other single-dose cephalosporin regimens (see above) OR
    - Spectinomycin, 2 g IM as single dose
- Disseminated gonococcal infection and gonococcal scalp abscesses in newborns:
  - Ceftriaxone, 25–50 mg/kg IV or IM QD for 7 days (10–14 if meningitis)

Q. How will you prevent ophthalmia neonatorum?

A. Erythromycin is the only antibiotic ointment recommended for use in neonates. Silver nitrate ointment (1%) is also effective (Crede's method).

Q. Would you prefer low dose ceftriaxone or high dose ceftriaxone and why?

A. A 500 mg dose of ceftriaxone is now recommended over a 125 mg dose given as:

- Increasingly wide geographic distribution of isolates demonstrating decreased susceptibility to cephalosporins in vitro,

- Reports of ceftriaxone treatment failures,
- Improved efficacy of ceftriaxone 500 mg in pharyngeal infection (which is often unrecognized), and
- The utility of having a simple and consistent recommendation for treatment regardless of the anatomic site involved.

Q. How will you investigate a case of urethral discharge?

A.

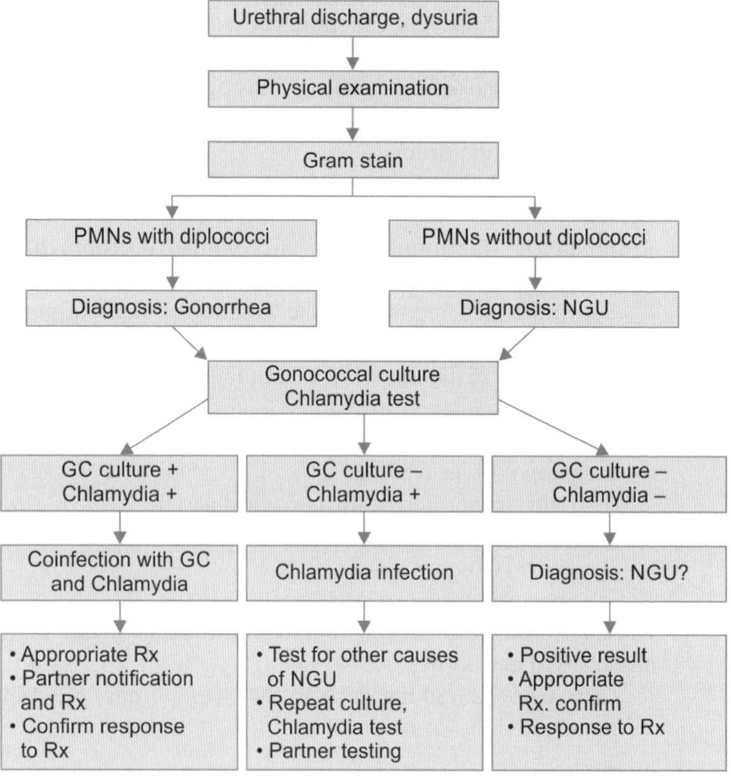

(Rx: treatment; NGU: nongonococcal urethritis; GC: gonococcal)

Q. What is the difference between gonococcal urethritis and non-gonococcal urethritis?

A.

Gonococcal urethritis	*Nongonococcal urethritis*
Thick purulent discharge	Thin mucoid discharge
Incubation period within a week	More than 2–4 weeks
More symptomatic	Less symptomatic
Associated with strangury	Pruritus

Q. What are the two varieties of resistant organisms encountered in gonorrhea?

A. • Penicillinase producing NG (PPNG)
- Quinolone resistant NG (QRNG)
- Due to the latter, nowadays fluoroquinolones are not used in gonorrhea)

Q. What are the other differential diagnosis of urethral discharge?

A. • Trauma/foreign body/stricture
- Intraurethral ulcers (chancre/chancroid/herpes simplex)
- Benign or malignant neoplasms
- Rarely tuberculosis

7 Hansen's Disease

CASE PROFORMA

History Taking in Leprosy

Name/Age/Sex/Occupation/Residing at ... /Hailing from ... /Marital status
Look at the occupation because occupations involving trauma to hands and feet can cause blisters or ulcerations due to anesthesia.

Chief complaints:

1. Light colored patches/noticed since___days/months (I/T/BT)
2. Multiple patches with tingling numbness in hands or feet (BT/BB/BL)
3. Stuffiness of nose/nasal bleeding/swelling of asymmetrical glove and stocking type of anesthesia since___ months (BL/LL)
4. Sudden redness and swelling and pain over pre-existing light colored lesions associated with fever since___ days (type I lepra reaction)
5. Tender raised transient painful lesions on bilateral shins, arms, face with fever and other constitutional symptoms since____ days (type II lepra reaction)
6. Deformity like claw hand/wrist drop/foot drop since ___ days (late stage of any advance disease)
7. Nonhealing ulcer since ___ days/weeks (advanced stage of disease)

ODP

Patient was apparently alright ____days/months ago.

1. TT/BT:
   - Patient then noticed light colored patch over the ___area of the body since ___ days/months.
   - The lesion was approximately pea sized and then gradually increased in size over ___time period to the present size.
   - The patient also noticed ___ (number) such similar lesions.
   - On enquiry patient reveals that there is decreased hair, decreased sweating and decreased sensations over that area
2. BL/LL:
   - Patient was apparently alright ___months ago.
   - Patient then developed bleeding from the nose/epistaxis

- Occasionally associated with stuffiness of the nose.
- Patient also C/O swelling over B/L ankle and feet which is more in the evening
- On enquiry patient also C/O dryness on both L/L
- Patient C/O asymptomatic skin colored/reddish/light colored lesions over the trunk since ___months
- The lesions gradually increased in number and in size to involve___ (areas of the body).
- Patient C/O of glove and stocking type of anesthesia since___ weeks/months.
- There is also decreased sensation over the palms and soles which has lead to unnoticed injury leading to nonhealing wounds.
- To rule out systemic involvement:
  - H/O eye involvement in the form of redness/irritation and increased lacrimation
  - H/O reduced libido
  - H/O swelling of the breast tissue in males
  - H/O infertility
  - H/O bone pains in the small bones of the hand and feet
  - H/S/O facial palsy
  - H/O hoarseness of voice
  - H/O alopecia
  - H/O inability to perceive smell (anosmia)
  - H/O dyspnea on exertion
  - H/O swelling of feet.

3. Type 1 reaction:
   - C/O redness, swelling and pain over the pre-existing lesions since___days.
   - H/O similar complaints in past. If yes—how many episodes
   - H/O associated fever
   - H/O associated weakness of hands and feet
   - H/S/O claw hand or foot drop or other deformities.
4. Type 2 reaction:
   - H/O fever—intermittent:
     - Low grade
     - More in the evening
   - H/O crops of red raised painful evanescent nodules over the B/L shins occurring since___days
   - H/O similar complaints in past. If yes—how many episodes
   - H/O joint pain/bone pain/muscle pain:
     - H/O epistaxis

  - H/O blurring of vision with deep pain in the eye with redness of eyes
  - H/O cloudy urine (proteinuria), flank pain

Rule out exacerbating factors that precipitate the reaction:

- Spontaneous
- H/O intercurrent infections
- H/O physical or mental stress
- H/O onset of puberty
- H/O pregnancy/parturition/lactation.
- H/O recent surgery
- H/O drugs like OCP, potassium iodide.
- H/O vaccinations.

5. Deformity:
   - H/O numbness over affected area since ___days.
   - H/O difficulty in doing fine movements like buttoning of shirt
   - H/O feeling like walking on cotton wool
   - H/O slipping of *chappals* while walking
   - H/O development of frank deformity like claw hand, wrist drop, claw toes, foot drop
6. Ulcer:
   - C/O nonhealing ulcer over the ball of the great toe since___days
   - H/O decreased sensations over the glove and stocking area since___weeks
   - H/O multiple unnoticed minor trauma
   - H/O fluid filled blister at the pressure points
   - Followed by development of an ulcer at the same site after ___ days.
   - No H/O pain over site of trauma.
7. Ask for:
   - H/O loss of lateral 1/3rd of the eyebrows
   - H/O drooping of eye lids
   - H/O hanging of ear lobes
   - H/O sagging of face
8. H/O treatment taken:
   - Rx. received in the form of blister combi packs?
   - Was the treatment taken in the form of monthly supervised dose as well as daily unsupervised doses?
   - Was the treatment taken regularly or not?
   - Rx. taken for how long?
   - Any untoward reaction during the course of treatment in the form of drug reaction or in the form of type 1 or type 2 reaction.

Past history:
H/O TB /DM/HT/Ischemic heart disease/Bronchial asthma

Personal history:
- Sleep
- Appetite
- Bowel/Bladder
- H/O addictions:
  - Alcohol,
  - *Beedi*/cigarettes,
  - Chewing beetle nut
- Menstrual history
- LMP:
  - 4 to 5 days
  - Regular cycle of 28 days
  - Normal bleeding
- Obstetric history:
  - G_P_A_L_
  - Contraceptive used
  - Tubal ligation done or not

Family history:
- H/O similar complaints in the family
- H/O TB in the family contacts

Quality of life:
- Personal—effect of disease on the interpersonal relationship with spouse and other family members
- Professional—effect of disease in terms of numbers of working days lost.

Socioeconomic status:
- Total monthly income of the family
- Total number of dependant family members
- Type of house—*pucca* house or hutment
- Sanitation facility

ON EXAMINATION

General Physical Examination

1. Patient is well oriented in time, place and person.
2. - Temperature
   - Pulse—increased in C/O reaction

- Blood pressure—increased in C/O renal involvement in LL or type 2 lepra reaction
- Pedal edema—in C/O LL and type 2 reaction
  (*Note*: Press on the lower tibia with the ball of your thumb for atleast 15 seconds to demonstrate pitting)
- Lymphadenopathy—seen in type 2 reaction, advanced LL
- Respiratory rate
- BMI

Cutaneous Examination

TT/BT:

1. Distribution of lesions—few/___ number of lesions over the ___ areas of the body
2. Arrangement—asymmetrical
3. Morphology:
   - Well defined skin colored/coppery/erythematous round to oval plaque measuring approximately ___ × ___cm with raised edge and flattened center (TT)
   - Well defined to ill-defined skin colored/coppery/erythematous round to oval plaque measuring approximately ___ × ___ cm with sloping edges. Few peripheral satellite lesions seen (BT)
4. The surface of the lesions show:
   - Hair—decreased
   - Sweating—decreased
   - Surface—dry
   - Sensation to cotton wool/hot and cold/pin prick reduced
5. Feeding nerve palpable or not
6. Tinel's sign—tingling pain on tapping of the feeding nerve.

BL/LL:

1. Distribution—multiple lesions scattered over almost the entire integument sparing the scalp and axillae
2. Arrangement—lesions are tending toward symmetry/or are symmetrical
3. Morphology:
   - Multiple, smooth, shiny and skin colored/erythematous nodules seen.
   - The hair/sweating and sensations over skin lesions are preserved.

Nerve Examination

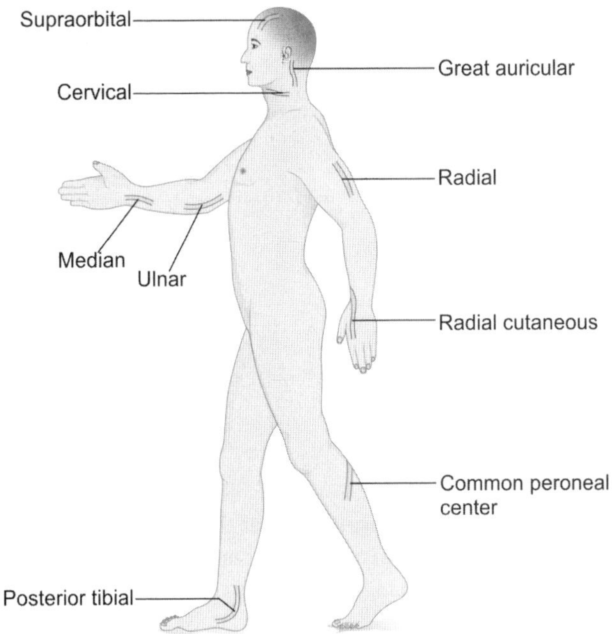

Look for the following points on palpation:

- Thickened +/-
- Tender +/-
- Nodules +/-

Nerve	***Right***	***Left***
Supraorbital		
Infraorbital		
Temporal		
Greater auricular		
Supraclavicular		
Infraclavicular		
Radial		
Ulnar		
Median		
Radial cutaneous		
Common peroneal		

Continued

Continued

Nerve	**Right**	**Left**
Anterior tibial		
Posterior tibial		
Sural		

Note: When there is no time, atleast palpate.

1. Temporal
2. Ulnar
3. Median
4. Radiocutaneous
5. Common peroneal
6. Post tibial
7. Sural

Sensory Examination

- Check for the loss of sensations over the lesions (the permissible limit for reference is 1 cm on hand, 2 cm on face and 7 cm on back)
- Check for glove and stocking anesthesia

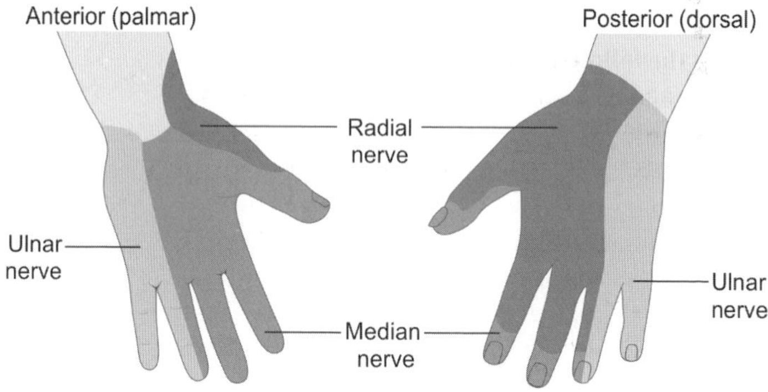

Cutaneous innervation of the foot
Saphenous nerve ①
Deep peroneal nerve ②
Superficial peroneal nerve ③
Medial plantar nerve ④
Lateral plantar nerve ⑤
Calcaneal branch (tibial nerve) ⑥
Sural nerve ⑦

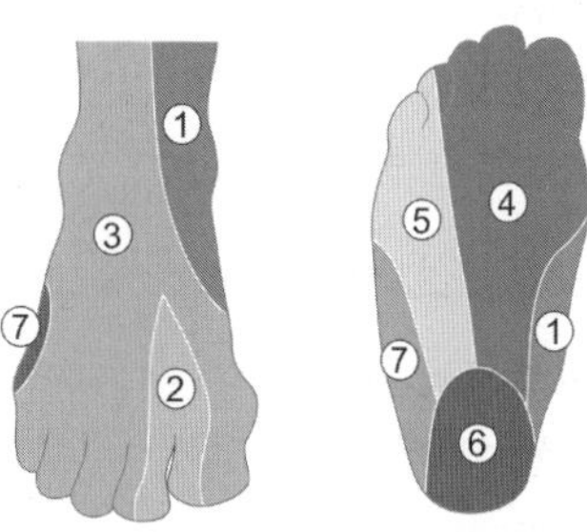

- Protective sensation over palms and soles (ideally with Semmes Weinstein filaments)
- Sensations over the dorsomedial forearm and anterolateral legs

Motor Examination

Ulnar:

- e/o wasting of thenar/hypothenar muscles
- e/o guttering over the palmar and dorsal interossei
- e/o failure of adducting fingers (palmar interossei)—card test/ Wartenberg's sign
- e/o failure of abduction of fingers (dorsal interosei)—unable to separate fingers against resistance
- e/o partial claw (lumbricals of little and ring finger)—ask patient to flex MP joint while extending IP joint against resistance
- Froment's book test—if book is held between thumb and index finger, the tip of the thumb flexes because the short flexor and adductors of thumb flexes because they are paralyzed and only way of tightening pinch is using FPL
- Muscle of forearm like FDP and FCU are paralyzed—e/o flattening of these muscles.

Median:

- Look for thenar wasting
- Pen test to check abductor pollicis brevis (ape thumb)
- Ask patient to stabilize hand and with the thumb parallel to the palm touch the tips of the other fingers—to check for opponens pollicis brevis
- Ask patient to flex at metacarpophalangeal joint with inter phalangeal joint extended—to check for the 1st and 2nd lumbricals
- Ochsner's clasping finger test, i.e., pointing index finger—to check for flexor digitorum superficialis and profundus.

Radial:

Ask patient to extend the wrist against resistance.

Superficial peroneal nerve:

- Look for e/o fanning of toes
- Ask patient to evert the foot against resistance

Anterior tibial nerve or deep peroneal nerve:

- Ask patient to dorsiflex, i.e., extend the foot against resistance
- Ask patient to invert the foot against resistance

Posterior tibial nerve:

- Ask patient to plantar flex, i.e., flex the foot against resistance.
- Ask patient to invert the foot against resistance.

Examine for Trophic Changes

- Asymptomatic, deep, nonhealing fissures on heels and toes
- Callosities on palms and soles
- Multiple spontaneous blisters on trauma prone areas
- Frank trophic ulcer

Short examination to test the nerves in the hands:

- Keep the hand flat on the table with palm upwards.
- Ask the patient to move the little finger outwards against resistance (if normal—ulnar nerve is unaffected)
- Make patient draw the thumb up and try to bring it down to level of other fingers against resistance. If able to do so—then median nerve is normal.
- Keep the arms straight outwards, and ask patient to dorsiflex the wrist. If possible—radial nerve is normal.

To test for nerves in the feet:

- Ask patient to keep the heel on the ground and dorsiflex the foot—if possible—lateral popliteal is normal
- Ask patient to dorsiflex the great toe, if possible—anterior tibial is normal
- Ask patient to plantar flex all together—off possible, post tibial is normal

Examination of Ulcer (If Present)

- Site
- Size
- Margin—elevated
- Edges—hypertrophic
- Floor—covered with slough
- Base—hard
- Local lymphadenopathy

Examination of Relevant Cranial Nerves

5th nerve:

Corneal reflex lost

7th nerve:

- Look for e/o ptosis or lagophthalmos
- e/o deviation of angle of mouth
- e/o dribbling of saliva
- e/o flattening of nasolabial groove.

Note: 1st nerve generally not tested but that is also involved.

Examination of Specific Deformities

- Madarosis
- Buddha ear
- Nose—epistaxis/nasal collapse
- Sagging of face
- Leonine facies
- Gynecomastia

Examination of Special Areas

Oral: Look for

- Papules over lips/macrocheilia
- Nodules over tongue/palate/uvula
- Perforation of the hard palate
- Loss of upper incisor teeth
  (Müller Christensen facies leprosa on radiology)

Nasal mucosa: Look for

- Nasal crusts that may lead to mouth breathing
- Insensitive, pale, thickened nasal mucosa
- Destruction of inferior turbinates

Eyes:

- Look for any skin lesions around periocular region
- Look for frequency of blinking, blink interval and blinking completeness (normal blinking is about 6/min)
- Look for photophobia, redness of eyes, watering of eyes
- Corneal reflex
- Light reflex
- Intraocular pressure by manual palpation

Digits:

- Tapering
- Deformity due to bone atrophy
- Add resorption

Nails:

- Dry
- Lustreless
- Shrunken
- Narrow
- Longitudinal ridges
- Inverse pterygium

External genitals:

- Size and consistency of the testicles
- Testicular sensation
- Tenderness

Systemic Examination

Respiratory system:

- Hoarseness of voice
- Dryness of throat
- R/O bronchopneumonia
- R/O tuberculosis

DIAGNOSIS

My patient ____, aged __, unmarried/married with __ kids is a case of mention the following points:

1. Hansen's or not
2. Active/Inactive—active means requiring MDT, inactive means patient has completed MDT and does not require it (this is as per definition of WHO)
3. Type of the disease—I/TT/BT/BL/LL/B
4. In reaction or not
5. In type 1 or 2 reaction
6. What grade of deformity/disability (Grade 0—no deformity, 1—non-visible deformity, i.e., anesthesia, 2—visible deformity)
7. Any ulcers
8. Has the patient been on regular treatment or not

Q. What are the diagnostic criteria?

A. There are 3 relative and 1 absolute criteria (slightly different from WHO):

Absolute criteria:

1. Presence of AFB is SSS

For diagnosis, absolute criteria itself is enough

2. Out of 3 relative criteria are enough for diagnosis
If only 1 is present, patient should be observed
Some people use nose for demonstrating AFB, but maybe cumbersome.

Q. What are the investigations to be done?

A. Routinely done:

- Slit skin smear
- Skin biopsy

Done only in doubtful cases:

- Histamine test
- Pilocarpine sweat test
- Nerve biopsy and USG nerves to study enlargement, structural abnormalities and vascularity.

Done rarely:

- Animal inoculation model
- Polymerase chain reaction
- Phenolic glycolipid-1 test

Q. Describe slit skin smear.

A. Take verbal consent:

- Area cleaned with spirit and allowed to dry.
- Firm pressure is applied with thumb and index finger so that skin blanches, for 30 seconds after this using a no. 15 blade used to make a 2–3 mm long 0.5 mm deep slit.
- Wipe if any blood is present. The blade is then turned 90° and the base of cut is scraped.
- The pulp is collected and smeared on a slide (circular fashion)
- Smear is then heat dried or air dried.
- The slit is sealed with Tincture benzoin
- Smear is stained with Z-N stain.

The sites used are: Both ears, forehead, skin lesion, elbow, knuckles
PB patients generally not smeared—either ear and skin lesion can be taken.

Q. What histopathological features are seen on skin biopsy?

A.
- Biopsy should be taken from active border of the skin, but normal skin should not be included.
- A deep biopsy should be taken.
- Slides should be stained with H&E and Fite-faraco stain (modified acid fast stain).
- Following features are observed:
  - In lepromatous leprosy—flattened epidermis, grenz zone present, foamy/Virchow/lepra cells seen (with globi in their

cytoplasm), destruction of cutaneous appendages, excessive inflammatory infiltrate.
  - In tuberculoid leprosy—dense lymphocytic infiltrate, absent grenz zone, large epithelioid cell granulomas, Langhan's giant cells, infiltration of dermal nerves
  - In borderline lepromatous—lymphocytes more prominent, perineural fibroblast proliferation (onion skin appearance), foamy cells are present but not prominent
  - In borderline tuberculoid—ill defined periappendageal granulomas, foreign body giant cells present
  - In upgrading type-1 reaction—granulomatous erosion of the epidermis, Langhan's giant cells are larger, sometimes fibrinoid necrosis within the granulomas
  - In downgrading type-1 reaction—necrosis less common, bacilli density increases over time
  - In type-2 reaction—foci of acute inflammation superimposed on chronic multibacillary leprosy, polymorph nuclear lymphocytic infiltrate, foamy macrophages

Q. What is histamine test?

A.
- Two symmetrical sites selected (test and control).
- One drop of histamine acid diphosphate on each site. Superficial prick made through each drop.
- Delayed and feeble flare in borderline and indeterminate leprosy, absent in tuberculoid.
- Flare indicates intact dermal nerves.

Q. What is sweat test?

A.
- 0.2 mL of 1 in 1,000 sol of pilocarpine nitrate is injected intradermally.
- Injection site is painted with iodine. Starch powder dusted over it.
- Sweating causes blue discoloration. Sweating indicates intact dermal nerves.
- For a more quantitative assessment, we can use a filter paper soaked in a dye called bromophenol. The paper initially is colorless shows multiple blue dots depending on number of functioning sweat glands.

Q. Comment on PCR and PGL-1 tests.

A.
- PCR is polymerase chain reaction for amplification of specific sequences of bacterial DNA. Subclinical cases can also be detected.
- PGL-1 stands for phenolic glycolipid-1 antigen present in *M. leprae*. This test lacks sensitivity and specificity.

Q. Comment on animal inoculation models.

A.
- Since *M. leprae* cannot be cultured in artificial medium, animal models have been used.
- Foot pad of mouse or nine banded armadillo used because of lower temperature (other animals used are Slender Indian Loris, Korean Chipmunk, Hedgehog).

Q. Differential diagnosis of a flat hypopigmented lesion.

A. Differentiate Hansen's from the following:
- Pityriasis versicolor—fine branny scaling, presence of fungal hyphae
- Vitiligo—depigmentation, leucotrichia, no thickened nerves, negative histamine test
- Pityriasis alba—ill-defined hypopigmented macules with scaling, associated features of atopy may be present
- Nevus depigmentosus
- Nevus anemicus
- Steroid induced hypopigmentation
- Idiopathic guttate hypomelanosis
- Post-kala-azar dermal leishmaniasis—hypopigmented macules over trunk and limbs, erythematous papules and nodules on face, facial erythema may be present, Leishman-Donovan bodies
- Onchocerciasis—depigmentation confined to pretibial regions, gastrointestinal symptoms present, stool examination positive
- Yaws—depigmentation over hairless areas of palms, hyperkeratosis of palms and soles, sabre tibiae, juxta-articular nodes, positive serological tests
- Morphea—may be slightly raised with purple edges, hair growth and sweating are lost

Q. Differential diagnosis of raised infiltrated lesion.

A. Differentiate Hansen's from the following:
- Tuberculosis verrucosa cutis—initially papule later thickened crusted sharply demarcated warty mostly at site of injury, mostly farmers and butchers
- Lupus vulgaris—lesions mimic lesions of tuberculoid form, erythematous indolent infiltrated asymptomatic, tendency to ulcerate, lesions heal at one edge v/s leprosy lesions which heal centrally, apple-jelly nodules on diascopy
- Lupus erythematosus—erythema, skin atrophy, follicular plugging, adherent scales
- Granuloma annulare—indolent asymptomatic papules or nodules in an annular pattern

- Granuloma multiforme—early papulonodular lesions later plaques, sensations preserved
- Pellagra—asymptomatic symmetrical patches with burnt-out appearance, associated dementia diarrhea may be present
- Annular syphilides—positive serological tests
- Seborrheic dermatitis—itchy scaly lesions, scalp may be involved, cardinal signs of leprosy absent
- Post-kala-azar dermal leishmaniasis—erythematous infiltrated raised lesions, LD bodies can be demonstrated
- Oriental sore—discoid infiltrated indurated plaques with central ulceration
- Tinea circinata—lesions are pruritic, fungal elements can be detected in the scrapings, raised erythematous edge with vesicles
- Sarcoidosis—sensations preserved, Kveim test positive, relatively uncommon in tropics
- Pityriasis rosea—erythematous plaques with collarette of fine scales, herald patch may be confused with tuberculoid Hansen's
- Psoriasis—erythematous scaly infiltrated plaques, Auspitz sign positive

Q. Differential diagnosis of nodular lesions.

A. Differentiate Hansen's from the following:

- Post-kala-azar dermal leishmaniasis—in advanced cases nodules on face neck extremities, absence of AFB, LD bodies diagnostic
- Cutaneous leishmaniasis—LD bodies diagnostic
- Syphilis—nodular and noduloulcerative lesions in late syphilis, absence of AFB, serological tests for syphilis positive
- Sarcoidosis
- Onchocerciasis
- Leukemia cutis—nodules with diffuse infiltration, leukemic nodules are bluish red, rubbery in consistency
- Mycosis fungoides—intensely pruritic plaques and red shiny tumors on face and trunk, presence of mycosis cells are diagnostic

Q. Differential diagnosis of sensory impairment with or without muscle wasting.

A. Following conditions should be ruled out:

- Neuropathy—think of the mnemonic DANG THE RAPIST (Dr Dang—the villain in a famous Hindi movie!)
- Diabetes

- Alcoholism
- Nutritional
- Guillain-Barré syndrome
- Toxic and drug induced
- Hereditary
- Refsum's disease
- Amyloidosis
- Periarteritis nodosa
- Infections (including leprosy and HIV)
- Systemic diseases (autoimmune)
- Tumors (carcinomatous neuropathy)

Of the above the following is discussed in some detail:

- Diabetes—very symmetrical glove and stocking anesthesia, accompanied by dysesthesia. Associated with cold, shiny and thinned out skin with loss of hair and anhidrosis. Loss of deep reflexes (usually never lost in leprosy). Nerve size normal.
- Alcoholic and nutritional—usually history, presence of calf tenderness, absence of thickened nerves.
- Hereditary sensory neuropathy—loss of sensation and sweating more in lower limbs. Motor function normal. Deep painless plantar ulcers, tendon reflexes lost. Nerves normal. Positive family history.
- Bernhardt-Roth syndrome—neuropathy of lateral femoral cutaneous nerve, due to pressure or edema of the femoral canal. Burning sensation and numbness over the lateral part of thigh. There may be slight reduction in hair. Nerves normal.

Q. Causes of thickened nerves without neurological deficit.

A. Following conditions should be ruled out:

- Excessive muscular development—in body builders or people with excessive muscle development nerves are thickened secondary to muscle hypertrophy
- Thin persons can have easily palpable nerves which may be mistaken for thickened nerve
- Traumatic neuropathy due to recurrent minor traumas, e.g., ulnar nerve of the right hand which is often subjected to minor injuries during the stress and strains of writing.
- Pachydermoperiostosis—clubbing of the nails, thickened skin of the forehead accompany thickened nerves
- Neurofibromatosis—neurofibromas, cafe-au-lait macules.
- Sarcoidosis—rare cause of thickened nerves.

Q. Causes of palpable nerves with some neurological deficit.

A. Following conditions should be ruled out:

- Primary amyloidosis—lower limbs, impaired sensation, muscle wasting, foot drop
- Familial hypertrophic interstitial neuropathy (Dejerine-Sottas) associated with muscular atrophy, claw hand, foot drop and loss of deep reflexes
- Peroneal muscular atrophy (Charcot-Marie-Tooth). Muscle weakness, hammer toes, callosities and reduced deep reflexes
- Endotoxic polyneuritis—cause unknown, adult onset, tendon reflexes absent

Q. Differential diagnosis of deformities.

A. Following conditions should be kept in mind:

- Dupuytren's contracture—due to involvement of palmar aponeurosis. Involves middle aged, usually diabetic males. Ring finger involved first. There is flexion of MCP joints but extension of IP joints (reverse of the claw hand found in leprosy)
- Syringomyelia—lesions only on upper limb. Touch sensation normal while there is inability to feel temperature. Associated with wasting of hand muscles. Nerves normal.
- Sclerodactyly—skin is edematous in early phases, later hide bound. Flexion deformities are found. Painful ulcers at tips of fingers. H/O Raynaud's phenomenon. Seen more in females. Similar appearance is found unilaterally due to cervical rib (thoracic outlet syndrome).
- Ainhum (saw)—seen in Africa. Painless constricting bands develop at base of little toes, leading to autoamputation. No sensory loss, no thickened nerves.
- Facial palsy—isolated facial palsy almost never due to leprosy. Bell's palsy is the common cause. Of the lower motor neuron type. Bell's phenomenon (upward rolling of the eyeball when attempting to close the eye) seen. Preceded by pain in the ear.

Q. Differential diagnosis of neuropathic ulcers.

A. Following conditions should be ruled out:

- Diabetes—same site as leprosy (under great toe). No thickened nerves.
- Tabes dorsalis and taboparesis—lightning pains, broad based gait, positive Romberg's sign, loss of knee reflexes, pupillary changes
  A mnemonic may help to remember signs of neurosyphilis.
  P: Personality changes

A: Depressed affect (emotional state)
R: Reflexes change (increased in paresis, decreased in tabes)
Eye changes sensorium altered
Impaired intelligence
Speech defects

- Syringomyelia, spina bifida, hereditary sensory neuropathy can lead to trophic ulcer
- Plantar corns—after excessively paring a corn, deep cavities can be left behind which can be mistaken for a plantar ulcers.
- Yaws—now rare. Painful hyperkeratotic ulcers over the palms and soles with fissuring called as crab yaws.

Q. Causes of Leonine facies.

A. Leonine facies can be seen in following conditions:

- Lepromatous leprosy
- Diffuse cutaneous Leishmaniasis
- Post kala azar dermal Leishmaniasis
- Sarcoidosis
- Primary systemic amyloidosis
- Scleremyxedema
- Pachydermoperiostosis
- Acromegaly
- Myxedema
- Actinic reticuloid
- Parthenium dermatitis
- Mycosis fungoides
- Leukemia cutis
- Sézary's syndrome

TREATMENT OF LEPROSY AND REACTIONS

Q. What is MDT?

A. It stands for multidrug therapy. In this multiple drugs are given at the same time in order to avoid resistance to any single drug.

Q. Which was the 1st MDT?

A. The 1st MDT was given in 1976 is Malta. The drug isoprodiaz (INH + prothionamide + dapsone) . It was combined with rifampicin but though effective, it was stopped due to unacceptably high hepatitis.

Q. When was WHO MDT introduced?

A. 1982.

Q. How is leprosy MDT given?

A. In an adult following regimen is followed:

Type of leprosy	*Monthly supervised*	*Daily self-administered*	*Duration of therapy*
Multibacillary	• Rifampicin: 600 mg • Dapsone: 100 mg • Clofazimine: 300 mg	• Dapsone: 100 mg • Clofazimine: 50 mg	1 year
Paucibacillary	• Rifampicin: 600 mg • Dapsone: 100 mg	Dapsone: 100 mg	6 months

Q. What are the pediatric doses?

A. In children following doses are given in a similar fashion:

Age group	*Drug doses*
<6 years	• Dapsone: 25 mg/day • Rifampicin: 150 mg/month • Clofazimine: 100 mg/month and 50 mg 2 times/week
6–12 years	• Dapsone: 50 mg/day • Clofazimine: 150 mg/month and 50 mg on alternate days • Rifampicin: 300 mg/month
12–15 years	• Rifampicin: 450 mg/month • Clofazimine: 200 mg/month and 50 mg/day • Dapsone: 50 mg/day
15–20 years	Same as adults

Today the WHO has recommended that MDT should be uniform in ALL patients. But, the duration should be 6 months for PB an 1 year for MB.

Q. Common side effects of MDT drugs.

A.

Drug	*Side effects*
Rifampicin	RIPAS: Respiratory symptoms, influenza-like symptoms, purpura, abdominal pain, shock (hypotension) hepatotoxicity, red discoloration of body fluids
Clofazimine	Pigmentation of initially infiltrated skin, GI symptoms, nephrotoxicity, ichthyosis, phototoxicity

Continued

Continued

Drug	**Side effects**
Dapsone	Hemolytic anemia in G6PD deficient patients, methemoglobinemia (treated with IV methylene blue), peripheral neuropathy, nephrotoxicity, hepatotoxicity, light headedness, dapsone syndrome

Q. What is ROM therapy?

A. Single dose of the following drug combination:

- Rifampicin: 600 mg (300 mg for children > 7 years)
- Ofloxacin: 400 mg (200 mg for children > 7 years)
- Minocycline: 100 mg (50 mg for children > 7 years)

Q. Treatment of type-2 lepra reaction.

A. Following drugs are used along with MDT:

- Aspirin: In a dose of 600 mg 3–4 times/day (in mild cases)
- Steroids: In a dose of 0.5–1 mg/kg/day (in a rapid taper over 2–3 weeks but may have to be used forlonger times severe cases, which may make the patient steroid dependent)
- Clofazimine: In a dose of 300 mg/day
- Thalidomide: In a dose of 100 mg 3–4 times/day
- Colchicine: In a dose of 0.6 mg/day
- Pentoxifylline: 400 mg TDS

Q. Treatment of type-1 lepra reaction.

A. Following drugs are used along with MDT:

- Steroids in a dose of 1 mg/kg/day to be tapered slowly over 6–9 weeks
- NSAIDs can be used in mild cases
- Chloroquine: 250 mg twice/day

Q. Treatment of neuritis.

A. Steroids, perineural injections (lignocaine + hyaluronidase + hydrocortisone), surgical decompression.

Q. Side effects of drug used in treatment of reactions.

A. Side effects are:

Drugs	**Side effects**
Steroids	Hypertension, diabetes, sodium retention, peptic ulcers
Thalidomide	Teratogenicity, infertility, constipation, drowsiness, peripheral neuritis

Continued

Continued

Drugs	***Side effects***
Colchicine	Diarrhea, abdominal pain, CNS depression, aplastic anemia
Clofazimine	As mentioned earlier
Aspirin	Internal bleeding, peptic ulceration, gastritis

Q. Management of other associated conditions.

A. The following conditions should be treated:

- Acute iridocyclitis—1% hydrocortisone eye drops
- Acute epididymo-orchitis—treated with prednisone and scrotal support
- Care of hands and feet—treatment of ulcers and deformities
- Management of rhinitis
- Care of the eyes—in case of lagophthalmos, artificial tear drops

Q. Should MDT be given in pregnancy?

A. Under any circumstances MDT should not be stopped.

Q. Leprosy and TB—How to treat together?

A. Start AKT in the proper doses. Start MDT for leprosy (without monthly rifampicin, since daily rifampicin is being given in daily regimen. After AKT is over start giving monthly rifampicin).

Q. Treatment of trophic ulcers.

A. Following points should be considered:

- Rest
- Leg elevation
- Eusol soaks
- Systemic antibiotics in case of secondary infections
- After infection subsides, below knee walking plasters
- Graded physical rehabilitation
- Preventive treatment through instituting gradually increasing walking, frequent stopping and resting, visual inspection and palpation of soles at night for wounds or warm areas (hot spots, indicative of necrosis under the skin), soak and scrape hyperkeratotic areas, use microcellular rubber *chappals* (MCR *chappals*).

  Most of them heal within 6 weeks, if not healing then suspect non-compliance, deep secondary infections, osteomyelitis, bony spurs, malignancy.

Prevention of trophic ulcers (tips of patients): 4 S's

- **S**ee—inspect feet at end of the day
- **S**oak—in luke warm water for 15 days
- **S**crape—callosities with scraper, pumice stone
- **S**mear—apply oil on extremity to soften and lubricate.

Q. What are the recent trends in treatment of leprosy?

A. In cases of rifampicin resistance:

Regimen I: Ofloxacin 400 mg, minocycline 100 mg and clofazimine 50 mg for 6 months.

Followed by ofloxacin 400 mg or minocycline 100 mg and clofazimine 50 mg for 18 months.

Regimen II: Minocycline 100 mg, moxifloxacin 400 mg, clarithromycin 500 mg, clofazimine 50 mg for 6 months.

Followed by a continuation phase with once a month dosing of minocycline 200 mg, moxifloxacin 400 m, clarithromycin 1000 mg for 18 months.

In rifampicin sensitive cases:

- Rifampicin 600 mg or rifapentine 900 mg,
- Moxifloxacin 400 mg,
- Clarithromycin 1000 mg,
- Minocycline 200 mg

All daily for 12 months.

8 Leg Ulcers

History

Name/Age/Sex/Occupation/Residing at ... /Hailing from ... /Marital status

Chief complaints:

- History of (H/O) red raw lesions on ... sites, since ...
- Where did it begin ... did it start like a red raised solid lesion/pus filled lesion/fluid filled lesion/swelling (gradual/rapid enlarging?)/ on preexisting scar?
- Spontaneous/post-trauma
- Is the ulcer painful?
- Is there any discharge?
- If yes ... Serum/pus/blood
- History of limb heaviness/aching/swelling.
- Is it worse at the end of the day/swelling relieved by leg elevation?
- Is there a history of prolonged standing?
- Does the shoes become more tightly fitting in the evening?
- H/O fever/joint pains/recurrent oral ulcers/photosensitivity/malar rash
- H/O sexual exposure
- Any associated diseases (tabes dorsalis/syringomyelia/transverse myelitis/peripheral neuritis/generalized TB/nephritis/DM/tertiary syphilis/autoimmune CTD/atherosclerotic cardiovascular disease
- Any similar family history
- Treatment history—topical/systemic
- Whether aggravated/relieved symptoms
- Personal—smoking/alcohol intake obstetric—H/O recurrent/ spontaneous abortions

Physical examination:

- General examination: General condition—fair
- Patient is conscious/cooperative/well oriented in time/place/ position
- Pallor/clubbing/cyanosis/icterus/lymphadenopathy/edema feet

- Lymphadenopathy (tuberculosis) look for nutrition/syphilitic stigma
- Check both limbs (Buerger's disease)
- Palpate the arteries for calcification
- Auscultate for carotid bruit
- Capillary refilling time should be within 2–3 seconds
- All peripheral pulsations to be felt

Local examination:
- Inspection
- *Size and shape*:
  - Oval/circular/semilunar/serpinginous/irregular
  - Measure the size—press a sterile gauze on the ulcer to get its measurement
  - Number of ulcers
  - Position of the ulcer (medial malleolus/lateral malleolus)
  - Edge (inflamed/edematous/blue zone/white zone)
  - Undermined/sloping/punched out/rolled out (everted)/raised and pearly white beaded
  - Floor—covered with red/pale/yellow granulation tissue
  - Wash leather slough (like wet chamois leather) on the floor (gummatous syphilis)
  - Is the bone forming the floor of the ulcer? (trophic ulcer)
  - Is there any black mass in the floor (malignant melanoma)
  - Discharge—character/amount/smell should be noted
  - Scanty serous/purulent/serosanguineous (malignant or tuberculosis)
  - Greenish discharge? (*B. pyocyanea*)

Surrounding area:
- Glossy, red, edematous (inflamed ulcer)
- Pigmentation/verrucous surface (stasis dermatitis—venous ulcer)
- Telangiectasia (atrophie blanche)
- Scar or wrinkling surrounding the ulcer (old case of tuberculosis)
- Fibrosis/necrosis/cellulitis
- Thin, atrophic, hairless dry skin
- Whole limb should be examined
- Deep vein thrombosis/varicose veins
- Neurological insufficiency (trophic)
- Presence of any hypopigmented anesthetic patches

Palpation:

- Tenderness (tender/slightly tender/never tender)
- Edge and margin—corroborate inspector findings
- Palpate edge and surrounding tissue—for marked induration (squamous cell carcinoma or adenocarcinoma)
- Slight induration in any other chronic ulcer except malignancy (gummatous/syphilitic/trophic)

Base:

- If an attempt is made to pick up the ulcer between the thumb and the index finger, base will be felt.
- Slight/marked induration depth
- Record in millimeters
- Check whether it reaches bone bleeding
- Bleeds to touch? (malignant)
- Relation with deeper structures
- The ulcer is made to move over the deeper structures to know whether its fixed to these structures (fixed—gummatous and malignant ulcers)
- Surrounding skin

Skin around the ulcer must be palpated and examined:

- Check temperature/tenderness
- Mobility of surrounding skin
- Loss of sensation or motor deficit
- Feel the peripheral nerves thickening for abnormal thickening/ tenderness
- Feel the main artery supplying the part
- State of vein around the ulcer (varicose veins)

Lymph node examination:

- Enlarged/tender/abscess?
- Matted/nonmatted?
- Stony hard and fixed to the neighboring structures

Examination for vascular insufficiency:

- Varicose veins
- Check for deep vein thrombosis
- Arteries proximal to ulcer

Examination for nerve lesion:

- Sensory/motor examination/palpation and testing of sensation of any erythematous plaques for Hansen's (peripheral neuropathy)
- Deep tendon reflexes

QUESTIONS

Q. What is an ulcer?

A. Ulcer is a break in the skin or mucous membranes with associated necrosis (cell death). An ulcer heals with scarring.

Q. What is an erosion?

A. Erosion is a break in skin or mucous membranes without associated necrosis. It heals without scarring.

Q. What are the common causes of leg ulcers as far as a dermatologist is concerned?

A. Venous, neuropathic (including due to diabetes or leprosy), arterial and vasculopathic (most important being pyoderma gangrenosum).

Q. What is Marjolin's ulcer?

A. Squamous cell carcinoma developing on pre-existing scar of a burn. It is more aggressive and metastasizes early.

Q. Differential diagnosis of tender ulcers.

A.
- Inflammatory ulcers (pyoderma gangrenosum, vasculitis, polyarteritis nodosa, Wegener's granulomatosis), panniculitis/erythema induratum/hypertensive ulcers:
    - Tuberculosis ulcers.
    - Malignant ulcers infiltrating structures supplied by pain nerve endings.

Q. Painless ulcers-DD.

A.
- Trophic ulcers (leprosy/tabes dorsalis/peripheral neuritis/transverse myelitis)
- Syphilitic ulcers
- Deep fungal infections
- Cutaneous tuberculosis
- Ulcerative DLE
- Squamous cell carcinoma, basal cell carcinoma
- Venous ulcers

Q. Why is the shape of ulcers important?

Shape	*Condition*
Oval/irregular crescentic border	Tuberculosis
Semilunar/circular/serpiginous	Syphilis
Vertically oval	Varicose ulcers
Irregular	Carcinomatous

Q. What information do you get by knowing the location of a particular ulcer?

Site	*Condition*
Medial malleolus	Varicose ulcer
Ball of foot/heel	Trophic
Tibia	Gummatous ulcer
Any where	Malignant ulcer
Pretibial area, breast, hand, neck, peristomal skin, head	Pyoderma gangrenosum

Q. What is the difference between edge and margin?

A. Margin is the junction between normal epithelium and the ulcer. So it is the boundary of the ulcer. Edge is the area between the margin and the floor of the ulcer.

Edge	*Condition*
Undermined	Tuberculosis
Punched out	Gummatous ulcer/deep trophic ulcer
Sloping	Healing/traumatic/venous ulcer
Raised/pearly white/ beaded	Rodent ulcer
Rolled out/everted	Squamous cell carcinoma/ulcerated adenocarcinoma
Inflamed and edematous red granulation tissue in center, toward periphery blue (growing epithelium) and a white zone (fibrosis)	Spreading ulcer healing ulcer

Q. Is base and floor the same?

A. Floor is the exposed surface of the ulcer which can be both seen and felt on palpation while base is the area on which the ulcer rests. It cannot be seen but only felt. Floor is exposed surface within the ulcer.

Q. What is importance of floor of ulcer?

Floor	*Condition*
Red granulation tissue	Healthy and healing
Pale and smooth granulation tissue	Slowly healing ulcer
Wash leather slough	Gummatous ulcer
Bone	Trophic ulcer
Black mass	Malignant melanoma

Q. What is importance of discharge of ulcer?

Discharge	*Condition*
Scanty serous discharge	Healing ulcer
Purulent discharge	Spreading and inflamed ulcer
Serosanguineous discharge	Tuberculous ulcer, malignant ulcer
Greenish discharge	B-pyocyanea

Q. Why do you get undermined edge in tuberculous ulcer?

A. Because tuberculosis spreads in and destroys the subcutaneous tissue faster than it destroys the skin. The overhanging skin is thin, friable, reddish blue and unhealthy. The other ulcer which is undermined is pyoderma gangrenosum.

Q. What do you mean by punched out edge?

A. The edge drops down at right angles to the skin surface as if it has been cut out with a punch.

Q. Why do you get everted edges in squamous cell carcinoma?

A. Fast growing cellular disease, growing portion at the edge of the ulcer heaps up and spills over the normal skin resulting in everted edge.

Q. Why should you look at the surrounding skin?

Surrounding skin	*Condition*
Glossy red and edematous	Acutely inflamed
Eczematous and pigmented	Venous ulcer (varicose)
Scarred or wrinkling skin	Tuberculosis

Q. Which conditions cause arterial/ischemic ulcer?

A.
- Atherosclerosis
- Raynaud's disease
- Buerger's disease

Q. What type of lymphadenopathy does one get in various conditions?

Lymph nodes	*Conditions*
Regional tender lymphadenitis	Acutely inflamed
Matted, enlarged, slightly tender	Tuberculous
Shotty, discrete, firm	Hunterian chancre
Not usually involved	Gummatous ulcer
Stony hard/fixed to neighboring stages (late stages)	Malignant ulcer

Q. What are the investigations done in case of ulcer?

A.
- Total count/DLC (lymphocyte count)/ESR
- Increased lymphocyte count and raised ESR for tuberculosis
- FBS/PLBS
- VDRL
- Urine for sugar
- Pus/discharge for culture and sensitivity (inflamed and spreading)
- Mantoux test
- Chest X-ray (tuberculous ulcers, metastatic deposits)
- Biopsy (malignancy from edge and surrounding healthy tissue)—type/invasiveness/differentiation
- X-ray of bone and joints
- New bone formation (gummatous ulcers and sabre tibia)
- Contrast radiography—arteriography
- Imaging techniques—Doppler (venous and arterial)

Q. Classification.

A.
- Clinical:
  - Spreading ulcer
  - Healing ulcer
  - Callus or chronic ulcer
- Pathological
- Nonspecific
- Specific
- Malignant

Q. What are the nonspecific ulcers?

A.
- Traumatic
- Arterial
- Venous
- Neurogenic
- Associated with other diseases
- Certain other types

Q. What are specific ulcers?

A.
- Tuberculosis
- Syphilitic
- Soft sores
- Actinomycosis

Q. Which are the malignancies causing ulcers?

A.
- Epithelioma
- Marjolin's ulcer
- Rodent ulcer
- Malignant melanoma

Q. What is Bazin's ulcer?

A. Found in obese adolescent girls particularly on the calves as purplish nodules followed by indolent ulcers.

Q. What is Martorell's ulcer?

A. Hypertensive patient with ulcer which affects legs where patches of skin necrosis are seen.

Q. Difference between arterial and venous ulcer and neuropathic ulcer.

Arterial	*Venous*	*Neuropathic*
Rare	Common	Common
Painful	Painless	Ulcer painless but paraesthesia of distal extremities
Small	Large	Large or small
On anterior and outer aspect of the leg/ dorsum of the foot/toes, ankle or the heel (above medial malleolus/bony prominences)	Medial aspect of the lower third of the lower limb (below medial malleolus)	Pressure sites (plantar surface overlying 1st and 5th metatarsal heads, plantar surface of great toe and heel)
Intermittent claudication/rest pain	No rest pain/ intermittent claudication	No pain
Punched out edges	Flat/sloping edges	Punched out
Base is dry, covered with necrotic debris tendons may be exposed	Base covered by healthy red granulation tissue	Bone
Surrounding skin— loss of hair, cold to touch, shiny, atrophic, dry skin, pallor, fissuring, thickening of nails	Eczema and pigmentation	Thick rim of callus. Dryness, fissuring because of autonomic involvement
–	Lipodermatosclerosis	–
Peripheral pulsations not felt	Peripheral pulsations felt	Felt

Continued

Continued

Arterial	***Venous***	***Neuropathic***
• Prolonged capillary refill time >3–4 secs • Pallor on leg elevation • Dependent rubor appears after a delay of normal 10–15 seconds in dependent position	Varicosities/ankle edema/lymphedema	Peripheral neuropathy/ decreased sensations/foot deformities
Audible bruit-femoral artery	–	–
Most common cause atherosclerosis	Most common cause is varicose vein/deep vein thrombosis	Leprosy/transvers myelitis/tabes dorsalis

Q. Which artery should always be felt when an arterial ulcer is suspected?

A. Dorsalis pedis artery and posterior tibial artery.

Q. What is the role of leg elevation in arterial ulcer?

A. If the leg is kept elevated above the heart level, there will be more pain and the ulcer will not heal.

Q. What is the gaiter area of the leg?

A. Extends from lower medial calf to just below the medial malleolus.

Q. What is a callus ulcer (trophic/neurogenic)?

A. It is an ulcer which starts with callosity under which suppuration takes place, the pus comes out and the central hole forms the ulcer with punched out corny edge.

Q. What is a tropical ulcer?

A.
- Tropical ulcers occur on the leg and feet of people in tropical countries, associated with malnutrition
- It is caused by vincent's organism (bacteroides fusiformis) refractory to heal.

Q. Why does a diabetic patient get an ulcer?

A.
- Diabetic neuropathy
- Diabetic atherosclerosis causing ischemia causing ulcer
- Glucose laden tissue is quiet vulnerable to infection

Q. What is the most characteristic feature of tuberculous ulcer?

A. It is its edge which is thin reddish blue and undermined.

Q. Which other skin disease is common in patients with chronic venous ulcers?

A. Allergic contact dermatitis.

Q. What is lipodermatosclerosis?

A.
- It represents fibrosed subcutaneous tissues (firm, indurated, woody).
- Early (acute)—diffuse indurated erythema, warm, tender.
- Advanced—inverted champagne bottle leg appearance.

Q. What is inverted champagne bottle leg appearance?

A. Proximal leg swells as a result of chronic venous obstruction and lower leg constricts because of fibrosis and loss of subcutaneous fat.

Q. What is atrophie blanche (livedoid vasculitis)?

A. Smooth ivory white atrophic plaques of sclerosis, multiple telangiectasias and surrounding brown discoloration (40% of cases with venous insufficiency/APLS like hypercoagulability states).

Q. What is lymphedema precox and tarda?

A. Lymphedema precox is at puberty while lymphedema tarda occurs after 35 years.

Q. What is Milroy's disease?

A. Congenital lymphedema.

Q. How do you differentiate lymphedema from lipedema?

A. Bilateral swelling of lower extremities but sparing of feet.

Q. What is Kaposi-Stemmer sign?

A. Inability to pinch the area between the 4th and the 5th toe characteristic of lymphedema.

Q. What is elephantiasis nostras verrucosa (mossy leg)?

A. *Nostra*- of our region.

It is a complication of chronic lymphedema characterized by hyperkeratosis, verrucous changes and fibrosis as well as massive enlargement of body part, usually scrotum or lower leg.

Q. What are the causes of secondary lymphedema?

A.
- Recurrent lymphangitis and cellulitis
- Parasitic infections (filariasis)
- Lymph node dissection (for melanoma/breast cancer)
- Rosaceous lymphedema
- Granulomatous disease
- Amyloidosis

- Malignant obstruction (lymphoma/Kaposi's sarcoma)
- Radiation injury
- Obesity

Q. What is yellow nail syndrome?

A. Yellow thickened nails with primary lymphedema of ankles and recurrent pleural effusion/bronchiectasis.

Q. What is intermittent claudication?

A.
- Pain in one or both legs, relieved by rest and is characteristic of arterial insufficiency.
- Rest pain in advanced disease and tend to keep limb in dependent position.

Q. How is capillary refill time measured?

A. It is obtained by compressing tip of the great toe until it blanches and then releasing the pressure.

Q. What is ankle brachial pressure index (ABI)?

A. Divide the ankle systolic pressure by the higher of the two systolic pressures obtained from brachial artery in both arms.

Normal >1

0.5–0.8 = occlusive arterial disease

<0.5 = severe occlusive disease (rest pain)

Q. False high index seen in ...

A.
- Diabetes
- Calcified vessels

Q. How will you check the sensory perception in a case of neuropathic ulcer?

A.
- Apart from the pin prick method, Semmes Weinstein monofilament is utilized to test sensory neuropathy. A 4.17 monofilament is normally felt (1 g of linear pressure)
- If a 5.07 monofilament (10 g linear pressure) cannot be detected, patient is said to have lost protective sensation.

Q. Why are the metatarsal heads more prominent in neuropathic ulcer?

A. Because motor neuropathy affects the small intrinsic muscles of the foot, the predominance of extrinsic muscles leads to cocked up toes and prominent metatarsal heads.

Q. What is acroangiodermatitis of mali?

A. Pseudo kaposi sarcoma in which violaceous patches and plaques on extensor surface of distal lower extremities and dorsal aspect of feet and is associated with venous hypertension/AV malformation or fistula.

Q. What is cryofibrinogenemia?

A.
- In cryofibrinogenemia there is a circulating protein that precipitates when the plasma is cooled. It may be idiopathic or secondary to malignancy/connective tissue disease/infection.
- It presents with purpura, livedo reticularis, ecchymoses or leg ulcers that are refractory to standard therapy.

Q. What is Buerger's disease?

A.
- Inflammatory and occlusive condition of medium sized arteries and veins caused by autoimmune process triggered by tobacco in young adults.
- Asymmetric coldness of extremities and decreased peripheral pulses.

Q. What is pyoderma gangrenosum?

A. Pyoderma gangrenosum (PG) is a primarily sterile inflammatory neutrophilic dermatosis characterized by recurrent very tender cutaneous ulcerations with mucopurulent or hemorrhagic exudate, undermined bluish borders and surrounding erythema.

Q. What is the initial lesion of pyoderma gangrenosum (PG)?

A. Pustule or papulopustule on an erythematous or violaceous base. Erythematous nodule/bulla.

Q. Variants of PG.

A.
- Ulcerative
- Bullous
- Pustular
- Superficial granulomatous

Q. Describe the ulcer of PG.

A. Ulcers are painful necrotic,undermined border with purulent or vegetative base on lower extremities (pretibial area) and rarely mucous membranes and peristomal sites.

Q. Histopath of PG.

A. A sterile dermal or appendageal abscess neutrophilic infiltrates.

Q. Which are the illnesses associated with PG?

A.
- Inflammatory bowel disease (ulcerative colitis, Crohn's disease)
- Arthritis
- Hepatitis C,
- Seronegative rheumatoid arthritis, spondylitis
- Lymphoproliferative disorders (monoclonal gammopathies, leukemia, lymphoma, and myelodysplastic syndrome)

Q. Which drugs cause pyoderma gangrenosum?

A.
- Propylthiouracil, pegfilgrastim—a granulocyte-stimulating factor
- Gefitinib—an inhibitor of epidermal growth factor receptor.

Q. What is PAPA syndrome?

A. The autosomal dominant inherited disease is characterized by familial recurrent nonaxial destructive arthritis, severe cystic acne and PC. PAPA syndrome is caused by mutations in the PSTPIP1 gene on chromosome 15 involved in regulation of inflammatory response.

Q. Why is history of joint pains important?

A. The PG-ulcers associated with arthritis (poorer prognosis), sickle cell anemia with crisis connective tissue disorder.

Q. Why is location of PG important to know?

A. PG involvement of the hands shows a higher percentage of lymphoproliferative than chronic inflammatory bowel disease.

Q. What are the extracutaneous manifestations of PG?

A. Involvement of upper airway mucosa, eye, genital mucosa, sterile pulmonary neutrophilic infiltrates or spleen infiltrates, and neutrophilic myositis. Sterile cortical osteolysis has been observed adjacent to PG ulcers as another extracutaneous manifestation of the disease.

Q. What is the differential diagnosis?

A.
a. Vascular occlusive or venous disease including calciphylaxis which is particularly painful and rapidly evolving.
b. Vasculitis. Differential diagnoses include Wegener's disease, anti, phospholipid syndrome, or in Adamantiades-Behçet's disease, etc.
c. Lymphomas or leukemia.
d. Infectious disease—ecthyma and deep (tropical) mycoses like sporotrichosis may resemble PG. The rapid onset of post-surgical PG often reminds of acute deep skin infection such as erysipelas or gangrene. Late syphilis has become more common again and may develop suppurative ulcerations. Deep viral herpetic infections can resemble PG.
e. Exogenous tissue injury—factitious panniculitis as a part of the Münchausen syndrome may masquerade as PG. Insect or spider bites can cause necrotizing skin ulcers.
f. Drug reactions—pustular drug reactions

Q. How do you treat PG?

A.
- Systemic glucocorticoids (0.5–1 mg/kg of prednisolone)
- Methyl prednisolone (1 g within 3–5 days)
- Immunosuppressants
- Sulfasalazine (1–4 g)
- Clofazimine
- Clochicine
- Infliximab

Q. What is the prognosis?

A.
- 70% better prognosis after steroids
- 66% after cyclosporine
- 30% mortality

Q. What is pathergy and in which diseases do you get pathergy?

A. Exaggerated,uncontrolled inflammatory response to a nonspecific stimulus as seen in:
- Pyoderma gangrenosum
- Behçet's disease

Q. Can PG lesions be painless?

A. Yes. Proliferating chronic ulcers of PG without the presence of an inflammatory halo, and slow evolution with marked tissue neutrophilia and usually without coexisting diseases.

Q. Can the ulcer be caused by necrobiosis lipoidica diabeticorum?

A.
- Ulcerative type of necrobiosis lipoidica diabeticorum can present with ulcers resistant to therapy and squamous cell carcinoma has been reported. Degenerative disease of collagen due to diabetic microangiopathy/immune complex disease/defective collagen synthesis.
- The immune reaction precedes and initiates the release of cytokines that finally cause the degeneration of collagen synthesis and granulomatous alterations.

Q. How do you differentiate such ulcers?

A. Presence of yellow-brown, atrophic, telangiectatic plaques surrounded by raised, violaceous rim in the legs. Giant ulcers with necrotic material and cribriform base with erythematous raised border have been reported.

Q. What are the factors causing NLD to ulcerate?

A. Trauma, the poor circulation over the pretibial area and an exaggerated immune response have been suggested as the causes of ulceration.

Q. What is a chronic leg ulcer?

A. Chronic leg ulcer is defined as a defect in the skin below the level of knee persisting for more than six weeks and shows no tendency to heal after three or more months. Chronic ulceration of the lower legs is a relatively common condition amongst adults, one that causes pain and social distress. The condition affects 1% of the adult population and 3.6% of people older than 65 years.

Q. Why ulceration occurs in gaiter area?

A. Patients with reduced mobility or obesity may develop ulceration in the gaiter area because of venous hypertension resulting from inadequate functioning of the calf muscle pump.

Q. Commonest cause of vasculitis ulcers.

A. The commonest causes of vasculitis ulcers are rheumatoid arthritis, systemic lupus, and polyarteritis nodosa.

Q. Enumerate hematological disorders associated with the development of leg ulcers.

A. Leukemia, hereditary spherocytosis, thrombotic thrombocytopenic purpura, granulocytopenia, sickle-cell disease, thalassemia, thrombocythemia, and polycythemia rubra vera and polyclonal dysproteinemia. Leg ulcers related to hematological disorders generally result from microcirculatory occlusion.

Q. Explain the three major theories of how venous ulceration develops.

A.
- Fibrin cuff theory—fibrinogen leaks from dilated capillaries of the epidermis forming a pericapillary fibrin cuff. This is then responsible for a reduced diffusion of oxygenated blood to the tissues resulting in ulceration.
- Leukocyte entrapment theory—venous hypertension reduces the pressure gradient between the arteriolar and venular end of the capillaries. This results in sluggish movement of the blood within these capillaries and increases the adherence of blood cells to the endothelium. Inflammatory mediators (ICAM-1, VCAM-1) and reactive oxygen species are then released resulting in the obliteration of functioning capillary loops aggravating ischemia and result in ulceration.
- Microangiopathy theory—it has been demonstrated that some of the capillaries in patients with venous leg ulcers are occluded by microthrombi or exhibit long intracapillary stasis. This in turn can reduce nutrition and oxygenation of the skin, predisposing to ulceration

Q. Enumerate mechanisms involved in the pathophysiology of ischemic leg ulcer.

A. (1) Extramural strangulation (2) Mural thickening or accretion, and (3) Intramural restriction of blood flow. There is often considerable overlap, and the exact pathogenesis cannot be always well defined. Most acute forms of vasculitis and some subacute and chronic forms are likely to cause leg ulceration due to tissue hypoxia and exudation of fibrin-like substances.

Q. Etiology of diabetic foot ulcers.

A. The major underlying causes are noted to be peripheral neuropathy and ischemia from peripheral vascular disease. Other factors in ulceration are trauma, deformity, callus formation, and edema.

Q. Complications of pressure ulcers.

A. Septicemia, osteomyelitis, and even death.

Q. Investigations in chronic leg ulcers.

A.
- The ankle brachial pressure index (ABPI) using a handheld Doppler ultrasound and sphygmomanometer can be carried out for more accurate assessment of arterial perfusion.
- Accurate and regular measurement of the wound is important to give an objective assessment of the effectiveness of the current management plan. The leg ulcer measurement tool (LUMT) is a validated tool that has been developed to quantify leg ulcer assessment and can be used to track change in wound status over time
- Blood investigations such as complete blood count, erythrocyte sedimentation rate, blood sugar, lipid profile, renal function tests, and liver function tests are essential in patients with chronic leg ulcers.
- The plain radiography of the foot along with CT and MRI should be done to rule out osteomyelitis and malignancy.
- Laboratory screening tests for vasculitis—urine analysis for proteinuria, hematuria, cylindruria, routine and immunohisto-pathology of skin biopsies, antinuclear antibodies, rheumatoid factor, complement C4, circulating immune complexes, para-proteins, immunoglobulin fractions, antineutrophil cytoplasmic antibodies, serological tests, and cultures for underlying infections
- Laboratory screening tests for clotting disorders—activated partial thromboplastin time, prothrombin time, thrombin time, factor V (Leiden) mutation (506R fi 506Q), factor II

(prothrombin) mutation (20210G fi 20210A), antithrombin III, protein C and protein S, and lupus anticoagulant anticardiolipin
- Venography may be performed as an investigational procedure prior to valvular surgery.
- Plethysmography and venous pressure data are important in determining the need for surgical bypass or valve replacement.
- A quantitative bacterial culture is more specific and should be performed once wound infection is suspected
- Ulcer biopsy is important in making a correct diagnosis and to rule out malignancy as these ulcers are prone to malignant transformation
- Gene variant analysis and evaluation in patients with venous leg ulcers

Q. Treatment options in venous ulcers.

A. Leg elevation, compression therapy, aspirin, pentoxifylline (Trental), surgical management.

Q. What is necrobiosis lipoidica diabeticorum?

A.
- Present in about 60% of diabetes patients
- Causative connection between necrobiosis lipoidica and diabetic microangiopathy
- Observed as ischemic ulceration
- Symmetrical on extensor sides of tibia
- In one-third of patients ulceration occurs
- It can ulcerate after a trauma
- Yellowish ulceration, fat ulcer bases
- Heals with difficulty

9 Lymphogranuloma Venerum

Q. What is lymphogranuloma venereum (LGV)?

A. Lymphogranuloma venereum is a STD caused by Chlamydia trachomatis serovars L1, L2, L3 that primarily affects lymphatics.

Q. LGV is also known as.

A.
- Durand-Nicolas-Favre disease-initially described in 1833 by Wallace, defined as a distinct clinical entity by Durand, Nicolas and Favre in 1913
- Climatic bubo

Q. How does the organism enter the skin and establish infection?

A. LGV affects mainly the lymphatic tissue in the genitorectal area. The organisms enter the body via microscopic defects in the mucosa or the skin. The microorganisms then enter the lymphatics, leading to lymphangitis, perilymphangitis and infection of lymph nodes. Over a period of many weeks to months, the inflammatory process expands and results in periadenitis, involvement of a few neighboring lymph nodes, the development of abscesses (which can rupture), and the formation of fistulae and strictures. Latent persistence of the microorganism within involved tissues may last for many years.

Q. What is the incubation period of LGV?

A. Incubation period is 3–12 days.

Q. Describe the stages of LGV.

A. The disease progresses through three stages:

1. *Primary stage*: Initial infection of the genital mucosa-characterized by the appearance of a transient herpetiform ulcer, heals rapidly leaving no scar.
2. *Secondary stage*:
   - Occurs after 2–6 weeks.
   - Classically described as the inguinal syndrome, and is characterized by tender, unilateral inguinal lymphadenitis resulting in suppurative buboes with fistulae and associated constitutional symptoms. Enlargement of the external iliac and inguinal lymph nodes separated by the inguinal ligament produces the 'sign of the groove' (Greenblatt sign).

- *Anorectal syndrome*: Patients complain of mucopurulent anal discharge, rectal pain and bleeding, tenesmus, constipation and ulcerative proctocolitis.

3. *Tertiary stage*: It may occur many years after the initial stages. The manifestations result from fibrosis and lymphatic obstruction. Elephantiasis of the external genitalia causes polypoid growths, fistulae, chronic ulceration, scarring and deformity.

Q. What is Grooves sign or Greenblatt sign?

A. In case of LGV the external iliac lymph node and the inguinal lymph nodes, both become enlarged, this will be separated by a groove formed by the inguinal ligament.

Note: In the most books, they give inguinal and femoral lymph node is written however it is not so.

Q. Describe the clinical manifestation in each stage of LGV.

A. Initial manifestations: 3–12 days
- Papule
- Erosion or ulcer
- Herpetiform vesicle
- Nonspecific urethritis or cervicitis
- Uncommonly, balanitis and nodular ulcerations.

Inguinal syndrome: 10–30 days up to 6 months
- Regional lymphadenopathy (mostly inguinal and femoral, also perirectal, deep iliac)
- Overlying erythema
- Constitutional symptoms
- Eruption of buboes
- Pelvic inflammatory disease.

Ano-genito-rectal syndrome: Months to years
- Proctocolitis
- Hyperplasia of intestinal and perirectal lymphatic tissue
- Perirectal abscesses
- Ischiorectal and rectovaginal fistulas
- Anal fistulas
- Rectal strictures and stenosis
- Frozen pelvis and infertility
- Esthiomene

Other manifestations:
- Urethro-genito-perineal syndrome
- Peno-scrotal elephantiasis
- Erythema nodosum

- Submaxillary or cervical lymphadenopathy associated with oropharyngeal lesions.

Q. What is bubonulus?

A. • Primary LGV associated with lymphangitis of the dorsal penis and formation of a large tender lymphangial nodule which is called bubonulus.
- Multiple tender nodules.

Q. What is esthiomene?

A. Esthiomene (Greek—eating away); a primary infection affecting the lymphatics of the scrotal, penis or vulva which may cause chronic progressing lymphangitis, chronic edema and sclerosing fibrosis of the subcutaneous tissues of these structures. This results in induration and enlargement of the affected parts and destructive ulceration.

Q. What is Fitz-Hugh-Curtis syndrome?

A. Fitz-Hugh-Curtis syndrome is inflammation of the liver capsule associated with genital tract infection associated with LGV. Classically presenting as sharp, pleuritic right upper quadrant pain.

Q. What is the difference between bubo and pseudobubo?

A.

Bubo	*Pseudobubo*
Enlarged lymph node	Subcutaneous nodules
Seen in chancroid, LGV	Seen in donovanosis

Q. What is the difference between bubo of chancroid and bubo of LGV?

A.

Bubo of chancroid	*Bubo of LGV*
Matted	Nonmatted
Unilocular (since single LN is involved)	Multilocular (since it involved multiple lymph nodes)
More tender	Less tender
Usually associated with genital ulcers	Not associated genital lesion
Bubo develops acutely	Bubo develops slowly
90% unilateral 10% bilateral	70% unilateral 30% bilateral
Shape of bubo-oval	Sausage shaped bubo is LGV

Continued

Continued

Bubo of chancroid	***Bubo of LGV***
Overlying skin is erythematous and thinned out	Overlying skin is purple, thickened, wrinkled
Bubo is of the same consistency throughout	Bubo is of different consistency in different phases (variegated)
Bubo ruptures with single opening	Ruptures with multiple openings
Discharge is thin, purulent	Discharge is thick, rope like
Giant chancroid develops at site of rupture	Multiple sinuses form without ulceration
Groove's sign (Greenblatt's sign)–ve	Groove's sign (Greenblatt's sign) +ve

Q. What is lymphorrohoids or perianal condylomas?

A. Obstruction of the lymphatics and venous drainage of the lower rectum produces perianal outgrowths of lymphatic tissues (that resemble hemorrhoids) are called lymphorrohoids or perianal condylomas.

Q. Which is the most sensitive method for diagnosis of LGV?

A. Polymerase chain reaction.

Q. What are the diagnostic modality of choice used in diagnosis of LGV?

A. The diagnostic method of choice is by nucleic acid amplification tests and confirmation by real-time PCR assays for LGV-specific DNA.

Q. What are the diagnostic modalities used in diagnosis of LGV?

A. Definitive diagnosis is by detection of the L serovar of *C. trachomatis* from the site of infection. Specimens may be obtained from ulcers and the rectum; or bubo aspirate:

- Nucleic acid amplification tests and confirmation by real-time PCR assays for LGV-specific DNA.
- The Frei intradermal test, which was based on a positive hypersensitivity reaction to a purified chlamydial antigen, is now only of historical interest.
- Imaging studies using CT or MRI scan may be useful if retroperitoneal adenitis or intra-abdominal abscess is suspected, and a barium enema may reveal the characteristic elongated stricture in rectal LGV.
- Screening for other sexually transmitted infections, including HIV, and viral hepatitis B and C, should be undertaken.

Q. What are the differential diagnosis of LGV?

A.
- Inguinal syndrome—syphilis, chancroid, granuloma inguinale, cat-scratch disease, tularemia, plague, mycobacterial disease and lymphoproliferative disorders.
- In women, pelvic inflammatory disease and tubo-ovarian abscess.
- Anogenital syndrome-enteric infections; other STIs caused by gonorrhea, oculogenital strains of *C. trachomatis*, herpes simplex virus and cytomegalovirus; and actinomycosis and schistosomiasis.

Q. What is treatment of LGV?

A.
- Recommended regimen: Doxycycline 100 mg orally twice a day for 21 days.
- Alternative regimen: Erythromycin base 500 mg orally four times a day for 21 days.

Q. How will you treat sex partners of LGV?

A. Persons who have had sexual contact with a patient who has LGV within the 60 days before onset of the patient's symptoms should be examined, tested for urethral or cervical chlamydial infection, and treated with a chlamydia regimen (azithromycin 1 g orally single dose or doxycycline 100 mg orally twice a day for 7 days).

Q. How will you treat LGV in pregnancy?

A. Pregnant and lactating women should be treated with erythromycin.

Q. How will you treat LGV in HIV?

A. Persons with both LGV and HIV infection should receive the same regimens as those who are HIV negative. Prolonged therapy might be required, and delay in resolution of symptoms might occur.

10 Pellagra

HISTORY TAKING

- Name/Age/Sex/Occupation/Residing at ... /Hailing from ... /Marital status:
    - More common in middle age persons
    - More common in low socioeconomic people, courier boys, salesman, farmer
    - Endemic in Deccan Plateau of India because they eat sorghum/ jowar as staple food

Chief complaints:

History of presenting complaints

- Did the rash start with redness/bullae/scaling?
- Onset, duration, sites involved (extensors/front and side of neck, back, buttocks, axillae, groins, pressure points)
- Progression—whether facial rash on and off (lupus erythematosus) or continuous (pellagra)
- History of diarrhea—duration, frequency, large/small volume, with or without blood.
- History of (H/O) episodes of sleeplessness/fear/anxiety
- History of redness in mouth/burning sensation aggravated while eating spicy food. Difficulty in eating
- History of photosensitivity—increased redness/burning/itching while exposure to sunlight.
- History of bloating, weight loss, aggravation of symptoms after taking specific food? (wheat, barley, oat), steatorrhea, anorexia, fatigue, abdominal pain, vomiting, dyspepsia (malabsorption)
- History of any abdominal surgery.
- History of any recurrent oral ulcers, joint pain, on and off rash over malar area, seizures, chest pain, difficulty in breathing (SLE)
- History of blistering, after minimal trauma, easy fragility, excessive hair over body (porphyria cutanea tarda)
- History of flushing, palpitations, giddiness and black out (low BP), aggravation of symptoms after eating cheese, chocolate (Carcinoid syndrome)
- History of tremors, inability to balance while walking, swaying to one side (Hartnup's disease)

Past history:

H/O any skin disease/major illness/sexual exposure.

Diet:

- Has he foregone meals?
- Bouts of vomiting
- Type of food (junk food/food fads)
- Breakfast/lunch/dinner veg/nonveg
- Staple diet-rice/maize
- Fruits and veg
- Total calorie intake
- Protein intake

Personal history:

- Habits—alcohol/smoking/recreational drugs
- Sleep/bowel/bladder habits

Socioeconomic history:

- Earning members
- Income
- Wife works or not
- Size of the room how much square feet?

QOL:

- Do fights lead to increased alcohol intake?
- Has the disease affected professional and sexual life?
- History of palpitations, loss of weight despite good appetite, intolerance to heat or cold, anxiety, insomnia, hairfall, muscle weakness, irregular menses (thyrotoxicosis).

Drug history:

Antiepileptic/antitubercular/oral contraceptive/antihypertensive.

Family history:

Any family member having similar disease (inborn errors in metabolism).

Menstrual and obstetric history (females):

- Menses regular/irregular.
- On-going pregnancy, if any.

General examination:

- General condition
- Conscious, cooperative, oriented to time, place and person, any evidence of dehydrated.
- Temperature/BP/PR/RR

- PR is significant for sign of dehydration.
- Are extremities cold and clammy?
- Pallor
- Icterus
- Clubbing
- Cyanosis
- Edema feet
- Lymphadenopathy

Cutaneous examination:

- Rash—symmetrical/asymmetrical, sites involved, present over photo-exposed area or not.
- Well-demarcated or ill demarcated from normal skin.
- Examine genitals. Are genitals involved? If yes, describe the rash.

Oral cavity and perioral area examination:

Dry, cracked and fissured lips; angular cheilitis, oral ulcer, tongue (tip and margin of tongue, papillae), gingivitis/nasolabial dyssebacia

Systemic examination:

- CNS examination:
  - Higher functions—consciousness (as clouding of consciousness can occur)
  - Memory (short term/recent memory)
  - Orientation
  - Cerebellar functions—incoordination, ataxia.
- *Per abdominal examination*—any organomegaly (liver—palpable/not, if palpable—liver span, tender or nontender). Any other sign of liver failure (flapping tremors, spider nevi, caput medusa).
- CVS examination—heart sounds.
- RS examination—any adventitious sound.
- Diagnosis—pellagra.

Q. What does the word pellagra mean?

A. "Pelle" is derived from Italian literature meaning skin, and "agra" meaning rough.

Q. What are the four D's of pellagra?

A. *D*iarrhea, *d*ermatitis, *d*ementia, and eventually *d*eath.

Q. Who described pellagra first ?

A.
- Gasper Casal described pellagra in 1762 in the Asturias region of northern Spain.
- He termed the disease as "mal de la rose" because all the affected patients had typical reddish and glossy rash on the dorsum of hands and feet.

Q. Who termed the word pellagra?

A. Frapolli named this disease as vulgo pelegrain and first used the term pellagra in 1771.

Q. Which regions is pellagra commonly found in?

A. Pellagra chiefly occurs in developing nations where corn and corn products are the major food source in ethnic populations with diets deficient in niacin/tryptophan.

Q. Who usually gets pellagra?

A.
- Jowar maize eating populations
- They have excess of leucine which interferers in conversion of tryptophan to niacin.

Q. What are the causes of pellagra?

A. Primary—tryptophan deficiency and niacin dietary deficiency.

Secondary:
- Inadequate diet—malnutrition, maize and jowar eating population. Washing corn with lime water (performed in mexico)—forestalling pellagra. Jowar—has adequate niacin but increased leucine that interfered in the niacin pathway—Sorghum vulgare.
- Prolonged diarrhea and malabsorption—gastroenterostomy, subtotal gastrectomy, Crohn's disease—there is impaired absorption of tryptophan and niacin, chronic colitis, severe ulcerative colitis
- Chronic alcoholism (poor diet and malabsorption)
- Metabolic derangement—Hartnup's disease and carcinoid syndrome
- Drug induced—isoniazid, 5-florouracil, 6-mercaptopurine, pyrazinamide, phenytoin, chloramphenicol, azathioprine, Phenobarbital
- Urocanic acid deficiency—protects the skin from UV light
- Hepatic cirrhosis
- Tuberculosis of GI tract
- HIV disease

Q. How does alcohol cause pellagra?

A.
- They can not afford the right type of food
- They do not buy the right food. Increased calories because of junk food increase the need of nicotinic acid
- Poor appetite because of gastritis
- Poor absorption in intestinal mucosa
- Decreased absorption of pyridoxine
- Improper metabolism of niacin due to liver dysfunction.

Q. Describe the pathogenesis of pellagra.

A.
- Primary pellagra results in deficiency of niacin, resulting from inadequate dietary nicotinic acid or its precursor essential amino acid tryptophan. Niacin is required for adequate cellular function and metabolism as an essential component in coenzyme 1 (NAD) and coenzyme 2 (NADP), these compounds are important co-enzymes for glycolysis, protein and amino acid metabolism, pyruvate metabolism, and maintains cellular energy levels.
- Cellular functions in multiple organs and tissues are affected by niacin deficiency, the clinical expression of pellagra is diverse.

Q. What are the early clinical symptoms of pellagra?

A. Lassitude, weakness, loss of appetite, mild digestive disturbance, psychiatric and emotional stress.

Q. Symptoms of pellagra.

A.
- Diarrhea is the first symptom
- Cutaneous manifestations—various types of dermatitis
- Photosensitive eruption, perineal lesions, thickening and pigmentation of skin over the bony prominences
- The dermatitis is bilaterally symmetrical at cutaneous sites of solar exposure.
- These are painful to touch (in the acute phase)
- It starts as an erythema changing to exudative eruption on the dorsum of hands, neck, face and chest with pruritus and burning. It becomes edematous, which forms a vesicle or bulla (acute pellagra/wet pellagra)/(Pemphigus pellagrosus) and eventually ruptures to form crusted erosions. This then leads to thickened, scaly and hyperpigmented skin.
- Characteristic well marginated eruption on the front of the neck (Casals necklace) on the C3 and C4 dermatome.
- On the face an erythematous rash extending from nose to the cheeks, chins, lips and may resemble lupus erythematous—Butterfly rash.
- Pellagra may also present as perineal lesions. Scrotal and perineal erythema with erosions are common.

Q. What are the GI features of pellagra?

A. Soreness of tongue and mouth, loss of appetite, indigestion and painful abdomen. Diarrhea may lead to nausea, vomiting which may in turn lead to malabsorption forming a vicious cycle.

Q. What are the neurologic features of pellagra?

A. • They occur late in the course of disease, early symptoms are insomnia, fatigue, nervousness, depression.
- Neurologic manifestations include sensorimotor neuropathy, parkinsonism, retinitis and optic atrophy.

Q. Enumerate the differential diagnosis of pellagrous skin lesions.

A. Porphyria cutanea tarda and variegate porphyria, Hartnup's syndrome and drug induced pellagroid reactions. Photoallergy reactions can be similar.

Q. What is Hartnup's disease?

A. • It is an autosomal recessive disease.
- Usually diagnosed between 3–9 years of age
- The primary defect is in the transport system for monoamine and monocarboxylic acid—malabsorption of amino acids (tryptophan)
- It has pellagra like changes
- Neurological changes—cerebellar ataxia and moderate mental retardation
- Diagnosis is confirmed on demonstration of aminoaciduria

Q. What is carcinoid syndrome?

A. • Carcinoid syndrome occurs when a rare neuroendocrine cancerous tumor (carcinoid tutor) secretes certain factors like biological active amines and peptides (including tryptophan and serotonin).
- These factors cause cutaneous flushing and telangiectasias.
- The tryptophan and serotonin secretion depressed the endogenous niacin production.
- This causes pellagrous dermatitis, sclerodermatoid thickening, pruritus and may lead to cutaneous metastasis.

Q. How is the diagnosis of pellagra established ?

A. Levels of urinary metabolites of N-methyl nicotinamide and N-methyl-2-pyridine-5-carboxamide are decreased in pellagra. Urinary levels of NMN below 0.8 mg indicate niacin deficiency.

Q. What is the treatment of pellagra?

A. • Oral administration of nicotinamide or niacin 100–300 mg/day in three separate doses.
- Mental changes disappear within 48 hours, but skin lesions take 4 weeks to respond, most patients need to be given riboflavin and pyridoxine also, and a diet rich in calories and proteins to address malnutrition.

Q. Histopathology of pellagra.

A.
- Pathological changes in the skin are relatively nonspecific.
- Vesicles, if present, may arise subepidermally as a result of vacuolar degeneration of the basal layer, or intraepidermal as a result of intense spongiosis. The upper half of the Malpighian layer may show striking vacuolar alteration. There is also perivascular lymphocytic infiltrate of the superficial vascular plexus.
- Older lesions may have epidermal hyperkeratosis and parakeratosis, with variable acanthosis. There is often increased epidermal basal layer melanin. Eventually, there may be epidermal atrophy overlying dermal fibrosis, sebaceous gland atrophy and a chronic lymphohistiocytic perivascular infiltrate.

Q. How can pellagra be prevented?

A.
- Pellagra can be prevented by intake of a protein-rich diet. Food sources of niacin, and/or tryptophan include nutritional yeast, eggs, bran, peanuts, meat, poultry, fish, red meat, whole-grain cereals, fortified grains, legumes and seeds. Recommended daily allowance are as follows: for infants 5–6 mg, children 9–13 mg, adults 13–20 mg, and pregnant and lactating mothers 17 mg and 20 mg, respectively.
- Optimal supplementation is 20–30 mg daily. Nutritional education can be important.
- Supplementation of grain cereals with niacin may be desirable. For secondary prevention one should avoid sun exposure during the active phase of the disease. Close dietary follow-up of the patient upon recovery helps prevent recurrence of pellagra.

11 Psoriasis

Vital Data

Name/Age/Sex/Religion/Occupation/Staying at/Hailing from/Marital status

CHIEF COMPLAINTS

Skin

- Red raised scaly/nonscaly lesions________days/weeks/months/ years on ... (knees/elbows)
- In psoriasis the lesions are usually present for a number of years but the patient usually comes when there is a flare ... So one can say that lesions are since________years but flared up since________days
- Symptoms: Usually a patient with psoriasis has mild-to-moderate itching or is asymptomatic.
- Patient may also have pain due to formation of pustules, or cracking of the lesions.

Joints

Which joints/pain-swelling-blocked movements/morning or evening stiffness.

Note: Morning stiffness is due to inflammatory joint involvements while evening pain is due to degenerative joint involvement.

Onset Duration Progress

- Patient was apparently all right________years back when he noticed reddish, scaly rash (peasized/coin sized/palm sized/dew drop sized), initially over the________. These then spread to involve ... (sequence of spread). There was H/O waxing and waning, with new lesions occurring in (seasonal variations). Some lesions healed on their own or with treatment to leave behind pale areas. The lesions slowly increased over the past few years but have rapidly increased since the past few days. Mention whether lesions are static/ progressive/regressing.
- Pruritus
  - Continuous/intermittent
  - Mild/moderate/severe—disturbing sleep or not

On Enquiry

- What was the odor/type/amount of scales?
- Loose (fall off easily) scales/adherent scales
- H/O etiology/trigger factors
- H/O trauma at the site of the initial site or did the subsequent lesions occur at sites of injury?
- H/O drug intake prior to onset of initial lesions or were the subsequent lesions associated with drugs (topical or systemic)?
- H/O any infections prior to onset of initial lesions or were subsequent lesions associated with any fever, sore throat, dental, gastrointestinal (GI) infection or other infections?
- H/O sexual exposure/diarrhea (protected or unprotected) (Reiter's disease, secondary syphilis)
- H/O recurrent oral ulcers and photosensitivity (for subacute lupus erythematosus)
- H/O stressful events before initial lesions
- History for complications
- *Joint problems*: H/O low back/hip/finger pain/swelling/morning or evening stiffness/difficulty in movement
- *GI problems*: H/O recurrent abdominal pain, swelling, bloating or irregular bowel movements [for inflammatory bowel disease (IBD)]
- H/O any chest pain, palpitations or breathlessness, rapid gain in weight (metabolic syndrome)
- H/O spread of lesions to entire body with or without pus filled lesions and fever (erythroderma or pustular psoriasis)

If female:

- Any relation with present or previous pregnancies?
- H/O treatment taken
- Topical agents
- Oral therapies/phototherapy

Past history

- H/O similar episodes earlier in the past
- H/O any skin problem

Drug history

- Personal
- Sleep, bowel, bladder disturbances
- Addictions: Alcohol, smoking

Medical history

- Hypertension/cardiovascular diseases/liver pathology/kidney diseases/hyperlipidemia/pain/morning stiffness/loss of range of motion usually of thoracic spine.

Family history

- Similar complaints/H/O rheumatoid arthritis

Quality of life: Interfering with function in workplace/relation with spouse/outdoor activities

ON EXAMINATION

- General constitution: Fair/poor afebrile/febrile
- Pulse/blood pressure/respiratory rate/abdominal girth/weight
- Pallor/clubbing/cyanosis/lymphadenopathy/edema feet

Cutaneous Examination

- Primary lesion: Papules/plaques/pustules
- Secondary lesions: Scales/crusts/any erosions
- Distribution: Symmetrical/asymmetrical
- Maximum involved sites:
- Relative sparing:
- Body surface area involved: (1 palm = 1%)

Description of Primary Lesion

- *Plaque*: Well defined, bilaterally symmetrical, erythematous (if salmon colored say so), scaly over extensors/flexors/scalp/palms/soles/face. Do the scaly plaques extend beyond frontal margin of scalp?

Scales

- Dry/Greasy
- Silvery white/yellowish hyperkeratotic/ostraceous/rupioid
- Do the scaly plaques extend beyond frontal margin
- Auspitz sign+/-

If positive:

- On removal of scales (grattage) with the pin head or side of a slide, Auspitz sign is elicited. Auspitz sign consists of the following components:
  - If scales are minimal on grafting the scales become more visible the scales are silvery, shiny, arranged in layers (micaceous) and easily removed due to parakeratosis.
    - On removal of all the scales a glistening shiny red membrane (Duncan bulkeley)is seen because of suprapapillary thinning of epidermis.
  - When this membrane is scraped off, pinpoint bleeding is seen because of rupture of thinned out, dilated and tortuous capillaries in papillary dermis.

Candle Wax Sign (Signe de la Tache de Bougie)

- On removal, scales are loose and accumulate of the sides of scraped area like wax accumulated of the sides of a candle.

Woronoff Ring

- Presence of hypopigmentation around a healing psoriatic plaque because of PGE_2 deficiency because of inhibitor of prostaglandin synthesis (vasoconstriction).

Note: Perilesional halo can be found also due to application of steroids.

- **Abramowitz sign**: The earliest lesions of psoriasis often appear on the gluteal cleft (gluteal pinky).
- Deep dermal tenderness (DDT) (Buschke-Ollendorff sign) is negative is psoriasis unline in secondary syphilis where it is positive
- **Deck Chair sign**: Sparing of abdominal folds (characteristic of papuloerythroderma of Ofuji)
- **Pavithran Nose sign**: Sparing of tip of nose in severe cases of erythroderma
    - If papules, are they guttate/scaly/on removal check whether they leave behind normal/shiny red surface (wafer like oblaten scale of pityriasis lichenoides chronica).
    - Do the papules have collarette of scaling and are in Christmas tree pattern? (for pityriasis rosea)
    - Look for the nature of scales
- Silvery white, moist, thick layer (ostraceous), crust mixed with sales (rupioid) greasy (seborrheic dermatitis)

PASI (Psoriasis Area and Severity Index) Score

On the basis of desquamation, induration and erythema.

Plaque characteristics	*Rating score*	*Head (A1)*	*Upper limbs (A2)*	*Trunk (A3)*	*Lower limbs (A4)*
Erythema (E)	0—None 1—Slight 2—Moderate 3—Severe 4—Very severe				
Induration (I)	Same as above				
Scaling (D-desquamation)	Same as above				

- Add together each of the 3 scores for each of the body regions to give 4 separate subtotals

- Head and neck—represent 10% of body surface area (BSA)
- Upper extremity—20% of BSA
- Trunk (includes axilla, groin, genitals)—30% of BSA
- Lower extremity (including buttocks)—40% of BSA
- So they are given corresponding weightage in scoring by multiplying their scores by 0.1,0.2,0.3 and 0.4 respectively.
    - 0—no involvement
    - 1—1-9%
    - 2—10-29%
    - 3—30-49%
    - 4—50-69%
    - 5—70-89%
    - 6—90-100%
- PASI= 0.1 (Eh + Ih + Dh) Ah + 0.2 (Eu + Iu + Du) Au + 0.3 (Et + It + Dt) At + 0.4 (El + Il + Dl) Al
- PASI varies between 0 and 72 in steps of 0.1

Also calculate BSA by rule of 9.

MUSCULOSKELETAL SYSTEM

- Joints: Hands/knees/elbows/wrists/ankles/sacroiliac/lumbosacral
- Check for pain/swelling/range of motion/deformities

Diagnosis

My patient is a________old (M/F) who has ... with mild (<5%)/moderate (5-10%)/severe psoriasis (>10%) psoriasis which is stable/unstable (new lesions appearing/not appearing) involving BSA ... with/without Auspitz sign+/Koebner with PASI score ... with or without joint involvement, with nail/scalp involvement/currently on/not on treatment.

Q. How will you manage this patient?

A. Though the diagnosis is clinical, it is always better to confirm diagnosis by skin biopsy.

- Investigate patient for underlying associated metabolic disorder:
    - BMI
    - Blood sugars
    - Serum lipids
    - ECG
    - USG abdomen for nonalcoholic fatty infiltration
- Investigate for treatment:
    - Complete blood count (CBC)
    - Hb

- Erythrocyte sedimentation rate (ESR)
- Liver function tests (LFT)
- Renal Function Test (RFT)
- Chest X-ray (CXR)
- Mantoux test
- Serum uric acid

Treatment can be divided according to body extend involvement:

- Less than 5%: Only topical therapy is enough
- 5–10%: Topical + phototherapy
- More than 10%: Systemic therapy (with or without topical and phototherapy)

Topical therapy

- Topical corticosteroids:
  - Superpotent for palms and soles (e.g., Halobetasol propionate and clobetasol propionate)
  - Moderately potent for arms legs and trunk (betamethasone dipropionate and mometasone furoate)
  - Mildly potent for face, groins and genitals (Desonide, hydrocortisone)
  - Steroids induce remission extremely fast, but relapses will also be faster. Moreover, there may be tachyphylaxis (decrease response with long use) and precipitation of pustular psoriasis.
- Calcipotriol 0.005%:
  - Acts slowly but, may give sustained relief.
  - Never use > 100 g/week (risk of hypercalcemia)
  - Also never use on groins, scrotum, genitals
  - Can be combined with topical steroids
- Emollients: Mainstay of topical therapy should be used liberally.
- Phototherapy—can be either Ultraviolet B (UVB) or Ultraviolet A (UVA). UVB is the safest type of therapy availing and can also be given in pregnancy and to small children. 311 nm is preferred, called Narrow band phototherapy. UVA therapy is not useful alone and should be combined with psoralen.

  Psoralen and UVA (PUVA) therapy has got several side effects and is not often used.
- Systemic therapy—should be used in patient with more than 10% involvement/pustular/erythrodermic psoriasis/psoriasis interfering with the patients occupational, social or personal life.

The common systemic therapies are:

- Methotrexate (slow acting, but cheap)
- Cyclosporine (fast acting, but expensive)
- Oral acitretin (slow acting, except in pustular psoriasis where it works very fast, also expensive)
- Combinations of the above.
- Especially can be started with cyclosporine and Retinoids, once patient is better, withdraw cyclosporine.

Q. Why is it psoriasis vulgaris?

A. In view of bilateral symmetrical well demarcated scaly erythematous (salmon coloured) plaques on the extensors of extremities/trunk/lumbosacral with silvery white scaling ... Auspitz positive.

Q. What will a skin biopsy show?

A. Parakeratosis, Munro's microabscess, hypogranulosis spongiform pustule of kogoj, suprapapillary thinning of epidermis, regular elongation of club shaped/camel foot rete ridges, dilated and tortuous capillaries in papillary dermis.

Q. What is the differential diagnosis?

A.
- Reiter's disease/reactive arthritis
- Seborrheic dermatitis
- Secondary syphilis
- Pityriasis lichenoides chronica
- Parapsoriasis
- Drug induced papulosquamous eruptions
- Subacute lupus erythematosus
- Lichen planus (guttate papulosquamous lesions)
- Lupus vulgaris

But it will vary according to patient.

Q. Why is it not Reiter's/Sexually acquired reactive arthritis (SARA)/ reactive arthritis?

A.
- There is no preceding H/O diarrhea/urethral discharge, absence of limpet such as crusts, circinate balanitis, keratoderma blenorrhagicum, tendon friction rubs and ocular complaints (uveitis).
- Reiter's often involves the axial joints

Q. Why is it not secondary syphilis?

A. There is no H/O sexual exposure, ulcer in the genitals, absence of pruritus, DDT positivity, epitrochlear lymphadenopathy, mucous patches, condyloma lata, pigmentation or papulosquamous lesions in the palms and soles, with collarette of scaling (Biette's collar).

Q. Why is it not pityriasis lichenoides chronica?

A. Lesions are not reddish brown papules with wafer like (oblaten) scales which on removal leaves behind glistening shiny surface. Sometimes DDT test may be positive. No scalp involvement/pitting nails.

Q. Difference between seborrheic dermatitis and psoriasis.

A.

	Seborrheic dermatitis	***Psoriasis***
Morphology	Greasy yellow scales	Silvery white scales, usually dry
Distribution	Flexural areas	Extensor areas
Scalp lesions extension	Scalp lesions do not extend beyond frontal margin (corona seborrhica)	They extend beyond frontal scalp margin (corona psoriatica)
Auspitz	Negative	Positive
Joint pains	Negative	Positive
Metabolic disease	Negative	Positive

Q. Does psoriasis remit in pregnancy?

A. Yes, except impetigo herpetiformis (variant of pustular psoriasis) which occurs in pregnancy.

Q. Which drugs aggravate psoriasis?

A. Naproxen, lithium, antimalarials (In psoriatic arthritis indomethacin is preferred).

Q. Why do you ask history of smoking?

A. Smoking increases psoriasis by two-fold.

Q. Why do you ask about alcoholism?

A.
- Facial psoriasis is more common in alcoholics
- If we want to start patient on methotrexate and retinoids.
- Alcohol increases the severity to psoriasis and also makes it refractory to treatment.

Q. What is the relation between human immunodeficiency virus (HIV) and psoriasis?

A. The frequency of psoriasis is same but severity will be more and there is increased incidence of arthritis, dactylitis or enthesitis.

Q. What is the relationship between psoriasis and pregnancy?

A. There can be decreased fertility and increased fetal loss (more in pustular psoriasis).

Q. What is the risk of malignancy in psoriasis?

A. Psoriatic skin is intrinsically resistant to malignancy because of low levels of aryl hydrocarbon hydroxylase.

Q. What is Renbeok phenomenon?

A. Psoriasis disappears in the area of wrist band. (Negative koebners renbeok-opposite of koebner).

Q. What is Brocq's phenomenon?

A. In lichen planus patients rub instead of scratching—diffuse bleeding and pain.

Q. Which diseases show Auspitzs sign positive?

A.
- Psoriasis
- Darier disease
- Actinic keratosis

Q. In a case of psoriasis, can you get Auspitz negative?

A. Yes. (Guttate/flexural/pustular/scalp/partially treated psoriasis)

Q. Which diseases show koebners phenomenon?

A.
- Psoriasis
- Lichen planus
- Verruca vulgaris
- Lichen nitidus

Q. Which conditions show Woronoffs ring?

A.
- Psoriasis
- Halo nevus
- Lichen planus

Q. Which type of psoriasis is exacerbated by smoking?

A. Palmoplantar psoriasis.

Q. Which type of psoriasis is exacerbated by alcohol?

A. Erythrodermic psoriasis.

Q. What is Boyd and Neldner classification of koebners phenomenon?

A.
- True koebners:
  - Psoriasis
  - Lichen planus
  - Vitiligo

- Pseudokoebners:
  - Molluscum contagiosum
  - Warts
  - Pyoderma gangrenosum
  - Sweets syndrome
- Reverse koebners:
  - Granuloma annulare
  - Kyrle's disease

  After systemic infections like enteric fever, psoriasis may disappear.

Q. In which disease sacral pinking is prominent?
A. Psoriasis (called as Abramowitz sign).

Q. What is the classic X-ray finding in psoriatic arthritis?
A. Opera glass deformity and sausage shaped fingers.

Q. How do you calculate BMI?
A. Weight in kg/[height in meters (m^2)]
- Normal—18.5–25 kg/m^2
- Overweight—25–30 kg/m^2
- Obesity—from 30 to over 40 kg/m^2

Q. In which diseases geographic tongue is seen?
A.
- Pustular psoriasis
- Reiter's
- Physiological
- Atopy

Q. What are types of mucous membrane involvement in psoriasis?
A.
- Geographic tongue
- Silvery white micaceous scales
- Solitary patch on glans penis
- Gingival lesions

Q. Nails in psoriasis.
A.

Nail matrix involvement	Nail bed involvement
Pitting/Crumbling	Subungual hyperkeratosis
Red lunula	Onycholysis
Leukonychia	Salmon patch/oil drop sign/splinter hemorrhages

Q. How do you differentiate pitting of alopecia areata and psoriasis?

A.

Alopecia areata	*Psoriasis*
Scotch grid pattern—arranged at regular intervals	Irregular arrangement
Shallow	Deep and shallow
Smaller	Larger

Q. In how many patients nail pitting is seen?

A. 10–50%.

Q. What does the number of nail pits signify?

A.
- More than 20 pits—psoriasis
- More than 30 pits—psoriatic arthropathy

Q. Causes of nail pitting.

A.
- Psoriasis
- Reiter's/SARA
- Alopecia areata
- Lichen planus
- Eczema
- Pityriasis rubra pilaris
- Systemic lupus erythematosus (SLE)
- Sarcoidosis
- Trauma
- Idiopathic

Q. Which are the drugs causing psoriasis?

A.
- HCQS
- Anticonvulsants
- Beta blockers and angiotensin-converting enzyme (ACE) inhibitors
- OHAs
- Non-steroidal anti-inflammatory drugs (NSAIDs)

Q. Which drugs cause exclusively nail changes in psoriasis?

A.
- Lithium
- Beta-blockers

Q. Which NSAID is preferred in psoriatic arthropathy?

A. Indomethacin.

Q. What is Caspar criteria for psoriatic arthritis?

A.
- Psoriatic nail dystrophy
- Past or family history of psoriasis

- Current or past history of dactylitis
- X-ray: New bone formation (juxtaarticular)
- Negative rheumatoid factor test

Q. How will you differentiate psoriasis from rheumatoid arthritis (RA)?

A.

Psoriatic arthritis	***Rheumatoid arthritis***
Usually distal interphalangeal joint	Proximal interphalangeal joint
Asymmetrical	Symmetrical
Oligoarthritis	Polyarthritis
No morning stiffness	Morning stiffness present
Sausage shaped deformity	Swan neck deformity
Enthesitis	Not common
X-ray: No osteopenia	X-ray: No osteopenia

Q. Do you get hair loss in psoriasis?

A. No hair loss except erythrodermic psoriasis and corona psoriatica. (Hair loss is present in tinea capitis)

Q. What is white psoriasis?

A. Interdigital psoriasis.

Q. What is elephantine psoriasis?

A. Diffuse circumferential involvement of the skin.

Q. How will you treat?

A.
- First line: Indomethacin
- Second line: Methotrexate, Acitretin, Sulfasalazine oral steroids [Generalized pustular psoriasis (GPP) of pregnancy] Ciclosporin, Leflunomide
- Third line: Infliximab, Etanercept

Q. What is the indication of systemic steroids in psoriasis?

A.
- Pustular psoriasis
- Erythrodermic psoriasis
- Psoriatic arthritis
- Psoriasis with metabolic disturbances

Q. What is ingram coal tar bath?

A. First give UVB then apply anthralin (0.05–0.1%) in ointment or Lassars paste.

Q. What is Lassars paste?

A.
- 0.2–0.8% dithranol
- 2% salicylic acid
- 24% zinc oxide and starch each
- 2.5% hard paraffin
- White soft paraffin

Q. What is Goeckerman regimen?

A. 1–5% coal tar paste to be applied and kept for 12–24 hours—then UVB.

Q. What is Miami university modification of Goeckerman regimen?

A. Keep coal tar paste (1–5%) only for 2 hours then have a bath followed by UVB.

Q. What is Stanford regimen?

A. Anthralin at night and topical steroids in the morning.

Q. What is holiday and weekend therapy?

A. Calcipotriol on weekdays and topical steroids in the weekends.

Q. What is short contact anthralin therapy (SCAT)?

A. SCAT 2–4% for 20 minutes.

Q. What is the maximum dose of superpotent topical corticosteroids (TCS)?

A. 45 g/week. Maximum 14 days it should be applied.

Q. What is the maximum dose of calcipotriol?

A. Should not exceed 100 g/week.

Q. What do you mean by metabolic disorder?

A.
- Hypertriglyceridemia [Triglycerides (TGL) >150, high-density lipoprotein (HDL) <40 in males and <50 in females)]
- Diabetes mellitus [fasting blood sugar (FBS) >100]
- Hypertension
- Obesity (Waist circumference >102 cm in males and >88 cm in females)
- Atherosclerosis
- Cardiac disease (coronary insufficiency)
- Nonalcoholic fatty infiltration

Q. What caution you should take when giving methotrexate to elderly people?

A. Start in low dose and look for nonalcoholic fatty liver disease (NAFLD).

Q. How much time does it take for methotrexate, cyclosporine and acitretin to start to act and when is the action near complete?

A.
- Methotrexate—starts within 6–8 weeks. Some show improvement in 72 hours.
- Cyclosporine—starts within 2 weeks
- Acitretin—starts within 4–8 months for psoriasis vulgaris.
- Takes 10 days for pustular psoriasis.

Q. What is the permissible maximum dose?

A. 20/25 mg weekly.

Q. How does acute toxicity of methotrexate (MTX) manifest?

A. Aphthous stomatitis because of thrombocytopenia.

Q. What is the alarming level of serum MTX?

A. The risk of potentially fatal toxicity is significantly increased with high-dose MTX in the setting of renal impairment and is related to prolonged periods of exposure due to elevated serum levels. At 24 and 48 hours, toxicity is greater if the serum levels are above 20 and 2 μmol/L, respectively.

Q. What are the noninvasive tests for MTX toxicity?

A. Aminoterminal propeptide of type 3 collagen levels (p III np) > 4.2 ng/mL indicate hepatotoxicity.

HMRS—proton magnetic resonance spectroscopy-measure fat content

PMRS—to estimate cell membrane turnover and fibrosis.

Q. How about MCV?

A.
- MCV doesn't decrease inspite of folic acid treatment
- If WBC < 3500, platelet <1 lakh persisting for > 1 week then need to decrease dose.

Q. Risk factors for cytopenia.

A.
- Daily MTX
- No folic acid
- Use of NSAIDs
- Sulphomethaxozole
- Trimethoprim
- Renal impairment

Q. How can you prevent MTX toxicity?

A. By giving folic acid on all days except the days of MTX.

Q. What is the dose of leucovorin and how is it administered?

A. 20 mg IV or higher than last dose of MTX within 4–6 hours and repeated after 6 hours if renal parameters abnormal to avoid precipitation of MTX in renal tubules and till serum MTX level <0.01 μmol/min.

Q. If renal impairment what will you do?

A. • Reduce by half dose
- Adequate hydration
- Alkalinization of urine with soda bicarbonate

Q. Why is folic acid given?

A. • Decreases myelosuppression
- Decreases macrocytosis seen with MTX
- Decreases nausea and vomiting and so increases tolerance.

Q. What are the main side effects of MTX?

A. • Thrombocytopenia
- Oral ulcers
- Ulcerations on psoriatic plaques

Q. What is the cumulative dose which can be given?

A. 4 g.

Q. What is type 1 and type 2 psoriasis?

Type 1	*Type 2*
Onset before 40 years	Onset after 40 years
Bimodal onset	Not bimodal
Severe and recurrent	Mild
First degree relatives affected	Not affected
Guttate psoriasis	Chronic plaque psoriasis

Q. How many patients have koebners in psoriasis?

A. 30% of psoriasis patients have koebners. It is associated with early onset of psoriasis. It is an indicator of disease activity and may have a prognostic value.

Q. What are signs of borderline psoriasis?

A. • Hyperkeratotic plaques without scaling on extensor surfaces.
- Severe dandruff
- Subungual hyperkeratosis and onycholysis without evidence of fungus.
- Nail pitting
- Sterile multiple paronychia
- Recalcitrant scaly otitis externa
- Keratolysis like lesions of palms and soles
- Eczematous lesions on palms and soles

- Penile lesion sharply marginated areas of erythema without evidence of fungus.
- Intertrigo with sharp margination of erythema.

Q. What is the hallmark of psoriatic lesions?
A. Sharply demarcated margins with clear cut borders.

Q. What does scaling indicate?
A. Stable chronic plaque psoriasis.

Q. What does erythema indicate?
A. Unstable progressing lesions.

Q. Name morphological types of psoriasis.
A.
- Plaque/pustular
- Nummular/guttate/gyrate
- Rupioid/elephantine/ostraceous

Q. What are the different patterns of psoriasis?
A.
- Extensors
- Inverse
- Sebopsoriasis
- Widespread

Q. Based on inflammation what are the types?
A.
- Inflammatory
- Hyperkeratotic

Q. Types based on time of first onset.
A. Early and late.

Q. Types based on velocity of propagation.
A.
- Stable
- Unstable
- Eruptive

Q. What is psoriatic leukoderma?
A. Hypopigmentation usually associated with clearing.

Q. What is the most common type of psoriasis?
A. Chronic plaque psoriasis.

Q. What is the most common exanthematic type of psoriasis?
A. Guttate psoriasis.

Q. What is the risk of developing chronic plaque psoriasis after the first episode of guttate psoriasis?
A. 40%.

Q. What is the age group of patients with guttate psoriasis?

A. Children and young adults with family history of psoriasis usually following streptococcal infections/stress.

Q. How many patients of psoriasis vulgaris can get pustular psoriasis?

A. 2–5%.

Q. How many patients of plaque type psoriasis can get occasional pustular lesions?

A. 20%.

Q. What are the nail changes in GPP?

A. Subungual pustules.

Q. What can you find in the oral cavity in GPP?

A. Acute geographic tongue.

Q. What is impetigo herpetiformis?

A. Generalized pustular psoriasis in pregnancy.

Q. What is mechanism of action of MTX?

A. MTX inhibits dihydrofolate reductase, an enzyme that reduces folic acid to tetrahydrofolic acid. This inhibition interferes with DNA synthesis and cell reproduction.

Q. What is the drug of choice of pustular psoriasis?

A. Oral retinoids (acitretin) except in pregnancy where oral steroids are used.

Q. What is the role of cyclosporine in pregnancy?

A. Cyclosporine is a selective immunosuppressant that has been effectively used in the treatment of generalized pustular psoriasis and is grouped into category C for pregnancy drug risks.

Q. What is the therapeutic wavelength of UVB in psoriasis?

A. 311 nm.

Q. What is narrow band UVB?

A. Wavelengths ranging from 308–311 nm are called narrow-band ultraviolet B (NB-UVB).

Q. Advantage of NB-UVB?

A. Shorter wavelengths of UVB are not very effective in psoriasis, also they carry a higher risk of phototoxicity and skin cancers. These risks are minimized with NB-UVB.

Q. Which type of lesions respond poorly?

A. Thick lesions over palms, soles and scalp lesions.

Q. How is the therapy scheduled?

A. Increasing suberythemogenic doses of UVB given thrice a week for 2–3 months followed by once a week for next 2–3 months. Initial dose is about 80% of MED, and is increased by 20% at each exposure till erythema is seen.

Q. Contraindications to UVB phototherapy.

A. Photosensitivity, patient on phototoxic medications, unstable psoriasis, past history of skin cancer.

Q. Oral psoralens used in PUVA therapy.

A. 8-methoxypsoralen, 5-methoxypsoralen.

Q. Mechanism of action of PUVA in psoriasis?

A. Interferes with DNA synthesis thereby decreasing cellular proliferation. Also causes localized immunosuppression by causing apoptosis of cutaneous lymphocytes.

Q. Most commonly employed regimen.

A. On alternate days 8-MOP in the dose of 0.6 mg/kg dose followed 2 hours later by UVA exposure.

Q. What is RE-PUVA?

A. Combination of etretinate or acitretin with PUVA.

Q. Which oral retinoid is commonly used in psoriasis?

A. Acitretin.

Q. Advantage of acitretin over etretinate.

A. Etretinate is more teratogenic, longer half-life and stored in fat for a longer duration.

Q. Mechanism of action of acitretin in psoriasis.

A. Binds to nuclear retinoid receptors, regulates gene transcription, modulates epidermal cell differentiation, decreases inflammation.

Q. Dosing of acitretin in psoriasis.

A. 25–50 mg/day with food for 3–6 months.

Q. Indications of using retinoids in psoriasis.

A. Erythrodermic psoriasis, pustular psoriasis, psoriasis associated with HIV infection.

Q. Indications of cyclosporine in psoriasis.

A. Erythrodermic psoriasis, pustular psoriasis, psoriatic arthropathy, nail psoriasis, scalp psoriasis.

Q. How to monitor a patient on cyclosporine?

A. Blood pressure monitoring, serum creatinine levels, serum potassium levels.

Q. Enumerate the biologic that can be used in treatment of psoriasis.

A.
- Biologics targeting T-lymphocytes and APCs: Efalizumab, alefacept
- Biologics targeting tumor necrosis factor (TNF)-alpha: Etanercept, infliximab, adalimumab

Q. Which of these biologics is used most commonly?

A. Etanercept.

Q. Dose and side effects of etanercept?

A. 25–50 mg twice weekly subcutaneously for 12 weeks. Most common side effects include injection site reaction, reactivation of TB, CNS demyelination, congestive heart failure.

12 Systemic Lupus Erythematosus

Name/Age/Sex/Occupation/Residing at/Hailing from/Marital status

CHIEF COMPLAINTS

- Joint pains
- Malar rash
- Oral ulcers
- Gradual onset
- C/o joint pains in ... joints which increased to involve ... joints with/without morning stiffness
- Associated with swelling/deformity
- Relieving/aggravating factors
- History of (H/O) photosensitivity (how severe, since when)
- Any relieving factors
- H/O blistering/rash/redness/scaling and face swelling
- H/O burning/pruritus/pain
- H/O oral ulcerations (painful/painless)
- Difficulty in eating/swallowing with/without burning sensation
- H/O hyperpigmentation and scaling lesion on face
- H/O psychosis/epileptic fits/mood changes/depression/hemiplegia/neuropathy/ataxia
- H/O chest pain/dyspnea/palpitations
- H/O fever/malaise/myalgia/tiredness
- H/O oliguria/pedal edema/hematuria
- H/O nausea/vomiting/diarrhea/vague abdominal pain
- H/O drug intake prior to symptoms
- H/O dryness in eyes, dry mouth, watering or burning, tightness of skin/dysphagia
- H/O Raynaud's phenomenon/proximal muscle weakness/swelling around eyes
- H/O drug intake for the above complaints H/O response to drugs
- H/O present complaints

Past History

- H/O TB/hypertension (HT)/ischemic heart disease (IHD)/bronchial asthma/drug allergy
- H/O medical and surgical illness

Personal History

- Sleep/bowel/bladder/appetite/addiction/menstrual history
- Obstetric history
- Family history

Quality of Life

- H/O interfering with work/social/interpersonal/sexual life

General Examination

- Patient is conscious cooperative well-oriented to times place and person.
- BP/PR/RR
- Pallor/cyanosis/clubbing/icterus/edema feet/lymphadenopathy

Cutaneous Examination

- Malar rash: Symmetrical erythema, edema, scaling on both cheeks, bridge of nose and forehead with ill defined borders sparing the nasolabial folds
- Involving/sparing the ears
- Involving/sparing V area of the neck

Rest of the Skin

- Any ulcers/telangiectasia/purpura/gangrene/erythema multiforme/abnormal pigmentation/calcinosis cutis/acanthosis nigricans/anetoderma/lichen planus/annular erythema/thrombophlebitis associated with APLA.
- Evidence of Raynaud's phenomena?
- Fingers—swelling/deformity/ulcers
- Nail changes
- Mucous membrane changes (Oral and genital)

Systemic Examination

- RS—crepts/any effusion/breath sounds
- CVS—S1, S2 normal, murmurs
- CNS—ataxia/hemiplegia/motor deficit
- P/A—soft/nontender

Diagnosis

- Acute/subacute SLE with/without complications, with/without flare on treatment well controlled/poorly controlled

Q. How will you manage this patient?

A. First confirm diagnosis clinically, histologically, serologically

- Based in clinical features—ARA fulfilment
- Hb/complete blood count (CBC)/erythrocyte sedimentation rate (ESR)/C-reactive protein (CRP)
- LFT [increased (SGOT)/(SGPT)]

- RFT (increased BUN, creatinine)
- Urine >0.5 g proteinuria, granular RBC casts
- Blood sugar
- USG of abdomen
- Chest X-ray, ECG
- Vision perimetry
- Slit lamp fundoscopy
- If any skin lesions biopsy:
    - Histopathology
    - Direct immunofluorescence (DIF)
    - Lupus band test (LBT)
- Serological:
    - ANA in high titer
    - DsDNA, anti-SM, antiU1RMP
    - Complement level C3 C4, APLA (if h/s/o thrombosis or bad obstetric history)

Q. In how many percent of patients do you get raised ANA and DsDNA?

A.
- 98% ANA
- 60% DsDNA

Q. What are the ARA criteria?

A. Use the mnemonic: **DAMP ASRHINA**

D—**D**iscoid rash
A—nonerosive **A**rthritis
M—**M**alar rash
P—**P**hotosensitivity
A—**A**NA positive
S—**S**erositis: Pleuritis/pericarditis
R—**R**enal involvement: Proteinuria > 0.5 g in 24 hours, or 3+ RBCs and epithelial casts
H—**H**ematological: thrombocytopenia, anemia, leukopenia, lymphopenia
I—**I**mmunological involvement: False positive venereal disease research laboratory (VDRL), AntidsDNA, antiSmith antibody
N—**N**eurological involvement: Psychosis/seizures
A—recurrent **A**phthous ulcers

Q. What is Gillians classification?

A. Gillians classification:

1. LE specific skin diseases characterized by interface dermatitis
    A. Chronic cutaneous LE (CCLE)
        1. Classic discoid lupus erythematosus (DLE)
            a. Localized DLE
            b. Generalized DLE

2. Hypertrophic or verrucous DLE
3. Lupus panniculitis/lupus profundus
4. Mucosal DLE
   a. Oral DLE
   b. Conjunctival
   c. Nasal
   d. Genital
5. LE tumidus/Papulomucinous LE
6. Chilblain LE
7. Lichenoid DLE (LE/LP overlap)

B. Subacute cutaneous lupus erythematosus (SCLE)
1. Annular
2. Papulosquamous/Psoriasiform
3. Vesicobullous annular SCLE
4. TEN like SCLE

C. Acute cutaneous LE (ACLE)
1. Localised ACLE (malar rash)
2. Generalised ACLE
3. TEN like

2. LE nonspecific skin diseases with no interface dermatitis

A. Cutaneous vascular disease
1. Small vessel cutaneous leukocytoclastic vasculitis secondary to LE
   a. Dependable palpable purpura
   b. Urticarial vasculitis
2. Vasculopathy
   a. Degos disease like lesion
   b. Secondary atrophic blanche
3. Periungual telangiectasia
4. Livedo reticularis
5. Thrombophlebitis
6. Raynaud's phenomenon
7. Erythromelalgia

B. Nonscarring alopecia
1. Lupus hair
2. Telogen effluvium
3. Alopecia areata

C. Sclerodactyly

D. Rheumatoid nodules

E. Calcinosis cutis

F. LE nonspecific bullous lesions

G. Urticaria

H. Papulonodular mucinosis

I. Cutis laxa

J. Acanthosis nigricans
K. Erythema multiforme
L. Leg ulcers
M. Lichen planus

Q. What is the most common vascular lesion in SLE?
A. Telangiectasia.

Q. How will you describe the malar rash?
A. A butterfly blush or discrete maculopapular eruption with fine scaling on the butterfly area of the cheeks or elsewhere.

Q. D/D's of malar rash.
A.
- DLE
- SLE
- Heliotrope rash of DMS
- Rosacea
- Seborrheic dermatitis
- Photodermatitis
- Erysipelas/cellulitis

Q. In how many patients can you get a generalized rash?
A. 5–10%.

Q. What are the clinical variants of LE?
A. Morbilliform/exanthematous/bullous/TEN like.

Q. Why does a patient get bullous lesions in LE?
A. Severe interface dermatitis and basal cell vacuolar degeneration.

Q. What is lupus band test?
A. Deposition of one or more immune reactants (IgG, IgM, IgA, C3 and complement components) found as a linear band at the basement membrane zone by DIF termed as lupus band test. Sensitivity 95% and specificity 87% and is a prognostic indicator.

Q. In which scenario can one get false negative lupus band test?
A. It is seen when high levels of extra vascular dermal IgG is present.

Q. Which are the conditions in which lupus band test is positive?
A.
- SLE
- Drug induced lupus
- PLE
- LP
- Rosacea
- Facial telangiectasias
- BP
- Porphyria

Q. What are the types and staining patterns of lupus band test?

A. Types

- Lesional
- Nonlesional

Patterns

- Under low power staining pattern is described as being granular
- Under high power it has been described as homogenous fibrillar stippled shaggy lumpy—bumpy, linear or thready, in a continuous fashion.

Q. In which condition discontinuous or interrupted LBT is seen?

A.
- Actinic keratosis
- Rosacea
- PLE
- Nonlesional sun exposed skin (80%)

Q. What are the clinical correlations of various patterns of LBT?

A.

Pattern	*Description*	*Condition*
Stippled pattern	Multiple small round points of fluorescence	Clinically normal skin of SLE
Homogenous	Solid/homogenous band of well demarcated bright fluorescence	Chronic atrophic and hypertrophic lesions
Thready	Short closely set bright threads or fibrils	Acute erythematous and edematous lesions

Q. What are the uses of LBT?

A.
- To diagnose LE
- To differentiate LE from other cutaneous disorders (PLE/jessners lymphocytic infiltrate/lymphocytoma cutis)
- To differentiate SLE from DLE
- Making a diagnosis of SLE in patients without cutaneous lesions
- To differentiate from other ANA positive diseases (drug induced LE, rheumatoid arthritis, scleroderma, DMS, MCTD)
- Prognostic significance (positive LBT from sun protected normal skin indicates decreased long-term survival it correlates positively with risk of developing nephritis)

Q. What is LE cell test?

A. LE cells are polymorphonuclear leukocytes which have ingested nuclear material from degenerative white cells in the presence of antibody to deoxyribonucleic acid (LE cell factor).

Q. What is rosette phenomenon?

A. Large masses of nuclear material are found extracellularly and with surrounding leukocytes form rosettes.

Q. In which conditions LE cell test is positive?

A.
- SLE
- Drug induced lupus
- Chronic DLE
- Systemic sclerosis
- Rheumatoid arthritis

Q. Name the specific antibodies for various CTDs?

A.

Antibodies	*CTDs*
Anti-dsDNA	SLE (Renal disease)
Anti-SM	SLE
Anti-Ro, anti-La	SCLE/neonatal lupus/drug induced lupus
Anti-SS DNA, anti-Ro, anti-LA	Sjögren's syndrome
Anti-U1RMP	MCTD
AP LA	Antiphospholipid syndrome (recurrent thrombosis)
Anti topoisomerases1 (anti-Scl-70)	Systemic sclerosis
Anti-Jo, anti-RNA synthetase	DMS
Anti centromere	CREST syndrome

Q. What are the different ANA patterns seen in various CTDs?

A.

ANA	*Conditions*
Homogenous pattern	Drug induced lupus/SLE
Speckled pattern	SLE/MCTD/SCLE
Nucleolar pattern	Systemic sclerosis/SLE
Peripheral/membranous pattern	SLE with renal involvement

Q. What are the trigger factors?

A. UV radiation (discos/fluorescent light/UVA from photocopiers).

Q. Differential diagnosis of edema face.

A.
- Dermatomyositis
- SLE
- Hansens in reaction

- Contact dermatitis
- Seborrheic eczema
- Erysipelas

Q. Differential diagnosis of follicular plugging.

A.
- SLE
- DLE
- Acne
- Phrynoderma
- Follicular LP
- Platelet-rich plasma
- Keratosis pilaris
- Seborrheic keratosis

Q. Differential diagnosis of red lunula.

A.
- SLE
- Alopecia areata
- Psoriasis
- Vitiligo
- Nail patella syndrome
- Glomus tumor
- Subungual myxoid tumor
- Repeated trauma
- Systemic causes: Renal/CVS/endocrinology

Q. Differential diagnosis of blue/Azure lunula.

A.
- Phenolphthalein (in laxatives)
- Silver
- Zidovudine
- Cytotoxic drugs

Q. Differential diagnosis of cribriform scars.

A.
- Pyoderma gangrenosum
- DLE

Q. In which condition do you get black lunula?

A. Subungual hemorrhage (black).

Q. Where do you look for telangiectasia?

A. Reticulate telangiectatic erythema on thenar and hypothenar eminences of the palms, pulp, dorsum of fingers, toes and over the lateral borders of feet and heels.

Q. Where do you look for vascular necrosis?

A. Tips of fingers and alongside the nails.

Q. What are the nail changes in SLE?

A. Splinter hemorrhages, pitting, ridging, onycholysis, striate Leukonychia, red lunula, hyperkeratotic nail folds and ragged cuticles, dilated nail fold capillaries, clubbing.

Q. What are the hand changes in SLE?

A. Sclerodactyly/palmar erythema/telangiectasias/above nail changes.

Q. Differentiate rheumatoid nodules and SLE.

A. SLE subcutaneous nodules will be superficial and nonerosive.

Q. What are the types of alopecia seen in lupus erythematosus?

A.
- Scarring alopecia
- Alopecia areata
- Diffuse alopecia
- Lupus hairs

Q. What is the most common musculoskeletal manifestation?

A. Arthralgia/myalgia.

Q. What is the most common joints involved?

A. Nonerosive arthritis in PIP, MCP, wrist, knee, elbow.

Q. What are the causes of myopathy?

A.
- Inflammatory
- Corticosteroids
- Antimalarials

Q. What are lupus hairs?

A. Short, unruly, coarse, fragile, dry, broken off hair mainly on frontal margin probably because of slowed anagen growth.

Q. Which are the drugs inducing SLE like syndrome?

A.
- Hydralazine
- Minocycline
- Isoniazid
- Penicillin
- Penicillamine
- Phenytoin
- Valproate
- Infliximab
- Procainamide
- Chlorpromazine
- Terbinafine

Q. How do you differentiate drug induced LE from spontaneous LE?

A. The drug induced SLE differs from spontaneous SLE in that
- Older age group

- Renal and CNS involvement (infrequent)
- Antihistone bodies are frequent
- AntiDNA antibodies are absent
- Serum complements are absent
- Pulmonary and joint involvement is common
- Skin lesion is uncommon

Q. How does hydralazine cause lupus?

A. It inhibits binding of complement component C4 with subsequent lack of control of complement activity.

Q. What is Rowells syndrome?

A. Lesions of SLE like erythema multiforme with speckled ANA pattern.

Q. What are the other cutaneous features of SLE?

A.
- Facial edema
- SCLE
- Chronic DLE
- Scarring DLE alopecia
- Non scarring alopecia
- Chilblain lupus
- Bullous eruptions
- Raynaud's phenomenon
- Chronic urticaria
- Urticarial vasculitis (hypocomplementemic)
- Livedo reticularis
- Papular and nodular mucinosis
- Episcleritis
- Cheilitis

Q. What is lupus erythematosus telangiectoides?

A. Disseminated variety of DLE results in a persistent blotchy reticulate telangiectasia, seen on face, neck, ears, dorsa of hands, breasts, heels and on sides of feet.

Q. What is lupus erythematosus gyratum repens?

A. An annular variant consists of a migratory gyrate annular erythema with the histological features of LE although LBT is negative. There may be an underlying carcinoma.

Q. What are the connective tissue changes in SLE?

A.
- Hardbound/thickened skin with pigmentation on face/limbs
- Subcutaneous nodules because of vasculitis and thrombosis (elbows/knees/back of proximal phalanges/wrists/occiput/flexor aspects of fingers)

- Calcinosis cutis
- Panniculitis
- Relapsing nasal and aural chondritis (cartilage not involved)

Q. Which are the other skin diseases seen with SLE?

A.
- Acanthosis nigricans
- Herpes zoster more frequent
- Scabies more severe and crusted
- Eruptive dermatofibromas
- Hyperkeratotic erythematous follicular papules on trunk and limbs (Chinese)

Q. What are the features of bullous SLE?

A. Bullous lesions occur on face, neck, upper trunk mainly which heal with milia and photosensitivity/mouth ulcers/EM like lesions may be present with glomerulonephritis. A form resembling EBA has been described.

Q. What are the drugs that can precipitate Bullous LE?

A.
- Hydralazine
- Gamma interferon

Q. What is Senear–Usher syndrome?

A. Erythematous, scaly crusted or hyperkeratotic lesions on seborrheic areas and butterfly area having immunological features of both SLE and pemphigus foliaceus. It occurs spontaneously or induced by drugs.

Q. What are the types of LE nephritis?

A. I: Minimal mesangial lupus (normal glomeruli by light microscopy but immune deposits on immunofluorescence)

II: Mesangial proliferative lupus nephritis (purely mesangial hypercellularity of any degree or mesangial matrix expansion onlight microscopy with mesangial immune deposits)

III: Focal lupus nephritis:

A. Active or inactive, segmental or global, endo or extracapillary

B. Glomerulonephritis <50% of all glomeruli typically with focal

C. Subendothelial deposits with or without mesangial alteration

Focal proliferative and sclerosing glomerulonephritis

IV: Diffuse lupus nephritis—50% of all glomeruli involved

V: Membranous lupus nephritis—global or segmental subepithelial immune deposits may show advanced sclerosis

VI: Advanced sclerotic lupus nephritis more than 90% glomeruli globally sclerosed.

Q. What is normal creatinine clearance?
A. Creatinine clearance—80-120 mL/min.

Q. How much percent of patients get renal involvement?
A. 50%.

Q. What is the risk of patient developing SLE in cutaneous lupus?
A. Patient with localized cutaneous lupus have less than 5%. But with widespread lesion, risk may go upto 25%.

Q. What is the risk of SLE patient have DLE lesions?
A. 15% of DLE patient.

Q. What is the role of smoking in patients of lupus?
A.
- The disease is more severe in smokers. Also, the disease becomes more refractory to treatment in smokers.
- Patients should stop smoking—it will definitely have a better response to the treatment.

Q. What is Tumid lupus erythematosus (TLE)?
A. It is a form of cutaneous lupus where the lesions do not scar or do not have atrophy. It is highly photosensitive.

Q. Differentials of lupus lesions according to the type.
A.
- Acute cutaneous lupus—rosacea, facial contact dermatitis, photodermatitis (toxic or allergic), seborrheic dermatitis, dermatomyositis, erysipelas, lupoid delusion (patient is convinced she has a butterfly rash, but there is no rash)
- Generalized acute cutaneous lupus—morbilliform drug eruption, erythema multiform, toxic epidermal necrolysis
- Subacute cutaneous lupus—psoriasis, PMLE, pityriasis lichenoides chronica, pityriasis rosea
- Annular type of subacute LE—tinea corporis granuloma annulare, erythema annulare centrifugum
- Chronic Lupus- PMLE, Jessner's lymphocytic infiltrate, granuloma faciale, perniosis, actinic keratosis, seborrheic dermatitis, tinea facei, lichen plans, lupus vulgaris, sarcoidosis

Q. How will you manage lupus?
A.
- Preventive measures: photoprotection—with clothing and broad spectrum sunscreens.
  - Sunscreen should be applied 30 minutes prior to anticipated sun exposure
  - All patient should be give vitamin D supplements. It helps in lupus and to prevent osteoporosis.
  - Encourage all patients to stop smoking.

- Topical therapy:
    - Topical steroids—mainstay of treatment.
    - Highly potent steroid are preferred even though side effects are obviously higher.
    - Topical calcineurin inhibitors: Tacrolimus—an alternative to steroids can be combined
    - Intralesional steroid—in selective cases, oral or intramuscular steroids can be given
- Systemic therapy:
    - Antimalarials—1st line systemic therapy in lupus:
        - Hydroxychloroquine (5 mg/kg) is the antimalarial of choice twice a day.
        - Sometimes switching therapy from one antimalarial to another can increase efficacy
    - Others—Chloroquine, mepacrine
    - It is recommended to do baseline ophthalmic examination which should be repeated every 5 weeks
    - Other S/E—lichenoid eruption, gastric intolerance, dizziness, headache, ototoxicity, darkening of the skin

Refractory patients: If not responding to above—

- Oral vitamin A derivatives like acitretin—(counsel about contraception being mandatory)
- Dapsone—especially in bullous lesions. It can be combined with other drugs
- Oral steroids at 1 mg/kg/day—can be used in flares of the disease as well as "Breach therapy" when it can be combined with steroid sparing agents.
- Methotrexate—15–20 mg/week. Can be combined with cyclosporine.
- Azathioprine: Safest of all antimetabolites in pregnancy.
- Other: Cyclophosphamide, mycophenolate and IVIg

Recent therapies in LE:

- B cell targeted therapies are useful, e.g., rituximab, belimumab—both these induce B cell suppression.
- Cytokine modulators—ustekinumab (IL-12 and IL-23 inhibitor)
- Thalidomide and its deviator lenalidomide
- Fumaric acid esters
- There are some nonpharmacological management of lupus, though paradoxical, pulse diode laser—although it may flare up the disease

13 Scleroderma

Vital Data
Name/Age/Sex/Occupation/Residing at/Hailing from/Marital status

CHIEF COMPLAINTS

- Tightness of skin/darkening of skin since ...
- Painful bluish discoloration of fingers on exposure to cold since ...
- Breathlessness/chest pain since ...
- Joint pains since ...
- Difficulty in swallowing since ...
- Abdominal bloating since ...

Onset, Duration and Progress
Skin tightness:
- Gradual/sudden
- Starting from ... progressing to ...
- History of (H/O) preceding swelling of hands (pitting/nonpitting)
- Thickening/pruritus
- Difficulty in movement/any deformity?
- Difficulty in opening mouth/eating/swallowing
- Any facial changes patient has noted (thinning of lips/shiny face)
- Any discoloration/pigmentary changes?
- Is there a H/O painful discoloration to blue of fingers on exposure to cold which reverts back on rewarming?
- Since when? How long does it last?
- How frequently it occurs?
- Any blackish discoloration (for gangrene)
- H/O digital ulcerations/loss of digits/tapering of digits/nail changes?
- H/O frothy urine-proteinuria joint pains since ...
- Which joints? How was the progression?
- Aggravating/relieving factors?

Any morning stiffness?
- Swelling/range of motion/deformities/weakness of muscles/ impairment of work
- H/O fever, bodyache, myalgia
- H/O any hard raised lesions with chalky discharge/ulcerations

For RS
- H/O difficulty in breathing on exertion/at rest
- H/O dry cough
- H/O chest pain/palpitations

For gastrointestinal tract
- H/O difficulty in swallowing/reflux/vomiting
- H/O bloating/postprandial/abdominal pain
- H/O constipation/incontinence/diarrhea
- H/O acute abdominal pain
- H/O stools floating in water/passing gas more frequently (suggestive of malabsorption)

For Renal
- H/O oliguria/edema feet/swelling around eyelids
- H/O leg cramps/frothy urine
- H/O headache/visual disturbances/seizures (malignant hypertension)

For Sjögren's syndrome
- H/O difficulty in speaking or taking frequent sips of water, cracking and fissuring at angles of mouth [(s)/dry mouth]
- H/O grittiness in eyes increased at the end of the day (dry eyes)
- H/O tingling numbness in hands and feet (peripheral neuropathy)

For Systemic lupus erythematosus (SLE)
- H/O photosensitivity/rash on the face/seizures/psychosis
- H/O oral ulcers

For DMS
- H/O swelling around the eyes/difficulty in standing from squatting position/combing hair.
- H/O any drugs taken in the past (ergot/OCs)
- H/O treatment taken for the above complaints did symptoms worsen/improve with treatment
- H/O any complications of treatment
- H/O headache (for migraine)

Quality of Life
- Has it impaired work/interpersonal relationships (sexual/social)

Past Medical History
- Any H/O DM/HTN/TB/bronchial asthma/IHD/drug allergy/surgical illnesses.

Personal History

- Sleep/bowel (constipation, rectal incontinence)/bladder (decreased urine output or frothy urine)/appetite (malnutrition)
- Smoking/alcohol/any other addictions

Menstrual History

- Regular monthly cycles/duration/mild, moderate or heavy flow (secondary amenorrhea)?

Obstetric History

- Gravida ... para ... live births ... abortions ...
- Normal/lower (uterine) segment Caesarean section (LSCS) mode of delivery
- Any complications (miscarriage/premature labor)?
- Any improvement (Raynaud's improves) or worsening [gastro-esophageal reflux disease (GERD) worsens] during previous pregnancies if female?
- H/O impotence if males?
- H/O contraception

Family History

- Any similar complaints in family?
- On the basis of history, my diagnosis is
- Limited/diffuse systemic sclerosis in ... stage (edema/induration/atrophic) with ... organ involvement/treated or untreated

General Examination

- Patient is conscious, cooperative, well-oriented in time, place and person.
- Averagely well built and well nourished.
- Pulse rate/BP/RR
- Weight/height/BMI
- Peripheral pulsations [to rule out thromboangitis obliterans (TAO)]
- Pallor/cyanosis/icterus/lymphadenopathy/edema feet

Cutaneous Examination

- Face: Tight, taut shiny skin on face-induration (inability to pinch skin)/forehead with decreased wrinkling/shininess/pigmentation (salt and pepper)
  - Inability to retract lower eyelid (Ingram sign)
  - Parrot beak/pinched beak like nose with loss of nasolabial folds.
  - Ask patient to open mouth wide and put her own fingers in the mouth
  - Normally atleast 3 fingers can be put in the mouth
  - Difficulty in mouth opening/purse string appearance

  - Rhagades (linear cracks or fissures in skin specialty angle of mouth
  - Mat like telangiectasias on cheeks/nose
  - Tongue protruding/dental caries
  - Ridging and tightness/salt and pepper pigmentation of neck (Barnett's neck sign)
- Hands: Tautness of skin on hands/sclerodactyly extending till what level?
  - Sausage shaped digits/flexion deformities of hands/loss of pulp of finger/stellate scars with/without active digital ulcers, nailfold changes (periungual telangiectasia), pallor, nail plate changes
  - Hair loss on skin
  - Loss of appendages
  - Any pigmentation of skin of hands.
  - Calcinosis cutis
  - Tendon friction rubs+/-Juxtaarticular tendon fibrosis
  - Do full movement of the joint and keep finger on joint-crepitations felt at wrist, MCP, and interphalangeal joints
  - Raynauds elicitable/nonelicitable
  - Peripheral nerves: Sensations/claw hand/deformity
- Hair: Telogen effluvium
- Nails: Pterygium inversum unguis
  - Nailfold capillary dilatation and dropouts
  - Telangiectasia
- Mucosa: Oral (dental caries/difficulty to protrude tongue)
  - Sensations
- Diagnosis: Limited/diffuse systemic sclerosis in edema/induration/atrophic stage with organ involvement ... treated/untreated

QUESTIONS

Q. European league against Rheumatism criteria for diagnosis of Sjögren's syndrome (SS)?

A. There are eight criteria. Each of them has a difference score.

1. Proximal skin involvement. Skin thickening proximal to MCP joint—Score 9
2. Skin thickening of the fingers only—
   a. Sclerodactyly distal to MCP joint—Score 4
   b. Puffy fingers—Score 2
3. Finger tip lesions—
   a. Ulcers—Score 2
   b. Scars—Score 3
4. Telangiectasia—Score 2
5. Capillary nail fold abnormality—Score 2

6. Pulmonary involvement or interstitial lung disease (ILD)—Score 2
7. Raynaud's phenomenon—Score 3
8. Autoantibodies-(anticentromere RNA topoisomerase or anti-RNA polymerase)—Score 3

Total score should be more than 9 for definitive diagnosis of SS

Q. Major subsets of systemic sclerosis.

A.
- Limited—in which there is distal systemic skin sclerosis, long history of Raynaud's, pulmonary arterial hypertension, severe gastrointestinal (GI) tract involvement
- Diffuse—proximal limb and trunk sclerosis, short history of Raynaud's, increased renal crisis, increased cardiac involvement, severe ILD

Q. Scleroderma sine sclerosis.

A. No skin thickening, Raynaud's phenomenon, typical capillaroscopy, typical autoantibodies.

Q. Overlap syndrome.

A. One of the above two subsets together with clinical or serological evidence of another autoimmune disease.

Q. Why is occupation important in systemic sclerosis?

A.
- A light job—warm atmosphere and to avoid minor trauma for the hands (e.g., typist, computer operators, pneumatic drills) for Raynaud's phenomenon.
- Working in plastic industry can predispose to vinyl chloride disease with mimics scleroderma.

Q. Is there any treatment to decrease perioral and facial tightening?

A. 0.025 to 0.5% tretinoin.

Q. How do you treat digital calcinosis?

A. CO_2 laser, surgical excision. But the average healing time was found to be 6 weeks after laser.

Q. Should you give nifedipine or losartan in CREST syndrome?

A. Nifedipine worsen esophageal symptoms so losartan is preferred.

Q. What is the normal chest expansion?

A. 3–5 cm at level of T_4.

Q. How do you test for microstomia?

A. Measure oral aperture—4 fingers insertion is normal.
- Grade 1—3 fingers
- Grade 2—2 fingers
- Grade 3—1 finger

Q. How do you test for tendon friction rubs?

A. Do full movement of joint and keep finger on joint-crepitations felt at wrist, metacarpophalangeal joint and interphalangeal joints because of juxtaarticular tendon fibrosis and edema.

Q. What are bowed fingers?

A. It is a helpful sign in the diagnosis of early systemic sclerosis characterized by cold flexed fingers but no acrosclerosis or systemic abnormality. Seen in second to fourth decade and Raynauds phenomenon is not invariable.

Q. On which sites are pitted scars seen in systemic sclerosis?

A. Tips of digits, ulnar border of thumb, radial border of index and middle finger, dorsa of hands over joints.

Q. Where do you check for telangiectasia?

A. Face, lips, mouth, palms, upper trunk, hands and upper thighs.

Q. What are the sites you should look for pigmentary changes?

A. Face, legs and thighs.

Q. What are the other skin findings of systemic sclerosis?

A. Besides skin thickening and hardening on the fingers, hands, and face which are generally the earliest areas of the body involved, edematous swelling and erythema may precede skin induration. Other prominent skin manifestations include:

- Pruritus in the early stages
- Edema in the early stages
- Sclerodactyly
- Digital ulcers
- Pitting at the fingertips and atrophy of finger pulp (Mizutani's sign)
- Telangiectasia
- Calcinosis cutis

Q. What is pterygium inversum unguis?

A. Fusion of hyponychium with proximal nail fold because of fibrosis. Seen in:

- SLE
- Scleroderma
- Neurofibromatosis
- Leprosy
- Raynauds

Q. Why is grip poor?

A. If induration severe then grip will be poor.

Q. What is Barnett's neck sign?

A. Ridging and tightness with salt and pepper pigmentation.

Q. Difference between primary Raynaud's (Raynaud's disease) and secondary Raynaud's phenomenon.

Features	*Primary Raynauds*	*Secondary Raynauds*
Sex (f : m)	20:1	4:1
Age at onset	Puberty	>25 years
Frequency of attacks	<5/day	>5–10/day
Precipitants	Cold, emotional stress	Cold
Ischemic injury	No	Yes
Abnormal capillaroscopy	Absent	Present
Other vasomotor phenomenon	Yes	Yes
ANA	Absent or low titres	90–95% present
Anticentromere antibodies	Absent	50–60% present
Anti-SCL-70 (Topoisomerase I antibody)	Absent	20–30% present
In vivo platelet activation	Absent	>75% present

Q. What is the difference between diffuse and limited systemic sclerosis?

A.

Disease characteristics	*Limited scleroderma*	*Diffuse scleroderma*
Skin involvement	Distal to MCP joints, knees, face	Distal and proximal extremities, face, trunk
Raynaud's phenomenon	May precede skin changes by many years	May occur simultaneously or a year or two prior to or after onset of skin disease
Internal organ involvement	GI' pulmonary hypertension	Interstitial lung disease, renal, GI cardiac
Nail fold capillaries	Dilatation without dropouts	Dilatation with dropouts
ANA	Anticentromere antibodies	Antitopoisomerase
Disease course and prognosis	Slowly progressive, better prognosis except if pulmonary hypertension occours	Aggressive course in majority with risk of visceral involvement early in the disease course

Q. What are the various antibodies in scleroderma?

A.

Antibodies	*Prevalence (%)*	*Clinical association*
Anticentromere	20–30	Limited scleroderma, CREST, pulmonary hypertension
Anti-SCL-70	15–20	Diffuse scleroderma, interstitial lung disease
Anti-PM-SCL	2–3	Polymyositis scleroderma overlap
Anti-RNA polymerase	20	Diffuse scleroderma
Anti-cardiolipin antibodies	20–25	Diffuse subsets or limited subset, features of secondary antiphospholipid antibody syndrome rare
Anti-SM, anti-U-1:RNP	Rare	Overlap syndrome with features of scleroderma

Q. What is the treatment of digital scars?

A. Laser.

Q. What are the phases of scleroderma?

A. Edema, induration and atrophy.

Q. Why do you get edema?

A.
- Dermal glycosaminoglycans deposits
- Vascular changes
- Hydrostatic changes
- Inflammation

Q. What is the differential diagnosis of mask like facies?

A.
- Systemic sclerosis
- Hypothyroidism
- Myxedema
- Parkinsonism
- B/L UMN facial palsy
- Depression
- Myasthenia gravis
- Dementia

Q. Differential diagnosis of deformed or mutilated fingers.

A.
- Lepromatous leprosy
- Systemic sclerosis
- Raynaud's disease or phenomenon

- Frost bite
- Vasculitis
- Buerger's disease (thromboangitis obliterans)
- Trauma
- Syringomyelia
- Dermatomyositis

Q. What are the types of telangiectasias seen?

A.
- Mat
- Punctuate
- Linear
- Stellate

Q. What is the treatment of telangiectasias?

A.
- Pulse dye laser
- Argon laser
- ND: YAG laser

Q. Mixed connective tissue disease (MCTD) has combination of which disease.

A.
- Scleroderma
- SLE
- Polymyositis/dermatomyositis
- RA

and presence of anti-U-1 RNP antibody positive

Q. How often do you get calcinosis in systemic sclerosis?

A. 25%.

Q. What are the types of calcification?

A.
- Dystrophic
- Metastatic
- Iatrogenic
- Idiopathic

Q. What are the bony changes in systemic sclerosis?

A.
- Osteoporosis
- Osteopoikilosis
- Avascular necrosis
- Penciling of the digits
- If acro-osteolysis: Bone resorption

Q. How is the gastrointestinal tract (GIT) involved?

A.
- Macroglossia
- Esophageal reflux/dysphagia/strictures
- Hiatus hernia/bleeding from telangiectasia in stomach

- Intestinal obstruction/malabsorption
- Paralytic ileus
- Dilated atonic colon/telangiectasia in colon—Duodenal strictures and ulcers

Q. Why does malabsorption occur?

A. Abnormal peristalsis causes stagnation which results in bacterial overgrowth cause malabsorption and it can be corrected with tetracycline.

Q. What is steatorrhea?

A. Foamy looking bulky stools due to fecal fat 4 g/24 h.

Q. What are the endoscopic findings in systemic sclerosis?

A.
- Barrett's esophagus
- Stricture esophagus
- Hiatus hernia
- Stack of coin appearance

Q. What are the symptoms of pulmonary hypertension?

A. It is either asymptomatic or exertion breathlessness. Rarely chest pain or syncope.

Q. What are the symptoms of pulmonary fibrosis?

A.
- Dyspnea-exertional
- Dry cough
- Chest pain
- Hemoptysis (rarely)

Q. What is scleroderma renal crisis?

A. Occurs in 5–10% of scleroderma patients and characterized by malignant hypertension with rapidly progressing renal failure.

Q. What are the risk factors for renal crisis?

A.
- Rapidly progressive diffuse skin thickening
- High dose corticosteroids (so should be avoided in early diffuse disease)

Q. What are the symptoms of renal crisis?

A. Headache (seizures, encephalopathy), vision disturbances (retinopathy), malignant hypertension, left ventricular hypertrophy (LVH), cramps, decreased urine output, hematuria, proteinuria, edema of feet.

Q. Explain the relationship between pregnancy and systemic sclerosis.

A. Systemic sclerosis usually remains unchanged during pregnancy but it may also precipitate the disease in some cases and improves

Raynauds. Pregnancy worsens esophageal reflux, renal crisis and pulmonary and cardiac manifestations.

There is a high risk of miscarriage in systemic sclerosis or premature birth because of decidual vasculopathy.

Peripheral gangrene may occur. Fertility may be impaired.

Q. How does systemic sclerosis in childhood differ?

A. Raynaud's phenomenon is less frequent and renal involvement is rare. Course is slower disability and visceral involvement is less severe.

Q. What are the various associations of systemic sclerosis?

A.
- Dermatomyositis/polymyositis
- Sjögren's syndrome
- Myasthenia gravis
- Temporal arteritis
- Malignant atrophic papulosis

Q. What is Kahn's criteria and Alarcón-Segovia criteria for MCTD?

Alarcón–Segovia criteria	*Kahn's criteria*
A. Serological criteria	
Anti RNP→1:1,600	High titre anti RNP corresponding to speckled ANA→1:1,200 titre
B. Clinical criteria	
Swollen hands	Swollen fingers
Synovitis	Synovitis
Myositis (biologically proven)	Myositis
Raynaud's phenomenon acrosclerosis	Raynaud's phenomenon absent
MCTD is present if criteria A is accompanied by 3 or more clinical criteria one of which must include myositis or synovitis	MCTD is present if criteria A is accompanied by Raynauds, phenomenon with ←2 out of the remaining 3

Q. How will you manage a case of systemic sclerosis?

A.
- Thorough history and clinical examination will clinch the diagnosis.
- First confirm the diagnosis of scleroderma
- Document the extent of systemic involvement
- Investigations to find out the general status of the patient

For confirmation:

- A skin biopsy should be done for purpose of accurate documentation and for excluding scleroderma mimics

- Skin ultrasonography to determine the extent and depth of sclerosis.
- Antinuclear antibody and its patterns should be tested at the time of presentation
- Specialized antibodies can be checked like anti-SCL-7 and anti-U1 RNP (to rule out MCTD)
- For systemic involvement and complications
- X-ray of hands for periarticular osteoporosis, joint space narrowing, erosive arthropathy with "pestle and mortar" deformity of the DIP joints, resorption of terminal phalanges, tufting of the tip of the fingers, presence of calcinosis.
- Lungs: X-ray chest PA, lung function tests including 6 minutes walk test, DLCO, forced expiratory volume in 1 second (FEV_1), VC
- Skin USG to know extent and depth of sclerosis
- Anti-SCL 70/urine/PFT/6 minutes walk test/FEV repeated every 6 months.
- SKIN: Sclerosis, pigmentation, telangiectasia
- MSK: Motor examination/X-ray of hands
- GIT: Esophagoscopy/proctoscopy/colonoscopy/USG/LFT/Barium swallow (stiff glass tube appearance)/esophageal manometry
- CVS: ECG/echo/chest X-ray (cardiomegaly/LVH)
- Lung: Chest X-ray/PFT/CT/HRCT

Q. What will be seen in skin biopsy?

A. Early—less inflammatory infiltrate around dermal vessels, eccrine coils and around the subcutaneous tissue. Vascular changes mild. Late—paucity of blood vessels, thickening and hyalinization of walls and narrowing of lumen. Thickened collagen bundles.

Q. What can be the changes in X-ray, PFT and HRCT?

A.
- Chest X-ray: Ground glass appearance bilateral reticular or nodular basilar shadows fibrosis/cardiomegaly/LVH
- PFT: DLCO decreased/FLVC decreased
- HRCT: Narrow ill defined crescent in the lower lobe
- Reticular nodular shadows: Honey comb pattern/large cystic airspace/mediastinal involvement and pleural involvement.

Q. What do you expect in the blood tests?

A.
- CBC—anemia (renal failure/GI bleed/malabsorption)
- ESR—increased
- LFT—primary biliary cirrhosis often associated
- 24 hours urinary protein—proteinuria (0.5 g/day)
- VDRL—false positive in 5% patients
- Creatinine clearance—depends on renal involvement

Q. What can happen to the heart in scleroderma?

A. Conduction disturbances/arrhythmia/myocardial involvement/cardiomegaly/LVH/AV block/secondary to lung and renal involvement.

Q. What is watermelon stomach?

A. It is a striped appearance of the stomach on endoscopy because of gastric antral vascular ectasia seen in systemic sclerosis.

Q. What are eye changes in systemic sclerosis?

A. Tightness of lids, diminished tear secretion, Keratoconjunctivitis sicca, retinopathy.

Q. What are principles of treatment?

A.
- Assess which stage the patient is presenting in (edematous/infiltrated/atrophic)
- If any overt impending risk of internal organ involvement

Q. What is the treatment of Raynaud's phenomenon and digital ulcers?

A.
- Avoid cold and smoking.
- Simply warming the hands in hot water for 5 to 10 minutes regularly reduces the number and severity of attacks.
- Calcium channel blockers like Nifedipine 10 mg tds or sustained released preparations, Amlodipine, Nicardipine, Diltiazem
- Losartan (angiotensin type II receptor blockers) 50 mg/day IV prostacyclin analogue (iloprost)
- Other drugs: Aspirin, dipyridamole, pentoxifylline, topical nitroglycerine.
- Sympathetic blocks: Chemical or surgical sympathectomy

Q. Can you predict which patients of Raynaud's phenomenon will go on to get systemic sclerosis?

A. Yes. Nailfold capillaroscopy shows enlarged or distorted capillaries/loss of capillaries/disruption of capillary bed may indicate.

Q. In which conditions is cobblestoning seen?

A.
- Darier white disease
- Systemic sclerosis (small papules of lymphangiectasia)

Q. What are the advantages of ACE inhibitors?

A.
- May improve renal function and if given prevents
- Controls blood pressure in most and relieves encephalopathy, renal failure and death
- Doesn't aggravate esophageal symptoms

Q. What is the role of low molecular weight (LMW) dextran?

A. In occasion patients there is healing of ulcer tips. But there is risk or renal failure. 10% dextran in 5% dextrose or in normal saline solution IV. First inject 20mL over 3 to 5 minutes to decrease the risk of anaphylaxis. Then infuse 20 to 30 mL/h. Dose is 500–1,000 mL over 4 hours on day 1. 500 mL on day 2. Then on alternate days for 10 days.

Q. What are the recent advances in the treatment of Raynauds and digital ulcers?

A.
- Endothelin receptor antagonists (bosentan).
- Phosphodiesterase inhibitors (sildenafil, tadanafil)
- IV iloprost (high cost, inconvenient method of administration)

Q. How will you administer Sildenafil?

A. Start with half tablet of 25 mg twice a day gradually increase to 25 mg thrice a day, check blood pressure in supine and sitting position to rule out hypotension if hypotension SSRI like fluoxetine 20 mg/day.

Q. What is the dose of Bosentan?

A. Bosentan 125 mg twice daily, helps in preventing new digital ulcers by 50%, specially in patients with more than or equal to three digital ulcers at baseline.

Q. Which is the best drug for pulmonary hypertension?

A. Bosentan because of oral dosaging and lack of serious injection related adverse effects.

Q. Role of cyclophosphamide.

A. Oral or pulse IV Improves lung function, dyspnea, skin thickening and health related QOL.

Q. What is QUINS trial?

A. Quinapril 80 mg/day in scleroderma for 3 years, which holds promise to replace ACE inhibitors in PSS.

Q. SCOT trial.

A. Scleroderma—Cyclophosphamide or autologous stem cell transplantation.

Q. How can you reduce the skin tightness?

A.
- D-penicillamine 125 mg every alternate day–doubtful effect.
- Interferon - modest role (flu like syndrome is a side effect).
- Cyclosporine (no visceral improvement) and Tacrolimus
- Recombinant human relaxin
- IV immunoglobulin, plasmapheresis

- Halofuginone
- Infliximab
- Ximedon
- UVA phototherapy
- PVAC (derived from deglycolipidated *Mycobacterium vaccae*)
- Urokinase therapy
- Isotretinoin 1 mg/kg/day, factor 13 IV (cutaneous sclerosis)

Q. Why is penicillamine no longer used?

A. Penicillamine causes blood and platelet dysplasia and hepatotoxicity, pemphigus, lupus like syndrome, etc., limiting its use.

Q. How will you monitor skin fibrosis?

A.
- Modified Rodnan score (mRSS) for skin thickness
- 20 MHz ultrasound determination of skin thickness.
- Plicometer (medical tool with pair of tongs to pinch skin which measures skin thickening)
- Durometer (handheld device which measures the hardness of the affected skin by applying pressure/indentation on the skins surface.
- Cutometer, elastometer for skin elasticity
- Vesmeter for skin hardness, elasticity and viscosity.
- MRI measures skin thickness but expensive mostly used to determine and score musculoskeletal improvement (myositis/arthritis/calcinosis cutis)

Q. How will you treat arthritis associated with scleroderma?

A.
- NSAIDs
- Low dose steroids 5–10 mg/day
- Methotrexate (for severe polyarthritis)
- Physiotherapy, splinting, surgical correction in contractures and disability occurs.

Q. Explain the management of myositis in scleroderma.

A. High dose steroids with addition of immunosuppressants (methotrexate or azathioprine).

Q. Management of organ damage.

A.

Manifestations	*Treatment*
Gastrointestinal involvement	Proton pump inhibitors, H_2 blockers, prokinetic agents calcium channel blockers

Continued

Continued

Manifestations	***Treatment***
Scleroderma renal crisis	• ACE inhibitors • Antihypertensives • Dialysis • Renal transplant
Pulmonary hypertension	• Calcium channel blockers • Prostacyclin/analogues • Endothelial receptor blockers • Phosphodiesterase inhibitors • Combination therapy • Imatinib • Lung transplant
Interstitial lung disease	• Breathing exercises, • Antibiotics (infection) • Immunosuppressives (steroids, cyclophosphamide) • Imatinib • Lung transplant
Advanced stage multisystem disease	• Immunosuppressives (azathioprine 150 mg/day, ATG, ALG and MMF) • Autologous stem cell transplant

Q. How does D-penicillamine work?

A. Interferes with intermolecular cross linking of collagen.

Q. When patient is on D-penicillamine what should you look out for?

A.
- Hematological abnormality
- Proteinuria
- Autoimmune phenomenon (pemphigus/myasthenia gravis)

Q. Where will you use steroids?

A.
- Early edematous phase
- Arthritis and serositis in low dose
- Myositis and myocarditis in higher doses
- IV methylprednisolone pulse therapy for ILD

Q. Would you give cyclosporine in scleroderma?

A. Limited use because cyclosporine (2.5–4 mg/kg) causes arterial hypertension and nephrotoxicity.

Q. What is Modified Rodnan score ?

A. Usually 17 sites are assessed and skin thickness is categorized to grade 0, 1, 2 or 3 corresponding to normal, mild moderate and severe. Areas examined are:

- Fingers (2)
- Forearms (2)
- Thighs (2)
- Feet (2)
- Anterior chest (1)
- Hands (2)
- Upper arms (2)
- Lower leg (2)
- Face (1)
- Abdomen (1)

Q. How do you treat salt and pepper pigmentation?

A.
- Tacrolimus with narrow band UVB and topical tacrolimus alone for hypopigmentation.
- Hydroquinone, retinoids, salicylic acid and chemical peeling for hyperpigmentation with sunscreens.
- Topical calcipotriol for both hyperpigmentation and hypopigmentation.

Q. What is atrophie blanche?

A. This is a livedoid vasculitis also called as livedo reticularis with summer ulceration. Favors distal lower extremities especially the ankles characterized by painful punched out ulcers, white round or stellate scars with peripheral telangiectasias, reticulated violaceous erythema may extend from the ulcers.

Q. In which condition do you see atrophie blanche?

A.
- Collagen vascular disease (SLE, APLA syndrome)
- Vasculitis (Wegener's granulomatosis, cryoglobulinemia)
- Coagulation defects (decreased protein C, decreased factor 12 and decreased antithrombin 3)
- Chronic venous hypertension and varicosities
- Malignancies, mycosis fungoides, lymphomas
- Idiopathic or primary

Q. What is Sneddon's syndrome?

A. Idiopathic livedo reticularis with transient ischemic attacks/strokes with hypertension and/or dementia.

Q. Where is nail fold capillary dilatation seen?

A.
- Systemic sclerosis (limited and diffuse)

- Dermatomyositis
- Raynaud's disease
- SLE

Q. Why is there difficulty in walking?

A.
- Dyspnea
- DMS
- Joint pain

Q. Which is the most common collagen vascular disease (CVD)?

A. Rheumatoid arthritis.

Q. What is the importance of wounds in toes/fingers?

A. Non-healing wounds may cause auto amputation, bony involvement, gangrene.

Q. What are scleroderma mimics (pseudoscleroderma)?

A.
- Scleredema adultorum of Buschke
- Scleromyxedema
- Eosinophilic fasciitis/eosinophilia myalgia syndrome
- Toxic oil syndrome
- Amyloidosis
- Drugs: Bleomycin/pentazocine/vinyl chloride

Q. How will you differentiate scleroderma from scleredema, scleromyxedema, eosinophilic fasciitis?

	Systemic sclerosis	*Scleredema*	*Scleromyxedema*	*Eosinophilic fasciitis*
Major clinical variants	• Limited diffuse	• Post infectious (type I) • Monoclonal gammopathy associated (type II) • Diabetes mellitus (type 3)	–	–
Raynaud's phenomenon	++	–	–	–
Symmetric induration	++	++	++	++
Sclerodactyly	++	–	–	–

Continued

Continued

	Systemic sclerosis	*Scleredema*	*Scleromyx-edema*	*Eosinophilic fasciitis*
Facial involvement	+	± (in type I and II) – (in type III)	+	–
Systemic involvement	++	–	++	+
ANA	++	–	–	–
Anti-centro-mere antibodies	+ (in limited)	–	–	–
Anti-topoi-somerase I antibodies	+ (in diffuse)	–	–	–

Q. What is scleroderma sine scleroderma?

A. It is characterized by internal organ involvement and serological abnormalities without skin involvement.

Q. What is Groove sign?

A. It is seen in:

- Lymphogranuloma venerum, and
- Shulmans' syndrome: Eosinophilic fasciitis, linear depressions where veins appear to be sunken within the indurated skin

Q. What is nephrogenic systemic fibrosis?

A.
- Seen commonly in dialysis dependant CRF.
- Exposure to gadolinium based contrast medium/thrombotic events/surgical procedure.
- Ill defined thick indurated plaques symmetrically on extremity and trunk with an ameboid appearance.

Q. What are the predictors of bad prognosis of scleroderma?

A.
- Males
- Extensive sclerosis of skin and visceral involvement
- Rapidly progressive disease
- Late onset in life
- Low Hb
- High ESR
- Proteinuria
- Decreased DLCO

- Decreased complement
- Lung disease
- Arrhythmia
- Decreased CMI
- HLA-B8

Q. What is the disease activity index of systemic sclerosis?

A.
- Skin thickening—0.5
- Digital necrosis—0.5
- Arthritis—0.5
- DLCO < 80% IE—0.5
- Hypocomplementemia—1
- ESR > 30—1.5
- Any deterioration as per patient within last month in skin—2, vessels—5, heart, lung—2
- Disease in considered active if value of items detected in patients is > 3. But it has low sensitivity

Q. What is the diagnostic criteria for renal involvement in systemic sclerosis?

A. GHAP Criteria:
- GFR reduced hypertension > 140/90 mm Hg
- Azotemia—BUN > 25 mg/dL
- Proteinuria > 1 g/24 h

Q. What are the causes of death in systemic sclerosis?

A.
- Inter-current infection
- Scleroderma renal crisis
- Cardiac failure
- Perforation of GIT
- Occasionally CA-lungs.

Q. Can ergots be given in a patient of systemic sclerosis with migraine?

A. No, since they will increase Raynaud's phenomenon.

Q. What is ACR criteria?

A.
- Major: Skin tightening proximal to MCD joints
- Minor:
  - Digital pitted scars or tissue loss of Volar Pads of finger tips.
  - Sclerodactyly
  - Bibasilar pulmonary fibrosis.

One major and two minor criteria should be present.

14 Vesicobullous Diseases

Vital Data

Name/Age/Sex/Occupation/Residing at ... /Hailing from ... /Marital status

CHIEF COMPLAINTS

- Fluid filled blisters /raw areas /crusted areas on the body________ days/years associated with itching/pain/burning
- Painful oral ulcers________days /years.
- Difficulty in swallowing since________days

Pemphigus Vulgaris

- Patient developed raw painful areas in the mouth since________ days. The lesions had little tendency to heal and gradually increased in size and number making swallowing difficult.
- Patient then developed multiple clear fluid filled lesions on________ parts of body.
- The blisters burst on it own to form raw areas within________days.
- These lesions showed little tendency to heal and gradually increased in size and number.

Bullous Pemphigoid

- Patient developed itching over the________areas of the body, associated with red raised lesions.
- This was followed by development of tense, clear fluid filled blisters
- These lesions remained intact and eventually burst to form raw areas. These raw areas showed a tendency to heal.
- The lesions healed with post inflammatory hyperpigmentation without tendency for scarring.

History of (H/O) Systemic Features

- Fever
- Joint pain
- Malaise

Negative History to Rule Out other Blistering Disorders

- H/O itching prior to the onset of lesions and associated with diarrhea—Dermatitis herpetiformis (DH)
- H/O lesions over the other mucosae, i.e., eyes/genitals also with scarring—Cerebral palsy (CP)
- H/O raw areas at trauma prone area without a positive family history of blistering disorders—Epidermolysis bullosa acquisita (EBA)
- H/O palm and sole involvement and H/O drug ingestion prior to onset of symptoms—Bullous erythema multiforme (EM)
- H/O drug ingestions/topical application of any irritants
- H/O photo sensitivity/joint pain/oral ulcers—Bullous Systemic lupus erythematosus (SLE)/pemphigus erythematosus/porphyria cutanea tarda
- H/O weight loss/rash/history to rule out any underlying malignancy—Paraneoplastic pemphigus
- H/O exacerbation on alcohol consumption—PCT
- H/O insect bite

History of Aggravating Factors

- Sun exposure
- Seasonal exacerbation
  - Drugs
  - Ingestion of excess garlic
  - Ingestion of iodides/fish

History of Relieving Factors

- Diet avoidance of wheat
- Avoidance of trauma

History of Medication Taken

- Describe the oral /topical treatment taken
- H/O any monthly 3 days admission for IV Rx—Pulse therapy
- Effect of the Rx
  - Decrease in no and size of lesions
  - No new lesions
- Rx taken
  - Since.....months/years
  - Last dose taken on ...

Personal History

- H/O—DM/HTN/TB/bronchial asthma/IHD/drug allergy
- H/O addictions:
  - Alcohol—which type,
    - How many pegs
    - How often

- Smoking—*Beedi*/Cigarette
  - How many day
  - Tobacco chewing
  - Using *Mishri*
- H/O food—Spicy
  - Onion/garlic consumption
  - Tomato/banana (phenol and tannins)
  - Wheat
  - Fish/salt (iodides)
- Sleep
- Appetite—difficulty in eating due to raw lesions in the mouth leading to decreased food intake.

Quality of Life

How the disease has affected the patient's life:

- Personal life—relation with spouse/other family members and friends
- Professional life—number of days lost from work due to the disease

Menstrual History

LMP:

- 4–5 days regular cycle with normal bleeding
- Cycle every 28 days

Obstetric History

- G_P_A_L_
- Family completed or not?
- Contraceptive used
- Tubal ligation done or not?

SUMMARY ON HISTORY

Pemphigus Vulgaris

Mr/Mrs________aged________ ________by occupation comes with multiple raw painful areas in the mouth since________months, followed by development of multiple fluid filled blisters and raw areas with little tendency to heal on the body since________months/years.

Bullous Pemphigoid

Mr/Mrs________aged________by occupation comes with multiple red raised itchy lesions over the________areas followed by development of tense fluid filled blisters which have a tendency toward healing.

On Examination

- Pallor
- Icterus
- Cyanosis
- Clubbing
- Edema
- Lymphadenopathy
- Weight
- BMI = Weight (Kg)
- Height (cm^2)
- T, P, R, BP

Cutaneous Examination

- Distribution of the lesions:
  - B/L symmetrical involvement involving_______areas of body, grouped lesions in linear IgA dermatoses and dermatitis herpetiformis
  - Sparing_______areas of body
  - With approximately_______% body surface area (BSA) involved
- Arrangement:
  - Tending toward symmetry
- Morphology: Vesicle
  - Multiple
  - Clear fluid filled vesicles/Bullae
  - Measurement: Smallest being____cm diameter and largest____ cm diameter
  - On a clear base or erythematous base
  - Which burst/do not burst easily
  - Wheals ± raw areas
  - Multiple erosions/ulcers
  - Covered with crusts (corn flake like/thick/adherent)
  - Having musty/mousy/foul
  - Odor
  - Lesions heal—with or without postinflammatory hyperpigmentation

  No scarring/milia formation
- Signs:
  - Nikolsky sign—direct and marginal
  - Nikolsky phenomenon
  - Modified Nikolsky (Bulla spread sign/Asboe Hansen's sign/ Leutz sign)
  - Pseudo Nikolsky sign

    - Pear sign
    - Sheklekoffs sign
    - Microscopic Nikolsky sign
- Oral:
    - Tongue/Buccal mucosa/palate—i.e., which are the areas involved
    - Multiple erosions measuring____cm covered with whitish slough
    - Oral hygiene—good/poor
    - Gums hygiene—good/poor
- Other mucosae:
    - Genitals
        - Erosions +/-
        - Scarring +/-
    - Eyes
        - Erosions/redness
        - Scarring/no scarring
- Nails
    - Paronychia +/-
        - Scarring +/-
- Palms and soles—Involved/spared
- Any other lesions:
    - Nevi/Sebaceous cyst/vitiligo (unrelated skin lesions)
- Bulla charting:
    - Number of vesicles, Bullae
    - Number of erosions, crusts

SUMMARY

Pemphigus Vulgaris

Mr/Mrs________, aged________ years,________by occupation comes with multiple raw painful areas in the mouth________months, followed by multiple fluid filled________and raw areas with________tendency to heal on body________months________scalp/trunk and sparing palms and soles.

On examination—multiple, symmetrically distributed clear fluid filled________on erythematous base/normal appearing skin with tendency/little tendency to heal and form erosions with crusting

- Nikolsky sign +/-
- Sheklakov's sign +/-
- Patient is treated/not treated with________medicines.

VIVA QUESTIONS

PEMPHIGUS VULGARIS

Q. Why is this a case of pemphigus vulgaris ?

A.
- Age (fourth to fifth decade)
- History of—asymptomatic blisters
  - are flaccid
  - are clear fluid filled
  - on an clear or on erythematous base
  - with tendency to burst
  - without tendency to heal
- Distribution and morphology—tendency to symmetry with involvement of mouth/other mucosa
- On examination—BSS +, Nikolsky +

Q. What are the bed side examinations for pemphigus vulgaris?

A.
- Bulla-Tzanck smear is done which shows: Acantholytic cell

Pemphigus foliaceus	*Pemphigus vulgaris*
Oval	Round
Condensed nucleus	Hypertrophic nucleus
Basophilic cytoplasm	Hyalinized cytoplasm

- Streptocytes—are filamentous lines of leukocytes
- Mourning edged cells
- Sertoli rosette

Q. Differential diagnosis of oral lesions in pemphigus vulgaris.

A.
- Aphthous ulcer
- EM
- Primary herpetic gingivostomatitis
- Erosive lichen planus
- Trauma
- Leukoplakia

Q. Which other mucosa can be involved in pemphigus vulgaris?

A. Any stratified squamous lined mucosa like esophagus, larynx, pharynx, conjunctiva, urethra, cervix and anus.

Q. What are histopathologic features of pemphigus vulgaris?

A. Tombstone appearance with a supra basal split.

Q. What does direct immunofluorescence (DIF) and indirect immunofluorescence (IIF) show in pemphigus?

A.
- The DIF shows fish net pattern of IgG and C3.
- IIF shows increase in Desmoglein (Dsg1) and Dsg 3 titres.

Q. What are the reasons for a false negative DIF?

A. In 10% of specimens, it may result from technical error (e.g., by using wrong or weak antisera), the presence of clinical or subclinical inflammation and early blister formation within the biopsy specimen (this is especially true in cases with PNP), or the use of a limited panel of antisera that does not include IgA antisera (for cases with IgA pemphigus).

Q. In which pemphigus DIF maybe "truly" negative?

A. In a rare case with drug induced pemphigus.

Q. Tests to check disease activity/progress of disease?

A.
- IIF—twofold increase in titre is a marker for relapse
- Enzyme-linked immunosorbent assay (ELISA) titers

Q. Diagnosis of pemphigus vulgaris.

A.
- To confirm is: Tzanck smear
- Skin biopsy If facilities available

DIF/IIF

- In view of Rx:
  - Hb, CBC
  - ESR
  - LFT
  - RFT
  - Blood sugar
    - Fasting,
    - Postprandial
  - Lipid profile
  - ECG
  - Chest X-ray PA view
  - Urine
    - Routine
    - Microscopy
  - Stool
    - Routine
    - Microscopy

Q. How do you do Tzanck?

A. In the case of blistering disorders, the intact roof of a blister is opened along one side, folded back and the floor is gently scraped. The material thus obtained is smeared onto a microscopic slide, allowed to air dry, and stained with Giemsa stain. The commercially available Giemsa stain solution is diluted in 1:10 ratio with distilled water, and the diluted solution is poured over the smear and kept for 15 minutes. Then it is washed with water and examined under the microscope. The stained nuclei may vary in color from reddish blue to purple to pink. The cytoplasm stains bluish.

Q. Describe a Tzanck cell.

A. A typical Tzanck cell is a large round keratinocyte with a hypertrophic nucleus, hazy or absent nucleoli, and abundant basophilic cytoplasm. The basophilic staining is deeper peripherally on the cell membrane ("mourning edged" cells) due to the cytoplasm's tendency to get condensed at the periphery, leading to a perinuclear halo.

Q. What is sertoli rosette and streptocytes?

A. A "Sertoli rosette" consists of cell aggregates with an epithelial cell at the center surrounded by a ring of Leukocytes. "Streptocytes" are adherent chains of leukocytes formed by filamentous, glue like substances.

Q. How will you take a biopsy?

A. Shave biopsy from a new blister.

Q. What are the types of Nikolskys sign?

A.
- Nikolsky sign: The sign is elicited by applying lateral pressure with the thumb on the skin over a bony prominence.
  - Direct—is over normal appearing skin at a distant site
  - Marginal—is close to an existing lesion

  Nikolsky sign is positive in pemphigus (active disease)
- Nikolsky phenomenon—i.e. the superficial layer of epidermis is thought to move over the the deeper layer, instead of immediately forming an erosion like in Nikolsky's sign.
- Modified Nikolsky's sign—is peripheral extension of blister on applying pressure on its surface. This is useful in patients in whom there is no new blister for biopsy
- Bulla spread sign/Leutz sign—Unidirectional pressure applied by a finger causes peripheral extension of the bulla beyond the marked margin.

- Bulla spread sign/Asboe Hansen's sign—modified bulla spread sign where pressure is applied to the center of the lesion.
    - Bulla spread sign is positive in all varieties of pemphigus and subepidermal blisters like BP, DH, EBA, MMP, dystrophic EB, SJS, TEN
- Pseudo Nikolsky sign/epidermal peeling sign—this is Nikolsky's sign elicited on erythematous skin.
    - It is positive in SJS, TEN, burns, bullous ichthyosiform erythroderma
    - It is due to necrosis of epidermal skin and not due to acantholysis.
- Pear sign—is pooling of the fluid at the base of the lesion due to gravity
- Sheklakov's sign/false nikolsky's sign—involves pulling of the remanant of the roof of the blister.
    - It is positive in subepidermal blisters like BP, MMP, herpes gestationis, liner IgA dermatosis, EBA, junctional and dystrophic EB, porphyrias and bullous SLE.
- Microscopic Nikolskys sign—is rubbing the surrounding normal appearing skin with an eraser to cause an microscopic split. This is useful for taking a biopsy.

Q. Treatment of pemphigus group.
A.

Control	*Consolidation*	*Maintenance*
(↑ intensity of treatment to get ↓ disease control =? 2 weeks)	(Maintain same intensity of treatment until 80% of lesions have healed =? few weeks)	(intensity of Rx gradually ↓ to the lowest level to prevent new lesions)

Q. How is disease severity graded?
A.

Mild	*Moderate*	*Severe*
Less than 10 skin lesion	10–30 skin lesion	More than 30 skin lesions
Less than 5 mucosal	5–15 mucosal lesions	More than 15 mucosal lesions
Rx:		

Continued

Continued

Mild	*Moderate*	*Severe*
Topical steroids	Oral steroids 1.5–2 mg/kg body weight	Oral steroids 1.5–2 mg/kg body weight
ILS	DCP	DCP
Tetracycline		
Dapsone		
Azathioprine, Cyclophosphamide, Mycophenolate mofetil		

* Newer advances in treatment
  - Immunoablative doses of cyclophosphamide
  - Rituximab (Ab against CD20)
  - Immunoadsorption

* Investigations done in view of long-term steroids treatment?
  a. Blood pressure
  b. Blood sugar
  c. Weight record
  d. Abdominal; girth record
  e. Rupture eye examination
  f. Dexa scan, X-ray pelvis both hips

Q. Causes of death in pemphigus?

A.
- Mortality has decreased from 73 to <5% after the use of systemic steroids
- Before the use of steroids, most common cause of death used to be septicemia due to streptococcal abd streptococci infection.
- However, now cause of death is most commonly iatrogenic.

PEMPHIGUS FOLIACEUS

Q. Why is this a case of *P. foliaceus*?

A. Chronic with:
- No oral involvement
- Seborrheic areas of body involved
- Flaccid vesicles which have tendency to heal spontaneously
- Erosions with corn flake like crusts and mousy odor

Q. Can pemphigus foliaceus become pemphigus vulgaris?

A. Yes, rarely due to epitope spreading.

Q. Prognosis of pemphigus foliaceus.

A.
- Better prognosis than pemphigus vulgaris
- General health not affected
- Benign course with intermittent crops of lesions

Q. Presentation of pemphigus foliaceus.

A.
- Seborrheic dermatitis like
- Erythroderma

PEMPHIGUS VEGETANS

Q. Why is this case of pemphigus vegetans?

A. Chronic VBD with primary presentation pustule (scalp)/vesicle
- Tumid, vegetating hypertrophic plaques in intertriginous areas
- Cerebriform tongue

Q. Types of pemphigus vegetans.

A.

Neumann type	***Hallopeau type***
Early type with vesiculopustular lesions	Later vegetating type

Q. Differential diagnosis of pemphigus vegetans.

A.
- Seborrheic dermatitis
- Hailey-Hailey
- HS
- Donovanosis
- Halogenodermas
- Amoebiasis

Q. What is the Premlata's sign?

A. Characteristic cerebriform tongue in pemphigus *vegetans.*

Q. Differential diagnosis scrotal tongue.

A.
- Melkersson-Rosenthal syndrome
- Familial
- Down's syndrome
- Pachyonychia congenita
- 50% of patients with scrotal tongue have geographic tongue

Q. What are Differential diagnosis of geographic tongue?

A.
- Atopic dermatitis
- Pustular psoriasis
- Reiter's syndrome
- Lithium therapy
- AIDS

PEMPHIGUS ERYTHEMATOSUS

Q. What is pemphigus erythematosus/senear usher syndrome?

A. • Localized variant of Pemphigus foliaceus
- Features of both pemphigus and LE lupus band test + in 80%
- ANA+ in 30%

Q. What is endemic pemphigus foliaceus or Fogo selvagem?

A. • Distinctive form of pemphigus foliaceus
- With burnt appearance on sun exposed areas
- May be an infection cause by a virus transmitted by black fly (*Simulium* pruinosum)

Q. What is Vieira sign?

A. Nail is initially yellow them becomes dark in color seen in pemphigus foliaceus.

Q. What is the neonatal pemphigus?

A. • A pregnant woman with pemphigus vulgaris may deliver a child with vesiculobullous lesion
- Self limited
- Regresses in 3–4 weeks
- To be distinguished from pemphigus neonatorum (severe impetigo)

Q. What is pemphigus herpetiformis?

A. • Pruritus is severe
- Papulovesicular lesions with central clearing arranged in annular form
- Histopathology shows: Eosinophils and neutrophils in addition to the features if pemphigus.
- May develop into pemphigus foliaceus or pemphigus vulgaris
- Rx: Dapsone/low doses of prednisolone

Q. What is immunoglobulin A (IgA) pemphigus?

A. • It is a type of sub corneal pustular dermatosis with vesicular pustular eruption and intraepidermal neutrophilic infiltration.
- Morphologically: Flaccid bullae on erythematous skin arranged in annular/flower like pattern

PARANEOPLASTIC PEMPHIGUS

Q. What is the other name for paraneoplastic pemphigus?

A. Paraneoplastic autoimmune multiorgan syndrome.

Q. What is diagnostic criteria of paraneoplastic pemphigus?

A. Camisa et al. criteria for diagnosis of paraneoplastic pemphigus is:

- *Major criteria*:
  - Polymorphous mucocutaneous eruption
  - Concurrent internal carcinoma
  - Characteristic serum immunoprecipitation findings
- *Minor criteria*:
  - Positive staining of rat bladder by IIF
  - Intercellular and BMZ reaction on DIF
  - Acantholysis an H/E

Q. What are the tumor associated with paraneoplastic pemphigus (PNP)?

A.
- Non-Hodgkin's lymphoma (NHL)
- Chronic lymphocytic leukemia (CLL)
- Castleman tumor
- Waldenstrom macroglobulinemia
- Thymoma
- Retroperitoneal sarcoma

Q. Which are the auto Ab associated with paraneoplastic pemphigus (PNP)?

A. Autoantibodies are directed against:

- Desmoplakin I 250 kDa ⎤
- Desmoplakin II 210 kDa ⎦ Desmosome
- Envoplakin 210 kDa ⎤
- Periplakin 190 kDa ⎦ Desmosome
- BP Ag 230 kDa Hemidesmosome
- Plectin
- DSG1-160 kDa ⎤
- DSG3-130 kDa ⎦ Lower epidermis

Q. What are differential diagnosis of annular lesions in VBD?

A.
- Pemphigus herpetiformis
- Linear IgA bullous dermatosis
- Sub corneal pustular dermatosis
- Hailey–Hailey disease

BULLOUS PEMPHIGOID

Q. Why is this a case of BP?

A.
- Older age group 60–80 years
- Transient /no oral lesions

- Multiple well defined erythematous plaques with itching associated with tense clear fluid filled bullae with little tendency to burst. After bursting the ulcers have a tendency to heal.
- Lower abdomen and LL areas of involved
- Absence of head and neck involvement
- Absence of mucosal involvement
- Absence of atrophic scar

Q. Differentiate between pemphigus vulgaris and BP.

A.

Pemphigus vulgaris	***BP***
40–60 years	60–80 years
M:F = 3:2	M:F = 1:1
Oral mucosal involvement ++	Transient oral mucosal involved in 40%
Trunk and seborrheic areas involved Nikolsky sign +	Lower abdomen and LL involved Nikolskys +/-
BSS +	BSS +/-
Pruritus usually absent	Present
Flaccid blisters which ruptures easily and have no tendency to heal	Tense blisters on erythema plaque which rupture to form erosions that heal easily
H/e suprabasal split with tomb stone appearance	H/e split in *lamina lucida* with eosinophil +
DIF- IgG and C3 in fish net pattern	DIF- Granular Linear IgG and C3 deposition
Nikolsky +	Nikolsky –

Q. What are the factors ppt BP?

A.
- UV light
- Surgery
- Adhesive dressing

Q. Types of BP.

A.
- Localized BP—pretibial
  - P and S dyshidrosiform
  - Vulval in young females
- Childhood BP
- Vesicular
- Vegetating
- Nodular
- Drug induced

- Erythrodermic
- Urticarial plaques of vesicle
- 105 kDA Ag anti-P-105 pemphigoid-widespread erosions like TEN or pemphigus vulgaris.

Q. What are the drugs causing bullous pemphigoid ?

A.
- Topical drugs like benzyl benzoate, 5FU, anthralin
- Penicillin, penicillamine, PUVA
- Antidiabetic
- Diuretic like furosemide
- Diclofenac

Q. What are the diseases associated with BP?

A.
- Lichen planus—lichen planus pemphigoides
- Malignancy—renal cell carcinoma, gallbladder CA, CA colon, breast CA, leukemia
- Diabetes
- Psoriasis
- Ulcerative colitis
- Multiple sclerosis
- Nephropathy
- Pernicious anemia
- Eosinophilia
- Elevated IgE

Q. Ix to confirm bullous pemphigoid.

A.
- H/P
- DIF
- IIF
- Saline split
- ELISA assay
- Newer Ix: Immunoblotting/western blot
  - Immunoprecipitation
  - Immunohistochemistry

Q. What is the course and prognosis of BP?

A.
- Benign self limited course from months and years
- Mortality rate reduced from 25% in presteroid era to 6% in the current steroid Rx era.

Q. What is the differential diagnosis of bullous pemphigoid ?

A.
- Pemphigus vulgaris
- Mucous membrane pemphigoid
- Linear IgA bullous dermatosis
- Other VBDs

MUCOUS MEMBRANE PEMPHIGOID

Q. How do you diagnose a case of mucous membrane pemphigoid?

A.
- Age group between 60 to 80 years
- Chronic inflammatory vesiculobullous diseases involving the mucus membrane with scarring
- Histopathology shows lesions and eosinophils with lymphocytes, in later lesions fibrosis seen
- DIF shows linear deposition of IgG, IgA, C3

Q. What are the types of mucus membrane pemphigoid?

A.
- Localized involvement:
  - Oral pemphigoid—desquamative gingivitis
  - Ocular pemphigoid
  - Nasopharyngeal involvement
  - Laryngeal involvement—hoarseness, chronic sore throat, laryngeal stenosis
  - Genital pemphigoid
- Extensive involvement of skin and mucosa

Q. What are the types of skin lesions in mucous membrane pemphigoid?

A.
- Scarring type, i.e., brunsting perry type which is localized, associated with atrophic Scarring. There is no mucosal involvement.
- Non-scarring type—bullous pemphigoid like. However itching is either absent or mild.

Q. Differential diagnosis of desquamative gingivitis.

A.
- Pemphigus vulgaris
- Bullous pemphigoid
- Mucous membrane pemphigoid
- Lichen planus
- Contact stomatitis
- Linear IgA bullous dermatosis in adults
- Erythema multiforme

Q. What is ocular pseudopemphigoid?

A.
- Mucous membrane pemphigoid like involvement of the eye associated with use of drugs like pilocarpine, epinephrine or timolol eye drops
- Here DIF is negative

Q. Which drug can induce mucus membrane pemphigoid?

A. Penicillamine.

Q. Rx of mucous membrane pemphigoid.

A. • Patient are divided as:
  ○ Low risk patient i.e., patients with oral diseases or both oral and skin diseases
  ○ High risk patient i.e., patients with ocular, genital, nasopharyngeal, esophageal or laryngeal mucosal involvement
  ○ The low risk patient are treated with:
    – Oral prednisolone/tetracycline + Nicotinamide/dapsone along with the topical corticosteroids
  ○ The high risk patients are treated with:
    – Oral prednisone (1 to 1.5 mg/kg/day)with or without cyclophosphamide or azathioprine (1 to 2 mg/kg/day)
    – Care of eyes and other mucosa to prevent development of synechia and strictures is a must.

Q. Newer Rx of MMP.

A. • IVIg
- Mycophenolate mofetil
- Etanercept, daclizumab

DERMATITIS HERPETIFORMIS

Q. How will you diagnose a c/o dermatitis herpetiformis?

A. • Usually in younger adults - second and third decade
- Intensely pruritic symmetrical papular or papulo vesicular eruption on bilateral extensors of limbs shoulders and buttocks
- Characteristics history of subepidermal blisters with neutrophilic inflammatory infiltrate.
- Granular IgA deposition at tips of dermal papilla on DIF (classically called picket fence pattern)
- Prompt relief in symptom on Rx with dapsone.

Q. In there mucosal involvement in DH?

A. • Rarely the oral mucosa may show maculopapular vesicles, ulceration which bleed and heal slowly
- Laryngeal lesion may lead to Hoarseness.

Q. What are Differential diagnosis for DH?

A. • Bullous pemphigoid
- Erythema multiforme
- Transient acantholytic dermatosis

- Papular uriticaria
- Scabies
- Neurotic excoriations

Q. What are associations of DH?

A.
- DH as associated with:
  - Gluten sensitive enteropathy
  - Diabetes mellitus
  - Collagen vascular diseases like LE, Sjögren's
  - Pernicious anemia
  - Biliary cirrhosis
  - Ulcerative colitis
  - Splenic atrophy

Q. Which Carcinomas may be associated with DH?
DH as associated with:

A.
- T-cell lymphoma
- Esophageal adenocarcinoma
- Non-Hodgkin's lymphoma
- Small bowel and stomach cancer

Q. What is the natural history of DH?

A. Majority of the patients have a life-long course with remissions and exacerbations 10 to 15 % of patients have spontaneous remission.

Q. How will you treat a C/O DH?

A.
- The mainstay of treatment induces:
  - Dapsone
  - Avoidance of gluten in diet
  - Dapsone is started in the dose of 100 mg/day. If there is no improvement, then the dose is increased by 50 mg every 2 weeks to a maximum of 300 mg/day
  - Gluten free diet—avoidance of Barley, Rye, oats, wheat, millet.
  - Rice and corn do not contain gluten and can be consumed
  - Other drugs like sulfasalasine, colchicin, cyclosporine, azathioprine and prednisolone have been tried.

LINEAR IGA BULLOUS DERMATOSIS (LABD)

Q. How will you diagnose a c/o LABD?

A.
- Bimodal onset adult onset, i.e., fifth decade and childhood, i.e., children <5 years age
- Sudden onset of tense bullae associated with mild pruritis.

- In children there is a "cluster of jewels" appearance, i.e., annular arrangement of new small tense blisters around a crusted healing erythematous plaque
- In adults the morphology may be:
  - Bullous pemphigoid like
  - Dermatitis herpetiformis like
- H/e showing subepidermal split with a sparse neutrophilic and eosinophilic infiltrate in upper dermis
- DIF shows linear IgA deposition along the DEJ
- IIF shows circulating IgA antiBMZ antibodies

Q. What is the mucosal involvement in LABD?

A.
- Oral mucosa is involved in 80% of patient
- Painful erosions or ulcers
- Desquamative gingivitis
- Other mucosa may be involved like:
  - Eye—irritation, redness, dryness, photosensitivity blurring of vision rarely conjunctival scarring and blindness
  - Nasal—stuffiness, crusting, bleeding
  - Laryngeal—hoarseness

Q. Association with LABD.

A. Other autoimmune disorders like SLE, dermatomyositis.

Q. Differential diagnosis for LABD.

A.

Childhood	*Adults*
Bullous impetigo	Bullous pemphigoid
Epidermolysis bullosa	Dermatitis herpetiformis
Porphyria	Erythema multiforme
	Eye involvement must be differentiated from mucus membrane pemphigoid

Q. How can one differentiate between BP and LABD?

A.

BP	*LABD*
Tense blisters on an erythematous base	Lesions may be BP like or DH like
H/P shows subepidermal split with intact epidermis. Dermal infiltrate consist of eosinophils, mononuclear cells and few neutrophilis	H/P shows subepidermal split. Dermal infiltrate is a spare and consist of neutrophils and few eosinophils

Continued

Continued

BP	*LABD*
DIF shows linear IgG and C3 deposits along BMZ	DIF shows linear IgA and C3 deposits along BMZ
In skin split D/f the IgG is found epidermal side	In skin split D/f the IgG is found epidermal side
IIF shows circulating antiBMZ IgG on epidermal side	IIF shows circulating antiBMZ IgG is found on epidermal side

Q. How will you differentiate between DH and LABD?

A.

DH	*LABD*
Group intensely pruritic papulovesicles on extensor surface of extremities	BP like or DH like
H/P–subepidermal split, neutrophilic micro abscess with few eosinophils seen in adjoining dermal papillae giving a multilocular appearance In older lesions the tips of dermal papillae separate and the blister becomes unilocular	Subepidermal split, sparse dermal infiltrate consisting of neutrophils and eosinophils
DIF granular IgA deposits giving a picket fence appearance	IgA linear deposits
Dramatic response to DDS	Steroid + DDS required

Q. Course and prognosis of LABD.

A.
- In 2/3 of children remission occurs in 4 years rarely disease may persist into adult hood.
- In adults diseases has a smouldering course but usually remits after 3 to 6 years.

Q. Pregnancy and LABD.

A.
- LABD usually remits after 2nd trimester
- No fetal abnormality associated

Q. Rx of LABD.

A.
- Mild cases can be managed with the topical corticosteroids
- Dapsone 1 to 2 mg/kg/day with or without prednisolone
- Other sulphonamides like: → sulfamethoxypyridazine (0.5 to 1.5 g/day) → sulfapyridine (1 to 2 g/day)
- Other immunomodulators like: Colchicine (2 mg/day), cyclosporine, tetracycline + nicotinamide, mycophenolate mofetil, erythromycin

SUBCORNEAL PUSTULAR DERMATOSES (SCPD)/ SNEDDON-WILKINSON DISEASE

Q. How will you diagnose a C/o SCPD?

A.
- Adult onset usually >40 years age
- Female preponderance M:F = 1:4
- Clinically multiple small flaccid pustules or vesicles that rapidly become pustular lesions on an erythematous base which usually occur in crops. The pustules may coalesce to form annular, circinate or serpiginous patterns. Lesions seen over flexural areas
- DIF and IIF are negative

Q. Associations of SCPD.

A.
- Elevated serum IgA
- IgA gammopathies—IgA myeloma, IgA paraproteinemia
- Collagen vascular diseases like SLE, RA

Q. What are culture reports form pustule ?

A. Sterile pustule.

Q. H/p finding of SCPD.

A.
- Subcorneal blister with neutrophils
- Absence of acantholysis

Q. Differential diagnosis.

A.
- Impetigo
- Dermatitis herpetiformis
- Subcorneal type of IgA pemphigus
- Pemphigus foliaceus
- Pustule psoriasis
- Glucagonoma syndrome
- Acute generalized exanthematous pustulosis

Q. Course and prognosis of SCPD.

A.
- SCPD is a benign condition with exacerbations, remissions, usually remits in 5 to 8 years.
- Appearance of myeloma is associated with poor prognosis.

Q. Rx of SCPD.

A.
- Sulfones such as:
  - Dapsone 50 to 1,500 mg/day
  - Sulfapyridine 1 to 3 g/day
- Systemic corticosteroids

- Acitretin
- Infliximab
- PUVA
- Milder cases may be managed worth topical corticosteroids or topical tacalcitol.

HAILEY–HAILEY DISEASE

Q. Incidence of Hailey–Hailey.

A. 1 in 50,000.

Q. Pathogenesis of Hailey–Hailey.

A.
- It is caused by a mutation of *ATP2C1* gene located on the long arm of chromosome 3.
- This gene encodes an enzyme calcium ATPase which is located on the Golgi apparatus. Mutation of this gene causes failure of calcium deposition in the Golgi apparatus.
- This results in defect in translocation of junctional proteins resulting in acantholysis.
- Loss of *ATP2C1* gene can cause oxidative stress which damages DNA.

Q. What are the causes of Hailey–Hailey disease?

A. Hailey–Hailey is an autosomal dominant inherited disease with complete penetrance but variable expressivity.

Q. Which is the gene involved in Hailey–Hailey diseases?

A. SERCA-1, i.e., sarco endoplasmic reticulum calcium ATPase 1 shows heterozygous mutations.

Q. How will you diagnose a c/o Hailey–Hailey disease?

A.
- Disease is more common in the third decade
- Autosomal dominant inheritance
- Clinically characterized by recurrent Vesiculobullous eruption over the flexures and groins.
- Nikolsky's sign is usually negative
- Aggravated by:
  - Heat
  - UV light
  - Mechanical friction
  - Infections like staph, strepto, proteus, pseudomonas, *candida albicans*

- Histological characterized by dilapidated brick wall appearance i.e., separated epidermal cells due to acantholysis with lymphocytic infiltrate
- Immunohistologically—negative

Q. Is there a clinical diagnostic test for Hailey-Hailey?

A. Yes, exposing the normal appearing skin of the back to UVA causes characteristic h/p change in 24 hours.

Q. What are the differential diagnosis for Hailey-Hailey?

A.
- D/D for crusted lesions—Impetigo
- D/D for annular lesions—Tinea circinata
- D/D for vegetating lesions—Pemphigoid vegetans, Dariers diseases

Q. What are the course and prognosis of Hailey-Hailey disease?

A.
- It has prolonged course of several weeks characterized by exacerbations and remissions
- The disease severity usually decreases with age.

Q. What is the treatment?

A. The acute flare of hailey and hailey can be treated with:
- Antibiotics like tetracycline—2 g/day followed by maintenance of 500 mg/day other systemic antibiotics like penicillin, erythromycin or minocycline have also been tried
- Systemic and topical corticosteroids
- Steroids sparing immunomodulatory drugs like dapsone in a loading dose of 100-200 mg/day till the flare subsides followed by maintenance of 50 mg/day
- Topical tacrolimus, calcitriol, tacalcitol
- UVA with psoralens
- The persistent recalcitrant cases can be treated with:
  - Split skin graft
  - Erbium Yag and Co_2 lesions

Q. Who were Hailey-Hailey?

A. Two dermatologist brothers Howard and Hugh hailey. They described the condition.

TRANSIENT ACANTHOLYTIC DERMATOSIS

Q. What is the etiology of TAD or grovers disease?

A.
- Sun exposure
- Heat and sweating

- Febrile or postoperative bed ridden patients
- Immunodeficiency like leukemia and lymphoma i.e., all these implicate an acrosyringeal involvement

Q. What is it clinically characterized by?

A.
- Usually seen in patient > 40 years M:F is 3:1 to 7:1
- Papules, Papulovesicles and nodules occur in crops which have variable pruritus

Q. What are clinically variants of TAD?

A.
- Transient eruptive, i.e., multiple itchy lesions that settle in a few weeks
- Persistent pruritic, i.e., cases with less severe pruritus than the earlier type but lesions persist for months to years showing only partial response to treatment
- Chronic asymptomatic, i.e., persistent truncal papules specially in inframammary region. These cases are more commonly seen in oncology patients.

Q. Grover's diseases is associated with which other skin conditions?

A.
- Eczema-asteatotic and seborrhea
- Allergic contact dermatitis
- Psoriasis
- Solar keratosis and other condition of actinic change

Q. What are the H/P findings of Grover's disease?

A. Acantholysis with vesicle formation is the characteristic epidermal change with five main patterns:

1. Pemphigus vulgaris like suprabasal acantholysis
2. Pemphigus foliaceus like superficial acantholysis
3. Hailey–Hailey like dilapidated brick wall appearance
4. Darier's like acantholytic dyskeratosis with corps ronds and grains
5. Eczema like spongiotic pattern

Q. What is the DIF and IIF?

A. Negative.

Q. What is differential diagnosis for Grover's disease?

A.
- Acne
- Acute febrile neutrophilic dermatosis
- Insect bite reaction
- Bullous impetigo

- Candidiasis
- Dermatitis herpetiformis
- Drug eruption
- Folliculitis
- Seborrheic dermatitis
- Scabies

Q. What are the histological differential diagnosis?

A.
- Pemphigus vulgaris
- Pemphigus foliaceus
- Hailey-Hailey diseases
- Darier's diseases
- Eczema

Q. Where is focal acantholytic dyskeratoses seen as a secondary feature?

A. Local secondary acantholysis is seen in:
- Herpes virus diseases
- Impetigo
- Solar keratosis
- Squamous cell carcinoma

But in Grover's disease it is seen as a primary pattern.

Q. What is treatment for Grover's diseases?

A. The patients of Grover's diseases can be divided as mild, moderate, severe disease depending upon the clinical involvement and can be treated accordingly.
- Mild diseases:
  - Avoidance of sun exposure and sweating
  - Using potent topical corticosteroids
  - Symptomatic Rx for pruritus
- Moderate and severe disease: When pruritus is severe and there is no improvement with topical line of management—
  - Oral vitamin A: (i) 50,000 IU TDS for 2 weeks (ii) f/b 50,000 IU OD for 12 weeks
  - Retinoids: (i) Acitretin 0.5 mg/kg/day (ii) Isotretinoin—40 mg/day tapered to 10 mg/day. Gradually over 12 weeks.
  - Dapsone
  - PUVA and NBUVB
  - Oral corticosteroids

EPIDERMOLYSIS BULLOSA

Q. What is the cause of epidermolysis bullosa?

A. It is genetically transmitted mechano bullous disorder.

Q. How is EB classified?

A. Depending upon the level of spilt:

- EB simplex—Intraepidermal split at the level of basal keratinocytes
- EB functional—Blister with in the BMZ
- Dystrophic EB—Blister beneath the BMZ

Q. Where is the mutation in EB ?

A.
- In EB simplex the mutation is at the genes encoding for keratin 5 and 14, plectin.
- In dystrophic EB, the mutation is in the laminin 5, collagen XVII, plectin
- In dystrophic EB, the mutation is in Collagen *vii* gene

Q. What are the types of EB simplex?

A.
1. Weber-Cockayne:
   - Most common type
   - Autosomal dominant
   - Manifests in infancy or early childhood
   - Hyperhidrosis of palms & soles
   - Thick walled blisters on palm and sales
   - Callosities
   - Hair/teeth/nail/mucous membrane are normal
2. Koebner EB:
   - Sporadic cases
   - Autosomal dominant
   - Manifests at birth or soon thereafter
   - Tense blisters which often heal with atrophic scaring seen on pressure and friction areas.
   - Nail involvement present but minimal.
   - Blistering tendency persists throughout life but tends to improve after puberty.
3. Dowling—Meara EBS or EB herpetiformis:
   - Autosomal dominant
   - Onset at birth or soon thereafter
   - Mucosal involvement, nail shedding and transient milia formation.

- Blistering tendency decreases after 6–7 years.
- Biopsy needed to differentiate from junctional and dystrophic forms.

4. EBS with muscular dystrophy—rare:
   - Autosomal recessive
   - Starts in early infancy
   - Blisters seen at trauma prone sites which heal with scarring and milia formation.
   - Muscular dystrophy can cause immobility and eventually death.
5. EB with mottled pigmentation—Autosomal dominant:
   - Manifests at birth or infancy.
   - Blisters may be localized or generalized and heal with mottled pigmentation.
6. EB simplex Ogna—Hemorrhagic blisters on hands and feet with Onychogryphosis.
7. EB simplex superficialis—autosomal dominant:
   - Manifests at birth

Q. What are junctional EB types?

A. 1. Herlitz junctional EB/EB lethalis:
   - Autosomal recessive
   - Manifests at birth
   - Skin is fragile. Skin involvement heals with minimal scarring.
   - Oral and pharyngeal involvement may be severe.
   - Painful corneal erosions
   - Teeth and nail involvement present.
   - 40% patients die at 1st year and most patients succumb in 1st 5 years.

2. Generalized non-Herlitz junctional EB/generalized trophic benign EB/Wolf-Hunter:
   - Manifests at birth
   - Generalized fragility
   - Significant nail, teeth and mucosal involvement but less severe than Herlitz.
3. Atrophic hair loss present. JEB with pyloric atresia:
   - Presents at birth
   - Nonbilious vomiting on attempt to feed should arouse suspicion.
   - Teeth and nail involvement
   - Death in few months

4. Inverse JEB:
   - Fragility and generalized blisters in neonate that localizes to intertriginous areas within several months.
5. Progressive JEB:
   - Delayed onset at 5–8 years.
   - Manifests as nail dystrophy and defective tooth enamel.
   - Partial deafness.
   - Blistering over the hands, feet, knees and elbows.

Q. What are the types of dystrophic EB?

A. 1. Dominant dystrophic EB (Cockayne-Touraine type) and Albopapuloid (Pasini type):
   - Autosomal dominant
   - Generalized blistering at birth at trauma prone sites.
   - Lesions heal with scarring and milia formation.
   - Nail dystrophy present
2. Pretibial dystrophic EB and EB pruriginosa:
   - EB pruriginosa
   - Autosomal dominant/recessive
   - Presents at birth
   - Intractable pruritis
   - Violaceous papules and plaques
   - Pretibial dystrophic EB
   - Autosomal dominant
   - Late onset
   - Itching bullae, atrophy and scaring on shins.
   - Mucosal involvement absent.
3. Autosomal recessive dystrophic EB/Hallopeau–Siemens:
   - At birth or infancy
   - Cutaneous as well as mucosal involvement.
   - Nikolsky's sign positive
   - Syndactyly leading to Mitten like appearance.
   - Flexural contracture.
   - Nail dystrophy
   - Scarring alopecia
   - Microstomia and Ankyloglossia
   - Hoarseness and aphonia may develop due to laryngeal involvement dysphagia due to oesophageal involvement.
   - Aspiration pneumonia
   - Anal stenosis and fecal retention.
   - Ocular involvement

- Urethral stenosis
- Anemia
- Growth retardation
- Multiple Squamous cell carcinomas in areas of repeated blistering.

Other types involve:

- Non-Hallopeau–Siemens recessive DEB.
- Transient bullous dermolysis of the new born
- Inverse recessive DEB

Q. In which types of Eb there is premature death?

A.
- Herlitz type JEB
- Hallopeau–Siemens RDEJ
- Dowling–Meara type of EBS

Q. What are the differential diagnosis for EB?

A.
- Herpes simplex
- Congenital syphilis
- Staphylococcal scalding skin syndrome
- Gunther's disease
- Neonatal pemphigus
- Incontinentia pigmenti
- Kindler syndrome
- Ichthyosis Bullosa of Siemens
- Bullous congenital ichthyosiform erythroderma
- Linear IgA disease
- Bullous pemphigoid
- Cicatricial pemphigoid
- Laryngo-onycho-cutaneous syndrome (Shabir's syndrome)

Q. How will you do the biopsy if there are no fresh blisters?

A. The skin that is clinically uninvolved but adjacent to a site where the patient usually blisters is selected (the palms and soles should be avoided because the increased skin thickness in these areas makes the identification of the cleavage site difficult). After preparation in a sterile manner a cotton-swab, pencil eraser, or gloved finger or thumb is used to apply a firm downward pressure to the skin and a traction is then exerted by twisting (at least 180 degrees each way), until erythema is produced. The development of erythema at the site is a good endpoint. For newborns or infants, a reasonable rule of thumb is to rub the selected area at least 20 times. Biopsies are performed at least 5 minutes after the induction of erythema to allow the development of a microscopically identifiable blister. The biopsy site is cleaned with an antiseptic solution (povidone iodine stings less than alcohol) and draped. Two separate biopsies from adjacent sites are taken. Most laboratories prefer punch biopsies over shave biopsies because punched specimens are easier to orient and embed for frozen sections.

Q. What are the contents of michel's media?

A. Ammonium sulfate, N-ethyl-maleimide, magnesium sulfate, potassium citrate buffer, and distilled water; the correct pH buffering is important. It is essential to avoid contamination of the IFM sample with formalin or TEM fixative to preserve antigen expression.

Q. What are the EM findings of EB?

A. Transmission electron microscopy (TEM) is time-consuming, labor-intensive, expensive, operator-dependent, potentially more subjective in its interpretation, and available only in a few specialized centers. However, TEM may be helpful for determining the level of skin separation and is used in some instances to confirm or refine the diagnosis obtained by immunofluorescence mapping (IFM). As an example, in milder forms of EB, particularly those inherited in a dominant manner, IFM may be normal, whereas TEM can identify microsplits and other ultrastructural abnormalities at the dermal-epidermal junction.

TEM utilizes a magnification of 3,000 to 30,000×, which allows the visualization of the level of skin cleavage and morphology of the structural components of the dermal-epidermal junction, including keratin intermediate filaments, hemidesmosomes, and anchoring fibrils. TEM is of particular use in diagnosing EB simplex Dowling-Meara, a subtype of EB simplex. In this form of EB, IFM may show no abnormality, except an intraepidermal split, whereas TEM demonstrates the characteristic aggregation of keratin intermediate filaments in the basal keratinocytes.

Q. What is the management of EB?

A. After confirming the diagnosis the following must be done:

- Genetic counseling
- Prenatal diagnosis with:
  - Chorionic villus sampling (10–12 weeks of gestation).
  - Amniocentesis (16–20 weeks of gestation) for successive pregnancies.

- Skin biopsy and blood sample from affected patient to confirm mutation.
- Fetal DNA-PCR

Treatment involves:

- Counselling the parents
- General skin care measures, i.e., avoid trauma, gentle handling of baby, prevent infections.
- General measures like air/water bed, loose soft clothing, soft leather shoes, air-conditioned low humidity cool environment, avoid band aids.
- Symptomatic treatment for painful blisters:
  - Amitriptyline
  - Phenytoin therapy
  - Vitamin E
  - Tetracyclines
  - Retinoids
  - Cyclosporine
  - PUVA
- Surgical management:
  - Split thickness skin grafting
  - Keratinocytes cultured in sheets
  - Tissue engineering

EPIDERMOLYSIS BULLOSA ACQUISITA

Q. How will you diagnose a case of EBA?

A. EBA is a diagnosis of exclusion:

- The Roegnic's criteria include:
  - Cutaneous lesions, i.e., erosions, blisters, milia, scars at trauma prone sites
  - Adult onset
  - H/E showing subepidermal split
  - Absence of family history of bullous disorders
  - Family history
  - DIF: Linear IgG and C3 deposition along DEJ
  - Exclusion of all other blistering diseases

Q. What are the clinic variants of EBA?

A.
- Noninflammatory, i.e., dermolytic pemphigoid which heals with scarring
- Inflammatory, i.e., generalized eruption similar to bullous pemphigoid.

Q. Differential diagnosis for EBA.

A.
- Bullous pemphigoid
- Cicatricial pemphigoid
- Dystrophic epidermolysis pemphigoid
- Linear IgA disease
- Dermatitis herpetiformis
- Porphyria cutanea tarda
- Bullous SLE

Q. How to differentiate between bullous SLE and EBA?

A.

Bullous SLE	*EBA*
No skin fragility	Generalized skin fragility
Photosensitivity present	No evidence of photosensitivity
Sun exposed areas involved in bullous SLE	Trauma prone areas involved in EBA
Dramatic response to dapsone	Dramatic improvement seen with corticosteroids

Q. Course and prognosis of EBA.

A. It has a chronic course with exacerbations and remissions. Rarely the disease may remit completely like bullous pemphigoid.

Q. Treatment of EBA.

A.
- Oral steroids: 0.5 to 1.5 mg/kg/day
- Dapsone
- Others: Azathioprine, IVIg, cyclophosphamide, mycophenolate mofetil
- Rituximab has been tried

SHORT CASES

1 Acanthosis Nigricans

Q. What is acanthosis nigricans (AN)?

A. Presence of bilaterally symmetrical, hyperpigmented, velvety plaques in the axillae, neck, groins.

Q. Is AN a misnomer?

A. Yes, there is neither acanthosis nor hyperpigmentation histologically. The excess melanin is in the stratum corneum.

Q. Classify AN.

A. Schwartz classification:

- Benign AN
- Obesity associated AN
- Syndromic associated AN
- Malignant AN
- Acral AN
- Unilateral AN
- Medication induced AN
- Mixed type AN—two types are present simultaneously

Q. What are the common sites of affection?

A. Acanthosis nigricans is commonly seen on axillae, neck, and groins. Other sites include the face, external genitalia, flexor and extensor surfaces of elbows and knees, dorsum of the hands and fingers, submammary, umbilicus, and perianal area.

Q. Enumerate a few endocrinopathies associated with AN.

A.
- Insulin-resistant diabetes mellitus
- Acromegaly
- Gigantism
- Cushing syndrome
- Addison's disease
- Polycystic ovary syndrome
- Hypothyroidism

Q. What is HAIR-AN syndrome?

A. Hyper-Androgenism Insulin Resistance–Acanthosis Nigricans in women.

Q. Which drugs can give rise to AN?

A. The following drugs can give rise to AN:

- Nicotinic acid
- Niacinamide
- Testosterone
- Diethylstilbestrol
- Oral contraceptives
- Protease inhibitor
- Triazinate
- Fusidic acid

Q. What is difference between benign and malignant AN?

A.
- Malignant AN starts suddenly, often pruritic, involved atypical areas and can involve the mucosal and palm (tripe palms)
- Benign is gradual, often present from young age and obesity associated, does not involve mucosa and not pruritic.

Q. What is the differential diagnosis?

- Terra firma-forme dermatosis (Duncan dirty dermatosis)—can be wiped off with alcohol
- Dowling-Degos' disease—soft fibromas with pitted acneiform scars periorally
- Gougerot-Carteaud syndrome—reticular pigmented papules in seborrheic areas
- Granular parakeratosis—hyperkeratotic papules/plaques, in patients who use deodorants, middle-aged women

Q. What is the Leser-Trelat sign?

A. Leser-Trelat sign is the rapid appearance or growth of multiple seborrheic keratoses along with AN. Its existence is controversial because eruptive seborrheic keratoses can also develop in erythrodermic patients who do not have an underlying malignancy.

Q. What are tripe palms?

A. Tripe (villous lining of ruminant stomach) palms, also known as acanthosis palmaris, are a manifestation of malignant AN and are characterized by thickened, velvety palms with thickening of the palmar dermatoglyphics (pachydermatoglyphy). Serum epidermal growth factor is elevated.

Q. Describe the histopathological findings.

A.
- Hyperkeratosis
- Irregular spiky papillomatosis
- Slight hyperpigmentation in the basal layer
- No acanthosis

Q. What is the pathogenesis of AN?

A. In benign forms, it probably results from keratinocyte and dermal fibroblast proliferation stimulated by insulin or insulin-like growth factor and stimulation of tyrosine kinase growth factor receptor. In malignant forms, transforming growth factors is involved.

Q. What are the malignant conditions associated with AN?

A. Most cases are associated with adenocarcinoma, especially of the gastrointestinal tract, particularly of the stomach; others being the lung, breast, gallbladder, pancreas, esophagus, liver, prostate, kidney, colon, rectum, uterus, and ovaries. Rarely, Hodgkin's disease.

Q. What is the treatment of AN?

A.
- If obese, then weight loss
- If malignancy is the cause, then removal of the tumor required
- Treatment of the underlying endocrinopathy
- Keratolytics—salicylic acid ointment, retinoic acid cream, oral isotretinoin or acitretin
- CO_2 or Alexandrite laser ablation

2 Acrochordon

Q. What is acrochordon?

A. It is a benign fibrous and fibrohistiocytic soft tissue tumor. It is the most common fibrous lesion of the skin and presents as a soft skin-colored to slightly hyperpigmented pedunculated papule, predominantly on the neck, axilla and groin.

Q. What are the synonyms of acrochordon?

A.
- Skin tag
- Fibroepithelial polyp
- Soft fibroma
- Papilloma colli
- Fibroma molluscum
- Fibroma pendulum

Q. What are the clinical features of acrochordon?

A. It presents as a soft skin-colored to slightly hyperpigmented, pedunculated papule, predominantly on the neck, axilla and groin, as well as scattered elsewhere. They are usually asymptomatic.

Q. What are the common sites for acrochordon?

A. Sides of neck, axilla, groins, eyelids.

Q. Which are the conditions associated with acrochordon?

A. Colonic polyps, diabetes, acromegaly. Most patients do not have any associated disease except obesity. They may also be associated with acanthosis nigricans.

Q. When can an acrochordon be painful?

A.
- When there is secondary infection
- When there is strangulation—the root can often be obstructed by a hair or a fabric thread. This can also be done by patient by applying a horse's hair

Sometimes the acrochordon becomes painful and falls off

Q. What are the histopathological findings?

A. Polypoid with variably loose to dense collagenous stroma with thin-walled, dilated blood vessels in the center.

Q. What are the differential diagnosis of acrochordon?

A.
- Seborrheic keratosis
- Nevus lipomatosus superficialis
- Angiofibroma
- Intradermal melanocytic nevus
- Pedunculated neurofibroma

Q. What is the treatment for acrochordon?

A. Unless irritated or infected, skin tags are more of a cosmetic issue than a clinical concern and can be easily removed by:
- Simple scissor excision
- Electrodesiccation
- Cryosurgery

3 Acne

Q. What are open and closed comedones?

A. Open comedones—they are 1-2 mm in diameter. They represent follicles with a widely dilated orifice. The black-head does not represent dirt, but it is due to oxidation of melanin and presence of certain lipids in the sebum.

Closed comedones—they are 1-3 mm diameter papular lesions without surrounding erythema. They represent follicles that have become dilated with cellular and lipid debris. They possess only a microscopic opening to skin surface. The lesions remain undetected unless the skin is stretched between the fingers to reveal it.

Q. What are types of comedones?

A.
- *Sandpaper comedones*: White heads, distributed on the forehead, produces gritty feel to the skin.
- *Macrocomedones*: These are closed or open comedones more than 1 mm in diameter.
- *Submarine-comedones*: They are deep seated and are the source of recurrent inflammatory nodular lesions.
- *Secondary comedones*: Produced after exposures to dioxins (chloracne), topical steroids, pomades.

Q. Are there any other conditions where comedones are present?

- Nevus comedonicus
- Hidradenitis suppurative

Q. What are grades of acne?

A. The severity of acne can be graded as under (Leid's classification):
- *Grade I (mild)*: Comedones and occasional papules are present.
- *Grade II (moderate)*: Comedones, many papules, few pustules.
- *Grade III (severe)*: Predominantly pustules nodules and abscesses.
- *Grade IV (nodulocystic)*: Mainly cysts or abscesses and wide spread scarring.

GLOBAL ACNE GRADING SYSTEM

Depending on the type of lesion present a score of 0–4 is given:
- No lesions
- For comedones
- Papules
- Pustules
- Nodules

The score does not change if there is more than one lesion and the lesion of highest score is taken and multiplied by the value for respective region:
- For nose
- For forehead
- For right cheek
- For left cheek
- For back

Q. What are variants of acne?

A. Acne can be classified as follows:
- Variants according to age:
  - Neonatal acne
  - Infantile acne
  - Childhood acne
  - Prepubertal acne (due to adrenal androgens)
  - Pubertal or classic acne
  - Acne in the early or late 20s often related to PCOS
  - Pregnancy acne
  - Premenopausal acne
  - Senile acne (misnomer)

Q. What are the various syndrome associated with acne?

A.
- MARSH syndrome—melasma, acne, rosacea, seborrhea and hirsutism
- SAPHO syndrome synovitis, acne, pustulosis, hyperostosis, osteitis
- PAPA syndrome sterile pyogenic arthritis, pyoderma gangrenosum, acne
- PAPASH syndrome
- PAPA + HS
- Polycystic ovary syndrome
- Abert's syndrome—acro-cephalo-syndactyly

Acne due to exogenous factors:
- Sunlight—acne aestivalis

- Helmet acne
- Mask acne (mascne)
- Acne mechanica
- Acne excrete
- Occupational acne
- Radiation acne
- McDonalds acne (due to working in hot humid environment of the kitchen of fast food companies)

Acne due to internal factors:

- Acne excoriee due to anxiety
- Drug indue to acne—remember mnemonic PIMPLES—phenytoin, INH, moisturisers, phenobarbitone, lithium, epidermal GF inhibitors, steroids
- Gram negative folliculitis
- Morbihan's disease—acne with solid facial edema
- Acne fulminant—acne, fever, LNpathy, leukocytosis

Q. What are different types of scars?

A. The different type of acne scars are:

- Ice pick scar—long narrow scar that extends deep into dermis, leaves a small yet obvious hole which looks as if it is pierced by an ice pick and caused by inflammatory break out, such as deep papule or cyst. Most commonly seen on cheeks.
- Rolling scars—a result of tethering of otherwise normal appearing skin to subcutaneous tissue below. The process gives skin a rolling or undulating appearance.
- Box scars—they are oval to round depressions 0.1–0.5 mm in depth that have sharp vertical edges, they do not taper to a point at the base.

Q. What is gram-negative folliculitis?

A. It is seen in patients with pre-existing acne vulgaris who are treated with long-term oral antibiotics especially tetracyclines. Patients give a history of initial reduction followed by worsening of the lesions. The lesions are papulopustules around the nose or deep-seated nodules. The organisms involved are *Enterobacter, Klebsiella, Escherichia* and *Proteus*. Treatment includes antimicrobials with Gram-negative coverage and resistant cases can be treated with oral isotretinoin for 4–5 months.

Q. What is hormone induced acne?

A. Acne with hormonal disturbances characterized by irregular menses, deepened voice, clitoromegaly, muscular habitus, androgenetic alopecia, increased libido, hirsutism, insulin resistance and acanthosis nigricans. Seen in patients with PCOS (Stein-Leventhal syndrome) and congenital adrenal hyperplasia and HAIR-AN syndrome. The acne in these patients is severe and more difficult to treat and onset is usually abrupt. Thorough history including age and pubertal status, physical examination, laboratory investigations like total and free testosterone, DHEAS, 17-hydroxyprogesterone. In patients of PCOD, FSH and LH should also be done.

Q. What are differential diagnosis of acne?

A.
- *Comedonal*:
  - Closed:
    - Milia
    - Osteoma cutis
    - Syringomas
    - Sebaceous hyperplasia trichoepithelioma
    - Eruptive vellus hair cyst,
    - Steatocystoma multiplex
    - Plane warts
    - Colloid milium
    - Follicular mucinosis
    - Trichodiscomas, fibrofolliculoma
  - Open comedones:
    - Trichostasis spinulosa
    - Favre-Racouchot disease
    - Nevus comedonicus
    - Basaloid follicular hamartoma syndrome
    - Dilated pore of Winer
    - Follicular spines (trichodysplasia spinulosa, type 6 PRP, multiple myeloma, demodicosis, lithium therapy)
- *Inflammatory type*:
  - Rosacea
  - Perioral dermatitis
  - Folliculitis
  - Acneiform eruption
  - Keratosis pilaris
  - Neutrophilic dermatosis
  - Furuncles/Carbuncle
  - Pseudofolliculitis barbae, acne keloidalis nuchae
  - Lupus miliaris disseminatus faciae
  - Follicular mycosis fungoides
  - Neurotic excoriations/faciei

- Neonatal acne (neonatal cephalic pustulosis):
  - Sebaceous hyperplasia
  - Milia
  - Candidiasis
  - Miliaria rubra (pustular variant)
  - Papular pustular eruption of hyper IgE syndrome
  - Vesiculopustular eruption of transient myeloproliferative disorder

Q. What is adrenarche?

A. Adrenarche is an early sexual maturation stage at around 6–8 years of age. During adrenarche, the adrenal cortex secretes increased levels of androgens such as DHEA and DHEAS, but without increase in cortisol levels. It is a result of development of new zone of adrenal cortex, the zona reticularis. It is a process related to puberty, but distinct from hypothalamic pituitary gonadal maturation and function.

Q. What is etiopathogenesis of acne?

A.
- Alteration in pattern of keratinization in sebaceous follicles
- Alteration in the circulating sex hormones
- Quality and quantity of sebum production
- Follicular microbial flora:
  - Resident bacterial flora includes *P. acnes, P. granulosum, Pityrosporum ovale.*
  - *P. acne* causes increase in lipase, protease, lecithinase which are proinflammatory.
- Mediation of inflammation:
  - Increase in interleukin 1 activity, ductal corneocyte produces IL-α, IL- 8 and TNF-α which causes inflammation.
- Environmental factors:
  - Hot humid climate.
  - Emotional stress.
  - External application of oil and pomades.
  - Diet with carbohydrates with high glycemic index.

Q. Diet in acne.

A. Avoid the food which is responsible for exacerbation or development of acne, like dairy containing food which is a key factor for inflammation. A balanced diet should be suggested. High glycemic food should be avoided as patients taking high protein diet, low glycemic index have less acne.

Q. How will you treat acne vulgaris?

A.

	Mild	***Mild***	***Moderate***	***Moderate***	***Severe***
	Comedonal	Papulopustular	Papulopustular	Nodular	Conglobata/Fulminans
1st line	Topical retinoid	Topical retinoid + Topical antimicrobial	Oral antibiotic + Topical retinoid +/– BPO	Oral antibiotic + Topical retinoid +/– BPO	Oral isotretinoin (may require concurrent oral corticosteroid, esp. for acne fulminans)
2nd line	Alternative topical retinoid Azelaic acid Salicylic acid	Alternative topical retinoid +Alternate topical anti-microbial azelaic acid salicylic acid	Alternative oral antibiotic‡ alt. topical retinoid ± BPO/ azelaic acid	Oral isotretinoin + Alternative oral antibiotic‡ alt. topical retinoid ± BPO/azelaic acid	Dapsone High dose oral antibiotic + topical retinoid + BPO
Options for female patient			Oral contraceptive/ antiandrogen	Oral contraceptive/anti-androgen	Oral contraceptive/anti-androgen
Surgical options	Comedone extraction		Comedone extraction	Comedone extraction + Intralesional corticosteroid	Intralesional corticosteroid

Continued

Continued

	Mild	***Mild***	***Moderate***	***Moderate***	***Severe***
Refractory to treatment		Exclude gram-negative folliculitis	Exclude gram-negative folliculitis		
			Female patient: • Exclude adrenal or ovarian dysfunction • Exclude use of anabolic steroid or other acne-exacerbating medication	*Female patient*: • Exclude adrenal or ovarian dysfunction • Exclude use of anabolic steroid or other acne-exacerbating medication	*Female patient*: • Exclude adrenal or ovarian dysfunction • Exclude use of anabolic steroid or other acne-exacerbating medication
Maintenance	Topical retinoid ± BPO	Topical retinoid ± BPO	Topical retinoid ± BPO	Topical retinoid ± BPO	Topical retinoid ± BPO

Q. What are the topical agents used in treatment of acne?

A. Topical agents available for acne treatment are:

- Topical retinoids.
- Benzoyl peroxide.
- Topical antibacterials.
- Sulfur, sodium sulfacetamide, resorcin and salicylic acid.
- Azelaic acid.
- Topical nicotinamide.

Q. Describe about topical retinoids.

A. Mechanism of action:

- Promote desquamation of follicular epithelium (reduces comedones and development of new lesions).
- Anti-inflammatory activity:
    - Agents available
    - Tretinoin (0.025% and 0.05%)
    - Adapalene (0.1%)
    - Tazarotene (0.05% and 0.1%)

Q. Describe about benzoyl peroxide.

A.
- Available in concentration (2.5%, 5%, and 10%). Wash formulations are also available which are utilized for truncal acne.
- Mechanism of action—antibacterial and decreases the likelihood of bacterial resistance.

Q. What are the topical antibiotic formulations available for treatment of acne?

A. Topical clindamycin, topical erythromycin, are available. Use of these is not recommended alone because of increasing antibiotic resistance.

Q. What is acne lotion?

A.
- Precipitated sulfur—3%
- Resorcinol—3%
- Zinc oxide—3%
- Glycerine—2 mL
- Methylated spirit—10 mL
- Rose water—to make 100 mL

It can be applied 2–3 times day but always shaking.

It is a traditional lotion used in treatment of acne from prebenzyl peroxide days. Still used for treatment of truncal acne.

Q. What is azelaic acid?

A. It is a 1:2 heptanedicarboxylic acid that has antimicrobial, anti-inflammatory and comedolytic effect. May lighten post-inflammatory hyperpigmentation. Available as 10% and 20%

formulations. Azelaic acid reduces comedones by normalizing the disturbed terminal differentiation of keratinocytes in the follicle infundibulum.

Q. What are the oral antibiotics available for acne?

A.

Tetracycline	*Doxycycline*	*Minocycline*	*Erythromycin*
250–500 mg 1–4 times a day on an empty stomach	50–100 mg once or twice a day	50–100 mg once or twice a day	250–500 mg 2–4 times a day
Side effects—nausea, vaginitis and perianal itching, staining of growing teeth, nephrotoxic, intracranial hypertension	Side effects—photosensitivity	Side effects—vertigo, pigmentation in areas of inflammation, oral mucosa, post acne osteomas or scars, in photodistributed pattern, on the shins, in sclera, nail bed, ear cartilage, teeth and lupus like hypersensitivity syndrome, intracranial hypertension	Side effects—gastrointestinal upset and vaginal itching

Q. What advice is to be given to a patient of acne?

A.
- Do not scrub as scrubbing the face increases irritation which worsens acne.
- Do not apply oil over scalp.
- A high glycemic diet may worsen acne.
- Use of only prescribed medications.
- Do not use harsh cleansers, antibacterial soaps, astringents.

Q. Topical agents used in acne.

A.
- Keratolytics—for example, sulfur, resorcinol, salicylic acid, glycol acid (peels)
- Comedolytics—for example, retinoid acid, adapalene, tazarotene
- Antibacterial—benzoyl peroxide, azelaic acid
- Antibiotics—clindamycin, azithromycin, nadifloxacin
- Anti-inflammatory—dapsone, nicotinamide

Q. What are the indications of oral isotretinoin?

A.
- Severe recalcitrant nodular acne (inflammatory lesions are > 5 mm in diameter and unresponsive to conventional therapy)
- Gram negative folliculitis

- Inflammatory rosacea
- Pyoderma faciale
- Acne fulminant
- Hidradenitis suppurativa

Q. What is the dose of isotretinoin?

A. 0.5–1 mg/kg/day in one or two daily doses. Duration of the course is 4–6 months. To obtain the greatest chance of prolonged remission, patients should receive 120–150 mg/kg over the treatment course.

Q. How will you monitor a patient on oral isotretinoin?

A. 1. *Baseline*:
   - Examination—careful history and physical examination.
   - Identify those patients at increased risk of toxicity or adverse effects.
   - *Laboratory*:
     - Pregnancy test (in women of child bearing age)
     - CBC with platelet count.
     - Liver function tests (AST, ALT, ALP, bilirubin)
     - Serum lipid profile.
     - Renal function tests (BUN and creatinine)
   - Special tests—consider baseline X-ray of wrists, ankles, or thoracic spine if planning for long term retinoid therapy.
   - Consider ophthalmologic examination if patient have history of cataracts or retinopathy.

2. *Follow ups*:
   - Examination—clinical evaluation monthly.
   - Assessment of patient response, improvement and complaints of adverse effects.
   - Laboratory—monthly:
     - CBC with platelets
     - LFT
     - Serum lipid profile
     - RFT
     - Pregnancy test for women in child bearing age
   - Special tests—as indicated by symptoms.

Q. Surgical treatment of acne.

A.
- Removal of comedones can be done physically by a comedone extractor.
- Cysts may require incision and drainage
- Surgical management of atrophic acne scars:
  - Punch excision—for ice pick scars
  - Elliptical excision

- ○ Skin grafting
- ○ Subcision—for rolling and depressed scars. It works by breaking the fibrous strands that binds the papillary dermis to deeper tissues

Q. Lasers and photodynamic therapy for acne.

A.
- Light therapy destroys propionibacteria by targeting porphyrins produced by these bacteria.
- They also suppress a range of proinflammatory cytokines.
- Various light therapies tried are—aminolevulinic acid (550–700 nm), methyl aminolevulinate and red light, and infrared laser therapy has been tried too for reducing inflammation.
- Light therapy may cause pain, erythema, crusting, edema, pigmentation and pustular eruptions.

4 Acne Excoriée

Q. What is acne excoriée?

A. Mild acne is accompanied by extensive excoriations and hyperpigmentation.

Q. What is acne excoriée also known as?

A. Acne excoriée des jeunes filles (excoriated acne of young girls).

Q. What is acne excoriée?

A.
- A subset of neurotic excoriations characterized by ritualistic picking of acne lesions. Often, mild acne is accompanied by extensive excoriations.
- Lesions can become so deep that scarring may occur.

Q. Is there any sex predilection for the disease?

A. Yes, it is frequently seen in young women.

Q. Who are at an increased risk of acquiring this disorder?

A. Patients with an anxiety disorder, obsessive—compulsive disorder or personality disorder are particularly at risk.

Q. What is the treatment?

A.
- Antidepressants
- Psychotherapy
- Trichloroacetic acid peels
- Skin lightening peels and also azelaic acid
- In severe cases, oral isotretinoin can be considered.

5 Acquired Melanocytic Nevus

Q. What are acquired melanocytic nevi?

A. They arise due to defects in the development of epidermal melanocytes, known as "nevus cells" and such nevus cells may also migrate into the dermis. Nevi are thought to be either developmental malformations (hamartomas) or benign proliferations.

Q. What is the routine word for acquired melanocytic nevus?

A. Acquired melanocytic nevus is commonly known as a "mole".

Q. How would you describe a typical melanocytic nevus?

A. A melanocytic nevus is well-defined, symmetrical round or oval, generally measuring 2–6 mm in diameter.

Q. What are the common varieties of acquired melanocytic nevi?

A.
- Junctional nevus
- Compound nevus
- Intradermal nevus

Q. What are junctional nevi?

A. A junctional nevus is a brown or dark brown, macular lesion with slight accentuation of skin markings generally appearing on any part of the body including mucocutaneous surfaces.

Q. How are junctional nevi differentiated from freckles?

A. Freckles have a predilection for sun-exposed areas and fade on sun protection, which is not a property of junctional nevi.

Q. What are compound nevi?

A. Compound nevi may be elevated lesions, their color being a lighter shade of brown then that of junctional nevi. Compound nevi have multiple round ovoid globules, sometimes forming a cobblestone pattern or they may be dome-shaped or papillomatous. They may contain coarse long hair in the center.

Q. What are dermal nevi?

A. Dermal nevi seen after adolescence are dome-shaped, smooth-surfaced, hemispherical nodules appearing on the face and the neck. Telangiectasias may be seen and impart an angiomatous appearance. The adult variety of dermal nevi consists of sessile or soft, wrinkled sac located in the flexures, which characteristically demonstrates the presence of cholinesterase in histochemical reactions.

Q. Do acquired melanocytic nevi have a potential for malignancy?

A. Yes, they have a tendency to develop malignant melanoma but very rarely (1:100,000). Most melanomas arise de novo. Pointers toward development of malignant melanoma are: diameter >7 mm, irregular edge, irregular pigmentation, inflammation, bleeding, crusting, and oozing.

Q. Which cytokines have a protective effect against malignant transformation of acquired melanocytic nevi?

A. Interleukin-1-alpha , IL-6 and TNF-alpha.

Q. What is pseudomelanoma?

A. Incomplete removal of the nevus by shaving or excision stimulates the remaining tissue to proliferate in a manner resembling melanoma. It has a "fried egg" appearance.

Q. What is the differential diagnosis of acquired melanocytic nevi?

A.
- Seborrheic keratotic—rough, verrucous surface, pseudo-horn cysts
- Dermatofibroma—firm consistency, dimpling, mostly on lower extremity
- Melanoma (look for ABCDE rule: A asymmetry, B border irregularity, C color variegation, D diameter > 7 mm, and E evolution changing morphology)
- Pigmented basal cell carcinoma—rolled out border
- Congenital nevus—history, often hairy

Q. What is the natural course of nevus?

A.
- Nevus cells are nothing but modified melanocytes. The only difference is that they tend to move while melanocytes are stable.
- Initially, some of the grouped melanocytes at the dermoepidermal junction " ABTROPFUNG" or "drop off" and then a compound nevus is formed. Gradually the melanocytes in dew disappear and only the dermal melanocyte.

Q. Pointers that they are developing melanoma.

A. Remember the ABCDE:

A: Asymmetrical shape

B: Border irregularity

C: Color variegation (multiple colors in the same region)

D: Diameter > 6 mm

E: Evolution that is change in the morphology

This is also called the ugly duckling sign where one nevus out of many appears different (derived from the story of Ugly Duckling). Late signs of melanoma—crusting, oozing, bleeding, inflammation and ulceration.

Q. What are the triggers for the development/growth of melanocytic nevi?

A.
- Sun exposure—autoimmune blistering disease
- Neonatal phototherapy
- Blistering process—TEN/SJS, epidermolysis bullosa, severe sunburn
- Scarring process—lichen sclerosus
- Chemotherapy
- Allogenic bone marrow transplantation
- Renal transplantation
- Chronic myelogenous leukemia
- Increased hormone levels in pregnancy
- Addison's disease
- Thyroid hormone
- Atopic dermatitis in children
- Postoperative fever

Q. What are the indications for removing acquired melanocytic nevi?

A.
- Changing lesion-size, shape and color
- Atypical appearance in suspicion of melanoma
- Cosmetic
- Repeated irritation and itching

6 Acrokeratosis Verruciformis of HOPF

Q. What is acrokeratosis verruciformis of HOPF?

A. Multiple skin colored, small, warty papules on the dorsal aspect of the hands and feet.

Q. Differential diagnosis?

A.
- Verruca plana
- Seborrheic keratosis
- Stucco keratosis
- Solar keratosis
- Arsenical keratosis (rarely)

Q. Etiology of acrokeratosis verruciformis of HOPF.

A. Autosomal dominant disorder due to mutation in the gene *ATP2A2*.

Q. What other disease is associated?

A. Darier disease.

Q. Describe histopathology.

A. Hyperkeratosis, papillomatosis and acanthosis, "Church spire" configuration (other causes of church spire appearance are verruca vulgaris, seborrheic keratosis, acanthosis nigricans).

Q. Treatment.

A.
- Electrodessication
- Cryosurgery
- Urea, lactic acid, alpha-hydroxy acids and retinoid preparations have also been tried.

7 Actinic Keratosis

Q. What do actinic keratosis represent?

A. They represent in situ dysplasias resulting from sun exposure.

Q. Differential diagnosis?

A.
- Seborrheic keratosis
- Squamous cell carcinoma
- Bowen's disease
- Superficial basal cell carcinoma (BCC)

Q. Where are they found?

A. Found chiefly on chronically sun exposed surfaces of face, ears, balding scalp, dorsal hands and forearms.

Q. Describe morphology of these lesions?

A. Multiple, discrete, flat or elevated verrucous or keratotic red pigmented or skin colored surface covered by adherent scale but sometimes smooth and shiny.

Q. How does it feel on palpation?

A. Surface is rough like sandpaper more easily felt than seen.

Q. Which are the most common epithelial precancerous lesions?

A. Actinic keratosis.

Q. Histological types of actinic keratosis.

A.
- Hypertrophic
- Atrophic
- Bowenoid
- Acantholytic
- Pigmented
- Lichenoid
- Epidermis may be—acantholytic or atrophic with overlying occasional parakeratosis
- Basal cells are dysplastic

Q. How can it be prevented?

A. Regular application of sunscreen and diet which is low in fats.

Q. Describe the hypertrophic type of actinic keratosis?

A. It leads to cutaneous horn formation most frequently present on dorsal forearms and hands.

Q. Difference between seborrheic and actinic keratosis?

A. Seborrheic keratosis are yellowish, have a stuck—on appearance and are sharply marginated as compared to actinic keratosis which are erythematous.

Q. Treatment.

A.
- Electrodessication, cryotherapy, excision.
- 5 FU, imiquimod.
- Photodynamic therapy can be given with blue light or red light.
- Systemic retinoids, oral nicotinamide, and oral vitamin D.

STUCCO KERATOSES/SEBORRHEIC KERATOSES

Q. What is seborrheic keratosis?

A. Oval, slightly raised, tan/light brown to black, sharply demarcated papules or plaques rarely > 3 cm in diameter 'stuck-on' lesions occurring on the lower legs especially in vicinity of Achilles tendon.

Q. What are the other names?

A. Stucco keratosis or keratoelastoidosis verrucosa of extremities.

Q. Differential diagnosis of seborrheic keratosis.

A.
- Verruca plana
- Basal cell carcinoma
- Squamous cell carcinoma
- Melanoma
- Bowen's disease

Q. Where else are they seen?

A. Instep, dorsum of feet, forearms, dorsal aspect of hands.

Q. Which areas are never affected?

A. Palms and soles.

Q. What is seen on histopathology of stucco keratosis?

A. Hyperkeratotic type of seborrheic keratosis with no hypergranulosis and no wart particles seen by electron microscopy.

Q. What is Leser–Trélat sign?

A. Sudden appearance of numerous seborrheic keratosis in an adult which may be the cutaneous finding of internal malignancy (commonly adenocarcinoma, primarily of the stomach). Acanthosis nigricans and tripe palms accompany seborrheic keratosis.

Q. How is seborrheic keratosis present over palms?
A. Eccrine poromas.

Q. What are dermatosis papulosa nigra?
A. A variant of seborrheic keratosis seen over the central face common in Africans, Americans and Asians.

Q. Six types of histopathology of seborrheic keratosis.
A. Types are:
1. Hyperkeratotic
2. Cloral
3. Adenoid
4. Acanthotic reticulated
5. Irritated
6. Melanoacanthoma

Q. What is the recent concept of etiology of seborrheic keratosis?
A. HPV-hence some believe it to be contagious.

Q. Can seborrheic keratosis turn malignant?
A. No, if there is malignancy it has to have been there from the beginning.

Q. Treatment of seborrheic keratosis.
A. Liquid nitrogen, curettage, electrofulguration, CO_2 laser vaporization and shave excision.

Q. Histopathology of seborrheic keratosis?
A. Hyperkeratosis, acanthosis, papillomatosis.

Q. Dermoscopy of seborrheic keratosis?
A. Comedone—like lesions, milia—like lesions, network—like pattern.

8 Alopecia Areata

Q. Why is this alopecia areata (AA)?

A. There is a well-defined area of hair loss, no scaling, no scarring, no breakage of hair at different length.

Q. Differential diagnosis.

A.
- Trichotillomania
- Tinea capitis (noninflammatory)
- Syphilis
- Androgenetic alopecia
- Pseudopelade of Brocq
- Telogen effluvium
- Traumatic alopecia
- Alopecia mucinosa
- Cong triangular alopecia
- Metastatic malignancies

Q. Classify alopecias.

A. Nonscarring:
- Diffuse:
  - AGA
  - Telogen effluvium
  - Postpartum alopecia
  - Neonatal alopecia
  - Anagen effluvium
  - Drug induced
  - Hair shaft disorders
  - Occasional AA
- Focal:
  - AA
  - Fungal, bacterial or viral infection
  - Trichotillomania
  - Traction alopecia
  - Tick bite alopecia

Scarring:
- Lymphocyte associate:
  - LPP

- Central centrifugal cicatricial alopecia
- Graham Little–Piccardi–Lassueur syndrome
- Pseudopelade of Brocq
- DLE

- Neutrophil associated:
  - Perifolliculitis capitis abscedens et suffodiens
  - Folliculitis decal vans
- Mixed type:
  - Acne keloidalis nuchae
  - Acne necrotica
  - Pustular dermatosis of scalp

Q. History of AA.

A.
- Hippocrates called alopecia, "Fox's disease"
- Alopecia areata was first described by Cornelius Celsus in AD30.
- Cornelius Celsus actually described two types of alopecia, alopecia totalis and alopecia ophiasis, which gives a "snake" like pattern. Celsus actually thought that alopecia ophiasis only occurred in children.

Q. What are the other names of alopecia areata?

A.
- Alopecia areata is sometimes known as "area celsi" in tribute to Cornelius Celsus.
- "Alopecia areata" was first used by Sauvages in his "Nosologica Medica", published in 1760 in Lyons, France.
- Also known as Pelade.

Q. Epidemiology of AA.

A.
- The prevalence of alopecia areata is 0.1 to 0.2%,
- With a calculated lifetime risk of 2%
- Family history positive in 10% AA patients

Q. Explain pathogenesis of AA.

A.
- "Immune privilege" becomes defective
- Genetic predisposition:
  - HLA haplotype; DR4, DQ3, DR11
  - Concordance seen in identical twins
  - Family history positive in 10%

Q. Animal models for AA.

A.
- Dundee experimental bald rat (DEBR)
- C3H/HeJ mouse

Q. IKEDAS classification.

A.
- Common type (81%):
  - Patchy pattern with short duration
- Atopic type (10%)
  - Ophiasis and reticular, 50% may go into totalis
- Prehypertensive type (4%):
  - Reticular
- Autoimmune type/endocrine type (5%):
  - Alopecia totalis

Q. Can we adapt it in an Indian setting.

A
- No, as the percentage of patients with prehypertensive group is very few, they should be classified as adult and childhood AA
- And further subdivided into—classical, atopic and autoimmune in both groups

Q. Classification by pattern.

A.
- Generalized: Universalis
- Totalis: Restricted to scalp
  - Patchy
  - Sisaipho
  - Diffuse
  - Totalis
  - Ophiasis
  - Reticulate
  - Subtotal

Q. What are the symptoms of AA?

A.
- Asymptomatic
- Patches of hairless on scalp or beard or anywhere on body usually noticed by a relative or the barber
- Overnight greying of hair
- Brittle nails with pitting

Q. Signs in hair.

A.
- Hair pull test—positive (take 20 hair and > 10% hair will get pulled)
- Exclamation mark hair
- Cadaver hair—broken hair seen over scalp as comedones (black dots)
- Follicular ostia—ostia are well preserved in alopecia areata, in contrast to the findings in scarring alopecia
- Depigmented hair
- Frayed rope appearance of free ends

- Coudability test—try to push hair toward scalp and it bends
- Dystrophic hair

Q. Explain exclamatory mark hair.

A.
- Anagen hair suffers defective keratinization and thinning and later turns into telogen, which causes narrowing of the shaft
- As this hair grows out it appears broad distally and thin proximally, appearing like an exclamatory mark
- This is seen in most severe form of injury

Q. What is dystrophic hair?

A.
- In least form of injury, the anlagen bulb does not go into telegenic but only changes to dystrophic anagen hair
- In moderate form of injury, we notice only a telegenic bulb on hair mount

Q. Changes in nails.

A.
- Scotch plaid nail pitting
- Trachyonychia (sandpaper like roughness because of excessive longitudinal ridging)
- Red or mottled lacunae
- Nail thinning and ridging
- Longitudinally arranged punctate leukonychia
- Dystrophy, onycholysis
- Few reports of cataracts have been reported

Q. What is the difference in nail pitting in psoriasis and AA?

A.
- AA: Regular pitting, superficial pitting, scotch plaid pattern
- Psoriasis: Irregular pitting, deep pitting

Q. Dermoscopy findings of AA.

A.
- Yellow dot—sebum collection in ostia
- Black dots—broken hair

Q. What are the scoring system in AA?

A. Severity of alopecia tool score (Salt Score).

Q. What are the associations of AA?

A.
- Down's syndrome
- Hashimoto's thyroiditis
- Addison's disease
- Pernicious anemia
- Vitiligo
- LP
- Morphea
- Lichen sclerosus et atrophicus

- Pemphigus foliaceus
- SLE
- Sjögren syndrome
- Ulcerative colitis
- Myasthenia gravis
- Autoimmune hemolytic anemia
- Diabetes mellitus
- Autoimmune testicular and ovarian disease
- Chronic mucocutaneous candidiasis with endocrinopathy

Q. What are the bad prognostic signs of AA?

A.
- Early age of onset
- Extensive scalp involvement
- Loss of eyebrows and eyelashes
- Alopecia totalis
- Alopecia universalis
- Recurrent episode
- Pattern—ophiasis, sisaphio, reticular
- Nail changes
- Associated systemic disorders
- Associated genetic disorders—Down's
- Patchy regrowth of terminal hairs
- Family history

Q. What are the lab tests for AA?

A.
- Fungal culture, skin biopsy, serology for lupus erythematosus or serology for syphilis.
- CBC for anemia
- Thyroid function tests

Q. What is the histopathology of AA?

A.
- Swarm of bees appearance
- Decrease in total number of follicles
- Increase in number of vellus hair

Q. Algorithm of treatment for AA.

A.
- If child < 10 years and extent < 50% → Topical mid potent steroids + 5% minoxidil solution
- If no response, you may add short contact Anthralin
- If child < 10 years and extent > 50% → Pulse steroids (5 mg betamethasone 2 times a week)
- If patient > 10 years of age, and extent of involvement is < 50%—intralesional steroids with/without 5% minoxidil with/without topical steroids

- If good response in 3 months, continue this.
- If poor response, 1% Anthralin, with or without 5% minoxidil.
- If patient > 50% involvement—1. topical immunotherapy, SADBE, JAK inhibitors with or without ILS—if no response, try immunotherapy.
- If extensive nonresponsive AA—consider scalp prosthesis.

Q. What if we do not treat AA?

A. Spontaneous remission occurs in up to 80% of patients with limited patchy hair loss of short duration (< 1 year). Such patients may be managed by reassurance alone, with advice that regrowth cannot be expected within 3 months of the development of any individual patch. The prognosis in long-standing extensive alopecia is poor and a wig may be an option.

Q. Explain contact immune therapy.

A.
- Contact immunotherapy was introduced by Rosenberg and Drake in 1976.
- The contact allergens used include:
    - 1-chloro, 2, 4, dinitrobenzene (DNCB); (Banned because mutagenic)
    - Squaric acid dibutylester (SADBE)
    - 2, 3-diphenylcyclopropenone (DPCP)
    - Initially patient is sensitized with higher concentration of allergen applied on forearm.
    - Later patient is challenged with very low concentration of allergens on the alopecic areas to maintain a brisk erythema over the lesion.

9 Aphthous Stomatitis

Q. What is aphthous stomatitis?

A. Presence of multiple, painful, round or ovoid ulcers with circumscribed margin, erythematous halo and a yellow or grey floor on oral mucous membrane, history of (H/O) recurrence, no other sites are involved.

Q. What is differential diagnosis of aphthous stomatitis?

A. Aphthous stomatitis must be differentiated from the following:

- Herpetic gingivostomatitis, recurrent herpes labialis
- Pemphigus
- Lichen planus
- Erythema multiforme
- Cicatricial pemphigoid
- Behçet's syndrome
- Candidiasis
- Avitaminosis like pellagra and scurvy
- Drug-induced

Q. What is etiology of aphthous ulcer?

A. Exact cause not known. The various etiologic agents are:

- Trauma such as self biting, tooth brush injury, dental procedures
- Spicy foods, citrus fruits
- Cessation of smoking (smoking is relatively beneficial in pemphigus, ulcerative colitis, though it is injurious to general health)
- Allergy
- Stress
- Heredity (one-third patients)
- Hormonal changes in women such as menstruation, pregnancy, menarche and menopause
- Hematological abnormality
- Infections and immunologic manifestations

Q. What is the pathogenesis behind aphthous ulcer?

A. The cause of recurrent aphthous ulcer is unknown but believed to be due to T-cell mediated localized destruction of oral mucosa associated with increased relative ratio of CD8+: CD 4+ T cell.

Q. What are most common sites of aphthous ulcers?

A. It mostly occurs as recurrent painful ulcers on buccal mucosa, labial mucosa and tongue, buccal and lingual sulci and soft palate. Involvement of heavily keratinized mucosa of the hard palate and gingiva is much less common.

Q. What is the classification and clinical features of aphthous ulcers?

A. Aphthous ulcers are classified into three forms:

1. Minor aphthous ulcer (Mikulicz ulcer) (80%)
2. Major aphthous ulcer (Sutton ulcer) (10%)
3. Herpetiform aphthous ulcer (10%)

1. **Minor aphthous ulcer**:
   - Most common, also called Mikulicz ulcer
   - It occurs mostly at age of 10–40 years
   - Prodromal stage of tingling and burning for 1 to 2 days
   - It begins with red discrete papules
   - They present as 1–5, round, painful, shallow ulcers measuring 2–4 mm and surrounded by erythematous halo and edema. The ulcer floor is covered with yellow gray pseudomembrane.
   - They tend to heal within 7–10 days without scarring
2. **Major aphthous ulcer**:
   - Also called as Sutton ulcers, mostly affects lips, soft palate and tongue
   - They are larger (> 1 cm), deeper with longer duration, more frequent in recurrence and more painful
   - They are round and oval with a raised irregular border with surrounding edema
   - They appear as group of ulcers 1–6 in number on any part of oral mucosa and heal in 10–20 days with scarring
3. **Herpetiform ulcer**:
   - It is seen in females of older age
   - Innumerable pinpoint vesicles about 1–3 mm, extremely painful and appear on any oral site
   - They enlarge to form large, irregular ulcers and heal in 10 days or more
   - Recurrence is frequent

Q. What are other diseases associated with aphthous ulcer?

A. Other conditions in which aphthous ulcer is seen are:

- Familial Mediterranean fever
- Hyperglobulinemia D
- Deficiency of interleukin—1 antagonist

- Behçet's syndrome
- HIV infection
- Malabsorption syndrome
- Ulcerative colitis
- Crohn's disease
- Pernicious anemia

Q. What are the histopathological findings of aphthous ulcers?

A.
- Lymphocytic infiltration
- Occasional plasma cells and eosinophils which suggest delayed hypersensitivity.

Q. Investigations to be done to confirm diagnosis.

A. Most of the times diagnosis is clinical:
- CBC
- Hemoglobin assay
- Differential WBC count
- RBC indices
- Iron studies
- Red cell folate levels
- Serum B12 levels
- Serum antiendomysial antibodies and IgA antitissue transglutaminase antibodies

Q. What is the management and treatment of aphthous ulcers?

A.
- No permanent cure is available
- *Good oral hygiene*: Use of hot saline mouthwashes and 0.2% aqueous chlorhexidine gluconate, 0.1% benzydamine mouthwash
- Lignocaine 5% viscous solution held in mouth for 5 minutes before meals is soothing
- Triggers like spicy foods, citrus fruits and dry fruits must be avoided
- Mechanical protection with a plastic guard
- Topical steroids like triamcinolone acetonide 0.1% in orabase or hydrocortisone hemisuccinate pellets four times a day. If no response, stronger topical steroids or topical tacrolimus may be used
- Topical tetracycline mouthwash or orally 250 mg tablet, dissolved in 10 mL of water and gargled for 3 minutes.
- Topical minocycline can also be used
- Rinses of hydrogen peroxide/water solution 1:4 strength
- Soothing applications of old tea bags to erosions

- Supplementation of folate, vitamin B12 and iron
- Oral corticosteroids for severe recurrent aphthous ulcer; e.g., prednisolone 40 mg for 5 days and then tapered by 5 mg every 2 days
- Thalidomide 300 mg/day, levamisol, dapsone, azathioprine, sucralfate, pentoxifylline, colchicine 0.5 mg TDS, thalidomide (50–300 mg daily) has been used
- T. Rebamipide—acts by decreasing the oxygen radicals, increases blood flow and increases protective prostaglandins. It is an amino acetyl analogue. Dose—100 mg TDS. Also used in Behçet's and stomatitis of nonspecific ethology. Its a category C drug. Side effects are very mild.

10 Asteatotic Eczema

Q. Synonyms.
A. Winter eczema, senile eczema, eczema craquele.

Q. Meaning of the word "asteatotic".
A. Decrease in lipid content.

Q. Define asteatotic eczema.
A. Asteatotic eczema is defined as a condition occurring in older age groups or in people with some underlying systemic disease or malignancy, characterized by dry scaly skin sometimes associated with fissuring and excoriations.

Q. Factors implicated in etiology.
A. Age related decrease in skin lipid content, dry weather, malnutrition, drugs, exposure to allergens and sensitizers, systemic diseases and malignancies.

Q. Which systemic diseases are associated with asteatotic eczema?
A. Hepatitis, cholestasis, uremia, hypothyroidism.

Q. Which drugs are implicated in etiology?
A. Diuretics, cimetidine, rarely topical corticosteroids (therapeutic paradox).

Q. Which internal malignancies are associated?
A. Malignant lymphoma, gastric adenocarcinoma, angio-immunoblastic lymphadenopathy, spheroidal cell carcinoma of breast.

Q. Describe the clinical features.
A. Dry, scaly skin. On the shin it gives "pavement stone" appearance called eczema craquele. Mostly extensor surfaces are involved. Sometimes generalized dryness can be present. Finger pulps become dry, cracked and parchment-like. Eczematous changes, fissuring, excoriations can occur as secondary changes.

Q. Histopathological features.
A. Mild hyperkeratosis, spongiosis, dermal infiltrate.

Q. How do you manage this condition?

A.
- General management—comfortable room temperature, decreased usage of soaps and detergents, avoid contact with allergens.
- Medical management—treat the underlying condition, sedative antihistaminics, topical immunomodulators, sedatives, UVB therapy, emulsifying ointment (emulsifying wax 20%, liquid paraffin 30% and white soft paraffin 50%) can be used as an emollient. In severe cases a mild steroid like triamcinolone can be added to it.

DIAPER DERMATITIS

Q. Synonyms.

A. Napkin dermatitis, napkin rash.

Q. Definition.

A. Its a type of irritant contact dermatitis developing in the diaper area in a newborn, due to various etiological factors.

Q. What are the etiological factors?

A.
- Friction—friction between skin and fabric.
- Water—hydration of skin increases susceptibility to frictional damage.
- Urine—ammonia and urinary degradation products cause irritation.
- Feces—various proteases and lipases have an irritant effect.
- Microorganisms—like *Candida albicans* and certain bacteria have a role.
- Topical antibiotics—broad spectrum antibiotics enhance growth of candida.
- Chemical irritants—like soaps, detergents, antiseptics have irritant effects

Q. What are the clinical features?

A. Lesions appear as areas of confluent erythema over the napkin area, i.e., buttocks, genitalia, lower abdomen, pubic areas and upper thighs. Deep groins and flexures are spared.

Q. Comment on incidence.

A. Most commonly in late infancy between 6–12 months of age. Less common in India. More common in affluent societies.

Q. What is meant by 'tide mark' dermatitis?

A. When lesions appear only on the margins of the napkin area.

Q. What is Jacquet's dermatitis?

A. Sometimes severe contact dermatitis occurs in the form of vesicles, erosions and ulcers, in a pattern like distribution, similar to diaper dermatitis.

Q. Can there be any variations in the clinical presentation?

A. Vesicles and pustules resembling herpes simplex, purple brown nodules along with rash known as infantile gluteal granuloma, sometimes dissemination to trunk and extremities as an ID reaction to *Candida albicans*.

Q. What is the differential diagnosis?

A.
- Napkin psoriasis
- Seborrhoeic dermatitis
- Acrodermatitis enteropathica
- Langerhans cell histiocytosis

Q. How do you manage this condition?

A.
- *General management*: Stop oil massage, stop using occlusive diapers, stop using irritant soaps and antiseptics.
- *Medical management*: Topical antibiotics/antifungals, topical steroids, emollients.

11 Atopic Dermatitis

Q. What is atopic dermatitis?

A.
- Presence of itchy papules which become excoriated and lichenified
- Flexural distribution (in adults or older children) or facial and extensor in infants.

Q. What does "Atopy" mean?

A. Atopy is derived from the Greek word 'atopos', meaning strange or unusual. The word atopy was coined by Coca.

Q. What is the triad of atopy?

A. Atopy is a triad of atopic dermatitis, bronchial asthma, allergic rhinitis.

Q. What is atopic dermatitis?

A.
- Atopic dermatitis is an itchy, chronic, or chronically relapsing, inflammatory skin condition characterized by itchy papules which become excoriated and lichenified
- Typically, have a flexural distribution, frequently associated with other atopic conditions in the individual or other family members.

Q. What are the diagnostic criterias for atopic dermatitis?

A. Hanifin and Rajka proposed the following criteria for atopic dermatitis.

- *Major criteria* (3 of 4 present):
  - Pruritus
  - Typical morphology and distribution of skin lesions
  - Chronic or chronically relapsing dermatitis
  - Personal or family history of atopy
- *Minor criteria* (3 of 23 present):
  - Xerosis
  - Ichthyosis/palmar hyperlinearity/keratosis pilaris
  - Immediate (type I) skin test reactivity
  - Elevated serum IgE
  - Early age of onset
  - Tendency toward cutaneous infections/impaired cell-mediated immunity

- Tendency toward nonspecific hand or foot dermatitis
- Nipple eczema
- Cheilitis
- Recurrent conjunctivitis
- Dennie–Morgan infraorbital fold
- Keratoconus
- Anterior subcapsular cataract
- Periorbital darkening
- Facial pallor/erythema
- Pityriasis alba
- Anterior neck darkening
- Pruritus when sweating
- Intolerance to wool and lipid solvents
- Perifollicular accentuation
- Food intolerance
- Course influenced by environmental/emotional factors
- White dermographism/delayed blanching

Q. What is refined Hanifin and Rajka's diagnostic criteria?

A. The UK refinement of Hanifin and Rajka's diagnostic criteria for atopic dermatitis. Scabies should be excluded.

In order to qualify as a case of atopic dermatitis with the UK diagnostic criteria, the child must have:

- An itchy skin condition (or parental report of scratching or rubbing in a child).

Plus three or more of the following:

1. Onset below age 2 years (not used if child is under 4 years).
2. History of skin crease involvement (including cheeks in children under 10 years).
3. History of a generally dry skin.
4. Personal history of other atopic disease (or history of any atopic disease in a first degree relative in children under 4 years).
5. Visible flexural dermatitis (or dermatitis of cheeks/forehead and limbs in children under 4 years).

Q. What are the three clinical stages of atopic dermatitis?

A.
1. Infantile Phase
2. Childhood Phase
3. Adult/Adolescent Phase

Q. What are the clinical features of infantile atopic dermatitis?

A. In the age group from birth to 2 years, lesions most frequently start on the face. When the child begins to crawl, the exposed surfaces, especially the extensor aspect of the knees, are most involved. The lesions consist of erythema and discrete or confluent edematous papules which are intensely itchy, may become exudative and crusted as a result of rubbing. Secondary infection and lymphadenopathy are common.

Q. What are the clinical features of childhood atopic dermatitis?

A. Age 2 to 12 years, involves most characteristically the elbow and knee flexures, sides of the neck, wrists and ankles. The sides of the neck may show a striking reticulate pigmentation (atopic dirty neck). The erythematous and edematous papules tend to be replaced by lichenification.

Q. What are the clinical features of adult atopic dermatitis?

A. In adults, AD is seen predominantly in a flexural distribution, but extensive areas of skin may be involved. Patients may present with head and neck, often with severe eyelid involvement OR may present with a chronic hand dermatitis components. In any stage of AD, the most severely affected individuals may evolve to generalized exfoliative erythroderma.

Q. What is Senile atopic dermatitis?

A. Occurs in age >60 years, characterized by marked xerosis.

Q. Name the regional variants of atopic dermatitis?

A.
- Cheilitis sicca
- Lip-lickers eczema
- Ear eczema
- Eyelid eczema
- Hand and neck dermatitis
- Juvenile plantar eczema
- Atopic hand eczema
- Dyshidrotic eczema

Q. What are Dennie–Morgan folds?

A. Symmetric, prominent fold (single or double) just beneath the margin of the lower eyelid is noted in many AD patients during infancy or childhood. The fold originates in or near the inner canthus and extends to affect one-half to two-thirds of the lower lid.

Q. Who are allergic shiners?

A. In patients of atopic dermatitis darkening under the eyes can be seen. Such patients are called allergic shiners.

Q. What is lichenification?

A. Lichenification refers to thickening and accentuation of skin markings due to epidermal proliferation. It is the late manifestation of atopic dermatitis because of chronic rubbing and scratching.

Q. What is Hertoghe's sign?

A. Absence or thinning of lateral eyebrows.

Q. What is white dermographism?

A. Stroking of skin leads to a white streak that reflects excessive vasoconstriction, most apparent on the forehead.

Q. How will you treat atopic dermatitis?

A. Treatment can be categorized into 2 broad groups.

A. *General measures*:
   - Breast-feed the baby as long as possible.
   - Avoidance of triggering factors like certain specific foods (egg white, shell fish, red meat, cow's milk, peanuts), dust, woolen clothes, carpets.

Bathing:
- Do not use harsh soaps and detergents
- Do not add any antiseptic to the bath water
- In acute phase—use no soaps
- Mild soap with pH near skin (Syndet) is advised
- Apply oil before bathing
- Bath with lukewarm water
- Pat dry immediately
- Use of moisturiser immediately
- Toys should not be furry
- Avoid pets.

B. *Local measures*:
   - Emollients
   - Topical steroids
   - Topical tacrolimus/pimecrolimus
   - Topical antibiotics
   - Phototherapy (UVA + UVB or NB - UVB)

C. *Systemic measures*:
   - Systemic corticosteroids
   - Oral cyclosporine (5 mg/kg then tapered to 2 mg/kg)
   - Azathioprine (2–3.5 mg/kg)
   - Mycophenolate mofetil (1–2.5 mg/kg)—antihistaminics (adjunctive therapy)

Q. What are bleach baths?

A.
- Bleach baths are used to reduce content of bacterial content on skin.
- Generally, we add one teaspoon of bleach in about 3.8 L of water.
- The child is soaked in this water for about 5 minutes. Afterwards, the skin is patted dry and moisturiser is applied. Usually, we do this twice a week.

Q. What are the complications associated with atopic dermatitis?

A.
- Infections—bacterial (impetiginization)
  Viral infections (eczema herpeticum, molluscum contagiosum)
- Ocular complication—atopic keratoconjunctivitis, vernal keratoconjunctivitis, subcapsular cataract, keratoconus.

Q. What are the various scores to assess the severity of atopic dermatitis?

A.
- EASI (Eczema Area Scoring Index)
- SCORAD (SCORing Atopic Dermatitis)
- POEM (Patient Oriented Eczema Measure).

12 Bacterial Infections Questions

Q. Classification on basis of depth of infection.

A.
- Superficial infection in epidermis—bullous and nonbullous impetigo, folliculitis, impetigo of Bockhart
- Infection at dermoepidermal level—ecthyma
- Infection in dermis—erysipelas, furuncle, carbuncle
- Deeper infection—cellulitis, abscess, necrotizing fasciitis, pyomyositis

Q. What is the normal bacterial flora of the skin?

A. Bacteria that are found regularly on skin form the normal flora. The normal flora has been classified in the following groups:
- *Resident flora*: The bacteria that grow on the skin and relatively stable in number and composition at particular sites. Increase in their numbers results from multiplication of those already present and not due to addition from outside
- *Transient flora*: The organisms that lie free on skin without attachment and are derived from exogenous sources. They are unable to multiply on skin. They disappear from skin within short time. For example, staphylococci, gram-negative bacilli
- *Aerobic bacteria*: Form microcolonies within the outer layers of the stratum corneum, whereas anaerobes are found in the deeper portions of hair follicle. The normal flora of moderately moist areas consists mainly of staphylococci. Lipid-rich areas contain mainly propionibacterium acnes. Very wet areas (axilla, toe webs) contain mainly lipophilic bacteria and other coryneforms. Certain areas like face may be contaminated by organisms from the nostrils and mouth (*Staphylococcus aureus,* beta hemolytic streptococci), but these are not part of normal facial flora.

Staphylococci and micrococci
- Gram positive, catalase-positive cocci
- They are divided into coagulase-positive *Staphylococcus aureus* and coagulase negative
- Coagulase-positive are pathogenic and transient residents on skin. They are found in the anterior nares and perineum

- Micrococci are much less frequently present than staphylococci. They are differentiated from the latter by their inability to produce acid anaerobically from glycerol in the presence of erythromycin.

Coryneform bacteria

- Recently these bacteria have been classified on the basis of presence and type of amino acid, mycolic acid and neutral sugars into following groups:
    - *Corynebacterium* species
    - *Brevibacterium* species: These are usually large colony coryneforms present in abundance in hyperhidrotics and in moist areas of skin. They are implicated in the production of odor in feet and resistant to penicillin
    - *Propionibacterium* species: (now called *Cutibacterium*) These are anaerobes. The commonest organism is *P. acnes,* which is abundant on scalp, forehead and back.

Gram-negative bacilli

- They die quickly on desiccation and are not part of resident flora
- The perianal region and perineum get contaminated from the gastrointestinal tract and they are transient flora.

Streptococci

They have been classified by Lancefield into 18 groups. Of these, group A, group B and C have dermatological significance.

Q. What are the degerming properties of skin?

A. Desiccation

- Hydration of the skin helps in bacterial growth on the skin surface
- A person has fewer bacteria on exposed parts such as the hands and forearms than on the axilla.

Resident flora

- These are the first line of defense against colonization and subsequent infection with pathogenic organisms.
- The phenomenon of bacterial interference is that the colonization of a site by one strain of bacterial interference that the subsequent colonization by another strain. A possible explanation is that these bacteria may be competing for the same nutrients, although it may also be due to production of antibiotics by resident skin bacteria which are capable of inhibiting other flora.

- Bacterial interference has been used therapeutically in patients with recurrent furunculosis.

Bacterial adherence

- The potential of an organism to colonize skin is related to its ability to adhere to the surface which varies in different individuals and at various skin sites.
- Adhesins of pathogenic staphylococci and streptococci are teichoic acids. If the skin or nasal mucus membrane is treated with teichoic acid, it blocks the epithelial receptors thus inhibiting colonization by *Staphylococcus aureus.*

Lipids

Sebum has a mild inhibitory effect on normal skin micro-organisms in vitro.

Desquamation

Surface bacteria that are unable to multiply (i.e., transients) are lost with the exfoliation of corneocytes.

Immune system

- In normal skin, IgG and IgA antibodies are secreted through eccrine sweat.
- Secretory IgA in sweat may explain the absence of bacterial colonization in eccrine ducts.

Acid mantle

Higher colonization by bacteria in patients with hemiplegia and diabetes was associated with high skin pH and this may contribute to endogenous infection in the ward. When the skin was cleaned with acidic mineral water, the skin surface pH was reduced and the frequency of bacterial infection was markedly decreased.

Q. What is folliculitis?

A.
- Folliculitis is defined histologically as the presence of inflammatory cells within the wall and ostia of the hair follicle, creating a follicular-based pustule.
- The inflammation can be either limited to the superficial aspect of the follicle with primary involvement of the infundibulum or the inflammation can affect both the superficial and deep aspect of the follicle.

Q. Clinical features of folliculitis?

A.
- Bacterial folliculitis frequently involved the face, chest, back, axillae or buttock.

- The appearance depends on the depth of follicular involvement.
- Lesions of superficial folliculitis (Bockhart's impetigo) are small, 1–4 mm pustules or crusted papules on an erythematous base.
- The lesions are frequently clustered and heal without scarring.
- Sycosis, a deep folliculitis, appears as large, tender, erythematous papules, often with a central pustule. The lesions may be pruritic and slightly tender.

Q. D/D of folliculitis?

A.
- Other forms of folliculitis, fungal or viral (molluscum can rarely cause folliculitis)
- Acne vulgaris
- Rosacea
- Chloracne
- Pseudofolliculitis barbae
- Keratosis pilaris

Q. Other name for impetigo?

A. Synonyms:
- Nonbullous impetigo
- Impetigo contagiosa
- Bullous impetigo
- Localized staphylococcal scalded skin syndrome
- Pemphigus neonatorum
- Staphylococcal impetigo

Q. What is impetigo?

A. Impetigo (latin word, means, to attack') is a common, highly contagious, superficial skin infection that primarily affects children. The condition presents in both nonbullous and bullous forms. The primary pathogens in nonbullous and bullous impetigo are *Staphylococcus aureus* and, less commonly, group A β-hemolytic *Streptococcus (Streptococcus pyogenes)*.

Q. D/D of impetigo?

A.
- Insect bites
- Eczematous dermatoses
- Infections—Tinea corporis
- Candidiasis
- Herpes simplex viral infection
- Varicella
- Infestations-Scabies
- Pediculosis

- Vesiculobullous disorders—pemphigus foliaceus
- Bullous pemphigoid
- Thermal burn
- Drug reactions—bullous erythema multiforme
- Stevens-Johnson syndrome

Q. What are the types of impetigo?

A. There are two forms of impetigo:

Nonbullous	*Bullous*
Caused by streptococci and staphylococci	Caused by staphylococci, usually *S. aureus*
Occurs in school going age	Occurs in neonates and infants
Starts as papules and evolve into small vesicles	Start as macules, evolve into flaccid vesicles which are fragile and contain yellow colored fluid
Sites are more on arms	Sites are more on face, neck, buttocks, and trunk
Lesions are covered with honey colored crust	Lesions covered with a varnish colored crust
Lymph nodes enlarged	LN may not be enlarged
No constitutional symptoms	Fever may be present

Q. Will impetigo leave scars?

A. NO. Because the crusts and blisters of impetigo are superficial, impetigo generally does not leave scars. Affected skin looks red for a while after the crusts go away, but this redness fades in a matter of days to weeks.

Q. What is the treatment of impetigo?

A. The treatment is divided into topical and systemic.

Topical: First line—mupirocin, fusidic acid.

Systemic:

First line:

- Dicloxacillin 250–500 mg QID for 5–7 days
- Amoxicillin plus clavulanic acid
- Cephalexin 25 mg/kg TID, 250–500 mg QID

Second line:

- Azithromycin 500 mg for 1 day then 250 mg daily for 4 days
- Clindamycin 15 mg/kg/day TID
- Erythromycin 250–500 mg QID for 5–7 days

Q. What is a furuncle?

A. Furuncle, is a deep folliculitis (furunculosis means petty thief). It is most commonly caused by infection by the bacterium *Staphylococcus aureus*, resulting in a painful swollen area on the skin caused by an accumulation of pus and dead tissue. Individual boils clustered together are called carbuncles. Most human infections are caused by coagulase-positive *S. aureus* strains, notable for the bacteria's ability to produce coagulase, an enzyme that can clot blood. Almost any organ system can be infected by *S. aureus*.

Q. What are the signs of furuncle?

A. They are pustules around a hair follicle that are tender, warm, and very painful. They range from pea-sized to golf ball-sized. In a severe infection, an individual may experience fever, swollen lymph nodes and fatigue. A recurring lesion is called chronic furunculosis. Skin infections tend to be recurrent in many patients and often spread to other family members. Systemic factors that lower resistance commonly are detectable, including: diabetes, obesity, and hematologic disorders.

Q. What are the risk factors for furuncle?

A. Risk factors for furunculosis include bacterial carriage in the nostrils, diabetes mellitus, obesity, lymphoproliferative neoplasms, malnutrition, and use of immunosuppressive drugs.

Q. Differential diagnosis.

A.
- Epidermal and pilar cysts (infected)
- Furuncular myiasis (due to maggots)

Q. What is carbuncle?

A. Carbuncle in Latin means "small piece of coal". It is an infection of multiple adjacent hair follicles and intervening tissue. It is a necrotizing swelling with high local temperature and pain. It is a tender firm to hard lump. Sites of involvement are neck, shoulder, hips, thighs. It has multiple sinuses in sieve pattern discharging pus. It is associated with diabetes mellitus, prolonged steroid therapy, immune-compromised status and exfoliative dermatitis.

Q. What is the management of recurrent furunculosis?

A.
- Careful evaluation of the underlying causes.
- Treatment of predisposing factors—poor hygiene, obesity, hyperhidrosis, ingrown hair, tight clothing.
- General care of skin—this is to reduce the number of *Staphylococcus aureus* on the skin. General care of both hands

and body with water and soap is important. The patient should avoid trauma to the skin as well as the potential skin irritant such as strong soaps and deodorant.

- Care of the dressing—dressing should be changed frequently if purulent drainage collects.
- Measures to eliminate nasal and skin carriage of *Staphylococcus aureus*:
    - Local use of ointment in nasal vestibule reduces the nasal carriage of *Staphylococcus aureus* and secondarily the shedding of the organism on skin. Intranasal application of 2% mupirocin contribute to reduce the recurrent furunculosis. Prophylaxis with fusidic acid ointment in nares twice a day every fourth week for patients and the family members have shown success.
    - Oral antibiotics: Rifampin 600 mg orally daily for 10 days. Other drugs used are dicloxacillin for methicillin susceptible *S. aureus*, trimethoprim-sulfamethoxazole, ciprofloxacin, or minocycline for methicillin resistant *S. aureus*.

Q. What is the interference therapy for treatment of recurrent furunculosis?

A.
- Bacterial interference therapy employs use of 502A strain of *Staphylococcus aureus* in treatment of recurrent furunculosis. By colonization of nose, it is hoped to interrupt the transfer the pathogenic staph from nasal mucosa to skin. Nasal colonization with 502A is achieved only in presence of the original resident *Staphylococcus aureus*.
- The 502A strain is transferred from a stock trypticase Soy Agar slant to trypticase Soy broth and incubated at 37° Celsius for eighteen hours. The dry sterile cotton swab dipped in diluted culture before implantation. A separate swab is used for each implantation site. A 502A implantation is performed every second or third day for 4 applications. Subsequently implantation is followed at weekly intervals.
- Dry sterile swab rotated in each nostrils to depth of 2 cm. Cultures of axilla, perineum and skin surface are made by scrubbing of these areas with dry cotton.

Q. What is ecthyma?

A. Ecthyma is an ulcerative pyoderma of the skin caused by bacteria such as *Pseudomonas, Streptococcus pyogenes*, and *Staphylococcus aureus*. Because ecthyma extends into the dermis, it is often referred to as a deeper form of impetigo.

Q. What is epidemiology of ecthyma?

A. Ecthyma has a predilection for children, elderly and diabetic individuals. Outbreaks have also been reported in young military trainees. Ecthyma usually arises on the lower extremities.

Q. What is the etiology?

A.
- Ecthyma can be seen in areas of previously sustained tissue injury (e.g., excoriations, insect bites, dermatitis), in patients who are immunocompromised (e.g., diabetes, neutropenia, HIV infection). Important factors contributing to the development of streptococcal pyodermas or ecthyma: High temperature and humidity, crowded living conditions, poor hygiene.
- Untreated impetigo that progresses to ecthyma most frequently occurs in patients with poor hygiene.
- Some strains of *Streptococcus pyogenes* have a high affinity for both pharyngeal mucosa and skin. Pharyngeal colonization of *S. pyogenes* has been documented in patients with ecthyma.

Q. What are the clinical features of ecthyma?

A.
- Ecthyma begins as a vesicle or pustule overlying an inflamed area of skin that deepens into a dermal ulceration with overlying crust
- The crust of ecthyma lesions is gray-yellow and is thicker and harder than the crust of impetigo
- A shallow, saucer-like ulceration is apparent when adherent crust is removed
- The dermal ulcer has a raised and indurated surrounding margin
- Ecthyma lesions can remain fixed in size (sometimes resolving without treatment) or can progressively enlarge to 0.5–3 cm in diameter
- Ecthyma heals slowly and commonly produces a scar. Regional lymphadenopathy is common, even with solitary lesions.

Q. What are the D/D's?

A.
- Ecthyma gangrenosum
- Insect bites
- Leishmaniasis
- Lymphomatoid papulosis
- *Mycobacterium marinum* infection of the skin
- Papulonecrotic tuberculid
- Pyoderma gangrenosum
- Sporotrichosis
- Tungiasis

Q. What is botryomycosis?

A. Greek word “Botyrs” means bunch of grapes. It is caused by *Staphylococcus aureus*. Two types of skin lesions are seen—cutaneous and subcutaneous nodules. There may be suppurative plaques, ulcers, abscess and sinus. Predisposing factors are trauma, alcoholism and diabetes mellitus. On histopathology granular bodies (club) are seen. It has basophilic center composed of cells, debris and bacteria. Eosinophilic rim of immune response is seen. This phenomenon is called Splendore Hoeppli’s phenomenon.

Q. What is acne keloidalis nuchae?

A.
- It is common on the nape of neck in males with curly hair or who shave hair often and close to scalp. Initially, itchy round small bumps appear associated with folliculitis. There is an acute perifollicular inflammation with weakening of follicular wall at lower infundibulum. Naked hair shaft is released in dermis acting as a foreign body, leading to acute or chronic granulomatous inflammation. Then fibroblasts deposits new collagen and fibrosis develops forming hypertrophic scar.
- It presents as a firm, dome shaped, follicular papule on occipital area with papules and pustules. These coalesce to form large plaque, ultimately forming keloid in band-like distribution. The lesions heal with scarring alopecia.

Q. What is Mudi-Chood?

A. It is a dermatoses affecting the nape of neck and upper back. It is caused by a folliculitis secondary to irritation by wet and oily hair in a hot and humid environment. It is seen in females and characterized by itchy pigmented follicular papule and pustules. It is quite common in the state of Kerala.

Q. Describe erysipelas.

A.
- Erysipelas is known as St Anthony fire/Ignis Sacer. It is caused by beta hemolytic group A *Streptococcus*. It is acute infection of superficial dermal lymphatics. Local redness, swelling with raised border. Margins are sharply demarcated. Prodromal symptoms of malaise, chills with fever, headache and vomiting are common. The spectrum of disease ranges from transient hyperemia with slight desquamation to intense inflammation with vesicles and bullae. Common over face and legs.
- On the face—the ear lobule is affected while it is spared in cellulitis (Million ear’s sign).
- Predisposing factors are operative wounds, fissure, obesity, abrasions, venous insufficiency, leg ulcers. Complications are septicemia, cellulitis, necrotizing fasciitis.

Q. How to treat erysipelas?

A.
- Treatment of erysipelas
- Erysipelas is treated with antibiotics including penicillin, dicloxacillin, cephalosporins, clindamycin, and erythromycin. Most cases of erysipelas can be treated with oral antibiotics. However, cases of sepsis, or infections that do not improve with oral antibiotics require IV antibiotics administered in the hospital.

Q. What is cellulitis?

A. It is a suppurative inflammation of subcutaneous tissue by *Streptococcus pyogenes* and rarely *Staphylococcus aureus*. It presents as a local erythema, tenderness, ill-defined borders, associated with malaise, chilly sensation. It can have vesicles or nodules that discharge pus with necrotic material. Complications are gangrene, abscess and sepsis. Associated with diabetes.

Q. What is MRSA?

A.
- Methicillin-resistant *Staphylococcus aureus* (MRSA) is a bacterium responsible for several difficult-to-treat infections in humans. It is also called multidrug-resistant *Staphylococcus aureus* and oxacillin-resistant *Staphylococcus aureus* (ORSA). MRSA is any strain of *Staphylococcus aureus* that has developed resistance to beta-lactam antibiotics, which include the penicillins (methicillin, dicloxacillin, nafcillin, oxacillin, etc.) and the cephalosporins. Strains unable to resist these antibiotics are classified as methicillin—sensitive *Staphylococcus aureus*, or MSSA.
- MRSA is especially troublesome in hospitals, prisons, schools, and nursing homes, where patients with open wounds, invasive devices, and weakened immune systems are at greater risk of infection than the general public.

Q. What are the risk factors for acquiring MRSA?

A.
- People with weak immune systems (people living with HIV/AIDS, people living with lupus, cancer patients, transplant recipients, severe asthmatics, etc.)
- Diabetics
- Intravenous drug users
- Users of quinolone antibiotics
- Young children
- Elderly
- College students living in dormitories

- People staying or working in a health care facility for an extended period of time
- People who spend time in coastal waters where MRSA is present
- People who spend time in confined spaces with other people, including occupants of homeless shelters and warming centers, prison inmates, military recruits in basic training, and individuals who spend considerable time in changing rooms or gyms.
- Veterinarians, Livestock handlers, and Pet owners.

Q. How is the diagnosis of MRSA made?

A.
- The bacterium generally must be cultured via blood, urine, sputum, or other body fluid cultures, and cultured in the lab in sufficient quantities to perform these confirmatory tests first. These techniques include real-time PCR and quantitative PCR and are increasingly being employed in clinical laboratories for the rapid detection and identification of MRSA strains.
- Another common laboratory test is a rapid latex agglutination test that detects the PBP2a protein.
- PBP2a is a variant penicillin-binding protein that imparts the ability of *S. aureus* to be resistant to oxacillin.

Q. Treatment of MRSA.

A.
- MRSA are resistant to traditional anti-staphylococcal beta-lactam antibiotics, such as cephalexin.
- MRSA has a greater spectrum of antimicrobial susceptibility, including to sulfa drugs (like cotrimoxazole/trimethoprim-sulfamethoxazole), tetracyclines (like doxycycline and minocycline) and clindamycin, but the drug of choice for treating CA-MRSA is now believed to be vancomycin.
- Linezolid is now felt to be the best drug for treating patients with MRSA pneumonia.
- Teicoplanin is a structural congener of vancomycin that has a similar activity spectrum but a longer half-life. Because the oral absorption of vancomycin and teicoplanin is very low, these agents must be administered intravenously to control systemic infections.
- Several newly discovered strains of MRSA show antibiotic resistance even to vancomycin and teicoplanin. These new evolutions of the MRSA bacterium have been dubbed vancomycin intermediate-resistant *Staphylococcus aureus* (VISA).

- Linezolid, quinupristin/dalfopristin, daptomycin, ceftaroline, and tigecycline are used to treat more severe infections that do not respond to glycopeptides such as vancomycin.
- There have been claims that bacteriophage can be used to cure MRSA.
- Cannabinoids, chemicals found in the Cannabis plant, are also suspected of being highly effective at killing MRSA.
- The psychedelic mushroom *Psilocybe semilanceata* has been shown to strongly inhibit the growth of *Staphylococcus aureus*.
- Hydrogen peroxide, tobramycin, chlorhexidine digluconate, chlorhexidine gluconate, levofloxacin, and silver sulphadiazine effective against MRSA topically.

Q. What are the infections caused by *Corynebacterium*?

A. Erythrasma, pitted keratolysis, trichomycosis axillaris. This is called as the *corynebacterium* triad.

Q. What is trichomycosis axillaris?

A. It is caused by *corynebacterium* tenuis. It is a superficial bacterial colonization of hair shaft in sweaty hair bearing areas in armpits, pubic areas. It presents as yellow, orange, black or red granular concretions coating hair shaft with malodor. Simple clipping of hair is effective.

Q. Describe pitted keratolysis.

A. It is an acquired, chronic, asymptomatic, superficial bacterial infection of the foot and occasionally of palms, characterized by discrete superficial crateriform pits and erosions with surrounding maceration. The lesions are shallow, circular with punched out appearance and coalesce to produce 0.5 to 7.0 mm in diameter pits and associated with hyperhidrosis and malodor. The patient may give a history of frequent immersion of hands and feet in water.

Q. What are the differential diagnosis?

A.
- Intertrigo
- Tinea pedis
- Hand eczema
- Keratolysis exfoliativa

Q. Causes of pits on palms and soles.

A.
- Pitted keratolysis
- Plantar warts
- Punctate keratoderma
- Pits of basal cell nevus syndrome

- Keratosis punctata
- Punctate porokeratosis
- Darier's disease
- Acropigmentation of Kitamura
- Arsenic poisoning

Q. Name the organisms causing pitted keratolysis.

A. *Micrococcus sedentarius* (*Kytococcus sedentarius*), *Dermatophilus congolensis*, and *Corynebacterium minutissimum*.

Q. What is the other name of pitted keratolysis?

A. Keratoma plantare sulcatum, ringed keratolysis.

Q. How does the infection occur?

A. Under prolonged hyperhidrosis and occlusion and contact with wet surface, the bacteria proliferate and release proteinases that destroy the stratum corneum. The malodor is caused by production of sulfur compounds such as thiols and thioesters.

Q. What do we see on histopathology of pitted keratolysis?

A. Presence of crater limited to stratum corneum, filaments and coccoid organisms can be seen at the base and margin, special stains such as Gram stain, PAS stain and methenamine silver stain can be used.

Q. How will you confirm the diagnosis?

A. Wood's lamp is negative. Scrapping of the lesions—gram staining, culture on brain heart infusion agar.

Q. How can one prevent pitted keratolysis?

A. Avoid using occlusive footwear, using absorbent cotton socks, avoid sharing footwear, cleaning the foot with antibacterial at the end of the day to remove dirt and debris from settling down.

Q. How can we treat pitted keratolysis?

A.
- Topical antibiotics such as erythromycin 1% gel twice daily, fusidic acid, mupirocin, etc.
- *Treatment of hyperhidrosis*:
    - Benzoic and salicylic acid ointment, Castellani's paint, clotrimazole cream, 2% miconazole nitrate cream, Whitfield's ointment.
    - Orally, macrolide antibiotics can be used.

Q. How does erythrasma present?

A. Dark discoloration of the skin folds which are moist and occluded. The duration is from months to years, mostly asymptomatic. Areas of involvement—axillae, genitocrural crease, web spaces in toes, inframammary area.

Q. Differential diagnosis of erythrasma.

A.
- Acanthosis nigricans
- Pityriasis versicolor
- Hailey-Hailey disease
- Candidiasis
- Contact dermatitis
- Intertrigo
- Flexural psoriasis
- Seborrheic dermatitis
- Tinea corporis
- Tinea cruris
- Tinea pedis

Q. Name the organism causing erythrasma.

A. *Corynebacterium minutissimum.*

Q. How does corynebacterium cause erythrasma?

A. The organism proliferates under heat and humidity. They are present between the intercellular spaces and dissolve keratin fibrils. The coral red fluorescence, seen under wood's light is created by the porphyrins produced by the diphtheroid and is diagnostic.

Q. Name dermatological and systemic associations in erythrasma.

A. Patients with erythrasma should be screened for pitted keratolysis and trichomycosis axillaris (corynebacterial triad). If extensive involvement of the body is noted, then diabetes mellitus should be excluded. Obesity and immune-suppressed states are predisposing factors for occurrence of erythrasma.

Q. Diagnosis of erythrasma on Wood's lamp.

A. Wood's lamp examination of erythrasma lesions reveals coral-red fluorescence of lesions. Results may be negative if the patient has had a bath prior to presentation. The cause of this color fluorescence has been attributed to excess coproporphyrin III synthesis by these organisms, which accumulates in cutaneous tissue and emits a coral-red fluorescence when exposed to a Wood's lamp.

Q. Name the antibiotics used in treatment of erythrasma.

A.
- Oral—erythromycin, clarithromycin
- Topical—fusidic acid, miconazole, clindamycin are effective.

Q. Prognosis.

A. Often recurrent if underlying factors like obesity are not controlled.

Q. Which bacterial infections are not pyoderma?

A. Rhinoscleroma, bacillary angiomatosis, erythrasma, trichomycosis axillaris.

Q. Which pyodermas are not bacterial infections?

A. Pyoderma gangrenosum, pyoderma faciale, pyoderma vegetans.

Q. Difference between primary and secondary pyoderma?

A.
- Primary—pre-existing skin is normal; caused by single organism; single antibody present
- Secondary—pre-existing skin disease present; caused by multiple organisms; multiple antibody present

Q. What is DCAP?

A. Dermatosis chronica atrophicans et pustulosa. It is chronic folliculitis of legs.

Q. What is hypopyon sign?

A. When a patient is made to sit or stand, semicircular meniscus of pus is formed in the lower part of bullae.

Q. What is follicular triad?

A. Hidradenitis suppurativa, nodulocystic acne (acne conglobata), dissecting cellulitis of scalp.

Q. What is follicular tetrad?

A. All of the above plus pilonidal sinus.

Q. Name the infections caused by pseudomonas.

A. Ecthyma gangrenosum, green nail syndrome, toe-web infection, blastomycosis-like pyoderma, hot-foot syndrome, pseudomonas folliculitis (hot-tub folliculitis or swimming pool rash, malignant otitis externa).

Q. Write about green nail syndrome?

A. It is onycholysis of distal portion of nail with greenish discoloration. It is caused by excessive contact of hands with water, use of detergents, soap, nail trauma and other causes of onycholysis. There is increased growth of pseudomonas aeruginosa which produces a blue-green pigment called pyocyanin. Diagnosis can be confirmed by Gram stain and culture. Differential diagnosis includes sub-ungual hematoma, melanocytic nevus, melanoma and aspergillus infection. Treatment is avoidance of predisposing factors and treatment with fluroquinolones and tobramycin orally and 1% acetic acid or Neosporin topically.

Q. What is hot tub folliculitis or swimming pool rash?

A. It is follicular maculopapular or vesicular or pustular lesion occurring 1–4 days after bathing in hot tub or public swimming pool. The organism gains entry through hair follicle or through break in skin. It resolves in 1–2 weeks. As the water temperature increases the chlorine content of water decreases and the number of bacteria increases. Diver's suit colonizes the bacteria, causing folliculitis on sides of trunk, axillae, buttocks, proximal extremities. Face and neck are usually spared. Associated symptoms are painful eyes, earaches, sore throat, headache, fever, painful swollen breasts, malaise, rhinorrhea, nausea, vomiting and abdominal pain. Differential diagnosis include *Staphylococcus aureus* folliculitis, insect bite, papular urticaria, Majocchi's granuloma, eosinophilic folliculitis, miliaria and acne vulgaris.

Q. What is hot foot syndrome?

A. Painful, erythematous plantar nodules or pustules on foot occurring after swimming in a pool containing *P. aeruginosa*. Systemic symptoms seen only in those who are severely infected. It is self-limiting and requires only symptomatic treatment.

Q. What is rhinoscleroma?

A. It is a chronic inflammatory granulomatous inflammation of upper respiratory tract, characterized by sclerosis and deformity. It is caused by *Klebsiella pneumoniae* rhinoscleromatis.

There are three stages:

1. Nasal catarrh,
2. Infliltrative stage,
3. Sclerotic stage

Q. What is the treatment of rhinoscleroma?

A.
- Surgery combined with antibiotic therapy is beneficial in patients with granulomatous disease and nasal or pharyngeal obstruction or nasal sinus involvement due to the proliferation of lesions.
- *Surgery*:
  - Tracheostomy in patients with laryngeal obstruction of the second degree (granulomatous stage) and above (sclerotic stage).
  - Plastic surgery in patients with cicatricial stenosis or when imperforation remains in the nasal cavity, pharynx, larynx, or trachea.
  - Surgery and laser therapy are required to treat airway compromise and tissue deformity.
  - Palatal symptoms may be relieved by means of uvulo-palato-pharyngoplasty.

- *Antibiotics*:
  - Tetracycline is the drug of choice.
  - Other antibiotics include ciprofloxacin and rifampicin, clindamycin and third-generation cephalosporins.
  - Sclerotic lesions respond well to treatment with ciprofloxacin. Ciprofloxacin has the following advantages: Its oral administration is convenient, it achieves good tissue penetration, it is concentrated in macrophages, and it may prove useful in the treatment of patients with rhinoscleroma.
- *Steroids*:
  - These agents have anti-inflammatory properties and cause profound and varied metabolic effects. Corticosteroids modify the body's immune response to diverse stimuli.
  - May decrease inflammation by reversing increased capillary permeability and suppressing PMN activity.

Q. What is infundibular folliculitis?

A.
- Called as disseminate and recurrent infundibular folliculitis described in 1968.
- Clinical presentation is like miliaria or keratosis pilaris. Generalized flesh-colored papules on chest, upper arm, back and the lesions are monomorphous. In a given area, all follicles are involved, without skipping of any follicle.

Q. What are the causes?

A. Hot, humid, tropical environment. Also common in atopics.

Q. D/D of infundibular folliculitis.

A.
- Keratosis pilaris
- Lichen nitidus
- Milia
- Pityriasis rosea
- Pityrosporum folliculitis
- Folliculitis
- Hypervitaminosis A

Q. Treatment of infundibular folliculitis?

A. Cooling, soothing agents like calamine and emollients. Topical steroids, PUVA and isotretinoin may be used in resistant cases.

Q. What are the topical antibacterials used in dermatology?

A.
- *Aminoglycosides*: Gentamicin 1% cream, Neomycin B and 3% Neomycin C, Framycetin 1% cream, Sisomicin 0.1% cream

- *Macrolides*: Erythromycin 1%, 2% gel, cream, lotion; Clarithromycin 1% cream
- *Lincosamides*: Clindamycin 1% gel, lotion, solution; Lincomycin 2% gel
- Fusidic acid 2% cream
- Mupirocin 2% cream
- *Fluoroquinolones*: Nadifloxacin 1% cream
- *Sulfonamides*: Silver sulfadiazine 1% cream
- *Metronidazole*: 0.75% gel, 1% cream
- *Benzoyl peroxide*: 2.5%, 4%, 5%, 10% gel or lotion
- Azelaic acid: 20% cream
- Polymyxin B

LUPUS MILIARIS DISSEMINATUS FACIEI (LMDF)

Q. Describe LMDF?

A. Uncommon, chronic, inflammatory, smooth surfaced, skin-colored papules, 1–3 mm in size, distributed symmetrically across the face, nose, eyelids and upper lip. Occasionally the lesions can appear on the trunk and extremities also. Most commonly seen in young adults.

Q. Differential diagnosis of LMDF?

A.
- Granulomatous rosacea
- Papular sarcoidosis
- Papular acne
- Acneiform drug eruption

Q. What is the etiology?

A. Exact etiology is unclear but many possible factors have been postulated to play a role. Some suggest a role of Demodex folliculorum, while others suggest it to be a granulomatous reaction to hair follicle destruction or ruptured epidermal cyst.

Q. Does scarring occur in LMDF?

A. Yes, the lesions regress over 12–18 months followed by scarring.

Q. Histopathology of LMDF.

A. Early lesions show superficial perivascular and periappendiceal lymphocytic infiltrates with a few histiocytes and neutrophils. Fully developed lesions show round granulomas, often with caseating necrosis. The changes mimic miliary tuberculosis (one of the few conditions showing caseation necrosis in skin is LMDF. Other tuberculosis lesions do not show it).

Q. Treatment of LMDF.

A. Reported therapy include:

- Oral prednisolone
- Isotretinoin
- Dapsone
- Tetracyclines
- Antimalarials
- Scar revision procedures (laser resurfacing, dermabrasion, chemical peel) may benefit patients after the disease has run its course. Treatment with the 1450 nm diode laser has been reported to be effective.

Q. What is FIGURE?

A. Facial Idiopathic Granuloma with Regressive Evolution.

13 Becker's Nevus

Q. What is the morphology of Becker's nevus?

A. Irregular, hyperpigmented, smooth macule on shoulder, anterior chest or scapular region with hypertrichosis.

Q. Differential diagnosis of Becker's nevus.

A.
- Café-au-lait macule (CALM)
- Congenital melanocytic nevus
- Plexiform neurofibroma
- Congenital smooth muscle hamartoma

Q. Synonyms of Becker's nevus.

A.
- Becker's melanosis
- Pigmented hairy epidermal nevus

Q. What is Becker's nevus?

A.
- It is a benign condition
- Organoid epithelial nevus

Q. What are the clinical features?

A.
- It presents as a macule growing in size to reach the size of a palm while acquiring thick dark hair
- The surface becomes thick and corrugated
- Firmness to palpation may point to an associated smooth muscle hamartoma
- Color fades with time
- It is a benign lesion

Q. What is the age and sex predisposition?

A.
- Adolescence
- Male predominance (5:1) due to androgen receptors being present on the surface

Q. What are the other coexisting conditions?

A.
- Connective tissue nevi
- Smooth muscle hamartoma
- Structural abnormalities of bone and soft tissues

Q. What is the pathogenesis?

A.
- Unclear
- Believed to be an organoid hamartoma of ectodermally and mesodermally-derived tissues
- An increase in androgen receptors and probable heightened sensitivity to androgens have been postulated

Q. Histopathological findings.

A.
- Papillomatosis, acanthosis, hyperkeratosis
- Increased melanin content of melanocytes
- Melanophages in papillary dermis
- Increased number of melanosomes
- Inreased number of smooth muscles (hamartoma)

Q. Treatment.

A.
- Not required
- Electrocautery
- Waxing for hair
- Camouflage, makeup
- Lasers: Q-switched Nd:YAG have been tried for cosmetic benefits

Q. What is Becker's nevus syndrome?

A. It is characterized by presence of a particular type of organoid epithelial nevus showing hyper pigmentation, increased hairness and hamartomatous augmentation of smooth muscle fibers and other ipsilateral hypoplasia of breast and skeletal anomalies.

14 Café–au–lait Macules

Q. What do you mean by café-au-lait?

A. It means Coffee with milk (light brown). If very dark, it is called café noire (black coffee), which is sometimes seen in Watson syndrome.

Q. Classical Café-au-lait macule (CALM).

A. A discrete, well circumscribed, uniformly light brown, round or oval macule of variable size.

Q. Pathogenesis of CALM.

A. Increased melanogenesis and increased melanin content within keratinocytes.

Q. Most common sites affected by CALM.

A. Head, neck, trunk and buttocks.

Q. Differential diagnosis of CALM.

A.
- Lentigines
- Pigmentary mosaicism
- Becker's nevus
- Postinflammatory hyperpigmentation
- Epidermal nevus
- Junctional nevus
- Nevus spilus
- Congenital melanocytic nevus
- Congenital smooth muscle hamartoma
- Mastocytoma
- Mosaic neurofibromatosis

Q. Age of appearance.

A. Usually soon after birth.

Q. Dermoscopic findings of CALM.

A.
- Homogenous brown patch with perifollicular hypopigmentation
- Faint reticular pattern

Q. Epidemiology of CALM.

A. Present at birth but become obvious during first year of life and increase in size proportionately with age.

Q. What is the frequency of solitary CALM in the normal population?
A. Found in 10–20% of normal population.

Q. Types of CALM.
A.
- Isolated CALM
- Multiple CALMs

Q. What is the difference between isolated and multiple CALMs?
A.
- Isolated CALM is an isolated phenomenon while multiple CALM is a marker of multisystemic disease.
- The number and size is larger in multiple CALM (>3 in number and >1.5 cm in size).

Q. What is Crowe's law?
A. Crowe stated that in an adult, if there are >6 macules of >15 mm diameter and in a child if there are 5 macules of >5 mm diameter, the diagnosis of neurofibromatosis can be presumed even if there are no neurofibromas at that time.

Q. Conditions associated with CALM?
A. Remember the pneumonic "BIT-CAFÉ CL"
- **B**: Blooms syndrome
- **I**: Idiopathic
- **T**: Tuberous sclerosis
- **C**: Dyskeratosis congenita
- **A**: Ataxia telangiectasia, Albright syndrome
- **F**: Fanconi's anemia
- **É**: Elephantiasis (neurofibromas)
- **C**: Carney complex
- **L**: LEOPARD syndrome

Q. Other causes of CALM.
A. Watson's syndrome (pulmonary stenosis), Russell–Silver syndrome (triangular face), Noonan syndrome (short stature), multiple endocrine neoplasia (MEN) syndrome.

Q. What is café-au-lait complexion?
A. Generalized light brown discoloration is often found in congenital syphilis, and rarely in chronic renal failure.

Q. What is the treatment of café-au-lait macules?
A.
- Q-switched ruby laser
- Frequency doubled Neodymium-doped yttrium aluminium garnet (Nd:YAG) laser
- Pulse dye laser
- Erbium-doped yttrium-aluminum-garnet (Er:YAG) laser

15 Corn (Clavus)

Q. Synonyms.

A. Corn, Halome.

Q. What is a corn?

A. It is a circumscribed, cone shaped, hyperkeratosis of the skin.

Q. What are the clinical features of corn?

A.
- The size varies from 1 mm to 2 cm in diameter
- The apex of this conical keratotic mass is pointed inwards and presses upon subjacent structures
- Pressure upon nerves can cause severe pain
- Dermatoglyphics are lost on the surface of the corn
- Vertical pressure on a corn causes severe pain while lateral doesn't cause any pain. While, a callus is generally not painful at all.

Q. What are the types of corn?

A. Hard corn, soft corn, vascular corn/clavus vasculare, neurofibrous corn, seed corn.

Q. What is a hard corn?

A. They are well circumscribed usually occurring on the dorsa of the toes (pressure areas, found in diabetics) and are painful. Surface is dry, smooth and slightly convex. When the upper portion is shaved off,the central yellowish white core is noted which is the hardest part. It is the apex of this core that presses on the nerves to cause severe pain.

Q. What is a soft corn?

A. It is also known as clavus molle, occurs in the interdigital spaces of the toes. Soft corns are soggy, and macerated so they appear white.

Q. What is a vascular corn?

A. Also known as clavus vascularae. It generally occurs on the sides of the foot along the junction of the plantar and the dorsal surface, but also occurs on distal ends of 4th and 5th toe. It is a modified hard corn in which superficial capillaries have involved the epidermis subjacent to the hyperplastic mass. Vascularity is presumed to be the result of repeated trauma to the corn. These corns are painful.

Q. What is a neurofibrous corn?

A. It is an advanced type of hard corn. There is underlying fibrosis and hypertrophy of nerve filaments that is associated with severe spasmodic pain. It is the most painful corn.

Q. What is seed corn?

A. Also known as clavi miliarae. They appear as multiple, asymptomatic, discrete, tiny (1–3 mm) sized, yellowish white papules on the plantar surface of the heel and fifth toe joint.

Q. What are the predisposing factors for corn?

A.
- Bony deformities like spurs
- Ill fitting occlusive footwear
- Improper walking
- Diabetes
- High heels

Q. How will you differentiate corn and callosity from plantar warts?

A.
- Callosities have no defined edge, while corns have well defined edge, so do warts.
- Callosities are not painful while the other two are. Corns are painful on vertical pressure while warts are painful on horizontal pressure.
- On paring callosity will disappear, corn shows a central yellowish white core while wart show Brown colored spot which are thrombosed capillaries.
- Dermatoglyphics markings are present in callosities and absent in other two.

Q. How is corn treated?

A.
- Palliative treatment—application of keratolytics such as 40% salicylic acid plaster. A solution of 17% salicylic acid and 17% lactic acid in flexible colloidal solution can be painted over the pared area and allowed to dry.
- Patient is advised to avoid ill fitting shoes.
- Surgical correction of bony or muscular defect.
- An intralesional injection of Triamcinolone acetonide may give relief from pain.

Q. What is the commonest cause of callosity in medical students?

A. Carrying heavy books.

16 Carcinomas

Q. What is basal cell carcinoma (BCC)?

A. Presence of pearly, waxy papules with central depression with rolled out or thready translucent border with erosion or ulceration, bleeding on slight injury, crusting and telangiectasia over the surface.

Q. Differential diagnosis (D/D) of ulcerative lesion on face.

A.
- Basal cell carcinoma
- Squamous cell carcinoma
- Keratoacanthoma
- Melanoma
- Leishmaniasis
- Syphilitic gumma
- Deep fungal infections

Q. Which is the commonest skin malignancy?

A. Basal cell carcinoma.

Q. Which is the commonest skin malignancy in immunocompromized?

A. Squamous cell carcinoma.

Q. What are the clinical types of BCC?

A.
- Nodular/nodulo-ulcerative BCC
- Pigmented
- Superficial
- Morphea-like
- Fibroepithelioma of Pinkus

Q. What is the fibroepithelioma of Pinkus?

A. Elevated, skin-colored, indolent, sessile lesion on lower trunk, lumbosacral areas, groin or thigh.

Q. Commonest BCC in HIV infected person.

A. Superficial type.

Q. Common syndromes associated with BCC.

A.
- Xeroderma pigmentosum
- Albinism

- Nevoid BCC (Gorlin syndrome)
- Bazex syndrome
- Rombo syndrome
- Rasmussen syndrome
- Linear unilateral basal cell nevi

Q. What is the etiology of BCC?

A.
- Ultraviolet radiation (UVB)—causes pyrimidine damage
- Ionizing radiation
- Arsenic exposure
- Immunosuppression
- H/O previous nonmelanoma skin cancer

Q. Cutaneous features of xeroderma pigmentosum.

A.
- Autosomal recessive (AR) type disorder
- Cutaneous features: Actinic keratosis/cheilitis, lentigines, atrophy, photosensitivity, mottled hyper/hypopigmentation
- Extracutaneous features: Photophobia, peripheral neuropathy, eye anomalies
- Neoplasm: Melanoma, SCC, brain and visceral neoplasms

Q. What is Bazex syndrome?

A.
- X-linked dominant condition
- Cutaneous features: Flexural hyperpigmentation, follicular atrophoderma, hypohidrosis, hypotrichosis, milia, trichoepithelioma

Q. What is Gorlin syndrome?

A. It is an autosomal dominant syndrome- *PTCH1* gene
- *Diagnostic criteria*:
  - Multiple BCC >5 or BCC before age of 30 years
  - Epidermoid cysts, Odontogenic keratocysts of jaws
  - Palmoplantar pits
  - Lamellar calcification of falx cerebri
  - First-degree relative with Nevoid basal cell carcinoma syndrome (NBCCS)
- *Minor criteria*:
  - Medulloblastoma, macrocephaly, cleft lip and palate, ocular abnormalities, rib abnormalities

Q. What is associated with multiple basal cell epithelioma?

A.
- Arsenic keratosis
- Chronic sunlight exposure immunosuppression
- BCC syndrome

Q. Histopathology of BCC.

A. Nest of basaloid tumor cells, retraction artefact, hyperchromatic nuclei, palisading of cells at periphery.

Q. Immunohistochemical markers for BCC.

A.
- Light weight keratin markers—BerEP4
- CK20—Positive in trichoepithelioma, trichoblastoma, fibroepithelioma

Q. What is Jacobi ulcer?

A.
- Also known as rodent ulcer
- Neglected BCC that has ulcerated

Q. Treatment of BCC.

A.
- Surgery: Curettage, electrosurgery, cryotherapy, excision
- Mohs micrographic surgery
- Radiotherapy
- Lasers: CO_2, Neodymium-doped yttrium aluminium garnet (Nd:YAG) laser
- Photodynamic therapy
- Medical treatment: Topical and intralesional 5-FU, 5% imiquimod, interferon α-2b.

Q. Do BCC metastasize?

A. Rarely metastasis, incidence is 0.0028–0.55%.

Q. Which variants of BCC metastasize?

A.
- Morpheiform
- Infiltrative
- Micronodular
- Basosquamous

Q. What is basosquamous BCC?

A. Basal cell carcinoma transition to squamous cell carcinoma, which is highly metastatic.

Q. What is collision tumor?

A.
- Two separate and distinct neoplasms which are in close proximity
- Nevus and BCC, nevus and seborrheic keratosis, BCC and melanoma, BCC and SCC

Q. What are the risk factors for metastatic BCC?

A. Large size >10 cm, long standing, recurrent lesion, aggressive histological pattern.

Q. What is retraction artefact?

A. While processing the sample, there is separation of the tumor mass from the dermis.

Q. Mohs micrographic surgery indications?

A. Indicated in large (>2 cm margin), ill-defined, incompletely excised, recurrent, and aggressive tumors, sites such as lips, eyes, nasal tip, fingers and toes, tumors with a high risk of recurrence, Immunocompromised patients, prior irradiated skin, genetic BCC syndromes.

Q. Hedgehog pathway inhibitors.

A. Vismodegib, inhibitor of SMO (smoothened), orally administered at a dose of 150 mg daily until disease progression stops.

Q. Why is this squamous cell carcinoma (SCC)?

A. Raised, firm, hard, pink to flesh-colored papules or plaque with telangiectasia, smooth or verrucous or papillated surface and indistinct margin and elevated base. It appears on normal skin and on premalignant skin conditions like actinic keratosis and arsenic keratosis. There is fixity to underlying structure. Surface becomes friable and undergoes central ulceration and hemorrhage and is painful. Common sites are face and back of hand.

Q. Different types of SCC.

A.
- Keratotic invasive SCC
- Nodular SCC
- Arsenic induced SCC
- Thermal SCC
- Radiation SCC
- Oral SCC
- Genital SCC
- SCC of lip
- Marjolin ulcer
- Periungual SCC
- Acantholytic SCC
- Verrucous carcinoma

Q. What is Marjolin ulcer?

A. Squamous cell carcinoma on site of chronic ulcer or scar.

Q. Etiology of SCC.

A.
- Cumulative lifetime sun exposure [ultraviolet B (UVB)]
- Ionizing radiation
- Syndromes of DNA repair failure such as xeroderma pigmentosum, bloom syndrome, ataxia telangiectasia fanconi syndrome

- Immunosuppressive therapy
- HPV Infection
- Chronic arsenicism
- Industrial, chemical
- Thermal exposure
- Chronic inflammation

Q. Mutations in SCC.

A.
- TP53 mutation caused by UVR leading to pyrimidine dimers—90% of SCCs
- Somatic mutations in NOTCH receptors—75% of SCCs

Q. Histopathology of SCC.

A. Keratinocyte dysplasia, nuclear atypia, loss of polarity, abnormal intercellular bridges, atypical mitosis, horn or keratin pearls.

Q. What are premalignant skin condition causing SCC?

A.
- Actinic keratosis
- Tar keratosis
- Arsenic keratosis
- Thermal keratosis
- Chromomycosis
- Bowen's disease (intraepidermal SCC)
- Erythroplasia of Queyrat

Q. What are skin condition causing SCC?

A.
- Scars
- Ulcerative oral lichen planus
- Chronic osteomyelitis
- EBDR (epidermolysis bullosa dystrophic recessive)
- Discoid lupus erythematosus
- Hidradenitis suppurativa

Q. Broder's system of classification of SCC.

A. Based on % of undifferentiated cells:
- <25%—grade 1
- <50%—grade 2
- <75%—grade 3
- >75%—grade 4

Q. What are the histopathological variant of SCC?

A.
- Keratoacanthoma-like
- Spindle cell
- Adenoid
- Mucinous SCC

- Papillary SCC
- Pseudovascular SCC
- Verrucous carcinoma
- Acantholytic SCC

Q. Treatment of SCC.

A.
- Electrodessication and curettage
- Mohs micrographic surgery
- Cryotherapy
- Radiotherapy
- Laser therapy
- Photodynamic therapy

Q. Other malignancy associated with SCC.

A. Respiratory cancer, buccal cavity, pharynx, small intestine, non-hodgkin lymphoma and leukemia.

17 Chickenpox

Q. Why is it a case of chickenpox?

A. They are pruritic vesicles, polymorphous rash in centripetal distribution which are present on an erythematous base giving dew drop on a rose petal appearance, umbilicated pustule or crust. Lesions arise in crops over 2–5 days.

Q. What is the differential diagnoses of chickenpox?

A. Disseminated herpes zoster, impetigo, insect bite, scabies, erythema multiforme, DH, drug eruption, secondary syphilis.

Q. What is chickenpox caused due to?

A. Varicella-zoster virus (VZV).

Q. What will you see on Tzanck smear?

A. Multinucleated giant cells, epithelial cells with acidophilic intranuclear inclusion bodies.

Q. What will you see on histopathology?

A. Ballooning degeneration of granular cells as well as cells of deeper layers like stratum spinosum.

Q. How will you manage?

A. Acyclovir 800 mg qid for 7 days in adults. In children 20 mg/kg qid for 5 days, if visceral cancer or immunocompromized; IV acyclovir or valacyclovir 1 g tds.

Q. What vaccines are available?

A. Live accentuated VZV vaccine (OKA stain) 0.5 mL subcutaneous 2 doses; 3 months apart at 1 year of age.

Q. What are the complications of Chickenpox?

A.
- Secondary bacterial infection
- Neurological complications such as acute cerebral ataxia, meningoencephalitis, transverse myelitis
- Reye's syndrome—Acute encephalopathy with fatty degeneration of liver
- Respiratory complications—Varicella pneumonia
- Others—Myocarditis, glomerulonephritis, keratitis, iritis

NEW MODALITY OF TREATMENT

In cases of inadvertent exposure to the virus, varicella-zoster immune globulin if given within 96 hours of initial contact can reduce the severity of the disease.

18 Congenital Melanocytic Nevus

Q. Why is it a congenital melanocytic nevus?

A. A pigmented, well-defined plaque with or without hypertrichosis present since birth.

Q. What are the synonyms?

A. Giant pigmented nevus, garment nevus, nevus pigmentosus et pilosus, giant hairy nevus, bathing trunk nevus.

Q. Pathogenesis.

A. It is a result of a developmental defect in neural crest-derived melanoblast occurring after 10 weeks in-utero but before 6th uterine month.

Q. Clinical features.

A.
- It is present at birth with both sexes having equal predilection seen in all races
- A plaque with or without coarse terminal dark brown or black hair, sharply demarcated or merging with surrounding skin, regular or irregular contour seen at any site
- Large nevus are wormy with smooth skin surface or pebbly, mamillated, rugose or cerebriform
- On dermoscopy-globules, a fine speckling of a darker hue with a lighter surrounding brown hue seen with follicular pigmentation, milia-like cyst

Q. Differential diagnosis.

A.
- Acquired melanocytic nevus
- Congenital blue nevus
- Nevus spilus
- Becker's nevus
- Pigmented epidermal nevi
- Café-au-lait macules
- Plexiform neurofibroma
- Congenital smooth muscle hamartoma
- Melanoma

Q. Histopathology.

A.
- Melanocytes occur as well ordered clusters (theques) in the epidermis and dermis as sheets, nests and cords. Nevus cells are

seen surrounding and within the blood vessels, appendages and nerves
- A diffuse infiltration of strands of nevomelanocytes in the lower one-third of the reticular dermis and subcutis is seen

Q. Treatment.

A.
- Surgical excision of the nevus.
- If <1.5 cm, observe the lesion since it has practically no chance of becoming malignant
- If 1.5–20 cm, slightly higher chance of malignancy, hence close and periodic observation and if on an amenable area, surgical excision is preferred
- If >20 cm, serial excision is advised (chances of malignant melanoma are around 5–13%)
- Even at present, dermabrasion or laser therapy is done, but these can lead to scarring, moreover, the deeper components of the nevi are not removed so the chances of malignancy are NOT reduced

Q. Newer modalities for congenital melanocytic nevus.

A.
- In order to minimize the length of the final scar, all incisions prior to the final excision, should be placed within the area to be excised. Intralesional excision is particularly important for pigmented lesions as it avoids any 'spill over' of the pigment on to the normal skin.
- Serial excision with the 'cogwheel pattern' method is simple, and it has many advantages. It can reduce the final scar length by avoiding the dog ear deformity. By suturing the superficial fascial layer and Z-plasty, it can prevent the occurrence of the 'stretch back' phenomenon. It can also have the possibility to decrease numbers of operation and lower the cost of the entire operation. All of these benefits are ultimately obtained with the 'cogwheel technique' serial excision. This new technique can be applied for treatment of nevus sebaceous, large skin scar, or any other nevi.

New technique: Full excision technique of the nevus tissue. The nevus tissue is then subjected though hydrostatic pressure thus inactivating it. Then replanting at the same site is done thereafter.

Drug: Trametinib—an NRAS inhibitor.

19 Cutaneous Manifestations of COVID-19

Q. What is COVID-19?

A.
- Coronavirus disease 2019 (COVID-19) is a global pandemic caused by the "severe acute respiratory syndrome coronavirus 2" (SARS-CoV-2), zoonotic RNA virus which was isolated for the first time in Wuhan (China) in December 2019. Common symptoms include fever, cough, fatigue, dyspnea and hypogeusia/hyposmia.
- Among extrapulmonary signs associated with COVID-19, dermatological manifestations have been increasingly reported.

Q. What are the cutaneous findings of COVID-19?

A. The polymorphic nature of COVID-19—associated cutaneous manifestations led our group to propose a classification, which distinguishes the following six main clinical patterns:
- Urticarial rash
- Confluent erythematous/maculopapular/morbilliform rash
- Papulovesicular exanthem
- Chilblain-like acral pattern
- Livedo reticularis/racemosa-like pattern
- Purpuric "vasculitic" pattern

Q. Describe the urticarial rash in COVID-19.

A.
- Urticaria-like eruptions have occurred in 15–20% of the cases.
- Urticarial lesions predominantly involved the trunk and limbs, relatively sparing the acral sites.
- Angioedema and urticarial vasculitis may also present.

Q. Describe the confluent erythematous/maculopapular/morbilliform rash in COVID-19.

A.
- Maculopapular eruptions accounted for 45–50% of all cutaneous manifestations who further subdivided this group of cutaneous lesions into macular erythema (13%), morbilliform exanthems (22%) and papulosquamous lesions (9%).
- Erythematous papules may also be arranged in a morbilliform pattern.

- The management of confluent erythematous/maculopapular/morbilliform rash varies according to the severity of the clinical picture. Topical corticosteroids can be sufficient in most cases, systemic corticosteroids deserving to be administered just in more severe and widespread presentations.

Q. Describe papulovesicular exanthem in COVID-19.

A.
- Two different morphological patterns were found: A widespread polymorphic pattern, more common and consisting of small papules, vesicles and pustules of different sizes, and a localized pattern, less frequent and consisting of monomorphic lesions, usually involving the mid chest/upper abdominal region or the back.
- No standardized treatments for COVID-19–related papulovesicular exanthem are available, also given that it is self-healing within a short time frame. Thus, a "wait-and-see" strategy may be recommended.

Q. Describe chilblain-like acral pattern in COVID-19.

A.
- Chilblain-like acral lesions associated with COVID-19 were depicted as erythematous-violaceous patches or plaques predominantly involving the feet and, to a lesser extent, hands.
- Pain/burning sensation as well as pruritus were commonly reported symptoms.
- In the absence of significant therapeutic options for chilblain-like acral lesions associated with COVID-19 and given their tendency to spontaneously heal, a "wait-and-see" strategy may be suggested.

Q. Describe the livedo reticularis/racemosa-like pattern in COVID-19.

A. Livedo describes a reticulate pattern of slow blood flow, with consequent desaturation of blood and bluish cutaneous discoloration. It has been divided into:
- Livedo reticularis, which develops as tight, symmetrical, lace-like, dusky patches forming complete rings surrounding a pale center, generally associated with cold-induced cutaneous vasoconstriction or vascular flow disturbances such as seen in polycythemia, and
- Livedo racemosa, characterized by larger, irregular and asymmetrical rings than seen in livedo reticularis, more frequently associated with focal impairment of blood flow

  In view of the absence of significant therapeutic options for livedo reticularis/racemosa-like lesions associated with COVID-19, a "wait-and-see" strategy may be suggested.

Q. What are the other dermatological conditions related to COVID-19 pandemic?

A.
- Mechanical injury/friction dermatitis—personal protective equipment (PPE)-induced skin injury is common, occurring in up to over 90% of healthcare workers. Long durations of PPE use (>6 hours/day) increase rates of skin damage. Masks, goggles, face shields, and gloves apply pressure, create abrasion, and retain moisture and can injure the nasal bridge, cheek, forehead, and hands. PPE-induced injuries include desquamation, erythema, maceration, fissuring, papules, and erosions, leading to itching and pain.
- Irritant and allergic contact dermatitis—due to rubber, adhesives, and formaldehyde, as well as irritant contact dermatitis due to pressure and friction, in healthcare workers wearing N95 or equivalent masks for >6 hours daily
- Facial dermatoses ("maskne")—New-onset or exacerbation of facial dermatoses, including acne ("maskne"), rosacea ("mask rosacea"), seborrheic dermatitis, periorificial dermatitis, and folliculitis, likely due to friction and occlusion, have been reported in persons wearing masks for >6 h/day.
- Mask-related Koebner phenomenon (trauma-induced development of lesions clinically similar to the underlying skin disease in previously uninvolved areas) has also been described in patients with a variety of skin disorders, including psoriasis, vitiligo, acne, and rosacea.

Q. Hair and nail manifestations of COVID-19.

A.
- Hair:
    - Alopecia areata
    - Telogen effluvium—2–3 moths after COVID.
    - Anagen effluvium
- These are more common in female patients. It maybe related to decreased expression of androgens. It maybe self limited, but may respond to PRP.
- Nail manifestations are nonspecific—onycholysis, white spots on nails and subungual hyperkeratosis

Q. What are the therapeutic considerations to be considered during the pandemic?

A. The COVID-19 pandemic has led to necessary adjustments to the therapeutic approach for some dermatologic diseases.
- Use of biologic and other immunosuppressive therapies—Biologic and immunosuppressive therapies play important roles

in the management of a wide variety of dermatologic diseases, such as psoriasis, atopic dermatitis, and other inflammatory or autoimmune conditions. Although it is generally accepted that most patients without COVID-19 who are already taking immunosuppressive drugs for dermatologic disease can continue therapy, a more cautious approach is typically taken for patients who have suspected or confirmed COVID-19 and patients who are considering starting a new immunosuppressive therapy.

The broad immunosuppression induced by small molecule immunosuppressants (e.g., cyclosporine, mycophenolate, azathioprine) may be of greater concern than the targeted immunosuppression induced by biologic drugs.

- Phototherapy—In-office phototherapy typically involves frequent clinic visits, potentially increasing exposure of patients and clinical staff to SARS-CoV-2. Thus, the risks and benefits of office-based phototherapy should be weighed carefully for individual patients.

  Home phototherapy is an alternative that may be the preferred method of phototherapy during the pandemic but may not be feasible for all patients. If in-office phototherapy is necessary, careful precautions, including screening for symptoms, limiting visitors, PPE use, and equipment disinfection, should be taken to reduce the risk of transmission of infection.
- Methotrexate and Janus kinase inhibitors (JAKi) treatments should held for 1 week after each vaccine dose, with no modification to vaccine timing.

Q. Post-COVID vaccine problems?

A.
- Antibody dependent enhancement and vaccine associated respiratory disease
- Urticarial rash
- Worsening of psoriasis, vitiligo, pityriasis rosea, platelet rich plasma (PRP)
- Vaccine toes-chilblain
- Lichenoid drug reaction
- Anlagen effluvium
- Frictional alopecia

Q. COVID vaccines.

A.
- mRNA vaccines—very safe, but require cold storage:
  - Moderna vaccine administered in 2 doses, 28 day interval
  - Pfizer vaccine
  - BioTech vaccine

- Nonreplicating viral vector vaccine—nonreplicating viral vector is used:
  - AstraZeneca (Covishield)—adenovirus vaccine
  - Janssen vaccine—adenovirus 26
- Recombinant protein vaccine:
  - Novavax—uses an insect virus
- Covaxin—inactivated
  - Sputnik—nonreplicating viral vector
  - Sinovac—inactivated vaccine

20 Contact Dermatitis

Q. Name two pathogenic types of contact dermatitis.

A. 1. Nonimmunologic irritant contact dermatitis

2. Immunologic allergic contact dermatitis

Q. Name two types of irritant contact dermatitis (ICD).

A. 1. Acute toxic eruptions

2. Chronic cumulative insult reactions

Q. Describe acute type of contact dermatitis.

A. Acute, toxic eruptions occur from a single exposure to a strong toxic chemical (acid/alkali) inducing erythema, vesicles, bullae or skin sloughing. The actions occur within minutes to hours after exposure, localized to the areas of maximum contact and have sharp borders. Healing occurs soon after exposure.

Q. Describe chronic cumulative insult subtype of ICD.

A. These are the more common type of ICD and are due to multiple exposures of many low level irritants such as soaps and shampoos over time. This may take weeks, months or even years to occur. It is characterized by erythema, scaling, fissuring, pruritus, lichenification and poor demarcation from surrounding skin.

Q. Why is the distribution of contact dermatitis rash important?

A. The location and distribution of the dermatitis are vital clues to the underlying culprit. For example, an eczematous dermatitis on the dorsum of the feet possibility of shoe dermatitis.

Q. Differences between irritant and allergic contact dermatitis.

A.

	Irritant	*Allergic*
Examples	Soap	Nickel, fragrance, hair dye
Number of compounds	Many	Fewer
Distribution of reaction	Localized	May spread beyond the area of maximal contact and become generalized

Continued

Continued

	Irritant	*Allergic*
Concentration of agent needed to elicit reaction	High	Can be in minute
Time course	Immediate to late	Sensitization in 2 weeks, elicitation takes 24–72 hours
Immunology	Nonspecific	Specific type IV delayed hypersensitivity reaction
Diagnostic test	None	Patch test
Prevalence	75%	25%

Q. How many percent of cases of contact dermatitis are ICD and how many ACD?
A. The 80% of ICD, 20% of ACD.

Q. Which is the only way to distinguish between ACD and ICD?
A. Patch testing.

Q. Which is the most common allergen overall?
A. Poison ivy (most common type IV allergen).

Q. Which is the most common allergen used in the tray of patch testing?
A. The metal nickel which is found commonly in costume jewellery.

Q. Why is nickel dermatitis more common in females?
A. There is a high rate of sensitization secondary to ear piercing hence it is more common in females.

Q. What causes nickel dermatitis in males?
A. In men, nickel dermatitis is predominantly of occupational origin.

Q. Which are the different agents which can cause eyelid dermatitis?
A. Nail polish, eye makeup and airborne allergens, false eyelashes.

Q. Suspicious agents involved in dermatitis of different areas?
A.

Location	*Suspicious agent*
Earlobes or neck	Metal jewellery
Forehead, scalp margin	Hair dye
Face	Cosmetic fragrances and preservatives, airborne allergens

Continued

Continued

Location	*Suspicious agent*
Axilla	Deodorants
Hands	Gloves, occupational contact
Waistband	Elastic
Dorsa of feet	Shoes

Q. What is the allergen causing contact dermatitis in the *bindi*?
A. Para-tertiary butylphenol (PTBP).

Q. What causes parthenium dermatitis?
A. Parthenium hysterophorus or photosensitizing weed.

Q. Which is an irritant and allergic sensitizer?
A. Turpentine.

Q. What allergy causes oral lichen planus?
A. Mercury in dental filling and gold.

Q. Differential diagnosis of contact dermatitis.
A. Contact dermatitis with its scaling, erythema, lichenification, and/or vesicles, belongs in the group of eczematous disorders. Other such conditions—atopic dermatitis, nummular eczema, neurodermatitis, stasis dermatitis, seborrheic dermatitis, photodermatoses, dermatophyte infections, drug eruptions, and dyshidrotic eczema (pompholyx) should always be considered when evaluating a prospective patient for contact dermatitis. A complete history including previous skin diseases, drug and exposure histories, location and course of the eruption, patch testing, and potassium hydroxide tests should help point to the diagnosis of contact dermatitis.

Q. If a change in skin care product does not lead to clearing of a patient's rash, does it mean that original product was not the culprit?
A. Not necessarily. Many commercial cosmetic and toiletry products contain the same allergens usually fragrances and preservatives. Many products contain cross-reacting agents that can exacerbate the original problem. For example, patients who are allergic to the hair dye allergen paraphenylenediamine will need to avoid over-the-counter topical anesthetic benzocaine. Both compounds belong to the para-amino group and can cross-react with one another.

Q. What substances are tested in the standard 'screening' patch test?

A.

Allergen	*Sources*
Benzocaine 5%	Topical anesthetic
Nickel sulphate 2.5%	Metal jewellery
Neomycin sulphate 20%	Topical antibiotics
Balsam of peru 25%	Perfume, medications
Formaldehyde 1%	Preservative, fabric finishes

Q. Management of contact dermatitis.

A.
- If the patient has allergic contact dermatitis (ACD) the allergen should be detected by patch testing and subsequently it should be thoroughly avoided—Sources of the allergen as well as cross-reacting agents should be explained to the patient. An acceptable nonsensitizing substitute should be offered.
- For ICD, avoidance of as many
- Irritants as possible is crucial. Frequent water exposure, which desiccates and chaps the skin should be kept to minimum. Frequent moisturization and hand protection with gloves are important. With contact dermatitis, systemic steroids should be used only in acute situations. Compresses may be helpful if vesicles are present. When the condition is chronic, topical steroids of appropriate strength and moisturizers are the mainstay of the therapy.
- Recently, the newer nonsteroidal macrolides, immunosuppressive agents such as azathioprine, methotrexate and cyclosporine, calcineurin inhibitors tacrolimus and pimecrolimus, have been used increasingly with good results. Lastly phototherapy and Grenz ray therapy has also been used in difficult cases.

Q. What is status cosmetics syndrome?

A.
- Status cosmetics syndrome is a cosmetic intolerance of the face to multiple types of cosmetics. This is often a mild irritant dermatits. The condition predisposing are—atopic dermatitis (AD), perioral dermatitis, seborrheic dermatitis (SD), rosacea.
- Common ingredients not tolerated—formaldehyde and Kathon CG
- These patients may often tolerate face powders, fragrance-free lipsticks, blush cosmetic and foundation lotions.

Q. What is 20th century disease syndrome?

A.
- AKA total allergy syndrome where patient claims to be hypersensitive to his entire environment and has multiple ill defined symptoms for which no organic cause can be found.
- It is accepted by many to be a psychiatric condition.

21 Cutaneous Tuberculosis

Q. What is the historical importance of cutaneous tuberculosis (TB) to a dermatologist?

A. Finsen, who used ultraviolet therapy (Finsen chambers) in 1903 for treatment of cutaneous TB, is the only dermatologist to have won a Nobel Prize to date.

Q. Classification of cutaneous tuberculosis.

A. Name—Bravo classification (analogous to classification of leprosy).

Multibacillary tuberculosis	By direct inoculation	Primary inoculation TB
	By continuity	Scrofuloderma
		Tuberculosis periorificial
	By hematogenous spreading	Acute military TB
		Gumma (cold abscess)
Paucibacillary tuberculosis	By direct inoculation (re-exposure)	Tuberculosis verrucosa cutis
		Lupus vulgaris
	By hematogenous spreading	Lupus vulgaris

- *Tuberculids*:
  - Micropapular
  - Papular
  - Nodular

Q. What is part of primary tuberculosis complex?

A.
- A painless red or brown papule—indurated nodule or plaque—ulcerates to form tuberculous chancre. This with prominent regional lymphadenopathy occasionally cold suppurative and draining lesions over lymph node complete the complex. It is often seen in physicians due to accidental inoculation.
- The complex is also called Ghon's focus.

Q. Differential diagnosis of primary inoculation tuberculosis.

A.
- Yaws
- Deep fungal infections
- Syphilis

- Atypical mycobacterial disease
- Blastomycosis
- Leishmaniasis

Q. What is the Prosector's wart?

A. Resulting from inoculation during an autopsy this is the prototype of tuberculosis verrucosa cutis. Also called anatomist.

Q. Morphology of tuberculosis verrucosa cutis.

A. Small papules which become hyperkeratotic resembling a wart. Lesion enlarges by peripheral expansion with or without central clearing. Fissuring may occur discharging purulent exudate mostly solitary.

Q. Frequent locations of tuberculosis verrucosa cutis.

A. Dorsa of fingers and hands in adults and buttocks in children

Q. Differential diagnosis of tuberculosis verrucosa cutis.

A.
- Verruca vulgaris (generally doesn't show atrophy or fissuring or purulent discharge)
- Atypical mycobacteriosis (caused by *Mycobacterium marinum*)
- Swimming pool granuloma
- Deep fungal infections
- Sporotrichosis
- Hypertrophic lichen planus
- Halogenodermas

Q. What is scrofuloderma?

A. It is tuberculous involvement of the skin by direct extension usually from underlying TB lymphadenitis.

Q. What is the meaning of scrofuloderma?

A. Scrofula—king's evil

Q. Differential diagnosis of scrofuloderma.

A.
- Cervicofacial actinomycosis
- Majocchi's granuloma
- Deep fungal infections

Q. Which is the condition in which caseation is seen in the skin?

A.
- In tuberculids, lupus miliaris disseminatus faciei—multiple caveating granuloma. Not relating to cutaneous TB, but maybe related to sarcoidosis.
- Can be related to syndrome called facial Afro-Caribbean childhood eruption. Also called chronic granulomatous periorificial dermatitis.

Q. What is the meaning of lupus vulgaris?

A. Lupus means wolf (refers to the mutilated appearance of the face as if bitten by a wolf) and; vulgaris means common.

Q. Describe lupus vulgaris.

A. Typically, a single plaque composed of grouped red brown papules which progress centrifugally and heal slowly in one area. Periphery has soft reddish brown papules which coalescing with slightly elevated soft scaly plaques. Regional lymph nodes maybe enlarged.

Q. Differential diagnosis of lupus vulgaris.

A.
- Rosacea
- Tertiary syphilis
- Sarcoidosis
- Leprosy
- Deep fungal infections
- Chronic discoid lupus erythematous
- Leishmaniasis
- Acne vulgaris

Q. What is diascopy?

A.
- Diascopy also called vitropressure is pressing a skin lesion to dry away the blood supply and manifest its actual color. When a lesion of lupus vulgaris is pressed with a slide, the yellowish brown nature of the lesion becomes apparent also known as Apple Jelly Nodules.
- Diascopy is also positive in sarcoidosis.
- One more test, rarely performed is to probe the lesion with a sterile probe, when it enters easily and there is a butter like consistency—Match stick sign.

Q. Histopathology of cutaneous TB.

A.
- Epidermal changes—hyperkeratosis, acanthosis, pseudoepitheliomatous hyperplasia. Rarely, atrophy
- Dermal changes—multiple noncaseating granuloma with lymphocytes, epithelioid cells, Langhans giant cells

Q. How will you investigate?

A.
- *Specific*:
  - Acid-fast bacteria (AFB) staining [very rarely positive in tuberculosis verrucosa cutis (TBVC) and lupus vulgaris. Often positive in scrofuloderma].
  - Culture—Löwenstein-Jensen (LJ) medium, or BACTEC
  - Skin biopsy—with hematoxylin and eosin (H&E), AFB staining and culturing LJ media
  - Polymerase chain reaction (PCR) to isolate *M. tuberculosis*

- *Nonspecific*:
  - Mantoux test or QuantiFERON TB Gold test—strongly positive in TBVC, moderately positive in lupus vulgaris, negative in scrofuloderma
  - CBC, ESR
  - Chest X-ray
  - USG abdomen

Q. Other lupus in dermatology.

A.
- Lupus erythematosus
- Lupus hair
- Lupus miliaris disseminatus faciei
- Lupus band test
- Lupus profundus/lupus panniculitis
- Lupus pernio
- Lupoid sycosis barbae
- Lupoid rosacea
- Lupoid leishmaniasis
- Lupus tumidus
- Lupoid sarcoidosis

Q. What is the treatment of cutaneous tuberculosis?

A.
- Patients with pulmonary or extrapulmonary TB need an adequate course of appropriate multi-drug anti-tuberculous treatment.
- This usually involves a combination of isoniazid 5 mg/kg, rifampicin 10 mg/kg, pyrazinamide 25 mg/kg, and ethambutol 15 mg/kg (4 HRZE + 2 HRE) given over a period of six months for a standard course.
- Multidrug resistant tuberculosis has become a significant problem worldwide.
- New anti-tuberculosis drugs are being developed, including bedaquiline which has FDA approval.
- Dosage—1st 2 weeks 400 mg PO once daily.
- Three weeks 200 mg 3 times/week.
- Total course—24 weeks
- Moxifloxacin—600 mg daily for 1st 2 weeks
- Clafazimine 100 mg daily
- Kanamycin 750 mg daily IM
- Delamanid—100 mg BD for 24 weeks

Note:
- MDR—resistant to INH and R
- XDR—resistant to injectable streptomycin + INH + R

Q. Side effects of AKT.

A.
- Rifamipicin—nephrotoxicity
- INH—peripheral neuropathy
- Pyrazinamide—hepatotoxicit
- Ethambutol—eye toxicity
- Bedaquiline and delaminid—QT prolongation

Q. What is DOTS?

A. Directly observed treatment short course.

Q. What were the drugs before AKT?

A.
- Injection vitamin D
- Phototherapy
- Sanatorium therapy—good diet, sunlight, rest

22 Darier's Disease

Q. Why is it a case of Darier's disease?

A. Lesions are present as keratotic red brown papules (greasy dirty warty follicular and nonfollicular keratotic papule papules) in 'seborrheic' distribution involving the trunk, scalp, face and lateral aspects of the neck.

- Despite its initial description as follicular dyskeratosis, the papules are not limited to a perifollicular location
- The lesions tend to become confluent and may form papillomatous masses
- Small (2–3 mm) hypomelanotic macules may be admixed with the keratotic papules occasionally are the predominant feature. Rarely, sterile vesicles or bullae are prominent, and, in these cases, herpetic infection (Kaposi varicelliform eruption) must be excluded
- There is mild flexural involvement. Moderate itching and malodour is fairly frequent.
- Nail changes include longitudinal red and/or white lines, 'v' shaped nicking of distal end and subungual hyperkeratosis.
- Flat, skin-colored or brownish papules resembling flat warts over dorsal aspect of hands and feet. Usually skin lesions are bilaterally symmetrical but rarely unilateral, arranged in a linear pattern.
- Palmoplantar involvement is in the form of punctate keratosis.
- Whitish papules over the palate, gingiva, buccal mucosa and tongue (cobblestone appearance) .

Q. What is the history of Darier's disease?

A. In 1889, the French dermatologist Jean Darier, at the Hôpital Saint-Louis in Paris, and James C White, Professor of Dermatology at Harvard University, independently reported a skin disease characterized by brown, crusted, malodorous lesions with a follicular distribution.

Q. What is the other name of Darier's disease?

A. Darier-White disease, keratosis follicularis, dyskeratosis follicularis.

Q. What is the epidemiology of Darier's disease?

A. The disease begins between the ages 6–20 years and peaks during puberty.

Q. What are the exacerbating factors?

A. It is worse in summer. Sweating, heat and occlusion and lithium precipitate the lesions.

Q. Prevalence.

A. One in 10 lakhs.

Q. What is the pathogenesis of Darier's disease?

A.
- Mutations in the *ATP2A2* gene which encodes an endoplasmic reticulum (ER) Ca^{2+} ATPase pump, SERCA2, leads to both acantholysis and apoptosis, accounting for the characteristic histologic finding of acantholytic dyskeratosis-mutant SERCA2 may exert a dominant negative effect by inducing ER stress and keratinocyte apoptosis
- *ATP2A2* mutations result in chronically low Ca^{2+} stores within the ER.
- This Ca^{2+} depletion leads to acantholysis.

Q. What are the symptoms?

A. Most patients complain of moderate itching. Equally distressing are the appearance and the odor, which can lead to social isolation

Q. What are the types of Darier's?

A.
- Classical Darier's
- Segmental/linear type 1—along Blaschko's lines
- Type 2—generalized
- Acral hemorrhagic type
- Bullous type

Q. What are the histopathology findings in Darier's disease?

A.
- The prominent histologic findings are acantholysis and dyskeratosis.
- Two types of dyrkeratotic cells are found—corps ronds and grains
- Corps ronds have a central homogenous basophilic pyknotic nucleus that is surrounded by a clear halo. This is seen in the upper stratum malpighian layer. The grains are small oval cells found in the horny layer and have elongated nuclei, eosinophilic cytoplasm and are surrounded by homogenous dyskeratotic material

- Other features present are papillomatosis, hyperkeratosis. There is mild to moderate perivascular inflammatory infiltrate in the superficial dermis

Q. What are the differential diagnosis of Darier's disease?

A.
- Acrokeratosis verruciformis of Hopf (flat wart like papules on the extremities).
- Seborrheic dermatitis
- Grovers disease (no palmoplantar involvement, nail changes and mucosal change)
- Pemphigus vegetans
- Hailey–Hailey disease
- Pyoderma vegetans

Q. What are the complications of Darier's disease?

A.
- Infections—Secondary bacterial infection with foul odor, fungi, Kaposi's varicelliform eruption due to HSV.
- Oral salivary gland obstruction with painful swelling
- Ocular complications like corneal ulceration or staphylococcal endophthalmitis

Q. What is course of Darier's disease?

A. It follows a chronic course without spontaneous remission. The disease severity can fluctuate over time with some patients reporting improvement and others deterioration over time.

Q. How will you manage a case of Darier's disease?

A.
- General measures—lightweight clothes, sunscreen.
  - Daily skin care includes the use of antimicrobial cleansers to prevent malodorous bacterial colonization and keratolytic emollients to reduce scaling and irritation.
  - Avoid heat humidity sunlight
- Topical therapy:
  - Topical retinoids—Adapalene, isotretinoin. Retinoid-associated irritation is common and can be reduced by alternate-day application liberal use of emollients and combination therapy with mid potency topical corticosteroids
  - Improvement following treatment with topical calcineurin inhibitors has also been reported
  - Treatment of infection with antibiotics and antifungals
  - Several case reports have suggested that topical 5-fluorouracil (1% or 5%) may be efficacious Benefit from topical application of diclofenac sodium 3% gel has also been described, and cyclooxygenase-2 (COX-2) inhibition

has been shown to rescue keratinocytes from UVB-induced downregulation of ATP2A2 expression

- Systemic management:
  - Oral isotretinoin and acitretin in severe disease unresponsive to topical therapy. It is not recommended in patients with predominantly bullous/intertriginous esions as it may aggravate the disease.
  - Cyclosporine in those who do not respond to oral retinoids
  - Doxycycline
- Surgical management:
  - It is done for focal recalcitrant lesions mainly in flexural and gluteal area.
  - Excision followed by split-thickness grafting, dermabrasion, or laser removal (CO_2 or Erbium:YAG or pulsed dye laser) may yield a long-term remission, botulinum toxin, electron beam radiation, PDT (photodynamic therapy)

Q. What are the odors in dermatology?

A.
- Mousy odor—pemphigus foliaceous, favus, phenylketonuria
- Rotten eggs—phagedenic infection
- Cheesy odor—coryneform
- Fishy odor—trimethylaminuria, bacterial vaginosis
- Grape juice like/mousy odor—pseudomonas pyoderma

23 Dermatofibroma

Q. Why is it a dermatofibroma?

A. Presence of mildly tender dome-shaped slightly erythematous dermal nodule with a button-like firm consistency seen usually on the extremities, sometimes tender with a dimple sign (on lateral pressure).

Q. Other names.

A. Solitary histiocytoma, Sclerosing hemangioma, benign fibrous histiocytomas of the skin.

Q. Pathogenesis.

A.
- Many think it is a late histiocytic reaction to an arthropod bite
- More often, there is no inciting event or trauma, and the dermatofibroma develops spontaneously
- Multiple eruptive DF can be associated with lupus erythematosus

Q. Clinical features.

A.
- Asymptomatic
- A solitary dome shaped papulo-nodular lesion with dull to shiny texture and ill-defined borders of 3–10 mm seen with color being variable from skin colored, pink, brown, tan to dark chocolate, center being dark fading to normal skin at periphery.
- Distribution—legs, arms, trunk.
- Dimple sign/Fitzpatrick sign—lateral compression with thumb and index finger produces a depression or dimple.
- Deep dermal tenderness positive

Q. Types of dermatofibroma.

A.
- Atrophic—classic
- Keloidal
- Eruptive

Q. Dermatoscopy.

A. Classical—with pigment network and central white patch.

Q. Histopathology.

A.
- Whorling fascicles of spindle cells with small amounts of pale blue cytoplasm and elongated nuclei seen (storiform pattern) epidermal hyperplasia is often seen.

- Localized proliferation of spindle-shaped fibrous cells admixed with histiocytoid cells within the dermis. This proliferation is usually nodular in appearance, with spiculated but moderately defined borders that may have a pushing appearance regarding the surrounding tissue.
- Trapped collagen bundles or “collagen balls” within and between the fascicles of spindled fibrous cells.
- Overlying epidermis is usually separated by a clearly delineated and unaffected zone of separation, the “Grenz-zone.”
- Epidermis shows hyperkeratosis and acanthosis elongated rete ridges diving into the dermis with hyperpigmented basal keratinocytes, referred to as the “dirty feet” sign.

Q. Differential diagnosis.

A.
- Papulonodular lesions containing mucin
- Scar
- Blue nevus
- Pilar cyst
- Metastatic cancer
- Kaposi sarcoma
- Dermatofibromsarcoma protuberans
- Basal cell carcinoma

Q. Treatment.

A. Cryosurgery, excision.

24 Dermatitis Artefacta

Q. Dermatitis artefacta is also known as.
A. Factitial dermatitis, dermatitis factitia.

Q. What is dermatitis artefacta?
A. Dermatitis artefacta is a psychocutaneous disorder in which patients self-inflict cutaneous lesions as a means to satisfy a psychological need, of which they are not always consciously aware.

Q. What are the clinical features of dermatitis artefacta?
A.
- The lesions of dermatitis artefacta can mimic any dermatoses.
- They can be single or multiple, unilateral or bilateral, and although usually within easy reach of the hands, the lesions may also be created by an external auxiliary agent.
- Lesions can range from vesicles to purpura to subcutaneous emphysema and can be caused by methods such as carving with sharp instruments, applying chemicals, injecting foreign substances, etc.

Q. Does dermatitis artefacta have any sex preponderance? In which age group is it more common?
A.
- Most frequently in adolescence and young adulthood, it can occur at any age.
- Female-male ratio of 8:1.

Q. What is the histopathology of dermatitis artefacta?
A.
- Hyperkeratosis
- Irregular acanthosis
- Irregular thinning and thickening of epidermis
- Keratinocytes showing dysplastic changes
- Blood vessel proliferation with extravasation of RBCs
- Sometimes polarizing exogenous material with a variable foreign body response is seen

Q. What is the differential diagnosis of dermatitis artefacta?
A.
- Primary skin disorders
- Monosymptomatic hypochondriacal psychosis [delusions of parasitosis (DOP)]
- Malingering
- Obsessive compulsive disorder

Q. What is the treatment?

A.
- Symptomatic
- Supportive
- Anti-anxiety
- Antidepressants
- Antipsychotics-dapsone

Q. Which age-group has the most favorable prognosis?

A.
- The most favorable prognosis exists for children or adults in whom the lesions represent a response to a transient stress.
- Difficult to treat in elderly

25 Dowling–Degos Disease

Q. What is it Dowling–Degos disease (DDD)?

A.
- Reticulate hyperpigmented macules affecting neck, axillae, submammary folds, flexors, elbows, knees and groin. Comedone-like papules on back and neck.
- Pitted perioral and facial scars and epidermoid cysts may be seen. Itching present.

Q. Synonym.

A. Reticulate and pigmented anomaly of the flexures.

Q. What is it?

A. Rare genodermatosis characterized by acquired reticulate pigmentation of the flexures.

Q. Mode of inheritance.

A. Autosomal dominant with variable penetration.

Q. Genetic defect.

A.
- Mutation in Keratin—5 gene located on chromosome 17
- POGLUT1 (protein O-glucosyltransferase 1), POFUT1 (protein O-fucosyltransferase 1)

Q. Prevalence.

A.
- Most cases reported from Asian and Mediterranean countries including India
- Both genders equally affected

Q. Differential diagnosis.

A.

Disease	*Clinical features*	*Histopathology*
Dowling–Degos disease (DDD)	• Pigmented reticulate macules in flexures • Comedo like lesions in neck and back • Pitted scar around the mouth	Antler like epidermal downgrowth with basal hyperpigmentation

Continued

Continued

Disease	*Clinical features*	*Histopathology*
Kitamura's reticulate acropigmentation	Reticulate depressed macules on acral areas accompanied by palmar pits	Epidermal atrophy, elongation of rete ridges, basal hyperpigmentation
Acanthosis nigricans	Velvety plaques on flexures	Hyperkeratosis and papillomatosis
Galli–Galli disease	Reticulated hyperpigmented scaly papules over flexures	Digitiform elongation of rete ridges with suprabasal focal acantholysis
Haber's syndrome	• Persistent red face with pitted scars • Pigmented keratitis papules on trunk and axilla	Downward budding of epidermis with follicular keratotic plugs

Q. Course.

A. Starts in early adult life (third to fourth decade). Slowly progressive.

Q. Histopathology.

A.
- Increased pigmentation of basal layer.
- Filiform elongation of rete ridges with suprapapillary thinning (antler-like pattern).
- Melanocyte proliferation, no melanin
- Incontinence

Q. Dermoscopy findings.

A. Irregular, brown, star-shaped figures overlying a red background.

Q. Relation with acropigmentation of Kitamura.

A.
- In many cases, features of both are observed. Some consider it to be varied presentation of same entity.
- In this, hyperpigmented macules appear during childhood on the dorsum of hands and feet in reticulate pattern and are atrophic. They are aggravated by sunlight.

Q. What is Galli–Galli disease?

A. Regarded as acantholytic variant of Dowling–Degos.

Q. Treatment.

A.
- Topical: Hydroquinone, tretinoin, adapalene, corticosteroids
- Lasers: Erbium-doped yttrium-aluminum-garnet (Er:YAG) lasers, intense pulsed light (IPL)

26 Epidermal Nevi

Q. What is a nevus?

A. It is a tumor like malformation, nonneoplastic, usually present from birth, consisting of abnormal proportions of normal cells indigenous to the tissue. The word "nevus" is derived from the word "materna."

Q. Why is this epidermal nevus?

A. The lesions are pigmented velvety streaks which were pink initially and gradually become brown and verrucous (wart-like) with age. The lesions follow the Blaschko's lines. These lesions do not cross the midline.

Q. What is the differential diagnosis of verrucous epidermal nevus?

A.
- Nevus sebaceous
- Lichen striatus—acquired condition, doesn't persist
- Verruca vulgaris—Koebner phenomenon +
- Linear lichen planus—violaceous, flat topped, severe pruritus
- Seborrhoeic keratosis
- Linear psoriasis
- Acrokeratosis verruciformis of Hopf
- Epidermodysplasia verruciformis
- Linear porokeratosis

Q. What are epidermal nevi?

A. Epidermal nevi can be—congenital lesions (birthmark) or a lesion arising early in life (1st year of life); a benign tumor of melanocytes; a hamartoma.

Q. Classify epidermal nevi.

A.
- *Keratinocytes*:
  - Verrucous epidermal nevus
  - Inflammatory linear verrucous epidermal nevus
- *Appendageal*:
  - Nevus sebaceous
  - Nevus comedonicus
  - Eccrine nevi
  - Apocrine nevi
- Epidermal nevus syndromes

Q. Where do epidermal nevi originate?

A. Epidermal nevi are thought to originate from the pluripotent stem cells in the basal layer of the embryonic epidermis.

Q. What is the pathogenesis of epidermal nevi?

A.
- Epidermal nevi display mosaicism—mutations of keratins 1 and 10, mutations in the *ATP2A2* gene.
- Yet another theory is that many of the nevi are caused by postzygotic mutations in fibroblast growth factor receptor 3 (FGFR3), which is a gain-of-function (activating) mutation. The hamartomatous process also involves a part of the dermis.

Q. What is nevus unius lateris and ichthyosis hystrix?

A.
- Nevus unius lateris is a variant in which there are extensive unilateral plaques, often involving trunk.
- Ichthyosis hystrix is a variant in which bilateral involvement on the trunk is seen. Hystrix means = porcupine.

Q. What is epidermal nevus syndrome?

A. Epidermal nevus seen with other developmental abnormalities such as kyphosis, scoliosis, atrophy or muscles.

Q. What are the complications of verrucous epidermal nevus?

A.
- The complications include: Maceration, infection, and paronychia
- Neoplasms like BCC, SCC and keratoacanthoma may rarely occur after puberty.

Q. What are the histopathological findings of verrucous epidermal nevus?

A. The histopathological findings consist of hyperkeratosis, acanthosis, and papillomatosis—“church-spire” pattern.

Q. How will you treat a case of verrucous epidermal nevus?

A.
- Cryotherapy—for small lesions
- Argon/CO_2 laser
- Full thickness surgical excision with grafting-definitive
- Topical therapy—corticosteroids, retinoic acid, tars, anthralin, 5-FU and podophyllin
- Oral therapy—retinoids

Q. Why is this inflammatory linear verrucous epidermal nevus (ILVEN)?

A. There are pruritic, unilateral, scaly, erythematous papules which coalesce to form a linear plaque, mostly on a limb and at times on the trunk.

Q. What are the differentials?

A.
- Congenital hemidysplasia with ichthyosiform nevus and limb defects (CHILD)
- Psoriasis superimposed on an epidermal nevus—micaceous scales (nevoid psoriasis)
- Lichenoid epidermal nevus—verrucous plaque

Q. What are other names of inflammatory linear verrucous epidermal nevus?

A. ILVEN is synonymous with dermatitic epidermal nevus and eczematous epidermal nevus.

Q. How is the pathogenesis of ILVEN different from that of psoriasis?

A.
- Involucrin, a structural component of mature squamous epithelium, is seen in large numbers in orthokeratotic epithelium of ILVEN, but is minimally expressed within the keratinocytes underlying areas of parakeratosis.
- However, in psoriasis, involucrin can be seen in all layers of the epidermis except for the basal layer.

Q. What are the clinical features of ILVEN?

A.
- Patients with ILVEN present before the age of six with pruritic, unilateral, scaly, erythematous papules which may coalesce to form a linear plaque, mostly on a limb and at times on the trunk.
- It has 4:1 female:male predilection and lesions resolved spontaneously by adulthood.

Q. Describe the histopathological findings.

A. The histopathological findings in ILVEN consists of elongation of rete ridges and broad zones of parakeratosis which alternate with depressed regions of orthokeratosis and hypergranulosis. Exocytosis of lymphocytes and neutrophils into the spongiotic epidermis may be seen.

Q. How will you treat a patient of ILVEN?

A.
- Surgical excision—results in scarring
- Pulsed-dye laser—destruction of small blood vessels in papillary dermis
- Topical tretinoin and 5-Fluorouracil cream combination therapy
- Topical calcipotriol
- Patients with arthritis may be treated with etanercept
- CO_2 Laser therapy for linear nevus

27 Erythema Multiforme

Q. What are the other names of erythema multiforme (EM)?

A. Erythema multiforme von Hebra, Erythema multiforme minor (also called as Erythema exudativum multiforme) and Herpes simplex associated erythema multiforme.

Q. Who first described EM?

A. Austrian dermatologist Ferdinand von Hebra in 1860.

Q. What are the important causes of EM?

A.
- *Infections*:
  - Herpes simplex associated EM
  - Mycoplasma induced EM
  - Histoplasma
  - Adenovirus
  - Cytomegalovirus
  - *Mycoplasma pneumoniae*
- Drug induced EM
- Radiation induced EM
- Exposure to poison ivy
- Systemic diseases (inflammatory bowels disease, LE, Behçet's syndrome, Sjögren's syndrome, dermatomyositis, rheumatoid arthritis)
- Idiopathic EM
- Internal malignancy
- Rarely, pregnancy

Q. Describe the classical lesion of EM?

A. Target or three zones are seen:
1. Central dusky purpura/bulla
2. Elevated pale ring (edematous)
3. Macular erythema

Q. What are the clinical features of EM minor?

A.
- EM minor is a self limiting recurrent disease of young adults lasting for 1–4 weeks. It is uncommon in childhood and shows slight male preponderance.

- Lesions begin as sharply marginated erythematous macule, which becomes raised edematous papule in 24–48 hours.
- Typical target lesions are seen. Lesions are symmetrical, acral and involve palms, soles and mostly dorsum of hands.

Q. Differences between EM minor, EM major and Stevens–Johnson syndrome (SJS).

A.

	EM minor	*EM major*	*SJS*
Type of skin lesions	Typical target	• Typical target • Atypical target • Occasional bullous lesions	• Dusky macules • Macular atypical target • Bullous lesions (>10% BSA)
Distribution	Extremities, face	Extremities, face	Trunk, face
Mucous involvement	Absent or mild	Severe	Severe
Systemic involvement	Absent	Present	Present
Progression to TEN	No	No	Yes
Precipitating factors	Infections	Infections and drugs	Drugs

Q. Is Koebner phenomenon seen in EM?

A. Yes.

Q. What is the classification of erythema multiforme?

A.
- Erythema multiforme minor
- Erythema multiforme major
- SJS
- Overlap syndrome
- Toxic epidermal necrolysis (TEN)

Q. Difference between drug associated, and infectious EM.

A.

Parameters	*Herpes*	*Mycoplasma*	*Drug*
Age	Young adults	Children and adolescents	Any age

Continued

Continued

Parameters	***Herpes***	***Mycoplasma***	***Drug***
Onset	1–3 weeks after attack	1–3 weeks after attack of respiratory infection	1–12 weeks after starting of drugs
Character-istic	EM minor lesions	Em major lesions	EM major lesions
Systemic symptoms	Minimal	Severe	Severe
Skin lesions	Target like lesions predominate	Bullae predominate	Both can occur
Mucosal lesions	Absent	Severe	Severe
Recurrences	Common	Unusual	Unusual

Q. What are the drugs causing EM?

A.
- Antibiotics: Penicillin and semi-synthetic penicillin, sulfonamides, tetracycline, chloramphenicol, streptomycin, griseofulvin.
- Anti tuberculosis: Rifampicin, isoniazid
- Anticonvulsants: Phenytoin, barbiturates
- NSAIDs: Acetylsalicylic acid, ibuprofen
- Others: Glucocorticoids, piroxicam, gold, cimetidine, methotrexate, digitalis
- Vaccination: BCG

Q. Which skin conditions can have EM as one of its manifestations?

A.
- Lupus erythematosus (LE) (Rowell's syndrome)
- Paraneoplastic pemphigus
- Sarcoidosis

Q. What is the histopathology of EM?

A.
- Normal basket weave stratum corneum
- Vacuolar interface dermatitis with vacuoles and foci of necrosis
- Mononuclear dermal infiltrate primarily in the upper dermis then at dermo-epidermal junction.
- T-lymphocytes seen
- Cytotoxic cells in the epidermis and helper cells in the dermis
- Edema of dermis seen

Q. What are histopathological differential diagnosis (D/D)?

A.
- Fixed drug eruption (FDE)
- Graft-versus-host disease
- Pityriasis lichenoides
- Lupus erythematosus

Q. What are the clinical D/D?

A.
- Bullous arthropod reaction
- Urticarial vasculitis
- Bullous pemphigoid
- Pemphigus vulgaris
- Paraneoplastic pemphigus
- Fixed drug eruption
- Lupus erythematosus
- Urticaria multiforme (has two zones instead of three)
- Erythema annulare centrifugum
- Erythema gyratum repens
- Erythema chronicum

Q. What is the treatment of EM?

A.
- In HSV induced EM—treatment with antiviral (acyclovir, valacyclovir, famciclovir)
- Prevent out breaks of HSV
- Use of sunscreen to prevent UVB-induced outbreak in HSV induced EM
- Topical steroids and oral antihistamines.
- In extensive disease—systemic steroids.

Q. What is severity-of-illness score for toxic epidermal necrolysis (SCORTEN)?

A. It is a severity-of-illness score to determine prognosis for cases of TEN based on 7 independent risk factors for death as assessed on the first day of hospitalization. It includes the following parameters:

1. Age > 40 years
2. Presence of malignancy
3. Epidermal detachment
4. Heart rate >120 beats/min
5. Bicarbonate < 20 mmol/L
6. Urea >10 mmol/L
7. Glycemia >14 mmol/L

Note: 1 point is awarded for each parameter, SCROTEN is then derived after totaling of scores.

Scorten	***Probability of death***
1	3
2	12
3	35
4	58
>5	90

Q. What is the prognosis and mortality rate of EM minor, EM major and SJS?

A.

	EM Minor	***EM Major***	***SJS***
Prognosis	Good	Good	Variable
Mortality	Low	Low	1–5%

28 Erythema Nodosum

Q. Define erythema nodosum (EN).

A. Erythema nodosum is a commonest type of septal panniculitis, which could be caused by internal infections, neoplasms, inflammatory multisystem diseases and drug induced.

Q. Why is this EN?

A. The lesions are erythematous, warm, painful nodules, 1–5 cm in diameter which is usually slightly elevated above the skin surface, occurs mostly on the lower extremities, particularly on anterior tibial surface and lateral shin.

Q. Differential diagnosis of EN.

A.
- Erythema induratum—seen on posterior calves, chronic course, possibility of ulceration and scaling often associated with tuberculosis more common in your females, also called erythema induratum of Bazin.
- Erythema nodosum leprosum (ulcerates, on face and trunk, heals in 24–48 hours)
- Syphilitic gumma—unilateral distribution
- Subcutaneous fat necrosis associated with pancreatitis and nodular vasculitis—associated clinical features and histopathology can be used to differentiate
- Cellulitis—unilateral associated with lymphadenopathy
- Erythema nodosum of Whitfield—associated with dermatophytes, most common on anterior shin.
- Sweet's syndrome—more commonly on face and neck, plum colored purple papule with pseudovesicular appearance
- Bruises—erythema contusiformis

Q. What is the etiology of EN?

A. Remember the mnemonic: "SORE SHINS"
- **S**: Streptococci
- **O**: Oral contraceptive pills
- **R**: Rickettsial
- **E**: Eponyms-Behçet's
- **S**: Sulfonamides
- **H**: Hansens disease

- **I**: Inflammatory bowel disease (IBD)–ulcerative colitis (UC), Crohn's
- **N**: Non-Hodgkin's lymphoma
- **S**: Sarcoidosis

The various causes of erythema nodosum are:

- Infections:
  - Bacterial:
    - Streptococcal infections, tuberculosis, *Yersinia enterocolitica, Mycoplasma pneumoniae*, lymphogranuloma venereum, leptospirosis.
  - Fungal:
    - Histoplasmosis, coccidioidomycosis
  - Parasitic:
    - Toxoplasmosis, amoebiasis, giardiasis
  - Viral:
    - Hepatitis B, C virus, herpes simplex virus (HSV)
- Drugs:
  - Sulfonamides, bromides, iodides, sulfonylurea, oral contraceptive pills (OCPs), penicillin, gold, infliximab
- Malignancies:
  - Hodgkin disease, non-Hodgkin lymphoma, acute myelogenous leukemia
- Granulomatous dermatosis:
  - Sarcoidosis
- Inflammatory bowel disease:
  - Ulcerative colitis, Crohn's disease
- Neutrophilic dermatosis: Behçet's disease, Sweet syndrome
- Pregnancy
- Reiter's disease

Q. In children, what is the most common cause?

A. The most common cause in children is streptococcal infection.

Q. Why is EN common in females?

A. In pregnancy and young females predisposition to high levels of estrogen favors EN.

Q. What are the clinical features of EN?

A.
- EN is most frequently seen in females in age group 20–30 years
- It appears as erythematous, warm, painful nodules, 1–5 cm in diameter which is usually slightly elevated above the skin surface which occurs mostly on the lower extremities particularly on anterior tibial surface and lateral shin

- Lesions are rarely seen on posterior calves, upper leg, extensor arms, neck and very rarely face
- Lesion change color in second week from bright red to bluish, which then fades to form the bruise that is called erythema contusiforme which disappears in 1–2 weeks
- The nodules usually don't ulcerate and subside within 2–6 weeks, without atrophy or scarring leaving behind hyperpigmentation

Q. What are the types of EN?

A. There are two types of EN:

1. Acute type: Fever, headache, episcleritis, conjunctivitis, malaise, joint pain, arthralgia occur in 50% cases. Erythema, swelling and tenderness, morning stiffness occur over joint. Any joint may be involved, but ankles, knees and wrist are most commonly affected
2. Chronic type: Also called erythema nodosum migrans (Vilanova disease), is a chronic form of panniculitis, that presents as asymptomatic or minimally painful nodules on leg. The lesion starts as nodules and form plaques. The plaques show peripheral extension and central clearing and last for months to years. Linear EN: A form of thrombophlebitis

Q. Difference between EN and erythema nodosum leprosum (ENL).

A.

ENL	*EN*
Lepromatous leprosy, on or not on treatment or post-treatment	Healthy patient
Trunk, face and limbs	Anterior shins
Nodules seen	Plaques, which later become nodules
Can ulcerate	Don't ulcerate
Heal in 48–72 hours (evanescent)	Takes weeks to months
HPE: Neutrophilic vasculitis, fibrinoid necrosis maybe present in vessels	HPE: • Thickened septum, neutrophils and lymphocytes • Miescher's granuloma being the hallmark

Q. In which condition does EN-like lesions are seen?

A. EN-like lesion are seen in helicobacter septicemia, brucellosis, cat scratch disease, Behçet's disease and Sweet's syndrome.

Q. What is histopathology of EN?

A. • It is a prototype of septal panniculitis
- In early stage, septal edema and lymphohistiocytic infiltrate with few neutrophils and eosinophilis
- In older lesions there is granulomatous infiltrate
- Miescher's radial granulomas are the hallmark of EN. These granuloma consist of small well defined aggregation of small histiocytes arranged radially around the central cleft
- There is also thickening of septa in late lesions due to fibrosis

Q. What are the investigations to be done for EN?

A. The following investigation should be done:
- ESR—ASO titer through a throat swab culture
- Preceding diarrhea history is suggestive of *Yersinia* infection
- Travel and exposure history for endemic fungal infections
- Chest X-ray and Mantoux test for tuberculosis or sarcoidosis
- Complete blood count and bone marrow studies for hematological disorders
- Colonoscopy and barium studies for patients with gastrointestinal symptoms

Q. What is the management and treatment of EN?

A. The treatment of EN consists of three components:
1. Identifying trigger
2. Rest and elevation of affected extremity
3. Specific anti-inflammatory medication

The following steps to be done:
1. Bed rest in most of the cases especially children.
2. Reducing vigorous exercise and restriction of physical activities
3. Diagnose and treat underlying cause
4. Compression therapy
5. Infection if any should be controlled to prevent prolongation of EN
6. NSAIDs like aspirin, indomethacin and naproxen should be given
7. Supersaturated solution of potassium iodide (KI), 5 drops three times a day, increasing per drop per dose everyday upto 30 drops three times a day (1 drop = 50 mg KI).
8. In tablet form, KI is 300 mg three times a day
9. HCQ's 200–400 mg can be given daily
10. Dapsone 50–100 mg can be given daily

11. Cyclosporine 3–5 mg/kg/day
12. Adalimumab and infliximab can be given
13. Intralesional steroids are given for persistent lesions
14. In acute lesion, colchicine 0.6 mg twice daily
15. Aspirin and potassium iodide are 2 drugs which cure and cause EN
16. Short course of steroids can be given

29 Fixed Drug Eruptions

Q. Who coined the term fixed drug eruption (FDE)?

A. Brocq termed fixed drug eruption.

Q. Why is this FDE?

A. History of drug intake, typical site—mucosal, genital are common sites, typical morphology—one or a few, round, sharply demarcated erythematous and edematous plaques are seen sometimes with a dusky, violaceous hue, central blister or detached epidermis. Heals with pigmentation.

Q. What are the various clinical variants of FDE?

A.
- Classical (pigmented)
- Generalized (pigmented)
- Localized Bullous
- Generalized Bullous
- Mucosal
- Purpuric
- Non pigmented—Large lesions heal without residue seen in the girdle region, usually seen with pseudoephedrine, phenylephrine, phenylpropylamine (3 Ps- all vasoconstrictive)
- It has two variants—pseudo-cellulitis or scarlatiniform type and baboon syndrome (symmetrical drug related intertriginous and flexural exanthema-SDRIFE).
- Wandering FDE—when FDE like lesions occur at a different site with every exposure

Q. What are the clinical features of FDE?

A.
- It starts as a red purple circular plaque with a gray center, most patients have 1-5 plaques. It targets area with thin skin, e.g., lips genitals mucosa and perianal area.
- Targets that are favored are the ones where there is previous trauma.
- The initial lesion occurs up to 1 week after drug ingestion. Subsequent lesions can occur up to 30 minutes after ingestion.
- It is usually mildly symptomatic and resolves with pigmentation which can last for a long time.

Q. Explain the differential diagnosis to be considered in a case of FDEs.

A.
- To differential generalized FDE from Stevens-Johnson syndrome/toxic epidermal necrolysis (SJS/TEN)
  - Extent of involvement <10% in generalized FDE, >10% in SJS/TEN.
  - Sizeable area between normal skin in FDE but less area of normal skin in SJS/TEN.
  - Erosive mucous involvement rare in FDE, while very common in SJS General health—not affected. Fever and other symptoms common in SJS
- Erythema multiforme—characteristic target lesions
- Localized contact dermatitis
- Phytophotodermatitis
- Herpes simplex viral infections

Q. Common medication according to site.

A.

Site	*Drug*
Oral	NSAIDs, cotrimoxazole
Male genital	Tetracycline, cotrimoxazole
Female genitals	Nonsteroidal anti-inflammatory drugs (NSAIDs)
Nonpigmenting	
Generalized bullous	Metronidazole, rifampicin, cotrimoxazole, NSAIDs

Q. Why is it called "fixed" drug eruption?

A. Fixed drug and fixed site.

Q. What are the various causative drugs responsible for FDEs?

A.
- Antibiotics—sulfonamides, tetracyclines (classically produces genital FDE), erythromycin
- NSAIDs—pyrazolone derivatives, paracetamol, naproxen, oxicams, mefanimicacid, acetaminophen, celecoxib
- Barbiturates
- Carbamazepine
- Phenolphthalein
- Cetirizine, hydroxyzine
- Dextromethorphan
- Quinine
- Lamotrigine
- Phenylpropanolamine

Q. What are the predisposing factors of FDE?

A. HLA-B22.

Q. What is the pathogenesis?

A. Supposed to be type IV hypersensitivity reaction. It can be reproduced by patch testing in some cases.

Q. Histological features seen in FDE lesions.

A. Interface dermatitis with subepidermal vesicle formation, necrosis of keratinocytes and a mixed superficial and deep infiltrate of neutrophils, eosinophils and mononuclear cells.

- Pigment incontinence is usually marked.
- The stratum corneum is normal.
- Papillary dermal fibrosis and deep perivascular pigment incontinence are commonly present from prior episodes

Q. How can you confirm the diagnosis?

A.
- Oral challenge test—giving 1/10th of the suspected drug to the patient (risk of flaring up of FDE exists)
- Patch testing over hyperpigmented area—it is a sensitive method, specially for NSAIDs.
- Lymphocyte transformation test
- Biopsy

Q. What is the treatment advised in a case of FDE?

A.
- Counselling—they should be told not to use the suspected drug again.
- The offending drug should be clearly mentioned in the case paper and should be explained to the patient.
- Symptomatic management of the disease—antihistaminics, steroids, topical antibiotic form the mainstay of treatment.
- Mild oral lesions—topical lignocaine, topical steroids or topical tacrolimus.
- Genital FDE—topical zinc paste
- Skin lesions—topical steroids
- In all cases—H1-antihistamines to be given
- For generalized and bullous—moderate oral steroids, cyclosporine

Q. What is the treatment for the pigmentation produced after FDE?

A. No treatment is known. It subsides with time.

Q. In which drug was this phenomenon 1st described?

A. With phenolphthalein, which was used as a laxative.

ACUTE GENERALIZED EXANTHEMATOUS PUSTULOSIS (AGEP)

Q. Why is it AGEP?

A.
- Nonfollicular pustules, >100 and <5 mm in diameter occurring on face and major skin creases
- Nikolsky's sign is positive
- Mucous membrane involvement is common

Q. Differential diagnosis (D/D) of AGEP.

A.
- Generalized pustular psoriasis
- Pustular psoriasis of pregnancy (impetigo herpetiformis)
- Subcorneal pustular dermatosis

Q. What is another name of AGEP?

A. Toxic pustuloderma, pustular drug eruption.

Q. What is the incidence of AGEP?

A. 1 to 5 cases/million/year.

Q. What is the most common cause of AGEP?

A. Drugs:
- Ampicillin, amoxicillin, cephalosporins, quinolones and hydroxychloroquine
- Sulfonamides, antibiotics, terbinafine, imatinib, corticosteroid, and macrolides
- Oxicam, NSAIDS and antiepileptics
- Mercury exposure, bacterial and viral infections (EBV, CMV)

Q. What are the associated abnormalities with AGEP?

A. Fever, facial edema and scarlatiniform rash (sheets of erythema). Laboratory abnormalities—leukocytosis, neutropenia, eosinophilia.

Q. What is the % of mortality in AGEP?

A. 5%.

Q. Diagnostic criteria.

A.
- Fever > 38°C
- Sudden onset of pustular eruptions
- Neutrophilic
- Sometimes eosinophilia
- Subcorneal pustules or intraepidermal pustules
- Spontaneous resolution within 2 weeks

Q. Histopathology of AGEP.

A. • Early lesion—marked papillary edema, neutrophilic clusters in dermal papillae and perivascular eosinophils
- Well developed lesion—marked intraepidermal or subcorneal pustulosis

Q. D/D of AGEP.

A. Stop the offending drug:
- Mostly topical steroids and antihistamines. Systemic steroids in the dose of 1 mg/kg/day.
- In severe cases—infiximab, etanercept. Cyclosporine may be used

LICHENOID DRUG ERUPTION

Q. How does lichenoid drug eruption differ from lichen planus (LP)?

A. • Lichenoid drug eruption has a later age of onset, more generalized involvement without flexural predilection on photo-exposed areas.
- Lichenoid drug eruption tends to be absent from the flexures of the wrist, genitals and mucous membrane unlike idiopathic LP
- Lichenoid drug eruption often occurs on sun exposed areas.
- Morphologically they are more eczematous, psoriasiform or pityriasis rosea like and Wickham's striae absent, mucous membrane are spared.

Q. How to differentiate them histologically?

A. • Difficult to distinguish but certain points maybe helpful
- Parakeratosis seen, spongiosis rarely seen, band like infiltrate consists of eosinophils and the basal cell degeneration is focal.

Q. Drugs causing lichenoid drug eruption.

A. • Gold, hydroxychloroquine, furosemide, NSAIDs, aspirin
- Angiotensin-converting enzyme (ACE) inhibitors, beta blockers, calcium channel blockers (CCBs)
- Anticonvulsants, antituberculosis, ketoconazole
- Antimalarials
- Hepatitis B vaccinations

Q. When does lichenoid eruption occurs?

A. Months to years after starting the offensive drug.

Q. Metal causing oral lichenoid eruption.

A. Mercury, gold, cobalt and nickel.

Q. What is the unusual form of eruption?

A. Drug-induced ulceration of lower lip.

Q. What is the treatment of lichenoid drug eruption?

A. Stop the offending drug:

- Oral antihistamines
- Topical steroid
- Tacrolimus
- Oral steroid like prednisolone
- Good oral hygiene to prevent secondary candidiasis

30 Freckles

Q. What are freckles?

A. Freckles are small, <0.5 cm, well-circumscribed light to dark brown macules that occur profusely on the sun exposed skin of the face, neck, shoulders and back of the hands appearing in the first 3 years of life in fair colored people. Autosomal dominant inheritance may be likely. Not found on mucous membranes. Decrease later in life.

Q. What is the pathogenesis of freckles?

A. It results from sun-induced melanogenesis and transport of an increased number of fully melanized melanosomes from melanocytes to keratinocytes.

Q. What are the predisposing factors for freckles?

A. Exposure to sun and positive family history.

Q. What is the other name for freckles?

A. Ephelides.

Q. Which population is more susceptible to freckles?

A. Blonds and red heads with blue eyes and of celtic origin.

Q. What are the differential diagnosis?

A. Simple lentigines, solar lentigines, café-au-lait macules (solitary and larger) and junctional nevi.

Q. How will you differentiate ephelides from lentigo simplex?

A.
- Lentigo simplex are benign, persistent, discrete, hyperpigmented macules, appearing at any age and on any part of the body, including the mucosa. The intensity of color is not dependent on sun exposure.
- Solar lentigo occurs at older age due to long standing exposure to sun. The back of hands and face are favored sites.

Q. How do you differentiate ephelides from solar lentigines?

A. They appear by third to fourth decade of life are larger in size seen on areas of chronic sun–exposure especially on dorsum of hand, not associated with any hair type more common in type 1 and type 2 skin, there is history of repeated sun exposure, are persistent for life, may darken in summer and not hereditary.

Q. What is the histology of ephelides and does it differ from lentigo?

A.
- The ephelides show increased production of melanin pigment by a normal number of melanocytes which are larger in size and have more branching dendrites. Epidermis is normal showing increased pigmentation in the basal layer.
- In lentigo, the number of melanocytes are increased and rete ridges are broader and deeper.

Q. What is the prevention and treatment for freckles?

A.
- Appropriate sun protection
- Topical retinoids, hydroquinone, cryotherapy and pulsed-dye lasers are effective in ephelides

Q. Newer modalities of treatment for freckles.

A.
- Using a fractional nonablative 2940 nm Erbium-doped yttrium-aluminum-garnet (Er:YAG) laser
- Superficial pigmented lesions, such as freckles, respond to variety of lasers.
- Most commonly used lasers are the pigment lasers, namely the frequency-doubled Q-switched (QS) Neodymium-doped yttrium aluminium garnet (Nd:YAG), QS ruby, Q-switched alexandrite laser (QSAL), and pulsed dye green laser.
- These work by targeting melanin, these lasers cause melanosome rupture, hence freckle lightening
- Ablative lasers such as the CO_2 laser have been used to nonspecifically damage the epidermis to remove pigmented lesions
- The advantage of CO_2 is that it achieves very good clearance rate with one or two sessions

31 Fox–Fordyce Disease

Q. Other name for Fox–Fordyce disease.

A. Apocrine miliaria.

Q. Definition.

A. Fox–Fordyce disease is a chronic, itchy, papular eruption involving apocrine gland-rich areas of the body characterized by numerous firm, flesh-colored, follicular-based papules arranged in a grouped configuration.

Q. Epidemiology.

A. Females between the ages of 13 and 35 years comprise >90% of cases. Fox–Fordyce disease is rarely reported before puberty or after menopause. There is no known racial predilection for the disease F:M = 13:1.

Q. Etiology.

A.
- It is unclear but the tendency of the disease to present at puberty and remit after menopause suggest hormonal component. Improved during pregnancy and with administration of oral contraceptive (OC) pills.
- Genetics likely play a role in Fox–Fordyce disease.
- It is thought that laser-induced thermal damage to the follicular infundibulum causes altered keratinocyte maturation and subsequent plugging of the apocrine gland duct insertion site.

Q. Cutaneous findings.

A. Fox–Fordyce lesions manifest as flesh colored grouped, symmetrically distributed, monomorphic, dome-shaped papules (1–3 mm) that are typically follicular based, flesh-colored to mildly erythematous, and intermittently pruritic. Excoriations and lichenification are often present secondary to scratching.

Q. Sites affected.

A. The axillae are most commonly affected. The pubic, perineal, areolar, umbilicus, and sternal areas also can be involved. Diminished sweat production is frequently observed in affected areas.

Q. Diagnosis.

A. Fox–Fordyce disease is a clinical diagnosis based on careful history and cutaneous findings. Histopathologic analysis can facilitate with diagnosis, but findings are variable and nonspecific.

Q. Differential diagnosis.

A. Irritant contact dermatitis, lichen amyloidosis, granular hyperkeratosis, lichen nitidus, eruptive syringoma, or infectious folliculitis, early stages of hidradenitis suppurativa, Darier's, Hailey–Hailey, pseudofolliculitis.

Q. Treatment.

A.
- *Symptomatic therapies*:
  - Oral antihistamines, low dose doxepin
- *Topical therapies*:
  - Topical steroid creams are first-line therapies
  - Intradermal triamcinolone
  - Topical calcineurin inhibitors (1% pimecrolimus cream, 0.1% tacrolimus)
  - Topical 0.1% adapalene gel
  - Topical clindamycin in propylene glycol solution
- *Oral therapies*:
  - Oral isotretinoin
  - Oral contraceptives
- *Procedural therapies*:
  - Intralesional steroid injection
  - Intralesional botulinum toxin injection
  - Surgical excision
  - Microwave thermal ablation

Q. What are the other conditions associated with Fox–Fordyce?

A. Impetigo Tilbury Fox.

32 Granuloma Annulare

Q. Enumerate other names of granuloma annulare (GA).

A. Pseudorheumatoid nodule—subcutaneous granuloma annulare variant, generalized granuloma annulare and disseminated granuloma annulare.

Q. Who discovered GA?

A. Calcott Fox first described "ringed eruption of fingers" in 1895. Radcliffe-Crocker called this entity granuloma annulare in 1902.

Q. Definition.

A. Its a necrobiotic disorder characterized by degenerative changes in the dermis which evokes a granulomatous response leading to a characteristic pathological appearance.

Q. Pathogenesis.

A. Believed to be a delayed hypersensitivity reaction to various etiological triggering factors.

Q. Various etiological factors.

A. Following factors have been implicated:

- Trauma
- Sunlight
- At sites of insect bite
- Various drugs—amlodipine, allopurinol, quinidine, gold
- Diabetes mellitus
- Familial
- BCG vaccination
- Various autoantibodies (antithyroid antibodies, antinuclear antibodies)
    - Viral infection—HIV
    - COVID vaccination

Q. Incidence.

A.
- Rare disorder
- More in children
- All age groups can be affected
- In adults, more common in females

Q. Classical lesion.

A.
- Asymptomatic or mildly pruritic, single or multiple, well defined closely set skin colored to erythematous papules arranged in an annular fashion, center of the lesion showing slight atrophy.
- Inverse koebnerization positive (injury causing healing).
- Average duration about 3 months to 2 years.

Q. Clinical variants.

A. Following variants are seen:
- Giant form
- Targetoid form
- Perforating granuloma
- Disseminated form
- Generalized GA
- Subcutaneous GA
- Malignancy associated GA

Q. What is Arcuate dermal erythema?

A. Arcuate dermal erythema: This is an uncommon form of granuloma annulare that manifests as infiltrated erythematous patches that may form large, hyperpigmented rings with central clearing.

Q. Associated condition.

A. DM, AIDS, internal malignancies, Mauriac's syndrome (poorly controlled type 1 diabetes mellitus), necrobiosis lipoidica, sarcoidosis, mycosis fungoides.

Q. Differential diagnosis.

A. Following conditions should be ruled out:
- Tuberculoid leprosy
- Lupus vulgaris
- Sarcoidosis
- Gumma
- Tinea circinata
- Erythema multiforme (for targetoid form)
- Rheumatic nodules (for subcutaneous GA)
- Lymphoma cutis (for disseminated GA)
- Erythema annulare centrifugum
- Tinea corporis

Q. Histopathology of GA.

A. Early interstitial or incomplete granuloma annulare lesions show an interstitial pattern characterized by lymphocytes around vessels of the superficial and deep plexuses and by macrophages scattered between reticular dermal collagen bundles that are separated by mucin within which mast cells may be found. Mucin in granuloma annulare is hyaluronic acid and is visible in sections stained with hematoxylin and eosin as faintly basophilic stringy material. Its presence can be confirmed by staining with colloidal iron or Alcian Blue at pH 2.5.

Q. Treatment.

A. Following treatment options:

- A skin biopsy can cause healing of lesion (inverse koebnerization).
- Corticosteroids
- Tacrolimus and pimecrolimus and imiquimod cream.
- Etretinate
- Isotretinoin
- Pentoxifylline
- Rifampin at 600 mg, ofloxacin at 400 mg, and minocycline hydrochloride at 100 mg monthly for 3 months (few studies in GA refractory to treatment)
- Potassium iodide
- Alkylating agents
- Chloroquine
- Hydroxychloroquine
- Niacinamide
- Cryotherapy
- Ultraviolet (UV) B, mostly narrowband UVB
- Photochemotherapy
- Lasers

Q. Role of pentoxifylline in GA.

A. The exact mechanism of action of pentoxifylline in granuloma annulare is not known. We postulate that, in granuloma annulare, pentoxifylline, probably with its tumor necrosis factor alpha (TNF-α) blocking action inhibits macrophage activation and hence the granulomatous inflammation. Moreover, with its anti-inflammatory action it may also reduce the vasculitis occurring in granuloma annulare.

Q. What is the recurrence rate of GA?

A.
- There is 40% recurrence rate. The recurrent lesions tend to occur at original sites, but clear more rapidly.

33 Hemangiomas

Q. Which is the most common benign vascular neoplasm of childhood?

A. Hemangioma of infancy (HOI-benign tumor of capillary endothelium).

Q. Prevalence of hemangioma.

A.
- 2–3% in neonates, 10% in infants. More in white races, more in premature babies.
- Mostly sporadic, rarely AD.

Q. Clinical subtypes of HOI.

A.
- Superficial (strawberry) 50–60%
- Deep (subcutaneous) 15%
- Mixed 25%

Q. What can a superficial HOI mimic?

A. Capillary malformations.

Q. How to different HOI and vascular malformations?

A.

HOI	*Vascular malformations*
Often not present at birth	Present at birth
Can grow out of proportion to child's growth	Grows in proportion to child's growth
Involute by 7–10 years	Do not involute
HP: Endothelial hyperplasia	HP: Normal endothelial cells
Doppler: High flow/normal flow	Doppler: Low flow or normal flow
GLUT (glucose uptake transponder) +	GLUT –

Q. What is the appearance/color of superficial HOI?

A. Bright red color with finely lobulated surface.

Q. What is the appearance of a deep HOI?

A. Soft skin colored to blue nodule with scattered telangiectasias.

Q. Discuss the natural history of hemangioma.

A.
- Hemangiomas can have a superficial, deep or both components.
- Very often precursor lesion is present at birth which are a cluster of telangiectasia or bluish gray macules.
- Later in the first 6 months of life, there is a proliferative phase, when the lesion are raised, well defined and nonblanchable, often surrounded by a zone of pallor
- The deep hemangiomas appear as compressible bluish nodules
- Mixed hemangiomas can have both these pictures.
- This proliferative phase is followed by a stable phase when the growth slows down and by 12 months most hemangiomas reach their maximum size.
- By about 18 months, hemangiomas start regressing. This is evidenced by grayish discoloration with softening and flattening.
- About 50% of hemangiomas involute by 5 years and 90% by 9 years.
- At least 20–50% will leave behind areas of scarring, atrophying fatty tissue.

Q. Are infantile hemangiomas present at birth?

A. Usually absent at birth, precursor lesions may be present at birth.

Q. How do the precursors look?

A. They can have a bruised appearance or can look like nevus anemicus or red telangiectatic patch.

Q. Problem with hemangioma on beard area.

A. It is associated with laryngeal hemangiomas.

Q. HOIs more common in which infants.

A.

Worrisome hemangiomas	***Why?***
Location	Complication/Risk
Beard hemangioma	Associated with laryngeal or subglottic hemangioma—obstruction, stridor
Around the mouth—perioral or anogenital	Ulceration, infection, scarring, feeding difficulty
Parotid, nose and lip	Can affect mandibular and external auditory canals (EAC)

Continued

Continued

Worrisome hemangiomas	*Why?*
Cervicofacial	PHACES syndrome
Lumbosacral	Dysraphism, tethering of the cord, renal involvement
Periorbital	Strabismus, astigmatism, amblyopia
Multiple (diffuse) hemangiomas	Visceral hemangiomas—liver, lung, brain, gastrointestinal tract (GIT)

Q. Acronymous hemangiomas.

A. • PHACES syndrome: Postcranial fossa abnormalities, hemangioma (segmental), arterial abnormalities, coarctation of aorta, eye abnormalities, spinal agensia
- PELVIS syndrome: Large Perianal hemangioma, external genitalia malformations, lipomyelomeningocoele, vesicorneal abnormalities, imperforate anus, skin tags
- RICH: Rapidly involuting congenital hemangiomas
- NICH: Noninvoluting congenital hemangiomas

Q. Histopathology of proliferating type.

A. • Endothelial cell hyperplasia
- Lobule formation
- Mast cells
- Prominent basement membrane
- Perineural invasion

Q. Histopathology of involuting type.

A. • Fibrofatty tissue replacement
- Decreased mast cells

Q. How does a hemangioma appear during involution?

A. Dull red or violaceous or gray color and softening of hemangioma.

Q. How do residues of hemangioma appear?

A. About 50% have normal skin; the other 50% show telangiectasias, atrophy, hypopigmentation fibrofatty deposition and if ulceration occurs then scarring.

Q. What are the segmental patterns of hemangiomas? (Topographical classification)

A. • S1: Frontotemporal
- S2: Maxillary prominence
- S3: Mandibular
- S4: Frontonasal

Q. Name complications of hemangiomas.

A.
- Obstruction of vital functions—seeing (vision), breathing, eating, urinating
- Ulceration followed by thrombosis, bleeding and infection
- High output cardiac failure
- Mutilation and scarring

Q. Most common complication.

A. Ulceration in diaper area.

Q. What is Kasabach–Merritt syndrome?

A. Platelet trapping and consumption coagulopathy, both associated with vascular tumor.

Q. Two vascular tumors associated with KMS (most commonly).

A. Kaposiform hemangioendothelioma and tufted angioma.

Q. Port wine stains and lymphangiomas are not neoplasms. What are they?

A. Vascular malformations.

Q. Are vascular malformations present at birth?

A. Yes, usually evident at birth.

Q. Do vascular birth marks involute or persist?

A.
- HOI: Spontaneous involution over years
- Vascular malformations: Persist into childhood and adulthood

Q. Where and in whom are cherry angiomas most commonly seen?

A. Cherry angiomas: 1.5 mm red to purple papules located primarily on the trunk and upper extremities commonly seen in the middle aged and elderly.

Q. What is cyrano nose?

A. Hemangioma of the tip of the nose is called cyrano nose which causes enlargement and obstruction of the nose and poor cosmetic outcome.

Q. Where do you find venous lakes?

A. Dark blue slightly raised papules on sun exposed skin surfaces of elderly patients most commonly on ears, lips and face.

Q. What is the most common presenting feature of pyogenic granuloma (PG)?

A. Pyogenic granulomas are 5–10 mm soft red papules that bleed easily with minor trauma Most commonly seen on skin; may also occur on mucous membranes or rarely blood vessels.

Q. What is granuloma gravidarum?
A. A variant of PG that occurs on gingiva during pregnancy.

Q. What are blue black hyperkeratotic vascular papules?
A. Angiokeratomas.

Q. Types of angiokeratoma.
A.
- Localized angiokeratoma—usually solitary found on extremity
- Angiokeratoma circumscriptum—unilateral plaques on extremity present at birth
- Angiokeratoma of Mibelli—dorsal surface of hands and feet develops in childhood or adolescence
- Angiokeratoma of Fordyce—common on scrotum
- Angiokeratoma corporis diffusum (Fabry disease)
- X-linked recessive disease resulting from deficiency of lysosomal enzyme and galactosidase. Accumulation of glycolipids in cells of various tissues

Q. Which benign acquired vascular disease is often initially confused with Kaposi's sarcoma?
A. Acroangiodermatitis (gravitational purpura)—eruption of purple macules, papules, plaques; usually associated with chronic venous insufficiency.

Q. What is Klippel-Trénaunay syndrome (KTS)?
A. Overgrowth of an extremity due to vascular malformation: Capillary (port wine stain), varicose veins and soft tissue and/or bony hypertrophy of extremity.

Q. What is Klippel-Trénaunay-Webber syndrome?
A. Same as KTS but with arteriovenous malformation.

Q. What is the biological classification of vascular birth marks?
A.
- Vascular tumors:
  - Infantile hemangioma
  - Congenital hemangioma
  - Kaposiform hemangioendothelioma
  - Tufted angioma
  - Spindle cell hemangioma
  - Pyogenic granuloma
  - Congenital hemangiopericytoma
- Vascular malformations:
  - Capillary malformations (slow flow)
  - Venous malformations (slow flow)

- ○ Typical/glomus cells
- ○ Arterial malformations
- ○ Lymphatic malformations (slow flow)
- ○ Macrocystic/microcystic
- ○ AV malformations (fast flow)
- ○ Combi malformations (slow flow)

Q. What vascular tumor is associated with Sucquet-Hoyer canal (SHC)?

A. Sucquet-Hoyer canal—arterial segment of glomus body and may give rise to glomus tumors.

Q. Where are angiolymphoid hyperplasia with eosinophilia lesions seen most commonly?

A. Clusters of grapes—head and neck (red brown papules).

Q. Which is the most prevalent tumor of infancy?

A. Hemangiomas of infancy.

Q. Histopathology of hobnail hemangioma.

A.
- Dilated blood vessels
- Big endothelial projection proceeds into vessel

Q. Treatment of hemangiomas.

A.
- Treatment is indicated for any infant for obstructive hemangiomas (airway, eye)
- Painful ulcerated hemangiomas
- Multiple hemangiomas
- Large hemangiomas
- Causing cardiac failure
- Hepatic hemangiomas
- Oral beta blockers: Propranolol (exert its effect by vasoconstriction of the blood vessels and also inhibit angiogenesis through inhibition of VEGF-A, matrix metalloproteins, suppressing renin production)
- Improvement seen within 24–48 hours of first dose
- Complete regression with in 6 months
- Dose: 2–3 mg/kg body weight in 3 divided doses
- Monitor: Blood glucose to prevent hypoglycemia
- Withheld the drug if there is wheezing or respiratory infection
- Follow-up: Monthly

Topical timolol:
- Strength: 0.25 and 0.5%
- Onset of action: Within 2 weeks

- %—6 months
- Under occlusion
- S/E: Sleep disturbance, psoriasiform lesions, urticaria
- Indications: Superficial hemangiomas and eyelid hemangiomas

Topical steroids:

- Stabilize the growth of hemangiomas but do not completely involute
- Acts on VEGF-A factor
- Dose: 2–3 mg/kg body weight

Steroids: Intralesional—periorbital hemangiomas

Systemic:

- Vincristine: Interferes with mitotic microtubules tumor cell apoptosis
- Severely complicated, HOI not responding to steroids
- IV weekly 0.5 mg/kg for 15 weeks
- 1 mg/m^2 for children
- Nearly 100% efficacy, regression in 3 weeks from starting treatment
- Side effects: Fatigue, alopecia, hematological toxicity, peripheral neuropathy
- Lasers: Flash pump pulsed-dye—superficial ulcerative hemangiomas, residual telangiectasia
- Nd:YAG laser: Periorbital hemangiomas

Q. Will you give propranolol in fibrofatty hamangiomas?

A. No, only laser or excision.

Q. What has to be done especially in perineal HOI?

A. If patient has perineal spreading hemangiomas, do pelvic MRI, spinal MRI even with no neurological symptoms.

Q. When will you give interferons?

A.
- Severely complicated, not responding to steroids.
- Interferon α: 2A + 2B (subcutaneous)—antiangiogenic
- 1–3 million units/m^2/day (no blood vessel formation).
- Fibroblast growth factor reduces: 6–12 months

Q. Most severe side effect of interferon alpha.

A. Spastic paralysis 10–30%.

Q. Commonest side effect of interferon alpha.
A. Fever, flu like symptoms (+hemat/hepat toxicity).

Q. Which laser works in hemangioma?
A. Pulse dye laser.

Q. What are the indications for surgery?
A.
- Pedunculated or exophytic HOI in which scarring is probable
- Ulcerated hemangiomas with severe pain
- Hemangiomas which lead to significant discrepancy
- Bleeding hemangiomas
- Nonregressing hemangiomas
- Laryngeal HOI

Q. When do you do late surgery?
A. To repair postregression residue.

Q. What is PHACES syndrome?
A.
- **P**: Posterior cranial fossa abnormalities
- **H**: Hemangioma (segmental)
- **A**: Arterial abnormalities
- **C**: Coarctation of the aorta
- **E**: Eye abnormalities
- **S**: Spinal agensia

Q. What is the PELVIS syndrome?
A.
- **P**: Large perianal hemangioma
- **E**: External genitilia malformations
- **L**: Lipomyelomeningocoele
- **V**: Vesicorneal abnormalities
- **I**: Imperforate anus
- **S**: Skin tag

Q. What is RICH and NICH?
A.
- RICH: Rapidly involuting congenital hemangioma
- NICH: Noninvoluting congenital hemangioma

Q. What is SACRAL?
A.
- **S**: Spinal dysraphism
- **A**: Anogenital anomalies
- **C**: Cutaneous abnormalities
- **R**: Renal and urologic anomalies
- **A and L**: Angioma of lumbosacral localization

Q. What is LUMBAR?

A.
- **L**: Lower body hemangioma
- **U**: Urogenital abnormalities
- **M**: Myelopathy
- **B**: Bony deformities
- **A**: Anorectal malformations; arterial anomalies
- **R**: Renal anomalies

Q. What are the other strawberries in dermatology?

A.
- Strawberry hemangioma seen in infantile hemangioma
- Strawberry tongue seen in Kawasaki's disease
- Strawberry cervix—*Trichomonas vaginalis*

34 Hailey–Hailey Disease

Q. Who were Hailey and Hailey?

A. Two brothers Howard and Hugh Hailey who described the disease first.

Q. Why is it a case of Hailey–Hailey?

A. Lesions start as flaccid vesicle which ruptures and gives rise to crusted erosions. Lesions are present in intertriginous areas (axilla and groins), perianal region. Malodorous vegetations are present. Nail involvement in form of longitudinal leuconychia. Lesions heal with hyperpigmentation. No scarring present. Pruritus—moderate to severe.

Q. What is the other name of Hailey–Hailey?

A. Benign familial chronic pemphigus.

Q. Why do you get Hailey–Hailey?

A.
- Keratinocytes are held together through desmosomes and adherens junctions. An overall defect in keratinocyte adhesion appears to be secondary to a primary defect in a calcium pump protein, ATP2C1.
- ATP2C1 encodes the secretory pathway Ca^{2+}/Mn^{2+}-ATPase (hSPCA1)

Q. What are the exacerbating factors?

A.
- Infections (including scabies)
- Heat
- Sweating
- Friction
- Pregnancy
- Menstruation
- Drugs like NSAID and efalizumab
- Sun exposure

Q. What are the uncommon presentations of Hailey–Hailey?

A.
- Facial lesions due to koebnerization on acne lesions
- Perianal lesions mimicking condylomata acuminata
- Psoriasiform lesions
- Lesions on non-intertriginous lesions

Q. What are the rare forms?

A.
- Type 1 segmental—due to postzygotic genetic mutations-localized unilateral blistering eruptions
- Type 2 segmental Hailey-Hailey—earlier age of onset and is more generalized due to loss of heterozygosity. Lesions are both segmental and nonsegmental. Adnexal involvement maybe seen.

Q. Dermoscopic findings of Hailey-Hailey.

A. Irregular pink and white areas are seen with pink furrows and polymorphous vessels.

Q. What is the differential diagnosis of Hailey-Hailey disease?

A.

Disease	*Clinical features*
Hailey–Hailey	Usually starts in third to fourth decade. Lesions in intertriginous areas, flaccid vesicles and blisters which become plaques and vegetation
Erythrasma	Middle aged diabetics. Inguinal axillary and interdigital folds. Well defined reddish brown plaques. Central clearing—rare
Tinea cruris	Any age. Annular plaques with central clearing. Peripheral borders may show vesicles and pustules
Candidiasis	Obese, diabetic. Axillary and inframammary areas. Erythematous plaques and pustules. Satellite pustules common
Acanthosis nigricans	Usually in obese people. Velvety plaques in axillary inguinal and cubital area. Usually nonpruritic
Seborrheic dermatitis	Usually older age groups. Erythematous with greasy scales. Scalp often involved
Atopic dermatitis	Lesions associated with pigmentation and lichenification. Highly pruritic
Inverse/Flexural psoriasis	Variable age. Sharply demarcated nonscaly erythematous plaques in any flexural areas
Darier's disease	Childhood onset. Intertriginous folds rarely. Nails and oral mucosa commonly involved. Greasy keratotic papules. Bullae and vesicles are rare. Foul odor

Continued

Continued

Disease	***Clinical features***
Pemphigus vegetans	Fourth and fifth decade. Intertriginous folds commonly involved. Starts as flaccid bullae or vesicles which rupture to form vegetative plaques. Foul odor
Granular parakeratosis	Variable age. Erythematous papules and plaques common in the axilla. No nail or mucous involvement
Fox–Fordyce disease	Almost exclusively in young females. Axilla show flat-topped papules with loss of hair. Highly pruritic
Galli–Galli disease	Variable age. Flexural involvement. Reticulate hyper pigmentation with erythematous macules and papules
Subcorneal pustular dermatosis (SCPD)	Middle aged. Obese females. Flaccid pustules with erosions in intertriginous area, Hypopyon sign present

Q. What is the course of Hailey–Hailey?

A. The course is characterized by exacerbations more in summer and remissions. Lesions rarely, subside on their own. The severity of the disease decreases with increasing age.

Q. What are the complications of Hailey–Hailey?

A.
- Infections—secondary bacterial infections, fungal and viral infections (Kaposi's varicelliform eruption)
- Poor wound healing.
- There are a few case reports of squamous cell carcinoma.

Q. What is the histopathology of Hailey–Hailey?

A. There is extensive but incomplete acantholysis in epidermis giving 'Dilapidated brick wall' appearance. Dermal papillae lined by single layer of basal cells protrude into blister cavities and are referred to as 'villi'. There is moderate perivascular infiltrate present in the superficial dermis.

Q. How will you manage a case of Hailey–Hailey?

A. General measures:
- Patient is advised to wear lightweight clothes to avoid friction and sweating
- Avoid occlusive and adhesive dressings.

- Microbial infections should be prevented and treated with Soothing compresses (aluminum acetate 1:40 dilution), povidone iodine and chlorhexidine.
- *Treatment of secondary infections*:
  - Topical therapy:
    - Topical steroids
    - Calcineurin inhibitors
    - Topics 5-FU—3 times a week for 1st 3 months and then once a week further.
    - Topical vitamin D twice daily
    - Cadexomer iodine topical
    - Topical aminoglycosides like gentamicin
  - Oral:
    - Dapsone—100 mg starting. Maintaining 50 mg
    - Doxycycline or minocycline 100 mg bd for 2 weeks f/b lower doses by further few months
    - Terbinafine 250 mg bd for 4 weeks
    - Penicillin, cephalexin, erythromycin
- Also, oral retinoids (acitretin), oral steroids—prednisolone, oral immunosuppressants (MTX, thalidomide, etanercept)
- Injections of botulinum toxin A can also be given
- In nonresponsive cases:
  - CO_2 or Erbium-doped yttrium-aluminum-garnet (Er:YAG) laser or pulsed dye laser
  - Also, photodynamic therapy with aminolevulinic acid (ALA).

Q. Newer therapies.

A.
- Oral vitamin D 800 IU daily
- Oral magnesium chloride 300 mg daily
- Oral Naltrexone 400 mg daily
- Oral Apremilast 30 mg daily
- Oral anticholinergic: Oxybutynin
- Subcutaneous alpha melantotide 60 mg sc.
- UVB therapy has also been tried

35 Halo Nevi

Q. What is a halo nevus?

A. It is a nevus with distinguishing feature of a surrounding hypochromic or achromic feature.

Q. What are the synonyms of halo nevus?

A. It is also known as Sutton nevus, perinevoid vitiligo and leukoderma acquisitum centrifugum.

Q. Describe the lesion of halo nevus.

A. The lesions are characterized by pigmented nevus, with a surrounding depigmented zone. Halo nevi tend to occur most frequently on the trunk, mostly in teenagers. The central nevus gradually loses its pigmentation, turns pink and then disappears. Over time, the area repigments. Darkening of the central nevus than lightening can be seen in association with halo phenomenon.

Q. What are the stages of evolution of halo nevus?

A. There are four stages in halo nevus evolution, which occurs over a period of months to ≥10 years:

- *Stage I*: Contains a central pigmented nevus outlined by a circular or oval hypo- or depigmented area;
- *Stage II*: The central nevus loses its color resulting in a pink-colored papule surrounded by the halo;
- *Stage III*: The central papule disappears and the depigmentation remains;
- *Stage IV*: Shows a partial or complete re-pigmentation of the skin.

Q. What are the lab diagnosis seen in halo nevus?

A. The infiltrate contains cytotoxic T-cells, and may represent immunologically induced rejection. The peripheral blood has also been shown to contain activated adhesive lymphocytes that disappear when the lesion is excised. Antibodies against melanocytes and cell mediated immunity to melanoma has also been demonstrated.

Q. What are the other lesions that can be seen with leukoderma?

A. Blue nevi and neurofibroma.

Q. What is the histology of halo nevi?

A. It demonstrates band of lymphocytes that extends throughout the lesion, intimately mingling with the melanocytes. The lymphoid infiltrate associated with melanoma tend to aggregate at the periphery of the lesion. Term Meyerson's nevus has been applied to eczematous change associated with a nevus. Hypopigmentation may be present.

Q. Name the other eponymous nevi.
(*source*: Our dermatology Online 2012) (alphabetically)

A.
- Clark's nevus—atypical, melanocytic nevi. It can overlap with dysplastic nevi which has a higher incidence of melanoma.
- Tièche-Jadassohn nevus—blue nevi
- Masson's nevus—the nevi cells have a spindle shaped (neuroid) appearance
- Meyerson's nevus—inflammations around the nevus. Sometimes it has a target like appearance called cockade nevus. sometimes such nevi has areas of hyperpigmentation. This is called as Bolognia sign.
- Miescher's nevus—this presents as firm brown dome shaped papule in which nevus cells project deep into the dermis. (endophytic arrangement)
- Nevus of Ito—dermal melanocytes nevi
- Nevus of Nanta—presence of ossification in the nevus cells
- Nevus of Ota—dermal melanocytes nevi
- Pointillist nevus—multiple variegated dots on the nevi
- Reed's nevus—pigmented spindle like cells of nevus
- Spitz nevus—spindle like epithelioid cells Kamino bodies
- Unna's nevus—soft exophytic bodies found on trunk and extremities.

Q. Treatment.

A. Ignore or excise.

36 Henoch–Schönlein Purpura

Q. Why is this Henoch-Schönlein purpura (HSP)?

A. Palpable purpura over the lower limbs and buttocks associated with abdominal pain, diarrhea, and polyarthralgia.

Q. Differential diagnosis (D/D) of HSP.

A.
- Subsiding drug rash
- Erythema multiforme
- Subsiding erythema nodosum
- Viral exanthem
- Idiopathic thrombocytopenic purpura
- Disseminated intravascular coagulation
- Subacute bacterial endocarditis

Q. What is Henoch's purpura?

A. Purpura with abdominal pain.

Q. What is Schönlein's purpura?

A. Purpura with arthritis.

Q. What is HSP?

A. It is small vessel vasculitis involving skin, joint, gastrointestinal tract and kidneys. There is IgA mediated vasculitis.

Q. Triad of HSP.

A.
- Palpable purpura
- Joint pain
- Abdominal pain

Q. What are the causes of HSP?

A.
- Infections: Epstein–Barr virus (EBV), varicella virus, parvovirus B19, *Campylobacter, Bartonella henselae*
- Vaccination: Typhoid, cholera, measles, yellow fever
- Drugs: Penicillin, aspirin, macrolides

Q. What are the clinical features of HSP?

A.
- Common in children in age group of 5–15 years
- Palpable purpura over the lower limbs and buttocks. Urticarial wheals, necrotic, bullous and hemorrhagic lesions also occur.

Skin lesions heal in 5 days. Associated with abdominal pain, diarrhea and polyarthralgia. Edema of the hands, feet, scalp and ears.

- Arthritis, most commonly involving the knees and ankles
- Abdominal tenderness
- Gastrointestinal bleeding
- Acute scrotal edema that may mimic testicular torsion

Q. What is the dreaded complication of HSP?

A. Renal involvement in form of proteinuria, hematuria, RBC casts.

Q. What are other names of HSP?

A.
- Anaphylactoid purpura
- Purpura rheumatica

Q. Histopathology of HSP.

A.
- Leukocytoclastic vasculitis features
- Small blood vessels (postcapillary venules) are infiltrated with neutrophils that show fragmented nuclei
- Swelling and fibrinoid degeneration of vascular walls
- Extravasation of RBC

Q. What are complications of HSP?

A. Henoch–Schönlein purpura can have complications which generally occur more frequently in children than in adults. These complications include severe abdominal pain and gastrointestinal bleeding. Adults can have extended kidney problems.

Q. What is the prognosis of HSP?

A.
- Henoch–Schönlein purpura is generally a benign disease with an excellent prognosis.
- More than 80% of patients have a single isolated episode lasting a few weeks
- Approximately 10–20% of patients have recurrences
- Fewer than 5% of patients develop chronic HSP
- Abdominal pain resolves spontaneously within 72 hours in most patients

Q. What is the variant of HSP in infancy and early childhood?

A. Acute hemorrhagic edema of infancy (Finkelstein's disease). Here there is facial edema and also targetoid lesions on extremities.

Q. Treatment of HSP.

A.
- HSP is benign and self limiting
- Rest and observation is needed

- Dapsone 50–200 mg/day, colchicine 0.6 mg/day, systemic steroids, IVIG are given for refractory cases
- Nonsteroidal anti-inflammatory drugs (NSAIDs) may help joint pain and do not seem to worsen the purpura. However, NSAIDs should be used cautiously in patients with renal insufficiency
- For abdominal pain, H2 blockers or systemic steroid (prednisolone 1 mg/kg) cyclophosphamide and dipyridamole can be used
- Other regimens include steroids/azathioprine, and steroids/cyclophosphamide (with or without heparin and warfarin)

37 Herpes Simplex Virus

Q. Enumerate all the herpes viruses.

A.
- Alpha *Herpesviridae*:
  - HSV-1, HSV-2, HSV-3
- Gamma *Herpesviridae*:
  - EBV (HSV-4), HSV-8
- Beta *Herpesviridae*:
  - Cytomegalovirus (HSV-5), HSV-6, HSV-7

Q. Historical aspects of herpes simplex virus (HSV).

A.
- The word Herpes means to creep or crawl.
- Lipschitz was first to suggest antigen differences between HSV-1 and HSV-2
- Hippocrates and Gallan have also described herpetic lesions.

Q. What are the clinical features of herpes simplex infection?

A. The characteristic lesions of herpes infection are grouped vesicles on an erythematous base filled with clear fluid which break down to form superficial erosions with characteristic scalloped borders. Sometimes only erosions or ulcerations are seen especially in herpetic gingivostomatitis.

Q. What is the differential diagnosis of herpes infection?

A.
- Genital herpes has to be differentiated from chancre, chancroid, mucus membrane pemphigus, candidiasis
- Oral herpes has to be differentiated from erosive or ulcerative lichen planus, erythema multiforme, streptococcal infections, mucus membrane pemphigus, aphthae, oral candidiasis, Behçet's disease.

Q. What are the type of herpes simplex virus?

A. Types of HSV viruses are HSV-1 and HSV-2. HSV-1 (Herpes labialis) is more common, 30–95% adults are seropositive for HSV-1 whereas HSV-2 (genital herpes) is less common, seroprevalence, as it appears at the age of onset of sexual activity, antibody to HSV-2 rarely found prior to adolescence.

Q. Epidemiology of HSV infection.

A. Children less than the age of 10 years get asymptomatic infection of HSV-1 type (80–90%). Up to 90% of adults have HSV-1 (20–40 years) and 70–90% of genital herpes infection in HSV-2.

Q. What is the mode of HSV transmission?

A. HSV-1 infection occurs through contaminated saliva and through direct contact and HSV-2, through sexual contact. Virus replicates at the site of infection (mucocutaneous) travels to dorsal root ganglia and establishing latency until reaction.

Q. What is primary HSV infection?

A. Primary infection refers to individuals who are exposed to the HSV virus for the 1st time, either type 1 or 2 at any site these patients are seronegative initially but subsequently develop HSV-specific antibodies.

Q. What about recurrent infection?

A. Recurrent HSV infection represents reactivation of the latent virus in the sensory ganglia "reactivated" virus particles migrate back along the nerves to the site in the skin where the primary infection occurred with subsequent viral replication and the development of the clinical lesions. The most common sites for recurrent herpes simplex infections are the lip (herpes labialis, cold sores), genitalial and sacral area.

Q. What is the difference between a primary and an initial HSV infection?

A. When an individual without preexisting antibodies to either HSV-1 or HSV-2 develops an infection with herpes (either type 1 or 2), it is referred to as primary infection. When an individual with preexisting antibodies to one type HSV then experiences an infection with the other HSV type, it is referred as the initial (or initial, nonprimary) infection.

Q. Define asymptomatic shedding.

A. In some cases recurrent infection, clinical lesions may not be visible, but virus can be covered if the skin or mucosal site is cultured and the virus can be transmitted to another person, the host immune response is believed to eliminate the focus of virus before full-fledged recurrence develops. Patient should be counselled regarding this.

Q. How long is HSV incubation period, the time from initial infection to appearance of the vesicles?

A. The time between exposure and development of primary disease is estimated to be 3–14 days.

Q. How is Tzanck smear performed?

A. In a Tzanck smear, the base of the suspected herpetic lesion is gently scraped, and the skin or mucosal cells removed are placed on a glass slide. The cells are stained and then examined by light microscopy for evidence of viral-induced cytologic change including the characteristics multinucleated giant cells. The technique cannot distinguish HSV from VZV.

Q. What is the histopathological features in herpes?

A.
- Epidermis-ballooning of cytoplasm of keratinocytes (earliest histopathological findings). Nuclei shows degeneration and margination if chromatin to form intranuclear inclusion bodies. Infected keratinocytes fuse and form multinucleate giant cells. Spongiosis +. Intracellular edema forms thick walled vesicles
- Dermis—dense infiltration of leukocytes, neutrophils and eosinophils +++

Q. Who gets herpetic whitlow?

A. Herpetic whitlow (HSV infection of the hand or fingers) was previously considered a disease of healthcare professionals which occurred as a result of contact with infected patients. In fact, as few as 10% of individuals with this disorder fall in that category. The remaining cases are seen in children and young adults and result from autoinoculation from another site of infection. In children the etiologic agent is generally HSV-1 while in adults its HSV-2.

Q. What is Kaposi's varicelliform eruption?

A. Eczema herpeticum, or Kaposi's varicelliform eruption, is an extensive, disseminated cutaneous infection with HSV occurs most commonly in patients with atopic dermatitis although it may also be associated with other dermatoses such as Darier's disease, pemphigus, severe Seborrheic dermatitis and psoriasis. Antiviral therapy is beneficial in this process.

Q. Can a baby get herpes? Is it a serious problem?

A. Neonatal herpes is one of the most critical problems associated with the increased incidence of genital herpes. Herpes infection is the neonatal period can be and often is devastating because of the inadequate immune response seen in neonates. In most cases, transmission of HSV to the neonate occurs by delivery through an infected birth canal. Postpartum acquisition occurs less commonly. Development of primary or initial nonprimary genital herpes by the mother at or near the time of delivery poses a significant risk for the infant, however most cases of neonatal herpes are the result of asymptomatic shedding in women with no history of genital herpes. The usual onset of neonatal herpes is 2–12 days following exposure. Approximately 80% of infected neonates have the least some characteristic skin lesions.

Q. What is herpetic sycosis?

A. It is the infection of the hair follicle. There are few eroded follicular papules or extensive lesions involving the beard area.

Q. What is herpes gladiatorum?

A. It is seen in wrestlers and boxers who are susceptible to HSV-1 infection and who come in contact with the infected individual with an active disease. The sites are lateral side of the neck, side of the face and forehead. Any wrestler with history of orolabial herpes should be put on suppressive therapy.

Q. Treatment of primary episode of HSV.

A.
- Acyclovir (ACV) 200 mg PO 5 times a day or 400 mg tid for 10 days.
- Valacyclovir (VAL) 1 g PO bid for 10 days
- Famciclovir (FAM) 250 mg PO tid for 5–10 days

Q. Treatment for recurrent episodes of HSV infection.

A.
- ACV 200 mg PO 5 times/day or 400 mg tid for 5–7 days
- VAL 500 mg PO for 5 days
- FAM 125 mg PO bid for 5 days

Q. What is the suppressive therapy for HSV infection?

A.
- ACV 200–400 mg bd
- VAL 500–1000 mg qd
- FAM 125–250 mg bid

Q. What is the treatment of HSV infection in immunosuppressed patients?

A.
- Primary/initial infection ACV 5–10 mg/kg IV q8h. If not severe 400 mg PO 5 times/dsy for 7–14 days
- VAL 1 g PO tid for 7 days
- FAM 500 mg PO bid for 7 days
- Suppressive therapy ACV 400–800 mg PO tid VAL 1 g PO tid
- FAM 500 mg PO bid.

Q. Histology of herpes simplex virus.

A.
- Enlarged slate gray keratinocyte nuclei with margination of chromatin.
- Acantholytic with distinct nuclei inclusions.

- Intraepidermal vesiculation with ballooning degeneration of keratinocytes.
- Multinucleated giant cells with eosinophilic intranuclear inclusion bodies (cowdry type A inclusions)
- Late epidermal necrosis or full thickness acantholysis.
- Epidermal necrosis, hemorrhagic necrosis, perivascular cuffing in the dermis.
- Perineural infiltration of lymphocytes and neutrophils in the dermis

Q. Laboratory tests for diagnosis of herpes simplex virus infection.

- Viral culture
- Direct fluorescence antibody assays
- Molecular techniques (PCR—more rapid, sensitive and specific for HSV DNA).
- Serology (Western blot—Gold standard).

Q. Complications of herpes simplex.

A.
- Skin complications:
  - Eczema herpeticum
  - Herpetic whitlow (involvement of the fingers)
  - Herpes gladiatorum
- Visceral infections—prostatitis, salpingitis, cervicitis.
- CNS involvement:
  - Aseptic meningitis
  - Ganglionitis and myelitis
  - Herpes simplex encephalitis
- Pregnancy complications:
  - Neonatal infection leading to uterine growth retardation and Premature birth
- Neonatal disease
- Increased risk of HIV infection
- Ocular infections:
  - Conjunctivitis
- Bacterial and fungal infection
- Recurrence

HERPES ZOSTER

Q. Why herpes zoster?

A. It is a localized eruption characterized by unilateral radicular pain and vesicles on an erythematous base limited to the dermatome innervated by a single spinal or cranial nerve sensory ganglion.

Q. What is the differential diagnosis?

A.
- HSV infection
  - H/O recurrent lesions at the same site
- Contact dermatitis
  - Direct fluorescent antibody (DFA) is negative and no multinucleated epithelial giant cells on Tzanck smear
- Bacterial infection
  - DFA is negative and no multinucleated epithelial giant cells on Tzanck smear.
- Insect bite and blister beetle bite (*Paederus*) dermatitis

Q. Causative organism.

A. It is caused by reactivation of varicella zoster virus.

Q. What is the meaning of herpes and zoster?

A. Herpes—to creep and zoster-girdle.

Q. How will you identify the level of involvement?

A.
- C4—at the clavicle
- T4—at the nipple
- T10—at the umbilicus
- L1—at the genitalia

Q. What is the etiopathogenesis?

A.
- During the course of the disease, varicella zoster virus passes from the lesions in the skin and mucosal surface into ending of sensory nerves and is transported centripetally up the sensory fibers to sensory ganglia where it remains latent in ganglia. Subclinical reactivation occurs in immunocompromised individuals. Clinical manifestation arises when the virus is reactivated. The newly synthesized virus is transported to the skin. There is unilateral vesicular eruption of one or two dermatomes along distribution of sensory nerves. Reactivation is triggered by trauma, sunburn, stress and old age.
- Spread of infection along the posterior nerve root to the meninges and the cord results in local leptomeningitis, cerebrospinal fluid pleocytosis and segmental myelitis.

Q. What are the clinical manifestations?

A.
- Prodromal symptoms such as fever, malaise, paresthesia, dysesthesia, pruritus, tingling, tenderness, intense pain before lesion erupt.
- The pre-eruptive pain of herpes zoster simulates pleurisy, myocardial infarction, duodenal ulcer, cholecystitis. Pruritus, tenderness, tingling or hyperesthesia are also seen.

- A few patient experience acute segmental neuralgia without ever developing a cutaneous eruption (zoster sine herpete). This is common with HIV patients.
- The rash is usually unilateral, dermatomal and does not cross the midline (but about 1 finger overlap can be seen in midline due to overlapping of nerves).
- The time between start of pain and onset of rash averages 1–3 days in trigeminal herpes zoster and 2–3 days of thoracic disease. Closely grouped red papules, appearing in continuous or interrupted band, rapidly become vesicular and then pustular. New vesicles continue to appear for days.
- The mucous membrane of affected dermatome is also involved. The lymph nodes in the affected area are also enlarged and tender.
- The area supplied by trigeminal area, particularly the ophthalmic division and trunk from T3 to L2 are mostly affected. The dermatome involved are thoracic 53%, cervical 4–20%, trigeminal including ophthalmic and lumbosacral 11%
- Ramsay–Hunt syndrome: From reactivation of the infection in the geniculate ganglion leading to involvement of facial and auditory nerves leading to facial palsy in the combination of vesicles in external ear with or without tinnitus, tongue (causes taste loss in anterior 2/3rd) and hard palate, dry mouth and eyes, vertigo and deafness.
- Immunocompromised patients may have usual course of disease or they may develop recurrent and severe disease which is prolonged and atypical, e.g., hyperkeratotic papules, bullous, ecthymatous lesions, lichenoid papules and follicular papules. Disseminated lesions (defined as >20 lesions outside the area of involvement) or visceral involvement is seen in 10% of patients.
- Chronic herpes zoster is characterized by long standing single or multiple pox-like lesions with periods of exacerbation and regression. It is usually associated with acyclovir resistance.
- Transplacental transmission of varicella zoster virus does not occur with maternal herpes zoster.

Q. What are the complications associated with herpes zoster?

A. Most patients recover from it without any complication.

- The complication may be cutaneous, ocular, visceral and neurologic.

- The cutaneous complications include bacterial infection, scarring, Ramsay-Hunt syndrome, zoster gangrenosum and cutaneous dissemination
- Visceral complication such as pneumonitis, hepatitis, esophagitis, pericarditis, gastritis, cystitis, arthritis.
- Neurological complications include postherpetic neuralgia, meningoencephalitis, transverse myelitis, peripheral cranial nerve palsies, deafness and ocular complications.
- Multidermatomal, disseminated herpes zoster tend to have higher complication rate.

Q. Gold standard for diagnosis or HSV infection.

A. Viral culture.

Q. What is postherpetic neuralgia?

A.
- It's the commonest complication defined as recurrence or persistence of pain in the affected area for a month after the lesion have healed. It frequently, affects patients above 60 years. Other risk factors are presence of severe pain, greater rash severity. It remits spontaneously.
- The pain has 2 forms—a continuous and spasmodic shooting type. The healed lesions may become hyperesthetic causing severe pain on light touch and even on contact with clothes (allodynia). In addition to pain, patient may complain of severe pruritis, dysesthesia, anesthesia.

Q. What are the ocular complications?

A. Involvement of nasociliary branch of fifth cranial may lead to ocular complication. This may be suspected when Hutchinson's sign is positive, which is involvement of the tip or the sides of nose with herpes zoster. Corneal damage and retinal artery occlusion leading to blindness.

Q. What are the dermatological complications?

A. Bacterial infection in affected dermatome is the commonest complication. Necrotizing fasciitis, herpes gangrenosum, keloid and pigmentary changes of dermatome are also seen.

Q. How do you diagnose herpes zoster?

A. History, physical examination and Tzanck smear (multinucleated giant cell) are usually done. DFA, viral culture, serology, PCR and biopsy may also be done to rule out herpes zoster.

Q. What is treatment of herpes zoster?

A.
- Antiviral agents like acyclovir 800 mg five times a day, valacyclovir (1 g thrice a day) or famciclovir 500 mg tds for 7–10 days.
- The duration of treatment is longer in immune compromized patient and depends on clinical response. The drug should be administered within 48–72 hours after appearance of rash.
- For postherpetic neuralgia, temporary relief by application of cold water or ice cubes. Topical lignocaine patches or local infiltration of lignocaine, topical capsaicin, gabapentin, pregabalin, oral analgesics and anti inflammatory drugs may provide relief in mild to moderate cases. In severe or persistant pain, systemic therapy with tricyclic antidepressants like amitriptyline 25–75 g day, antiepileptics like carbmazepine (600 mg to 1,000 g) or phenytoin (300 mg/day). Combination of antiepileptics and antidepressants are also useful. The live attenuated varicella vaccine has been approved by FDA as a prophylaxis for persons of 60 years and above without history of herpes zoster.

Q. Vaccines useful in herpes zoster.

A.
- Live attenuated zoster vaccine
- Adjuvanted glycoprotein E subunit zoster vaccine

38 Hidradenitis Suppurativa

Q. What is hidradenitis suppurativa?

A. It is a chronic inflammatory disease believed to be due to occlusion of hair follicles (not of apocrine glands) characterized by double (sister) comedones, deep sinuses and abscesses and clinically characterized by painful subcutaneous nodules. It is more common in females and improves in pregnancy.

Q. What are the other names of HS?

A. Apocrine acne, acne inversa, apocrinitis, Verneuil's disease, pyoderma fistulans significa.

Q. Differential diagnosis.

A.
- Chronic furunculosis
- Scrofuloderma
- Cutaneous Crohn's disease
- Mycetoma
- Donovanosis
- Elephantiasis nostras verrucosa cutis.

Q. Can HS be seen in children?

A. HS starts at or after puberty. Children are not affected unless they develop precocious puberty.

Q. What are the sites of HS?

A. Axilla, groins, inframammary, inguinal, perianal, periareolar and posterior auricular.

Q. What is Hurley's classification?

A.
- *Stage 1*: Abscess formation but without sinuses or scarring.
- *Stage 2*: One or more widely separated abscess with sinuses and scarring.
- *Stage 3*: Multiple interconnected abscess with sinuses involving the entire area.

Q. What is follicular occlusion triad and tetrad?

A.
- *Triad*: Hidradenitis suppurativa, acne conglobata and dissecting cellulitis of the scalp
- *Tetrad*: HS, acne conglobata, dissecting cellulitis of scalp and pilonidal sinus.

Q. What are the conditions associated with HS?

A.
- *Common*: Obesity, Crohn's disease
- *Rare*: Acanthosis nigricans, Fox Fordyce, KID syndrome, pachyonychia congenita, Dowling-Degos, SAPHO and PAPA syndrome.

Q. What are the complications of HS?

A. Strictures, fistulae, scarring, anemia, malnutrition, cutaneous SCC, sacral osteomyelitis, lumbosacral abscess and cutaneous amyloidosis.

Q. What is the treatment of HS?

A.
- *Topical*: Topical antibiotics like clindamycin
- *Systemic treatment*: Oral tetracycline, rifampicin, minocycline, dapsone, isotretinoin, acitretin (high doses), cyproterone acetate and ethinyl estradiol, finasteride (high doses), low dose steroids, cyclosporine, biologicals like infliximab, etanercept, botulinum toxin, radiotherapy and light therapy
- *Surgical*:
  - Radical excision—perianal and axillary areas shows good results
  - Incision and drainage—opening of sinuses and allowing them to heal by secondary intention
    - Approach:
      - Stage1—systemic antibiotics + ILS
      - Stage 2—long term immunosuppressive therapy and limited surgical treatment
      - Stage 3—wide surgical excision of skin, radiation therapy and immunosuppressive therapy.

39 Ichthyosis

Q. Definition.

A. Disorder of keratinization resulting from abnormal epidermal differentiation or metabolism.

Q. Word derivation.

A. Ichthys = fish (greek); because disease is characterized by fish-like scales.

Q. Classification.

A.
- Congenital ichthyosis
- Acquired ichthyosis
- Ichthyosiform syndromes

Q. Classify congenital ichthyosis.

A. Classified as follows:
- Autosomal dominant:
  - Ichthyosis vulgaris
  - Bullous ichthyosiform erythroderma
  - Ichthyosis bullosa of Siemens
- Autosomal recessive:
  - Lamellar ichthyosis
  - Nonbullous ichthyosiform erythroderma
- X-linked—X-linked recessive ichthyosis.

Q. Classify acquired ichthyosis.

A.
- Malignancy associated—Hodgkin's lymphoma, multiple myeloma, solid organ malignancy
- Infections—leprosy, AIDS
- Metabolic—malnutrition, renal failure
- Endocrine disorders—diabetes, hypothyroidism
- Connective tissue disorder—SLE, dermatomyositis
- Granulomatous disorder—sarcoidosis
- Drug induced—statins, clofazimine, cimetidine.

Q. Name ichthyosiform syndromes?

A. BIDS syndrome, KID syndrome, CHILD syndrome, Netherton's syndrome, Refsum's disease, Sjögren-Larsson syndrome.

Q. Differentiate between three major types of congenital ichthyosis?

A.

Features	***Icthyosis vulgaris***	***X- linked recessive icthyosis***	***Lamellar icthyosis***
Synonyms	Ichthyosis simplex, autosomal dominant ichthyosis	Steroid sulfatase deficiency	Nonerythrodermic autosomal recessive lamellar ichthyosis, ichthyosis congenita type 2
Pathogenesis	Histidine reduced, defective filaggrin	Steroid sulfatase deficiency, corneocyte retention	Tg 1 mutation, deficient cell to cell cross linking
Onset	After 3 months of life	Within 3 months of life	At birth
Sites involved	Extensors more involved	Flexors involved	Flexors, palms and soles
Type of scale	Dry skin, fine white flaky scales, pasted on large scales	Smaller darker brown adherent scales, dirty neck appearance. Periauricular involvement is characteristic	Large quadrilateral, brown scales free at edges, stuck in center
Associated/ special feature	Hyperkeratosis of palms and soles, associated keratosis pilaris	Only in males. Extracutaneous features like cryptorchidism, corneal opacities	Most babies encased in collodion membrane. Dry shiny facial skin, ectropion, sometimes maceration over flexures, nails involved. Heat intolerance
Course/ prognosis:	Improves with age	Does not improve with age	Remains lifelong
Histopathology	Hyperkeratosis, follicular plugging, hypogranulosis	Stratum corneum thickening, hypergranulosis infiltrate	Hyperkeratosis, hypergranulosis, mitotic figures
Treatment	Emollients, urea, salicylic acid, ammonium lactate	Oral retinoids, emollients, urea, propylene glycol	MTX, isotretinoin, calcipotriol, salicylic acid, emollients

Q. Synonym of bullous ichthyosiform erythroderma.

A. Epidermolytic hyperkeratosis.

Q. Extracutaneous findings.

A.
- Intellectual disability
- Microcephaly
- Ataxia
- Di or tetraplegia
- Cataract
- Corneal opacity
- Anosmia
- Neonatal respiratory distress
- Cardiac defects
- Hepatomegaly
- Chronic diarrhea
- Elevated IgE
- Hearing impairment
- Neuropathy, myopathy
- Stippled epiphyses
- Hypogonadism/Cryptorchidism

Q. BIDS syndrome.

A. **B** – Brittleness of hair
I – Ichthyosis
D – Decreased fertility
S – Short stature

Q. KID syndrome.

A. **K** – Keratosis
I – Ichthyosis
D – Deafness

Q. CHILD syndrome.

A. **C** – Congenital
H – Hemidysplasia
I – Ichthyosiform erythroderma
L – Limb
D – Defects

40 Idiopathic Guttate Hypomelanosis

Q. What is idiopathic guttate hypomelanosis?

A. It is a common acquired condition seen in elderly of both the sexes most common in females, characterized by asymptomatic hypomelanotic to amelanotic macules all over the body. It is a common sign of aging.

Q. What is the other name for idiopathic guttate hypomelanosis?

A. Leukopathia symmetrica progressiva.

Q. Describe the clinical appearance of idiopathic guttate hypomelanosis.

A. Individual lesions are small hypopigmented to depigmented macules averagely 2 to 5 mm in size distributed chiefly on the shin and forearms. The average number is between 10 to 30. They spare face and trunk regions. The lesions are irregularly shaped and very sharply defined like depigmented ephelides.

Q. What is the histology of idiopathic guttate hypomelanosis?

A.
- Epidermal atrophy and reduced number of hypoactive melanocytes
- Flattening of dermal-epidermal junction
- Moderate to marked reduction focal absence of melanin granules in the basal and suprabasal layers
- Basket weave hyperkeratosis.

Q. What are the differential diagnosis for idiopathic guttate hypomelanosis?

A.
- Pityriasis versicolor
- Postinflammatory hypopigmentation.

Q. What are the factors responsible for idiopathic guttate hypomelanosis?

A.
- Chronic sun exposure
- Genetic influence
- Trauma

Q. What is the pathogenesis of idiopathic guttate hypomelanosis?

A.
- DOPA reaction is decreased or absent
- Deficient epidermal melanin
- Decreased number of melanocyte and incompletely melanized melanosomes have been seen.

Q. What is the treatment for idiopathic guttate hypomelanosis?

A.
- Superficial dermabrasion
- Cryotherapy

41 Incontinentia Pigmenti

Q. What is incontinentia pigmenti also known as?
A. Bloch–Sulzberger syndrome; Bloch–Siemens syndrome.

Q. What is incontinentia pigmenti?
A. X-linked dominant disease, lethal in male fetuses and is caused by mutations in the *NEMO* gene (NF-kB essential modulator) on Xq28.

Q. Describe the cutaneous lesions of incontinentia pigmenti?
A. Cutaneous lesions tend to follow the lines of Blaschko, and occur in four classic phases:

1. *Vesicular stage*: Yellow or clear vesicles in linear and whorled streaks, most prominently distributed on the lower extremities.
2. *Verrucous phase*: Hyperkeratotic linear plaques.
3. *Linear and whorled hyperpigmentation*: Occurs most often over the trunk. There are lines of reticulate hyperpigmentation, the scalloped edges of the lesions are consistent with growth of normal keratinocytes into the damaged areas.
4. *Atrophic, hypopigmented thin streaks*: May persist indefinitely.

Q. What are the other cutaneous lesions of incontinentia pigmenti?
A.
- Patchy scarring alopecia
- Woolly hair nevi
- Nail dystrophy
- Anhidrosis in atrophic streaks
- Asymmetric breasts and supernumerary nipple

Q. What are the extracutaneous manifestation of incontinentia pigmenti?
A.
- Dental abnormalities—partial anodontia and conical or peg-shaped teeth
- CNS abnormalities—seizures, delayed psychomotor development, mental retardation and spastic hemiplegia
- Ocular disease—abnormalities, microphthalmia, pseudoglioma, cataract, optic atrophy and eventually blindness
- Skeletal—skull anomalies, scoliosis
- Pulmonary hypertension.

Q. What is the pathology of incontinentia pigmenti?

A. • *Stage 1*: Eosinophilic spongiosis and scattered dyskeratotic keratinocytes
- *Stage 2*: The epidermis is acanthotic with hyperkeratosis and foci of dyskeratosis
- *Stage 3*: Pigmentary incontinence
- *Stage 4*: Thinned epidermis and dermis devoid of appendages

Q. What are the differential diagnosis of incontinentia pigmenti?

A. • Neonatal incontinentia pigmenti-infectious causes (e.g., herpes zoster, varicella or herpes simplex or other viral infections)
- Linear and whorled nevoid hypermelanosis and hypomelanosis of Ito

Q. How will you manage incontinentia pigmenti?

A. • The cutaneous lesions generally do not require therapy. Treatment is symptomatic.
- Keep the skin cool and dry during all the stages for the first year to avoid any secondary infections. All affected infants should be referred for a baseline ophthalmologic examination and should have periodic neurodevelopmental and dental evaluation.

42 Keloid

Q. What is a keloid?

A. A firm irregularly shaped fibrous hyperpigmented, pink or red papule or plaque.

Q. What is the origin of keloid?

A. Growth occurs over a cut, laceration or burn or less often an acne pustule over chest or upper back, spreads beyond limits of original injury and often sends out claw like projections (keloid = chela= claw).

Q. Describe a typical lesion.

A. Overlying epidermis is smooth glistening and thinned from pressure. Can be surrounded by erythematous halo, have consistency of rubber mostly linear with bulbous ends. Keloid may be telangiectatic.

Q. What are the symptoms?

A. Lesions may be tender, painful, pruritic may rarely ulcerate or develop draining sinus tracts.

Q. Common locations of keloids.

A. Commonest—chest (sternal region), neck, ears (earlobes), extremities, trunk, rarer on face, palms and soles, eyelids and genitals.

Q. Keloids are common in which race?

A. Blacks (and in them, they are larger in proportion).

Q. Epidemiology.

A.
- Prevalence higher in younger female than in males
- Occurs most commonly in adults aged 10–30 years

Q. Histopathology of keloid.

A. Dense, sharply defined nodular growth of myofibroblasts and collagen with a whorl like arrangement. Central thickened hyalinized bundles of collagen and paucity of elastic tissue. By pressure, tumor causes thinning of normal papillary dermis and atrophy of adjacent appendages. Mast cells are present.

Q. Differential diagnosis of keloid.

A.
- Hypertrophic scar
- Carcinoma en cuirasse
- Dermatofibrosarcoma protuberans
- Keloidal blastomycosis (lobomycosis)
- Keloidal scleroderma (a type of morphea)

Q. Treatment of keloid.

A.
- Intralesional injection of triamcinolone initially 40 mg/mL, later 10–20 mg/mL—cryotherapy
- Flash lamp pulsed dye laser
- 5-Fluorouracil
- Calcium channel blockers
- Surgical excision
- Verapamil

Q. Difference between keloid and hypertrophic scar.

A.
- *Keloids*:
  - Itch and pain
  - Do not cross joint creases
  - Need not have history of injury
  - Is racial/familial
  - Recur after excision.
- *Hypertrophic scar*:
  - Asymptomatic
  - May cross joint creases
  - Have history of injury
  - Is not familial and racial
  - Itching present
  - Pain present
  - Occurs over the lines of tension
  - There need not be any history of (H/O) injury
  - Often racial and familial
  - Invariably recurs after excision
  - Stops growing after 6 months.

Q. Prognosis.

A. Rarely resolve spontaneously, with treatment they become softer, less tender, less painful and less pruritic.

43 Keratolysis Exfoliativa

Q. What are the other names of keratolysis exfoliativa?

A. Lamellar dyshidrosis, recurrent palmar peeling.

Q. What is keratolysis exfoliativa?

A.
- It is a superficial exfoliative dermatosis of the palms and soles. Clinically there is no inflammation, there is occurrence of white spots and these white spots spread towards the periphery. The lesions rupture to produce an annular adherent collarette. The lesions are asymptomatic
- The condition is exacerbated by environmental factors, the patients may also have atopy. The condition can also be identified as subclinical eczema.

Q. How can the condition be differentiated from dermatophyte infection?

A. Because of the scaling, the lesion has to be differentiated from dermatophyte infection, hence, a KOH mount is useful.

Q. How can we treat keratolysis exfoliativa?

A. Treatment is by use of urea, ammonium lactate and salicylic acid. Topical corticosteroids can be used when dermatitis is present.

44 Keratosis Pilaris

Q. What is the mode of inheritance?

A. Autosomal dominant, sporadic and acquired in some cases.

Q. Classical lesions of keratosis pilaris.

A. Multiple, discrete, skin colored to hypopigmented, goose-flesh like, horny follicular micropapules. They are better felt than seen.

Q. Commonly involved sites.

A. Shoulders, upper arms, lateral aspect of thighs, buttocks, upper back, sometimes legs.

Q. Age group affected.

A.
- Manifests by 2–3 years of age.
- Remains until adulthood; subsides gradually after that

Q. Associations.

A.
- Ichthyosis vulgaris
- Atopic diathesis (one of the minor criterias).

Q. Comment on the general health of the patient.

A. Usually unaffected.

Q. Histopathology.

A.
- Orthokeratotic keratin plugs in follicular orifices, which may contain twisted hair, dilate the infundibulum, creating the papules of KP
- Epidermis—hyperkeratosis, hypogranulosis, and follicular plugging
- Dermis—upper dermis and perifollicular areas contain mild perivascular lymphohistiocytic infiltrates

Q. Dermoscopy findings.

A. Widened follicular orifices, hyperpigmentation, perifollicular erythema, scaling, and thin and short hair shafts in lesional skin.

Q. Differential diagnosis.

A.
- Lichen spinulosus
- Lichen striatus
- Phrynoderma

- Pityriasis rubra pilaris
- Lichen nitidus
- Atopic dermatitis

Q. Medications causing keratosis pilaris-like eruptions.
A. Cyclosporine, vemurafenib, nilotinib, dasatinib.

Q. Treatment.
A. Mild topical keratolytics—3% salicylic acid. 0.1% tretinoin.

45 Lentigo

Q. What are different types of lentigo?

A.
- *Types*:
  - Lentigo simplex
  - Solar lentigo (lentigo senilis)
  - PUVA lentigines
  - Ink spot lentigo (sunburn lentigo)
  - Labial, penile and vulvar melanosis (melanotic macules, mucosal lentigines)
- *Syndromes associated with lentigo*:
  - Multiple lentigines syndrome
  - Moynahan syndrome
  - Generalized lentiginosis
  - Centrofacial lentiginosis
  - Carney complex
  - Inherited patterned lentiginosis in black
  - Partial unilateral lentiginosis
  - Peutz-Jeghers syndrome
  - LEOPARD syndrome

Q. What is lentigo simplex?

A.
- These lesions occur as sharply defined, round to oval, brown or black macules
- Seen in childhood but may appear at any age
- No predilection for areas of sun exposure
- No racial predilection
- Increase in number during childhood or puberty
- Eruptive form is called as lentiginosis

Q. What are oral melanotic macules?

A. They are found mainly in the fifth decade on the vermilion border, gingival, buccal mucosa, and palate.

Q. What is the histology of lentigo simplex?

A.
- Hyperpigmentation of the basilar keratinocytes
- Increase in number of melanocytes in the basal layer
- Melanophages are present in upper dermis.

Q. What is the other name for solar lentigo?

A. Lentigo senilis/liver spots.

Q. Describe the morphology of solar lentigines.

A.
- Persistent, benign, discrete, hyperpigmented round to oval macules occurring on the sun damaged skin
- Most commonly occur on back of the hands, cheek and forehead
- They may be accompanied by depigmented macules, actinic purpura, and other chronic degenerative changes in the skin
- They may evolve into benign lichenoid keratosis and reticulated seborrhoeic keratosis.

Q. What is the histology of solar lentigines?

A.
- Rete ridges show club shaped or narrow, budlike extension.
- Marked increase in pigmentation in the basal cell layer especially at the tip of bulbous rete.
- Number of melanocytes is increased.
- Upper dermis contains melanophages.

Q. What is the treatment of solar lentigines?

A.
- Sun protection
- Bleaching creams containing 4% or 5% hydroquinone
- Chemical peels, local dermabrasion, topical tretinoin, adapalene
- Combination of 2% 4-HA and 0.01% tretinoin
- Liquid nitrogen
- Cryotherapy
- Argon, Q-switched Nd:YAG, frequency doubled Nd:YAG laser.

Q. What is PUVA lentigines?

A. Individuals receiving oral methoxsalen photochemotherapy may develop persistent pigmented macules in which there may be melanocytic atypia. These lesions occur in sites normally protected from sunlight.

Q. Ink spot lentigo?

A.
- Synonym-sunburn lentigo.
- These lesions commonly occur on the shoulders as small markedly irregular, reticulated, gray black macules resembling spots of ink on skin.

Q. What is the histology of ink spot lentigo?

A. Histologically, there is mild increase in number of melanocytes and increased melanin in both the basilar keratinocytes and stratum corneum.

Q. What is labial, penile and vulvar melanosis?

A.
- Melanocytic macules are usually light brown on oral labial mucosa but may be strikingly irregular and darkly pigmented in the genitalia.
- Sites of predilection in females is labia minora, and in males is glans.

Q. What is the histology of labial, penile, vulvar melanosis?

A. Histologically these lesions demonstrate broad "box car" rete ridges with prominent basilar hyperpigmentation and a normal to slightly increased number of melanocytes. The melanocytes are morphologically normal.

Q. Multiple lentigen syndrome.

A. These lesions appear shortly after birth and develop a distinctive speckled appearance.

Q. What is LEOPARD syndrome?

A.
- **L**entigines
- **E**lectrocardiographic abnormalities
- **O**cular hypertelorism
- **P**ulmonary stenosis
- **A**bnormalities of genitalia
- **R**etardation of growth
- **D**eafness:
  - It is due to mutation in *PTPN11* gene
  - Clinically cafe noir spots, (black spots) are noted in these patients

Q. What is Moynahan syndrome?

A. It consists of multiple lentigines, congenital mitral stenosis, dwarfism, genital hypoplasia and mental deficiency.

Q. What is centrofacial lentiginosis?

A.
- It is characterized by lentigines on the nose and adjacent cheeks, associated with status dystrophic, multiple skeletal anomalies and central nervous system disorder.
- Mucous membranes are spared.
- Onset is in the first year of life.

Q. What is Carney complex?

A. Synonyms are:
- NAME (Nevi, Atrial myxomas, Myxoid neurofibroma and Ephelides) syndrome
- LAMB (Lentigines, Atrial myxoma, Mucocutaneous myxoma and Blue nevi) syndrome

Q. What is inherited patterned lentiginosis in black person?

A.
- These are seen in light complexion black patients with autosomal dominant lentigines beginning in infancy or early childhood, without internal abnormalities
- Distribution over central face and lips with variable involvement of dorsal hands and feet, elbow, buttocks

Q. What is partial unilateral lentiginosis?

A.
- There is presence of simple lentigines, wholly and partially involving half of the body
- Conjunctival involvement present

Q. What is Peutz–Jeghers syndrome?

A.
- It is an autosomal dominant syndrome consisting of pigmented macules on the lips, oral mucosa and perioral and acral areas
- Gastrointestinal polyps especially prominent in jejunum are frequently associated with it.
- It can present with bleeding per rectal

Q. What is Laugier–Hunziker syndrome?

A. Distribution similar to Peutz–Jeghers, but also includes melanonychia and genital melanosis.

Q. Treatment modalities of lentigo.

A.
- *Prevention*: The application of sunscreen helps decrease the rate of appearance and the darkening of solar lentigines.

Topical
- Tretinoin cream and hydroquinone cream
- TCA 50% solution
- Triple combination cream with fluocinolone acetonide 0.01%, hydroquinone 4%, and tretinoin 0.05%
- Bleaching solution containing 2% mequinol (4-hydroxyanisole, 4HA)
- Imiquimod 3.75% cream has been suggested as possibly efficacious

Cryotherapy
- Lasers—doubled, Q-switched Nd:YAG laser, the HGM K1 krypton laser, and the 532 nm diode-pumped vanadate laser are all used with success. 1064 nm Q-switched neodymium-doped yttrium aluminum garnet (QS Nd:YAG) laser
- Intense pulsed-light (IPL) treatment is another option.

46 Lichen Planus

Q. Why is this lichen planus (LP)?

A.
- Presence of violaceous, flat topped, papules and plaques with scant, adherent scales.
- On the surface, gray or white puncta or streaks (Wickham's striae) cross the lesion.

Q. What is the history of LP?

A. The term lichen planus was initially introduced by Erasmus Wilson in 1869 to describe the condition that had been previously named lichen ruber by Hebra.

Q. What are the differentials?

A.
- LE
- Lichenoid eruption
- Lichen nitidus
- Lichen striatus
- Lichen sclerosus
- PR
- Ashy dermatosis
- Psoriasis
- Lichenoid GVHD
- Secondary syphilis
- Paraneoplastic pemphigus

Q. Explain the primary lesion of LP.

A. The primary lesion consists of (The "P's" of LP):
- Purple (violaceous)
- Plane (flat topped)
- Polygonal
- Pruritic
- Papules
- Plaques
- Persistent
- Found on penis
- Responds to prednisolone (steroids)
- Heals with pigmentation
- Associated with pterygium

- The lesion is initially erythematous pin point papules but the well developed lesions become violaceous 0.5–1.5 cm plaques and the resolving lesions are often hyperpigmented. The surface is glistening and dry, with scanty adherent scales.
- On the surface, gray or white puncta or streaks (Wickham's striae) cross the lesion.
- Areas of predilection—flexor wrists, trunk, medial thighs, shins, dorsal hands, glans penis. They rarely occur on the face (over the eyelids or lips).
- Koebner phenomenon occurs in LP.

Q. Other name.
A. Lichen ruber planus or Erasmus Wilson's disease.

Q. What is meaning of "lichen"?
A. Lichen—moss, planus—flat topped.

Q. What is Broq's phenomenon?
A. A patient with LP reacts to the itching by rubbing rather than scratching and consequently scratch marks are usually not present.

Q. What is Grinspan syndrome?
A. Grinspan syndrome is a syndromic complex which comprises a triad of hypertension, diabetes, and oral lichen planus.

Q. Explain the nail changes in LP.
A.
- Longitudinal ridging and splitting
- Onycholysis and the lunula may be red
- Pterygium formation is very characteristic (the proximal nailfold fuses with the proximal portion of the nail bed)
- In nail bed LP there may be onychopapilloma, a localized distal subungual hyperkeratosis.

Q. Enumerate the various types of LP.
A
- Actinic LP
- Acute LP
- Annular LP
- Atrophic LP
- Bullous LP and LP pemphigoid
- Hypertrophic LP
- Inverse LP
- LP pigmentosus
- Lichen planopilaris
- Linear LP
- LP—lupus erythematosus overlap syndrome

- Nail LP
- Oral LP
- Ulcerative LP
- Vulvovaginal LP
- Lichenoid drug eruption

Q. Explain actinic LP.

A.
- Other names LP actinicus, LP subtropicus, LP tropicus and lichenoid melanodermatitis.
- Most patients are young adults or children. There is no predilection for either sex. The onset of this variant is during the spring and summer and the lesions primarily involve sun-exposed skin of the forehead and face followed by the dorsal surfaces of the arms, hands and the neck. The lesions usually consist of red-brown plaques with an annular configuration, but melasma-like hyperpigmented patches have been observed. Summertime actinic lichenoid eruption has sometimes been regarded as a variant of or synonymous with actinic LP.

Q. Explain acute LP.

A.
- Lesions are usually widely distributed and disseminate rapidly.
- This form is also known as exanthematous or eruptive LP. The commonly affected areas include the trunk, the inner aspects of the wrists and the dorsal aspect of the feet.
- The clinical course is usually self-limited and, in general, lesions resolve with hyperpigmentation within 3 to 9 months.

Q. Explain annular LP.

A.
- This form is thought to occur when papules spread peripherally and the central area resolves.
- The annular edge is slightly raised and typically purple to white in color, while the central portion is hyperpigmented or skin-colored associated scale in annular LP.
- The most common site of involvement is the axilla, followed by the penis, extremities and groin.
- Most patients are asymptomatic, while some have pruritus.

Q. Explain atrophic LP.

A.
- Atrophic LP may represent a resolving phase of LP, given the history of the lesions, papules coalesce to form larger plaques that often, over time, become centrally depressed and atrophic with residual hyperpigmentation
- The clinical appearance of atrophic LP is likely a result of thinning of the epidermis rather than degeneration of elastic fibers

- The epidermal atrophy may be accentuated by the use of potent topical corticosteroids
- The most common site of involvement is the lower extremity

Q. Explain bullous LP and LP pemphigoids.

A. Bullous or vesiculobullous lesions can develop just within pre-existing LP lesions or more randomly, including on previously uninvolved skin. The former is called bullous LP, while the latter is referred to as LP pemphigoides.

Q. Explain hypertrophic LP.

A.
- Also referred to as LP verrucosus.
- Extremely pruritic, thick hyperkeratotic plaques are on the shins or dorsal aspect of the foot and may be covered by a fine adherent scale. The lesions are usually symmetric and tend to be chronic because of repetitive scratching. The average duration of hypertrophic LP reported to be 6 years. Chronic venous stasis frequently contributes to the development of this condition. Squamous cell carcinoma, which must be distinguished from pseudoepitheliomatous hyperplasia has been reported to arise within these lesions.

Q. Explain inverse LP.

A.
- In this unusual variant, an inverse distribution pattern is observed. Violaceous papules and plaques appear in intertriginous zones (axillae> inguinal and inframammary folds) and less often in the popliteal and antecubital fossae. Occasionally, LP lesions occur elsewhere on the body.
- Hyperpigmentation is usually present as well and it may be the sole manifestation, leading to overlap with LP pigmentosus.

Q. Explain LP pigmentosus.

A. LP pigmentosus typically presents in individuals with skin types III and IV as brown to gray-brown macules over sun-exposed areas of the face and neck, usually with no preceding erythema and often evolving into diffuse or reticulated pigmentation. Involvement of intertriginous sites is occasionally observed, and a linear distribution following Blaschko's lines has also been described.

Q. Explain lichen plano pilaris.

A.
- In lichen planopilaris, involvement of the hair follicle is observed, both clinically and histologically. This variant is also called follicular LP and LP cuminatus.
- Multiple keratotic plugs surrounded by a narrow violaceous rim are observed primarily on the scalp, although other hair-bearing areas can also be affected.

- The inflammatory process may result in scarring and loss of follicular structure, i.e. a permanent alopecia. Over time, the central areas of the scalp often 'burn out' and are indistinguishable from other causes of 'end-stage' cicatricial alopecia. However, examination of the periphery may reveal the primary lesions. Women are more frequently affected than men and this form may occur alone or with typical LP lesions elsewhere. A variant of lichen planopilaris known as Graham Little–Piccardi–Lassueur syndrome is characterized by the triad of: (1) noncicatricial loss of pubic and axillary hairs and disseminated spinous or acuminated follicular papules; (2) typical cutaneous or mucosal LP; and (3) scarring alopecia of the scalp with or without atrophy. These features need not be present simultaneously.

Q. Explain linear LP.

A. Although linear lesions frequently occur in sites of scratching or trauma in patients with LP (as a result of the Koebner phenomenon), the term linear LP is usually reserved for lesions that appear spontaneously within the lines of Blaschko. Although linear LP is usually seen in patients in their late 20s or early 30s, the initial presentation can be in the first to eighth decades. Presumably this pattern reflects somatic mosaicism but how the involved and uninvolved skin differ is not known.

Q. Explain LP-lupus erythematosus overlap.

A. Patients whose lesions have overlapping features of both LP and lupus erythematosus (LE) have been reported. These lesions are preferentially located in acral sites. Histologic and direct immunofluorescence (DIF) microscopic findings show features of both LP and LE.

Q. Explain nail LP.

A. The nails are affected in approximately 10% of patients with LP; usually, several nails are affected. The characteristic nail abnormalities include lateral thinning, longitudinal ridging, and fissuring. These changes are manifestations of matrix damage, which can lead to scarring and dorsal pterygium formation if left untreated. Nonspecific changes in the nail bed include yellow discoloration, onycholysis and subungual hyperkeratosis. In some patients, twenty-nail dystrophy may represent a variant of LP. Nail LP presenting as twenty-nail dystrophy is much more common in children than in adults.

Q. Explain oral LP.

A. Oral LP can appear in at least seven forms, which occur separately or simultaneously—atrophic, bullous, erosive, papular, pigmented, plaque like and reticular. The most common and characteristic form of oral LP is the reticular pattern. It is characterized by slightly raised whitish linear lines in Alace-like pattern or in rings with short radiating spines. This form is usually asymptomatic and the most common site of involvement is the buccal mucosa; lesions are often bilateral and symmetric. Gingival involvement is common, and oral LP affecting the gingivae exclusively is seen in approximately 10% of cases. It typically presents as chronic desquamative gingivitis. Atrophic, erosive and bullous lesions are associated with symptoms ranging from mild discomfort to severe pain. There is a higher incidence of plaque-like lesions amongst tobacco smokers. For unknown reasons, oral LP is very uncommon in young patients and in some studies, women have been affected about twice as often as men. Patients with oral LP should be questioned about symptoms related to esophageal involvement and examined for other mucosal lesions, particularly genital lesions, and vice versa because 70% of the patients with mucosal vulvovaginal LP have clinical signs of oral LP. It has been reported that the erosive or ulcerative type of oral LP is less frequently associated with cutaneous LP than are all other types of oral LP. Such mucous membrane lesions are more therapy-resistant and less likely to spontaneously remit than cutaneous lesions. Malignant transformation of longstanding, nonhealing oral LP has been reported. Several studies have reported a relationship between oral LP and chronic liver disease, particularly that due to HCV infection 3,4.

Q. Explain ulcerative LP.

A. Also called as Cram's disease. Ulcerations can occur within palmoplantar lesions of LP, particularly those on the soles. Palmoplantar LP is not as rare as was once thought and usually appears between the third and fifth decade of life. Although palmoplantar LP is more common in men than in women, ulcerative LP prevails in female patients. Typical LP lesions may be present on other parts of the body. The ulcers are intensely painful and often recalcitrant to conventional therapy. Chronic ulcerative lesions are at risk of developing squamous cell carcinoma.

Q. Explain vulvovaginal LP.

A. LP of the vulva can present with several clinical variants, but the most common appears to be erosive disease. Vaginal involvement occurs in up to 70% of women with erosive vulvar LP, and because there is often oral mucosal involvement as well, the term 'vulvovaginal gingival syndrome' has been introduced.

Q. What is the difference between LP and lichen nitidus?

A.

	Lichen nitidus	*LP*
Size	Pin head	Pin head to plaques
Color	Skin colored	Erythematosus-violaceous
Number	Multiple	Multiple
Sites	All over except oral cavity, nail involved in 5–10%	Oral cavity also involved. Nail involvement in 10%
Wickhams striae	Absent	Common
Hyperpigmentation	Unusual	Common
Hypopigmentation	Common	Unusual
Koebnerization	Common	Common
Pruritus	Uncommon	Common
Histology	Parakeratotic cap, absent or thin granular layer, lymphocytes, epitheloid cells, occasional Langhans giant cells, Ball and claw appearance. No immunoreactants seen	Hypergranulosis, band like infiltrate of lymphocytes, deposits of IgG, IgA, IgM and C3 in the epidermis

Q. Explain the treatment of lichen planus.

A.
- Chronic—topical steroids, intralesional steroids injections, biologicals (alefacept, efalizumab)
- Apremilast has been used with success in treatment of LP
- NB-UVB
- UVA1 therapy combined with oral psoralen consists of oral psoralen 1.5–2 hours before ultraviolet light
- PUVA
- Isotretinoin, Acitretin are also found to be effective in some cases
- LMW heparin 3 mg injected subcutaneously once a week led to remission of cutaneous and reticulate oral LP
- For erosive skin lesions tacrolimus, pimecrolimus is effective

- Mycophenolate mofetil can induce remission in some cases
- For oral lesions super potent steroids in gel form are used. Other options include oral or topical retinoids
- Sulfasalazine shows improvement in lesions and pruritus in patients with generalized lichen planus
- In patients with vulvovaginal LP topical clobetasol is used. ILs may be used in nonresponsive cases
- Along with this supportive therapy like antihistaminics for itching can be used
- Acute-systemic steroids, cyclosporine.

Q. Why violaceous hue in LP?

A. Due to tyndall effect (diffraction of light—the same effect which makes the sky look blue).

Q. Why Wickham's striae are seen?

A. Due to focal hypergranulosis.

Q. Why is there itching in LP?

A. Due to band like infiltrate which releases cytokines.

Q. Histology.

A.
- Orthokeratosis
- Wedge shaped hypergranulosis
- Saw toothed rete ridges with irregular acanthosis
- Diffuse vacuolar degeneration of basal layer
- Civatte bodies/Colloid bodies (degenerated basal cells)
- Max Joseph space (artifact created due to degeneration of basal layer)
- Band like lymphocytic infiltrate at DEJ
- Melanin incontinence

Q. Drugs causing LP.

A.
- Antitubercular drugs (rifampicin)
- Anticonvulsants (phenytoin)
- Antipsychotics (carbamazepine)
- Diuretics (thiazide diuretics)
- NSAIDs (ibuprofen)
- Antidiabetics (sulfonylureas)
- Antimalarials (chloroquine)
- Heavy metals (gold)
- Sildenafil
- Therapeutic paradox (Griseofulvin and antimalarials).

Q. Which viruses are implicated in LP?

A.
- Hepatitis C
- Hepatitis B
- Various herpes viruses (HHV6,7, HSV and VZV)
- Transfusion transmitted viruses (TTV)
- Vaccines for viruses (HBV).

47 Lichen Planus Pigmentosus

Q. Definition.

A. Its a type of lichen planus characterized by slate gray pigmented macules and patches over sun exposed areas, trunk and flexures.

Q. Differential diagnosis.

A. Ashy dermatosis, frictional dermatosis, other causes of hyperpigmented macules.

Q. Racial variation.

A. More common among darker races.

Q. Classical lesion.

A.
- Asymptomatic, single or multiple, well defined, slate gray macules coalescing together to form larger patches.
- Pigmentation may be patchy, follicular or diffuse.

Q. Difference between erythema dyschromia perstans and LPP.

A.

Feature	*Erythema dyschromicum perstans*	*Lichen planus pigmentosus*
Synonym	Ashy dermatosis	Lichen dyschromicum perstans
Etiology	Ammonium nitrate ingestion, whip worm infestation	Autoimmune (similar to lichen planus)
Clinical features	Asymptomatic ash or blue-gray colored macules coalescing to form larger patches with an active raised erythematous border mostly affecting children and young adults	Asymptomatic or pruritic hyperpigmented to brown or slate gray colored macules and patches present in a reticular, diffuse or follicular pattern
Sites affected	Trunk, limbs, face	Exposed areas, face
Histopathology	Increased epidermal pigmentation, basal layer vacuolar degeneration, pigment incontinence, lymphohistiocytic infiltrate	Basal layer vacuolar degeneration, colloid bodies, pigment incontinence, band like infiltrate
Treatment	No effective treatment	Topical steroids

48 Lichen Simplex Chrnoicus

Q. Why is this lichen simplex chronicus (LSC)?

A. Single or multiple well defined plaques showing features of lichenification in areas easy to scratch, like: Occipital and nuchal areas, wrists, legs, perineum, scrotum and vulva.

Q. Differential diagnosis.

A. Following conditions should be kept in mind:
- Psoriasis
- Hypertrophic lichen planus
- Prurigo nodularis
- Atopic dermatitis
- Chronic allergic contact dermatitis
- Chronic eczema

Q. What is meant by lichenification?

A. It is characterized by:
- Thickening of the skin
- Increased skin markings
- Hyperpigmentation

Q. Etiology.

A. Itching and subsequent chronic scratching (itch-scratch cycle) leads to lichenification of the skin. Following causes of itching are suspected:
- Atopic disorders
- Psychological factors
- Site of pre-existing dermatosis
- Allergic contact dermatitis

Q. Epidemiology.

A.
- More in women
- Rare in children
- More between 30–50 years of age

Q. Clinical features.

A. Excessive itching, more at night and in free time, relieved only when lesion starts paining.

Q. Giant lichenification of Pautrier's.

A. Solid tumor like lichenified plaques are formed due to chronic scratching in areas where subcutaneous tissues are lax, e.g., Genitocrural regions.

Q. Histopathology.

A.
- Hyperkeratosis
- Acanthosis
- Irregular elongation of rete ridges
- Wedge shaped hypergranulosis
- Broadening of dermal papillae
- Mild perivascular dermal infiltrate
- Increased number of fibroblasts
- Vertically oriented collagen bundles in dermis

Q. Treatment.

A. Following options considered:
- Topical steroids
- Intralesional steroids
- Emollients
- Sedative antihistaminics
- Anxiolytics
- Botox injections
- Topical aspirin-dichloromethane
- Doxepin and capsaicin also can be used
- Phototherapy with UVA and/or UVB exposure therapy, as well as photochemotherapy, may be used for severe cases, except in case of genital involvement
- Psychological treatment—antianxiety medications
- Cryosurgery or surgical excision of small, localized lesions.

49 Lichen Spinulosus

Q. Why is this lichen spinulosus?

A. Lichen spinulosus is a clinically distinctive variant of keratosis pilaris. It is characterized by solitary or multiple patches of minute follicular papules, each centered by a horny spine, which may occur on any part of the body.

Q. Other name of lichen spinulosus.

A. Keratosis spinulosa.

Q. Signs and symptoms of lichen spinulosus.

A.
- Lichen spinulosus occurs during childhood to young adulthood
- It tends to have a sudden onset
- The follicular papules are small rough bumps that appear in round or oval patches, which extend and spread rapidly over a few days to affect large areas of skin
- Patch when rubbed gently with the fingers has been linked to the feel of brushing your fingers over a nutmeg grater.

Q. Sites involved.

A. Patches develop symmetrically at intervals on the neck, buttocks, thighs, abdomen, knees and extensor surfaces of the arms.

Q. Cause of lichen spinulosus.

A. The cause of lichen spinulosus is unknown. Several possible causes have been postulated but none have been confirmed. These include:
- Reaction to an unidentified infection
- Association with atopy (inherited, familial tendency towards some form of allergy such as eczema, asthma or hay fever)
- Genetic predisposition

Q. What are the differential diagnosis?

A.
- Keratosis pilaris, phrynoderma
- Lichen nitidus
- Lichen striatus
- Pityriasis rubra pilaris

Q. What is the underlying pathology?

A. There is abnormal keratinization of the pilosebaceous unit resulting in keratotic follicular papules.

Q. What are the histopathological features?

A.
- Dilated hair follicle with keratin plug
- Mild perifollicular infiltrate

Q. How do you treat this condition?

A. There is no specific treatment for lichen spinulosus and in most cases it resolves spontaneously within 1–2 years:
- Topical salicylic acid (3% oint)
- Topical tretinoin (0.025%) (for the first few weeks of treatment, redness and peeling of the treated areas can be expected. Topical retinoids should not be used in pregnancy)
- Ammonium lactate (12% lotion)
- Laser assisted hair removal may also be of benefit in some cases

50 Lichen Sclerosus Et Atrophicus

Q. Why the lesion is of lichen sclerosus?

A. White polygonal, flat topped papules, plaques or atrophic plaques surrounded by erythema or a violaceous halo:

- In atrophic lesion, skin is smooth wrinkled, soft and white.
- Bulla, purpura or telangiectasia can appear on the patch.
- Mostly seen on genitalia.

Q. What are the genital and extragenital D/D?

A. Genital D/D.

- Morphea
- Erosive lichen planus
- Sexual abuse (in children)
- Erythroplasia of Queyrat (Bowen disease of the glans penis)
- Balanitis circumscripta plasma-cellularis LSC

Extragenital D/D:

- Lichen nitidus
- Oral leukoplakia
- Vitiligo
- Anetoderma
- Atrophoderma of Pasini and Pierini

Q. What are the synonyms?

A.
- Kraurosis vulvae (in females)
- Balanitis xerotica obliterans (in males)
- Csillag's disease
- Circumscribed scleroderma
- Lichen album
- White spot disease
- Weissflecken dermatoses

Q. What is the epidemiology?

A.
- Seen in both childhood and old age
- More common in white
- Females are 6–10 times more affected than males
- Prevalence 1 in 30 older women
- 1 in 900 prepubertal girls
- Ethnicity—Caucasian

Q. What is this the etiology?

A.
- Cause unknown
- Possible theories are:
  - Hereditary: HLA class 2 antigen-DQ7
  - Autoimmune infectious: Borrelia constant friction
  - Autoantibodies against extracellular matrix protein 1
  - Infection with microorganisms like Borrelia Borrelia burgdorferi, atypical mycobacterium, HPV, hepatitis C virus

Q. What is the age of onset in females?

A. It has a bimodal distribution—prepubertal and postmenopausal.

Q. Describe the lesion of lichen sclerosus?

A.
- White polygonal, flat topped papules that coalesce into smooth, porcelain white/ivory white plaques or atrophic plaques which have a cigarette paper like texture with wrinkled and fragile surface
- Lesion surrounded by erythema or a violaceous halo
- In atrophic lesion, skin is smooth and wrinkled. Soft and white Bulla, purpura or telangiectasia can appear on the patch
- Mostly seen on genitalia, itching is severe with erosions
- Increased dysuria, urethral/vaginal discharge, dyspareunia and burning sensation are the complications
- Children may present with urinary and bowel complaints
- Normal anatomical structures obliterated

Q. What are the complications of genital LS?

A.
- Fusion of the labia minora with labia majora with burying of clitoral hood and urethral meatus
- Introital stenosis with fusion

Q. What is "figure of 8" or "hour glass" appearance?

A. In women, if the perianal area with vulvar and perineal area is involved, it leads to stenosis and fusion which looks like figure of 8 appearance.

Q. Is mucosa involved?

A. Vaginal and cervical mucosa not involved. This differentiates it from lichen planus (mucosa involved).

Q. What are the clinical features in prepubertal girls?

A. Infantile perineal protrusion refers to pyramidal soft tissue swelling covered by red or rose colored skin along medial perineal raphe.

Q. What is the effect of pregnancy?

A. Pregnancy leads to complete improvement and complete resolution.

Q. What is the role of OCPs?

A. OCPs are antiandrogenic, so increase in lesions is seen in pre-menopausal women.

Q. What are the histopathological findings?

A. Trizonal appearance:

- *Zone 1*:
  - Compact orthokeratosis, thinned epidermis
  - Follicular plugging
  - Vacuolization of the basal layer
- *Zone 2*: Remarkable edema in the papillary (upper) dermis is replaced by a dense, homogenous fibrosis as the lesion matures
- *Zone 3*: Lichenoid infiltrate below the zone of edema

Q. What are the sites involved in males?

A. Glans penis, penile shaft and scrotum.

Q. What are the complications in males?

A.
- Recurrent balanitis
- Poor urinary stream
- Phimosis and paraphimosis
- Dyspareunia

Q. Where are the extragenital lichen sclerosus lesions seen?

A.
- Mostly seen in upper back, chest, breast and wrist. Mostly asymptomatic, but can be pruritic.
- Associated with morphea with lichen sclerosus like lesion.
- Lichen sclerosus usually begins as white, polygonal papules that coalesce into plaques.
- Evenly spaced dells or comedone-like plugs correspond to obliterated appendiceal ostia. With time, the plugs and dells will disappear and leave a smooth, porcelain-white plaque. Skin color is white, often with a shiny porcelain appearance.
- Telangiectases and follicular plugs may be seen.
- The size of the plaque or plaques may vary widely.

Q. What is the prognosis?

A. The disease can last for a considerably long time. Occasionally, "spontaneous cure" may ensue, particularly in young girls. Lichen sclerosus is associated with a higher risk of squamous cell carcinoma (12–15%-genital LSA).

Q. What is the treatment?

A.
- Superpotent topical steroids daily once or twice a day or weekend therapy for 3 months

- Topical tacrolimus (0.1 to 0.03%)
- Topical pimecrolimus (1%)
- Gabapentin, duloxetine hydrochloride for vulvodynia
- HCQs, calcitriol, calcipotriol, tretinoin, cyclosporine, hydroxyurea in refractory cases
- Topical androgens
- Topical progesterone
- Cryotherapy
- Photodynamic therapy
- CO_2 ablation
- Surgical correction in females
- Circumcision in males

51 Lichen Striatus

Q. Why is this lichen striatus?

A. There are small, erythematous, scaly, 1 to 3 mm, papules that coalesce to form plaque, either continuous or interrupted.

Q. What is the differential diagnosis?

A.
- Lichen planus
- Linear psoriasis
- Inflammatory linear verrucous epidermal nevi
- Verruca plana
- Linear porokeratosis
- Linear Darier's
- Linear lichen nitidus
- Adult blaschkitis

Q. What is the age of onset?

A. Young children (mean age 3 years).

Q. What is lichen striatus?

A. Lichen striatus (also known as "Blaschko linear acquired inflammatory skin eruption"(BLAISE) and "Linear lichenoid dermatosis") is an uncommon skin condition that is seen primarily in children, most frequently appearing ages 5–15.

Q. Is there any gender variation?

A. Girls are affected more than boys.

Q. What is the pattern of the lesion?

A. Linear pattern, along the lines of Blaschko.

Q. What are lines of Blaschko?

A.
- German dermatologist Alfred Blaschko is credited for the first demonstration of these lines in 1901
- Blaschko's lines are skin lines invisible under normal conditions. They become apparent when some diseases of the skin or mucosa manifest themselves according to a specific pattern
- They follow a "V" shape over the back, "S" shaped whorls over the chest, stomach, and sides, and wavy shapes on the head

- The lines are believed to trace the migration of embryonic cells. The stripes are a type of genetic mosaicism
- They do not correspond to nervous, muscular, or lymphatic systems
- The lines can be observed in other animals such as cats and dogs.

Q. Is the lesion symptomatic?
A. Mostly asymptomatic, occasionally pruritic.

Q. What are the nail changes?
A. Only nails aligned with the skin lesions are affected. There is:
- Thinning
- Ridging
- Horizontal splitting and nail bed hyperkeratosis
- Dystrophy
- Total nail loss

Q. How do lesions heal?
A.
- Mostly, lesions heal spontaneously with hypopigmentation.
- In < 5%, hyperpigmentation is seen.

Q. What are the histological features?
A.
- Granulomatous infiltrate may be seen
- Band-like dermal infiltrate with necrotic keratinocytes at dermo-epidermal junction
- Dense lymphoid infiltrate around eccrine sweat glands and ducts

Q. Is Koebner's phenomenon seen?
A. Yes.

Q. What is Grosshan's Marot disease?
A. Synonym Adult blaschkitis.

Q. How do adult and children blaschkitis differ?
A.
- In adult blaschkitis, papulovesicular lesions are seen
- Multiple areas are affected
- Resolves rapidly and relapses are common
- On histopathology, more of spongiosis

Q. What is the treatment of lichen striatus?
A.
- Counseling of the patient about the chronicity of the disease and benign course
- Topical steroids
- Topical tacrolimus 0.1% or pimecrolimus 1%
- Antihistamines for symptomatic relief

52 Linear and Whorled Nevoid Hyperpigmentation

Q. Why is it called linear nevoid hyperpigmentation?

A. Hyperpigmentation is characteristically symmetrical, linear and has a dermatomal distribution following lines of Blaschko producing a Zebra like appearance.

Q. What is it?

A. A syndrome consisting of congenital anomalies and patterned melanocytic hyperpigmentation of the trunk and extremities.

Q. Synonyms.

A.
- Reticulate and zosteriform hyperpigmentation
- Reticulate hyperpigmentation of Iijima and Naito
- Zebra-like hyperpigmentation.

Q. What are the associated congenital abnormalities?

A.
- Atrial septal defect
- Dextrocardia
- Orbicular atresia
- Deafness
- Growth retardation

Q. Course of disease.

A.
- Lesions increase after birth
- Become stable, usually fades spontaneously. Other abnormalities can be surgically corrected.

Q. Differential diagnosis.

A.
- Incontinentia pigmenti
- Linear epidermal nevus
- Hypomelanosis of Ito
- Goltz syndrome

Q. Any relation to incontinentia pigmenti.

A. Some authors consider it as a variation of incontinentia pigmenti.

Q. Histopathology.

A.
- Hyperpigmentation of basal keratinocytes
- Prominent melanocytes
- Mild elongation of rete ridges
- Pigmentary incontinence with melanophages in papillary dermis

Q. Treatment.

A. Q-switched lasers have been tried.

53 Lipoma

Q. What do you find on examination?

A. A painless (rarely painful) swelling with normal overlying skin with no increase in temperature, no tenderness, smooth lobulated surface, soft edges and compressible, slipping away from fingers, nonfluctuating and freely mobile over deeper structures.

Q. Differential diagnosis.

A.
- Leiomyoma
- Fibroma
- Dermoid cyst
- Hibernoma
- Liposarcoma
- Lymphatic tumor
- Neurofibroma
- Rheumatic nodules
- Sebaceous cyst

Q. What is the cause of pain in lipoma?

A.
- Trauma or manipulation on part of the patient
- Secondary infection
- Angiolipoma
- Hemorrhage in the lipoma—malignancy (rare)

Q. D/D of tender tumors.

A. "BLEND AN EGG":

B: Blue rubber bleb nevi
L: Leiomyoma
E: Eccrine spiroadenoma
N: Neurilemmoma
D: Dermatofibroma
A: Angiolipoma
N: Neuroma
E: Endometrioma
G: Glomus cell tumor
G: Granular cell tumor

Q. What is it also called as?

A.
- Universal tumor
- Ubiquitous tumor

Q. What is the etiology of lipoma?

A. Chromosome 12q 13–15.

Q. What are the clinical features?

A.
- Seen in adults of age group 40–60 years.
- No gender predilection.
- Lipomas can occur almost anywhere on the body, but are most commonly found on the trunk, shoulders, neck, and armpits.
- Lipomas can also form in muscles and internal organs.
- Patient comes with a painless slowly enlarging mass on any of the above sites.

Q. Histopathological findings.

A.
- Epidermis normal
- Dermis normal
- Subcutaneous tissue—adipocytes are univacuolated and mature with eccentrically placed and compressed nuclei. Signet ring cells seen.
- Histopathology of hibernoma, on the other hand, shows multiple cells with small vacuoles of fat giving a granular appearance (brown fat).

Q. What is the treatment of lipoma?

A.
- Excision of the lipoma cleanly at first operation to prevent recurrence.
- Liposuction.

Q. What is Bannayan-Riley-Ruvalcaba syndrome?

A. Bannayan-Riley-Ruvalcaba syndrome is an autosomal dominant disorder consisting of constellation of:
- Multiple lipomas
- Macrocephaly
- Lymphangiomas
- Hemangiomas

Q. What are the other disorders related to lipoma?

A. Other disorders include:
- Adiposis dolorosa
- Madelung disease
- Cowden syndrome
- Gardner's syndrome

- Dercum's disease
- Hereditary multiple lipomatosis
- Proteus syndrome
- Multiple endocrine neoplasia type 1

Q. What are the types of lipoma?

A.
- Angiolipoma
- Fibrolipoma
- Hibernoma
- Myelolipoma
- Spindle cell
- Pleomorphic

54 Lipodermatosclerosis

Q. Why is it called lipodermatosclerosis?

A. Marked woody induration in a stocking distribution results in calves that resembles an inverted champagne bottle.

Q. What is lipodermatosclerosis also called as?

A. Hypodermitis, sclerodermiformis, stasis panniculitis.

Q. Age and sex of predilection.

A. Women older than 40 years with an above average body mass index.

Q. What is designated as sclerosing panniculitis?

A. Areas of fat necrosis are larger and present as tender erythematous subcutaneous nodules or plaques.

Q. What are ghost cells?

A. Pale cell walls with no nuclei due to ischemic necrosis of fat globules.

Q. Differential diagnosis of lipodermatosclerosis.

A.
- Morphea
- DM scleromyxedema
- Panniculitis
- Liposarcoma
- Erythema nodosum
- Diabetic dermopathy
- Cellulitis
- Scleroderma

Q. What is lipodermatosclerosis also called as?

A. Hypodermitis, sclerodermiformis.

Q. Distribution of lesions.

A. Predilection for medial lower third of lower legs. Bilateral, if unilateral either left leg is only affected or is more severe, if right leg is affected deep venous thrombosis currently or in past or we suspect venous injury to right leg.

Q. What are the phases of LDS?

A.
- Acute phase—affected area is red to violaceous, tender and warm

- Chronic phase—inverted champagne bottle appearance and dull aching pain
- In about 10% cases, ulceration follows the chronic phase.

Q. Pathogenesis of LDS.

A. There is inflammation as well as abnormal fibrinolysis, leading to microthrombi formation. The former, causes activation of WBCs, while latter causes tissue hypoxia. Both cause increasing levels of TGF beta 1, and then increased levels of fibroblasts expressing pro collagen 1. This causes skin hardening and fibrosis.

Q. What is hypodermitis sclerodermiformis?

A.
- Marked woody induration in stocking distribution results in calves that resemble inverted champagne bottle induration is due to fibrosis of subcutaneous fat without primary inflammatory panniculitis occurring multifocally and microscopically throughout affected area.
- Sometimes there maybe areas of fat necrosis.

Q. What is pseudocellulitis?

A. There are several entities resembling cellulitis including—Acute lymphedema (specially filarial), superficial venous thrombosis, allergic contact dermatitis, stasis dermatitis, erythema nodosum, gout and bursitis.

Q. Treatment of LDS.

A.
- Graded compression stockings—specially when ulcers are present. This can come as elasticized socks, stockings or tights. They are classified according to the pressure applied at the ankle. The pressure varies from 15–20 (class I), 20–30 (class II), 30–40 (class III). Lighter compression therapies are better tolerated. But higher compression therapy are better
- Leg elevation
- Pressure dressings like Unna boot (temporary but dramatic results)
- Unna boot with Coban and a foam buttress (bolster material to apply extra pressure to red inflamed areas)
- Anabolic steroids stanozolol 2–5 mg, it increases fibrinolytic action
- Danazol—modified testosterone derived 100–200 mg BD
- Oxandrolone 10 mg (twice a day)
- Less conventional options—Pentoxifylline 400–800 mg (three times a day), ILS, surgical excision of the LDS tissue, topical capsaicin 0.75%, Colchicine, Niacinamide, Sirolimus, Thalidomide.

55 Macular and Lichen Amyloidosis

Q. Why is it called macular amyloidosis?

A. Hyperpigmented macules showing rippled appearance on extensor aspect of arms and lateral aspect of lower legs.

Q. Why is it lichen amyloidosis?

A. Hyperpigmented plaques with acuminate papules and excoriation marks.

Q. What are the differential diagnosis of macular amyloidosis?

A.
- Atopic dermatitis
- Poikiloderma of civatte
- Postinflammatory hyperpigmentation
- Phototoxic contact dermatitis
- Erythema dyschromicum perstans
- Pityriasis versicolor
- Atrophic lichen planus
- Notalgia paraesthetica

Q. What are the differential diagnosis of lichen amyloidosis?

A.
- Prurigo nodularis
- Neurodermatitis
- Lichen simplex chronicus
- Scleroderma
- Pretibial myxedema

Q. What is amyloid?

A. Ultrastructurally, amyloid is composed of nonbranching fibrils, measuring 6–10 nm in diameter. The amyloid protein has an anti-parallel, beta pleated sheet configuration. It is composed of a non-fibrillary protein known as the amyloid P component and a fibrillary component.

Q. How is amyloid identified?

A.
- In light microscopy it appears as amorphous, hyaline-like, eosinophilic deposits
- With congo red stain—green birefringence
- With crystal violet—reddish metachromasia
- With thioflavin-T stain—yellow green fluorescence

Q. Clinical classification of amyloidosis.

A.

Primary systemic amyloidosis: • Plasma cell dyscrasias • Multiple myeloma associated *Secondary systemic amyloidosis*: • Chronic inflammation (rheumatoid arthritis) • Chronic infection (tuberculosis)	*Cutaneous*: • Primary—macular, lichen, biphasic, dyschromic, nodular • Secondary—within skin tumors Endocrine—medullary, carcinoma of thyroid, insulinoma, type 2 diabetes mellitus (T2DM)

Q. What is primary cutaneous amyloidosis?

A. It is associated with deposition of amyloid in skin only.

Q. What is the clinical presentation of localized cutaneous amyloidosis?

A.
- Macular amyloidosis:
  - May be pruritic and lesions are hyperpigmented in a confluent or rippled manner.
  - Sites of involvement are—upper back, scapula, extensor surfaces of extremities.
  - Presents in early adulthood affecting women > men.
- Lichen amyloidosis:
  - Persistent pruritic papules on the shins or other extensor surface of extremities. Initial lesions are discrete, firm, scaly, skin colored or hyperpigmented papules which later coalesce into plaques that often have a rippled or ridged pattern.
  - If both macular and lichen amyloidosis is present in a single patient then the term biphasic amyloidosis can be used.
  - Biphasic amyloidosis—fine papular lesions are superimposed upon a background of hyperpigmentation.

Q. What is friction amyloidosis?

A. Friction from brushes, towels, loofahs and coconut coir can produce macular amyloidosis.

Q. What is the histopathological findings in localized amyloidosis?

A.
- In lichen amyloidosis, deposits expand the papillae and displace the elongated rete ridges.
- Amyloid deposits are restricted to upper dermis in macular and lichen amyloidosis.
- Epidermis is acanthotic and hyperkeratotic.
- Pigment incontinence and perivascular lymphohistiocytic infiltrate is noted.

Q. Describe the different treatment methods for cutaneous amyloidosis.

A.
- Patients should be advised against frequent and chronic rubbing with brushes, towels and loofahs during or after bathing
- Topical application of potent corticosteroids under occlusion
- A mild keratolytic agent can also be used
- Topical calcineurin inhibitors
- Intralesional corticosteroids
- Phototherapy
- Dermabrasion
- CO_2 laser
- Cyclosporine
- Systemic retinoids.

56 Miliaria

Q. Why is it called miliaria?

A.
- Small superficial vesicles with no inflammatory reaction (miliaria crystallina).
- Pruritic, discrete, erythematous papulovesicles accompanied by sensations of prickling, burning or tingling which later, become confluent on the bed of erythema (miliaria rubra).
- Pustules are distinct, superficial, and independent of hair follicles (miliaria pustulosa).
- Most common sites of predilection are antecubital, fossa popliteal fossa, trunk, inframammary areas, abdomen (especially waistline), inguinal regions.
- Miliaria profunda a variant caused by even deeper obstruction of the eccrine duct, is very rare in infants which occurs in the form of asymptomatic nodules.

Q. What is the differential diagnosis (DD) of miliaria?

A.
- Depends on the type of miliaria.
- In case of miliaria rubra:
  - Grover's disease is an important DD.
- In case of miliaria pustulosa:
  - Acute generalized exanthematic pustulosis, where there are nonfollicular pustules, but also systemic symptoms like fever and a history of (H/O) exposure to drugs like antibiotics.
- In case of miliaria profunda:
  - Furuncles and other pyodermas have to be differentiated.

Q. What is miliaria?

A. It is the retention of the sweat as a result of occlusion of eccrine sweat ducts which produces an eruption that is common in hot, humid climates, such as in tropics, hot summer months and in temperate climates.

Q. Which organism can exacerbate miliaria?

A. Staphylococcal epidermidis.

Q. How is miliaria caused?

A. The polysaccharide substance may obstruct the delivery of sweat to the skin surface. The occlusion prevents normal secretions from the sweat glands and eventually pressure causes rupture of the sweat glands or ducts at different levels. The escape of substance in adjacent tissue produces miliaria.

- Possible irritant/toxin:
  - Occlusive clothing and overheating
  - Adhesive tape
  - Ultraviolet and infrared radiation
  - Aluminum chloride

Q. What are the different types of miliaria?

A.
- Miliaria crystallina (sudamina)
- Miliaria rubra (prickly heat)
- Miliaria pustulosa
- Miliaria profunda
- Postmiliarial hypohidrosis
- Tropical anhidrotic asthenia

Q. What is morphology and clinical features of miliaria crystallina?

A.
- It is characterized by small superficial vesicles with no inflammatory reaction.
- It appears in bedridden patients in whom fever produces increased perspiration
- Sweat collects beneath the stratum corneum, causing clear, small, flaccid vesicles that are often likened to "dew drops"
- Situations in which clothing prevents dissipation of heat and moisture, as in bundled children.
- Lesions are generally asymptomatic and their duration is short lived as they tend to rupture due to slight trauma.
- Lesions are self-limiting and resolve spontaneously.

Q. Name the drugs precipitating miliaria.

A. Isotretinoin, bethanechol, doxorubicin.

Q. What is the morphology and clinical features of miliaria rubra?

A.
- They appear as extremely pruritic, discrete, erythematous papulovesicles accompanied by sensations of prickling, burning or tingling. They later become confluent on the bed of erythema.

- Most common sites of predilection are antecubital, popliteal fossa, trunk, inframammary areas, abdomen (especially waistline), inguinal regions.
- Due to impending evaporation of moisture, there is maceration of these areas.

Q. At what level sweat gland is injured in miliaria rubra?

A. Prickle cell layer, where spongiosis is produced.

Q. What is the morphology and clinical feature of miliaria pustulosa?

A.
- Pustules are distinct, superficial, and independent of hair follicles.
- Pruritic pustules occur most commonly on extremities, scrotum and back of bedridden patients.

Q. Which diseases are associated with miliaria pustulosa?

A. Contact dermatitis, lichen simplex chronicus and intertrigo which occur several weeks after the disease is subsided.

Q. What is complication of miliaria pustulosa?

A. Recurrent episodes may be the sign of type 1 pseudohypoaldosteronism, as salt losing crisis may precipitate miliaria pustulosa or rubra with resolution after stabilization.

Q. What is the morphology and clinical features of miliaria profunda?

A.
- Nonpruritic, flesh colored, deep seated whitish papules characterize this form of miliaria
- Usually asymptomatic
- Lasts for mostly 1 hour after the heating has subsided
- Sites are trunk and extremities

Q. What is the site of injury of the sweat gland in miliaria profunda?

A. The occlusion is in upper dermis.

Q. What is postmiliarial hypohidrosis?

A. It results from occlusion of sweat ducts and pores and may be severe enough to impair individual's ability to perform sustained work in hot environment.

Q. What are the clinical features of postmiliarial hypohidrosis?

A.
- Decreasing efficiency
- Irritability

- Anorexia
- Drowsiness
- Vertigo
- Headache
- The duration and severity of hypohidrosis is related to degree of miliaria

Q. What is tropical anhidrotic asthenia?

A.
- This is a rare form of miliaria with long lasting portal occlusion, which produces anhidrosis and heat retention
- It occurs in people who are accustomed to temperate climates but then suddenly put in a tropical environment in which they have to do a lot of physical work (e.g., soldiers)

Q. What is the treatment given for miliaria?

A.
- Place the patient in cool environment
- Circulating air fans to cool the skin
- Anhydrous lanolin application
- Hydrophilic ointment
- Soothing cooling bath containing colloidal oatmeal or corn-starch is beneficial
- Dusting powder
- Miliaria resolves without treatment.
- Prevention is accomplished by avoidance of overheating and excessive swaddling when feasible.

57 Milium

Q. Why is this milia?

A.
- Small, translucent, yellowish white papules develop on areas exposed to sunlight, especially around the orbits, dorsa of the hands, back and sides of the neck and the ears.
- They may originate from the infundibulum of hair follicles or from eccrine ducts, and in the mouth from minor salivary gland ducts or from epithelium. Milia present as 1–2 mm, firm, white to yellow, subepidermal papules.

Q. Differential diagnosis of milium.

A.
- Trichoepithelioma
- Tuberous sclerosis
- Hidrocystoma

Q. What is milium?

A. It is a degenerative change occurring in the skin.

Q. What are the different types of milium?

A.
- Juvenile type
- Adult type
- Primary
- Secondary

Q. What is the etiology of milium?

A.
- Juvenile form is familial and begins before puberty.
- Adult form is due to trauma, exposure to sunlight, photodynamic effects of phenol in gas fuel, prolonged application of hydroquinone bleaching cream.

Q. What are primary and secondary milia?

A.
- Primary milia are derived from the lowest portion of the infundibulum of the vellus hair at the level of the sebaceous duct. They represent a keratinizing type of benign tumor and seen in the epidermis.
- Secondary milia may arise from hair follicle, sweat duct, sebaceous duct or epidermis. They are seen in various blistering disorders like bullous pemphigoid, dystrophic epidermolysis bullosa, PCT, after dermabrasion or other trauma. They represent retention cyst and are subepidermal.

Q. What are Bohn's nodules and Epstein's pearls?

A.
- 40–50% infants show milia which resolve in the first 4 weeks.
- Bohn's nodules are milia on the hard palate
- Epstein's pearls are milia on the gum margins.

Q. What is milia en plaque?

A. It is characterized by multiple milia within an erythematous edematous plaque, often seen in the postauricular area, may also be seen on anterior part of ear.

Q. In which condition are widespread milia seen?

A.
- Marie-Unna hypotrichosis
- Oral-facial-digital syndrome.

Q. What are the other associated symptoms with milium?

A.
- Basal cell carcinoma (BCC) associated syndromes
- Rombo syndrome
- Bazex–Dupré–Christol syndrome
- Loeys–Dietz syndrome
- Basaloid follicular hamartoma syndrome
- Basan syndrome
- Subset of Brooke–Spiegler syndrome (Rasmussen syndrome).

Q. Describe the histology of milium.

A.
- Colloid globules can be seen on the tip of dermal papillae.
- Fissured masses of colloid occur in the mid dermis surrounded by collagen.
- In adult type, the colloid is separated from the epidermis by a band of collagen and elastolysis is present.
- In juvenile type, elastolysis is absent and colloid is seen in the epidermis and immature civatte bodies are also present.

Q. What is the treatment of colloid milium?

A.
- Topical tretinoin
- Mechanical expression
- Electrodessication
- Dermabrasion
- Erbium:YAG laser
- Cryotherapy
- Chemical peels
- Resurfacing techniques

Q. How can milium be prevented?

A.
- Protection against sun, by use of sunscreens, covering the face before going into the sun.
- Regular use of emollients or moisturizing creams on areas of sun damage.
- Lower concentrations of alpha-hydroxy acids helps to improve skin texture.

58 Melasma

Q. Why is it called melasma?

A. Presence of symmetrically distributed light to dark brown macules and patches with defined borders over sun exposed areas.

Q. Differential diagnosis.

A.
- Rash of lupus erythematosus (LE)
- Drug induced pigmentation, e.g., due to antimalarials, chlorpromazine, antidiabetics, clofazimine, amiodarone, phenytoin, ingestion of silver (argyria)
- Acanthosis nigricans in men (seborrheic melanosis)
- Pigmentory demarcation lines (Voight lines)
- Lichen planus pigmentosus (LPP)
- Actinic lichen planus (LP)
- Riehl's melanosis
- Exogenous ochronosis
- Erythema dyschromicum perstans
- Pregnancy induced hypertension (PIH)
- Frictional melanosis
- Mastocytosis
- Nevi of Ito and Ota
- Pigmented contact dermatitis
- Poikiloderma of Civatte

Q. Incidence.

A.
- More in females, South Indians, Asians.
- More in darker individuals
- Rare before puberty and more common in reproductive years.
- Present in 15% to 50% of pregnant patients.

Q. Etiology.

A. Following factors:
- Sunlight
- Hormones
- Genetic
- Toxic (cosmetics)
- Drugs (most commonly phenytoin)

Q. Histopathology.

A.
- Melanocytes increased in number and activity.
- Increased size and melanization of melanosomes.
- In dermal melasma, melanophages are increased in the papillary dermis.

Q. Classification.

A. As following:
- Clinical classification:
  - According to distribution
    - Centro-facial
    - Malar
    - Mandibular
  - By Wood's lamp examination
    - Epidermal
    - Dermal
    - Mixed
- Histopathological classification:
  - Epidermal type (melanin basal and suprabasal layers)
  - Dermal type (melanin-laden macrophages in upper and mid dermis)

Q. Clinical features.

A. Well-defined, multiple hyperpigmented macules coalescing together to form larger patches, present over the forehead, nose, cheeks (mostly sun exposed areas).

Q. Dermoscopy findings.

A. Globules of pigmented areas arranged in a reticular or net like pattern.

Q. Treatment.

A. Following options considered:
- Sunscreens
- Modified Kligman's formula
- Tretinoin
- Azelaic acid
- Glycolic acid
- Kojic acid
- Superficial chemical peels
- Lasers

Q. What is modified Kligman's formula?

A. It contains:

- Retinoic acid (0.1%)
- Hydroquinone (2% or 4%)
- Steroids (triamcinolone, mometasone, fluticasone)

Q. What is original Kilgman's formula?

A.
- Hydroquinone 5%
- Retinoic acid 0.1%
- Dexamethasone 0.1%

Q. Which lasers are effective?

A. Following have been tried with success:

- Q-switched ruby laser
- Nd:YAG laser
- Alexandrite

Q. Prognosis.

A.
- Epidermal type responds well to therapy.
- Dermal type difficult to treat.

Q. What is exogenous ochronosis?

A. Due to prolonged use of topical high concentration hydroquinone, globules of homogentisic acid, a derivative of hydroquinone gets deposited in the dermis (banana bodies).

Q. Why is monobenzyl ether of hydroquinone (MBEH) not used?

A. It causes irreversible depigmentation in a characteristic speckled pattern.

59 Morphea

Q. Types of morphea.

A.

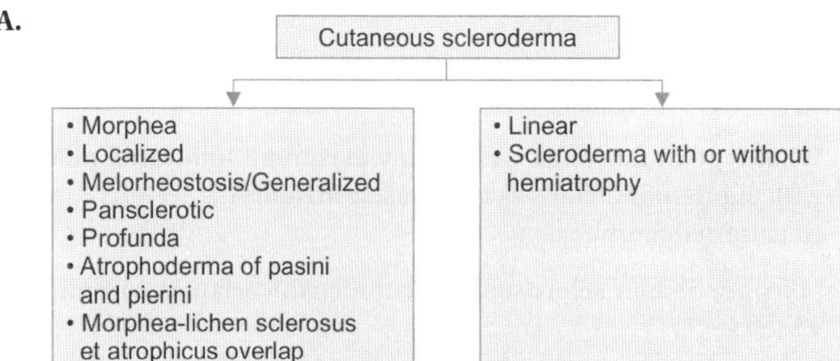

Q. What is the ratio of men is to women in localized morphea?

A. 1:2.

Q. Age group and sites affected with localized morphea.

A. In childhood and in adults, more over the trunk than extremities.

Q. Describe clinical course.

A.
- Rose/Violaceous macules appear first followed by smooth hard somewhat depressed yellowish white to ivory lesions.
- An inflammatory phase—pink, purple or bruise-like patches
- Sclerosis—the skin becomes hard, thickened, bound down, shiny, ivory white, and may have a purple border of surrounding inflammation
- Dyspigmentation and atrophy—this develops after a variable time period (usually months or years); hyperpigmentation is more common than hypopigmentation. Superficial (dermal) atrophy is seen as shiny skin, often with visible blood vessels. Deeper atrophy affecting fat, muscle or bone presents as concave indentations or discrepancies of limb circumference.

Q. Why is it called hidebound skin?

A. If skin is pinched or picked up between thumb and index finger, it is rigid and difficult to pick.

Q. Why is the skin said to have a pig skin appearance?

A. As follicular openings are more prominent like in pig skin.

Q. Discuss morphology of guttate morphea.

A. Multiple small chalk white flat or slightly depressed macules over chest, neck, shoulders, and upper back.

Q. What are the manifestations of pansclerotic morphea?

A. It involves dermis, panniculus, fascia, muscles, bones and joints (disabling, limiting motion).

Q. What does morphea profunda have an overlap with?

A.
- Eosinophilic fasciitis
- Eosinophilia myalgia
- Spanish toxic oil syndrome

Q. What type of morphea will show widespread indurated plaques with pigmentary changes and muscle atrophy?

A. Generalized morphea.

Q. Morphea-lichen sclerosus et atrophicus overlap is common in which sex?

A. Women.

Q. Differentiate between eosinophilic fasciitis and morphea profunda.

A.

Eosinophilic fasciitis	*Morphea Profunda*
Increased response to corticosteroids	Less response
Chronic debilitating course not present	Chronic debilitating course

Q. What is linear atrophoderma of moulin?

A. A variant of atrophoderma in which induration and pigmentary changes follow lines of Blaschko.

Q. Describe atrophoderma of Pasini and Pierini.

A. Brownish gray oval, round or irregular smooth atrophic lesions depressed below level of skin with sharp sloping borders.

Q. In atrophoderma of Pasini and Pierini, why do we take a perilesional biopsy?

A. Because changes are subtle, perilesional biopsy allows us to compare to normal skin.

Q. Describe the lesions of en coup de sabre.

A. Induration and depression parasagitally along the parting extending way down the forehead. May be associated with cicatricial alopecia.

Q. What does "en coup de sabre" mean?

A. Cut of the sword.

Q. Which morphea is difficult to differentiate from lichen sclerosus et atrophicus?

A. Guttate morphea as lesions are less firm.

Q. What is the histopathology?

A. The histopathology of morphea:

- Sharply squared-off biopsy ('cookie cutter' sign)
- Thick, closely packed, hyalinized collagen bundles in the lower dermis.
- Loss of adventitial fat resulting in trapped eccrine glands
- Sparse deep lymphoplasmacytic infiltrate
- Reduced number of CD34+ cells in the dermis.
- Superficial dermal pallor may be present, but the vacuolar interface dermatitis and lymphoid band of lichen sclerosus are lacking

Q. What is the treatment?

A. Local

- Topical corticosteroids
- Intralesional corticosteroids
- Topical calcineurin inhibitors
- Vitamin A analog
- Vitamin D analog

Systemic

- Penicillin
- Hydroxychloroquine or chloroquine
- Corticosteroids
- Vitamin A analogs
- Vitamin D analogs
- Cyclosporine
- Methotrexate

Phototherapy

- Oral photochemotherapy
- Bath photochemotherapy
- Cream photochemotherapy
- UVA1 +++ 2 ++ 2
- Photodynamic therapy + 3 ++ 3
- Extracorporeal photopheresis + 3 No experience
- Others CO_2 laser No experience ++ 3
- Surgery selected patients
- Physical therapy

60 Mycetoma

Q. Define mycetoma (Madura foot).

A.
- It is a chronic, slowly progressive, granulomatous disease characterized by triad of: (i) painless subcutaneous mass (ii) multiple sinuses (iii) seropurulent discharge containing grains.
- It may spread to involve the skin and the deep structures resulting in destruction, deformity and loss of function. It can sometimes also affect muscles, bones, tendons, and joints.

Q. Who recognized mycetoma first?

A. Gill, who worked at a dispensary in the southern province of Madura, first recognized mycetoma as a disease entity in 1842.

Q. What is the mycetoma belt?

A. The mycetoma belt stretches in a band between the latitudes of 150 South and 300 North. The belt includes Sudan, Somalia, Senegal, India, Yemen, Mexico among others.

Q. What is the incubation period?

A. Unknown but after animal inoculation, found to be 3 weeks.

Q. Why is occupation and residence important?

A.
- Mycetomas are mainly but not exclusively found in the dry tropics where there is a low annual rainfall. It is a disease of poverty, most commonly affecting agricultural workers and people who are habitually walk barefoot.
- In India, actinomycotic mycetoma is more commonly encountered than eumycotic mycetoma. However, eumycotic mycetoma is common in North India.

Q. What is Chalmers and Archibald classification?

A.
- Group 1—maduramycosis, caused by true fungi exhibiting septate filaments usually with chlamydospores.
- Group 2—actinomycosis, caused by delicate nonseptate filaments of the actinomyces which belong to higher bacteria.

Q. Why is socioeconomic history important?

A. Since it mostly affects young men, it has a socioeconomic effect on dependent family members.

Q. Name common causative agents of actinomycotic-mycetoma.

A.

Agent	**Grain color**
Nocardia asteroides	White
Nocardia brasiliensis	White
Nocardia otitidiscaviarum	White
Actinomadura madurae	White
Actinomadura pelletieri	Red to pink
Streptomyces somaliensis	White to yellow

Q. Common causative agents of eumycotic mycetoma.

Agent	**Grain color**
Madurella mycetomatis	Black to brown
Madurella grisea	Black to brown
Leptosphaeria senegalensis	Black
Curvularia lunata	Black
Neotestidina rosatii	Yellow
Acremonium species	White to yellow
Fusarium species	White to pale yellow
Scedosporium apiospermum	White to pale yellow
Pseudallescheria boydii	White

Q. What is the reason of the persistence of organism after an initial inoculation?

A. It appears to be related to its ability to evade host defences through a variety of adaptations such as cell wall thickening and melanin production.

Q. What are types of clinical material used for diagnosis?

A. Serosanguinous fluid or seropurulent fluid, scrapings of sinuses, tissue biopsy or excised sinus should be examined for the presence of grains. Saline dressings applied overnight over the swelling can also be observed for the presence of grains.

Q. Why is mycetoma painless?

A. It has been suggested that mycetoma produces substances that have an anesthetic action.

Q. Why do you get pain in mycetoma?

A.
- Expansion of bone with the mycetoma granuloma and grains
- Secondary bacterial infection

Q. Why are areas of local hyperhidrosis seen over the mycetoma lesion?

A. They are either due to sympathetic overstimulation or increased local temperature due to increased arterial blood flow caused by the chronic inflammation.

Q. Why are neurological and trophic changes rare until late in the disease process?

A. Because the tendons and the nerves are curiously spared, neurological and trophic changes are rare. The absence of the trophic changes may be explained by the adequate blood supply in the mycetoma.

Q. Difference between eumycetoma and actinomycetoma.

A.

	Eumycetoma	*Actinomycetoma*
Multiple punched out cavities throughout the bone	Larger in size, few in number, well-defined margins. Osteolytic lesions in bones	• Usually smaller in size. Numerous and have no definite margins • Both osteolytic and osteosclerotic lesions seen
USG	• Produce numerous sharp brightly reflective echoes (grains) • Multiple thick walled cavities with absent acoustic enhancement	Less distinct due to their smaller size and consistency. Individual embedding of the grains or the absence of cement substances in few of them
Cause	Fungus	Filamentous bacteria from the order, actinomycetes
Invasion into deeper tissue	Gradual and delayed	Earlier and extensive

Q. What are the causes of enlarged regional lymph node?

A.
- Secondary bacterial infection
- Genuine mycetoma lymphatic spread
- Local immune responses to mycetoma

Q. What are differential diagnosis (DD) of shotty lymphadenopathy?

A.
- Secondary syphilis
- Mycetoma

Q. What is the DD?

A.
- Osteomyelitis (bacterial or tubercular)
- Actinomycosis

- Botryomycosis
- Chromoblastomycosis
- Sporotrichosis
- Atypical mycobacterial infection

Q. Complications.

A.
- Secondary bacterial infection
- Cachexia
- Anemia (due to malnutrition, sepsis, and mental depression)
- Disfigurement/Deformities/Ankylosis
- Amputation (chronic neglected infection)
- Invasive infection (immunocompromized patients)
- Lymphoedema (lymphatic obstruction and fibrosis)
- Toxicity due to prolonged antimicrobial or antifungal therapy
- Osteomyelitis (bacterial or tubercular)

Q. What are the causes of death in mycetoma?

A.
- Cranial mycetoma
- Sepsis

Q. What are the common sites involved?

A. The foot (70%), especially the dorsal aspect of the forefoot. The left foot is affected more. The hand (12%) knee, arm, leg, head and neck, thigh and the perineum.

Q. What is the mode of spread of mycetoma?

A.
- Along the fascial planes
- Along the lymphatics to the regional lymph nodes
- Blood borne spread

Q. Clinical features.

A.
- Mycetoma starts as a localized swelling on an exposed site; two-thirds arise on the foot.
- The affected area has normal skin temperature and is often hyperpigmented.
- Multiple firm nodules appear and start to drain spontaneously or following pressure.
- The fluid discharged from sinus tract can contain the characteristic granular grains.
- Local pain is mild or absent, and it worsens only in later stages with more subcutaneous tissue damage or with secondary bacterial infection.

Q. Why, in mycetoma, surgery under local anesthesia is contra-indicated?

A. The apparent clinical features of mycetoma are not always a reliable indicator of the extent and spread of the disease, as some small lesions with few sinuses may have many deep connecting tracts, through which the disease has spread quite extensively.

Q. What is the DD?

A.
- Kaposi's sarcoma
- Malignant melanoma
- Fibroma
- Thorn and foreign body granuloma
- Tuberculosis (the presence of bone destruction in the absence of sinuses)

Q. Primary osseous mycetoma—DD.

A.
- Chronic osteomyelitis
- Osteoclastoma
- Bone cysts
- Syphilitic osteitis

Q. Why are pathological fractures rare in mycetoma?

A. They are rare because the cavities are usually filled with solid masses of grains and fibrous tissue, which provides bone support.

Q. Where are the bony changes unique?

A. In the skull. Purely sclerotic changes with dense bone formation and loss of trabeculation. The cause of this is unclear.

Q. What is Codman triangle?

A. Periosteal new bone spicules are laid down at right angles to the cortex to create a sun-ray appearance and Codman triangle; an appearance that may be indistinguishable from that of primary osteogenic sarcoma.

Q. What are the other X-ray changes?

A.
- In the early stage, a soft tissue granuloma is seen as a dense shadow or as scattered multiple soft tissue shadows.
- Calcification and obliteration of the fascial planes may sometimes be seen.
- As the disease progresses, the cortex may be compressed from outside by the granuloma leading to bone scalloping.

Q. Advantages of USG.

A.
- Differentiates between eumycetoma and actinomycetoma as well as between mycetoma and other conditions.

- The size and extent of the lesion can be accurately determined ultrasonically and this is useful in planning surgical incisions and procedures
- Safe, simple, noninvasive

Q. Advantages of MRI.

A. Visualization of the extension of bone destruction, periosteal reaction and soft tissue involvement. Assessment of the extent of mycetoma in the soft tissues.

Q. What is "dot-in-circle sign"?

A. MRI usually shows multiple 2–5 mm lesions of high signal intensity, which indicates the granuloma, interspersed within a low-intensity matrix which is the fibrous tissue. The "dot-in-circle sign", which indicates the presence of grains, is characteristic of mycetoma and it is highly specific.

Q. What is the DD of mycetoma on MRI?

A. Chronic osteomyelitis, granulomas, soft tissue tumors, bone tuberculosis, and cold abscesses.

Q. What is the role of CT scan?

A. Not specific but are helpful to detect early bone involvement.

Q. How should you do a biopsy?

A. It always needs surgical biopsy which should be a deep biopsy done under general or regional anesthesia. The chance of local spread with the surgical biopsy is high.

Q. What are the different types of stainings or procedures done on biopsy used?

A.
- Hematoxylin and eosin (H&E) stain
- Immunofluorescent
- Antibody immunohistochemistry techniques.

There are three types of host tissue reaction against the organism:

Type I tissue reaction, the grains are usually surrounded by a layer of polymorphonuclear leukocytes. The hyphae and cement substance disappear and only remnants of brown pigmented cement are left behind. Outside the neutrophils zone there is granulation tissue containing macrophages, lymphocytes, plasma cells and a few neutrophils. The outermost zone of the lesion consists of fibrous tissue.

Type II tissue reaction, the neutrophils largely disappear and are replaced by macrophages and multinucleated giant cells. The latter engulfs the grain material. This consists largely of pigmented cement substance although hyphae are sometimes identified.

Type III reaction, is characterized by the formation of a well-organized epithelioid granuloma with Langhan's type of giant cells. The centre of the granuloma sometimes contains remnants of fungal material.

Q. Role of fine needle aspiration cytology.

A. Fine needle aspiration cytology allows morphological identification of mycetoma and its classification into eumycetoma and actinomycetoma. The technique is simple, rapid, sensitive and can be tolerated by patients.

Q. What is the best way to obtain grains for culture?

A. Deep surgical biopsy. The grains extracted through the sinuses are usually contaminated and not viable and hence should be avoided.

Q. Which are the media used to isolate organisms?

A. Several media like Malt extract, Sabouraud's, and Glucose nutrient.

Q. Disadvantages of culture.

A. The culture technique is cumbersome and time consuming with chance of contamination happening which may give a false positive result. It also requires experience to identify the causative organisms.

Q. Any recent diagnostic techniques.

A. A specific PCR test amplifying a region of the internal transcribed spacer in the ribosomal gene complex is now available for molecular detection and identification of the causative organism to understand the disease etiology, epidemiology and organisms taxonomy, which ultimately improves patients' care.

Q. Explain serodiagnosis in mycetoma.

A. In the absence of the classical triad of mycetoma, the demonstration of significant antibodies titres against the causative organism may be of diagnostic and prognostic value. The common serodiagnostic techniques in use are counter-immunopheresis and ELISA. These tests are tedious, need purified antigens and hence it is time consuming with cross reactivity between the different organisms commonly occurring.

Q. How do you manage mycetoma?

A.
- Combined medical and surgical treatment is the gold standard in mycetoma. This regimen facilitates surgery, accelerates healing and reduces the chance of relapse. Combined drug therapy is always recommended to avoid drug resistance and for disease eradication.

- They are given in a form of cycles; each one consists of amikacin sulfate in a dose of 15 mg/kg twice daily for 3 weeks and Co-trimoxazole in a dose of 1.5 mg/kg twice daily for 5 weeks; the cycles are repeated till cure. The number of cycles ranges between 5 and 10 cycles.
- *Second line of treatment*: Amoxicillin-clavulanic acid, rifampicin, sulphonamides, gentamicin, and kanamycin. However, these drugs take a long time to achieve cure, the mean duration is around one year and the recurrence rate was high.

Q. Treatment of eumycetoma.

A.
- 400–800 mg/day ketoconazole,
- 200–400 mg/day itraconazole or 300–400 mg/day voriconazole 9–12 months.

Q. Why is ketoconazole not used these days?

A. Its because of side effects like hepatotoxicity, gynecomastia, lip dryness and ulceration, skin darkness and decreased libido.

Q. Is ketoconazole and itraconazole curative?

A. In most eumycetoma patients they only help in localizing the disease by forming well localized, thickly encapsulated lesions which are easily excised surgically.

Q. What is the duration of treatment?

A. Medical treatment for both types of mycetoma must continue until the patient is clinically, radiologically, ultrasonically, and cytologically cured.

Q. What will suggest radiological cure?

A. Reappearance of normal bone pattern and the disappearance of the soft tissue mass.

Q. What are the indications of surgery for mycetoma?

A.
- Small localized lesions
- Resistance to medical treatment
- For better response to medical treatment in patients with massive disease.

Q. What are the surgical options?

A.
- Wide local and debulking excisions
- Amputations.

Q. When is amputation indicated?

A. In advanced mycetoma not responding to medical treatment with severe secondary bacterial infection. As it can be a life saving procedure. The amputation rate ranges from 10–25%.

Q. Why is local anesthesia contraindicated in mycetoma?

A. It is because the disease extension along tissue planes is usually massive and unpredictable.

Q. Why is it mandatory to use a tourniquet when operating?

A. A bloodless operative field using a tourniquet is mandatory to identify the lesion margins to avoid bursting, which will facilitate local disease spread. The latter is an important cause of recurrence.

Q. What is the cause of recurrence in mycetoma?

A. The postoperative recurrence rate varies from 25 to 50% and this can be local or distant at the regional lymph nodes. This could be due to the disease biology and behavior, inadequate surgical excision due to the use of local anesthesia and lack of surgical experience and drug compliance due to financial reasons and/or lack of health education.

Q. Why is postoperative medical treatment essential?

A. Because if the treatment is stopped after apparent cure, recurrence may be immediate. Follow-up of patients with mycetoma must be long enough to detect early recurrence and to advise early treatment.

61 Nevus Comedonicus

Q. What is the other name of nevus comedonicus?

A.
- It is also known as comedo nevus
- It is a rare hamartoma of the pilosebaceous unit, resulting in numerous dilated keratin filled comedones

Q. Describe the epidemiology of nevus comedonicus.

A.
- Most of the cases are evident at birth, with others appearing during childhood, usually before 10 years of age
- Onset in adulthood is associated with trauma, or a dermatosis such as herpes zoster, lichen planus, and pyoderma.
- There is no racial or sexual predilection

Q. Comedo nevus syndrome.

A.
- They are usually solitary but may be part of a comedo nevus syndrome with associated skeletal, central nervous system, ocular, and other cutaneous abnormalities
- Skeleton—syndactyly, supernumerary digits, scoliosis, and spina bifida
- Central nervous system—seizures, developmental delay, microcephaly, transverse myelitis, and EEG abnormalities
- Eye—usually cataract
- Dentition—usually oligodontia
- Skin—verrucous epidermal nevus, hidradenitis suppurativa, basal cell carcinoma, squamous cell carcinoma, linear morphea, lichen striatus

Q. Distribution pattern.

A.
- Linear
- Interrupted
- Unilateral
- Bilateral
- Blaschkoid, i.e., following Blaschko lines.

Q. What is the pathogenesis behind development of nevus comedonicus?

A.
- It is thought to represent growth dysregulation affecting the mesodermal portion of the pilosebaceous unit

- The epithelial lined invaginations, are incapable of forming mature terminal hairs and sebaceous glands. This results in accumulation of a soft cornified ostial product resulting in a comedo-like plug
- A *FGFR2* mutation was also detected in the nevus skin.

Q. What are the clinical features of nevus comedonicus?

A.
- Single circumscribed area or linear streak composed of clusters of dilated follicular ostia containing firm darkly pigmented, cornified material
- Multiple linear plaques may be seen with midline demarcation
- Size ranges from few centimeters to extensive lesions covering half of the body
- Sites—face, trunk, neck, and upper limb
- Hormonal influence on the nevus can worsen the presentation

Q. What is the histopathology?

A.
- Underdeveloped hair follicles
- Dilated invaginations filled with cornified debris devoid of hair shafts
- Epidermolytic hyperkeratosis may be seen

Q. What is the differential diagnosis?

A.
- Familial dyskeratotic comedones is a rare autosomal dominant disorder in which comedones arise during childhood and are widely scattered on the trunk and are not linear
- Dilated pore nevus resembles nevus comedonicus clinically but differs histologically by containing dilated follicular cysts
- Acne neonatorum
- Keratosis pilaris
- Comedonal acne
- Chloracne
- Other epidermal nevi

Q. What is the treatment of nevus comedonicus?

A.
- Localized lesions can be surgically excised—it is difficult to excise larger lesions
- Manual comedo extraction
- Dermabrasion
- Keratolytic agents (salicylic acid, tretinoin, and ammonium lactate).
- Isotretinoin is not beneficial except for preventing cyst formation

Q. What are the other names of epidermal cyst?

A. Epidermoid cyst, infundibular cyst, epidermal inclusion cyst.

Q. Describe epidermoid cyst.

A.
- Well demarcated dermal nodules which have a visible central punctum representing the follicle from which cyst is derived, in size they are a few, mm – cm in size
- Tiny cysts are also known as milia
- They may be primary or secondary to disrupted follicular structures or traumatically implanted epithelium. Multiple epidermoid cyst can occur in individuals with acne vulgaris
- Rupture of cyst can be painful
- Development of basal cell carcinoma is rare

Q. What is the histopathology of epidermoid cyst?

A.
- Cystic cavity is filled with laminated keratin lined by stratified squamous epithelium including a granular layer
- In individuals with Gardner syndrome, some cysts show columns of pilomatricoma like shadow cells projecting into the cyst cavity

Q. What is the treatment?

A.
- Removal by excision is curative
- Incision and expression of the cyst contents is done
- If the entire cyst wall is not removed it may recur
- Inflamed lesions require intralesional triamcinolone and also excision with antibiotic therapy

62 Nevus Depigmentosus

Q. Why is this nevus depigmentosus?

A. Asymptomatic depigmented macule of a variable size with regular or serrated borders found on the trunk, neck, face and proximal part of extremities and it does not cross the midline.

Q. Differential diagnosis.

A.
- Nevus anemicus (diascopy is positive)
- Ash leaf macule
- Aplasia cutis (lesion is atrophic)
- Vitiligo
- In older children–segmental vitiligo and leprosy to be ruled out.

Q. What is nevus depigmentosus?

A. The disorder represents a congenital, stable, and leukodermic macular lesion that may occur in all races in both sexes.

Q. What are the clinical features of nevus depigmentosus?

A. It is an asymptomatic depigmented macule of a variable size with regular or serrated borders present on any region of the body, but is commonly found on the trunk, neck, face, and proximal part of extremities. It does not cross the midline. It may be focal, segmental or generalized in distribution.

Q. What is the pathology of nevus depigmentosus?

A. It is condition due to aggravation of melanosomes in melanocytes and a defect in transfer of melanosomes to keratinocytes.

Q. Describe the histology of nevus depigmentosus.

A. A normal to reduced number of melanocytes may be observed, but dihydroxyphenylalanine (DOPA) reaction shows them to be less reactive.

Q. What is the electron microscopy of nevus depigmentosus?

A. It shows stubby dendrites of melanocytes containing autophagosomes with aggregates of melanosomes.

Q. What is the treatment of nevus depigmentosus?

A.
- No treatment is necessary.
- PUVA
- Excimer laser
- Surgical grafting methods
- For small lesions, plastic surgery may be considered.

63 Nevus of Ota and Ito

Q. What is the classical presentation of a patient with nevus of Ota?

A. The presenting feature is a unilateral patch of speckled brown, blue, black or purple discoloration in the periorbital, temple, forehead, malar, earlobe or nose regions.

Q. What are nevus of Ota and Ito?

A. These are dermal melanocytic nevi arising due to the failure of complete migration of melanocytes into the epidermis.

Q. Other names.

A.
- Nevus fuscoceruleus ophthalmo-maxillaris—nevus Ota
- Nevus fuscoceruleus acromiodeltoideus—nevus of Ito

Q. What can be the differentials for these two conditions?

A.
- Mongolian spot—seen in infants over sacral region
- Blue nevus—can be found in oral mucosa, uterine cervix, prostate
- Melasma—brown, sparing of sun-protected sites, no mucus membrane involved
- Hori's nevus

Q. Why is there a characteristic blue color imparted to the lesions?

A. The blue color is due to melanin producing melanocytes in the dermis, in which the Tyndall effect occurs.

Q. The lesions are located in the distribution of which nerve?

A. Ophthalmic and maxillary divisions of the trigeminal nerve.

Q. Tanino's classification.

A.
- According to extent of cutaneous involvement:
  - I: IA—eyelids, periorbital, temporal region
    IB—infraorbital, nasolabial fold, zygomatic region
    IC—forehead
    ID—nasal region
  - II: Eyelids, periorbital, temporal, zygomatic cheek, temporal region
  - III: Scalp, forehead, eyebrow, nose region
  - IV: Bilateral

Q. What is the morphological classification?

A.
- Homogenous
- Speckled
- Mixed

Q. Describe the lesions in the eye.

A. The ipsilateral eye shows a diffuse bluish discoloration of the sclera and a patchy brownish color of the conjunctiva.

Q. Which ophthalmological condition may be associated with nevus of Ota?

A. Glaucoma may be seen in 10% of patients with nevus of Ota.

Q. How does nevus of Ito differ from nevus of Ota?

A.
- Nevus of Ito differs from nevus of Ota in terms of area of involvement
- Nevus of Ito involves the supraclavicular, scapular, and deltoid regions, which are not involved in nevus of Ota.

Q. What is Hori's nevus?

A. Hori's nevus is characterized by bilateral blue-gray to gray-brown macules of the zygomatic region, forehead, upper outer eyelids, and nose.

Q. What are the histopathological findings in nevus of Ota?

A. The noninfiltrated areas show pigmented, elongated, stellate, dendritic melanocytes scattered among the collagen bundles.

Q. What are the treatment options for a patient with nevus of Ota and Ito?

A.
- Cosmetic camouflage
- CO_2 snow alone or with dermabrasion
- Liquid nitrogen therapy
- Pulsed Q-switch ruby, alexandrite, and Nd:Yag lasers

Q. What is Panda's sign?

A. Post laser treatment the periorbital pigmentation remains looking like a Panda's eyes. Hence the name Panda's sign.

64 Nevus Sebaceous

Q. Why is it called nevus sebaceous?

A. Yellowish lobulated plaque with areas of alopecia.

Q. Who described nevus sebaceous?

A.
- First described by Jadassohn and is also known as organoid nevus
- It is not a sebaceous malformation, but a hamartoma that exhibits follicular, sebaceous, and apocrine malformation.

Q. What are the clinical features of nevus sebaceous?

A.
- It is a congenital malformation, the lesion is only slightly raised.
- It involves the scalp, neck, and rarely trunk.
- The lesions are distributed along the lines of Blaschko.
- When present on scalp, the area involved is hairless.
- Upon reaching adolescence, there is thickening and pebbling of the surface and lesions may also become verrucous.
- Secondary neoplasms may also occur, 1% of cases develop basal cell carcinoma.
- Other neoplasms are trichilemmoma, sebaceous adenoma, apocrine adenoma, and poroma.

Q. What is the histopathology?

A.
- Papillated epidermal hyperplasia, inter-anastamosis of rete and a coarsely fibrotic papillary dermis. There are enlarged sebaceous lobules and buds of follicular germinative cells.
- The verrucous surface of nevus sebaceous is histologically similar to verruca vulgaris.

Q. What is the treatment?

A.
- A conservative complete excision can be done for the cosmetic purpose as verrucous lesions are highly unsightly.
- Removal by shave or laser ablation is usually not successful. It is one of the lesions where early excision is recommended though the chances of malignancy are rather low.

65 Nevus Spilus

Q. What is nevus spilus?

A. It's a usually unilateral, segmental tan patch with superimposed speckles, that develop over time (spilus = speckled).

Q. What are the differential diagnosis?

A. Agminated nevi [junctional, compound, spitz, blue nevi].

Q. What is the etiology of nevus spilus?

A. There is controversy whether it is congenital or acquired, however, there is evidence that it is a congenital melanocytic nevus.

Q. What is the pathogenesis of nevus spilus?

A.
- It may have segmental or zosteriform distribution suggesting a localized 'field defect'.
- A nevus spilus has been linked to a garden of melanocytes in which any type of nevus can develop, simultaneously or sequentially.

Q. What are the clinical features of nevus spilus?

A.
- These lesions most commonly affect the trunk and extremities.
- The tan macular area commonly ranges from 1 to 4 cm in diameter.
- The darker speckles are approximately 1 to 6 mm in greatest diameter and may be macular or papular.
- Larger varieties of nevus spilus may be unilateral, segmental or follow Blaschko's lines.

Q. What is the histopathological findings in nevus spilus?

A.
- Lentiginous melanocytic hyperplasia
- Elongated epidermal rete ridges
- The papular foci represent junctional, compound, blue, spitz, and/or atypical nevi.

Q. What is the treatment of nevus spilus?

A.
- Individuals be followed on a periodic basis
- Areas of change or atypicality in a nevus spilus should be evaluated by biopsy or excision

66 Neurofibromatosis

Q. Define neurofibromatosis.

A. Autosomal-dominantly inherited neurocutaneous disorder or phakomatoses characterized by cutaneous lesions as well as central nervous system (CNS) and peripheral nervous system neoplasm.

Q. Define phakomatoses.

A. Inherited disorders of CNS that have congenital retinal tumors and cutaneous involvement.

Includes:

- Neurofibromatosis
- Tuberous sclerosis (epiloia, Bourneville's disease)
- Ataxia telangiectasia
- Von Hippel-Lindau disease (angiomatosis retinae)
- Sturge–Weber syndrome
- Nevoid basal cell carcinoma syndrome
- Nevus sebaceous syndrome
- Epidermal nevus syndromes

Q. Classify neurofibromatosis.

A. Riccardi classification:

- NF1: Von Recklinghausen disease
- NF2: Bilateral acoustic schwannoma
- NF3: Mixed
- NF4: Variant
- NF5: Segmental Café-au-lait macules or neurofibromas or both in one or more dermatome (segmental NF-1)
- NF6: Café-au-lait macules only
- NF7: Late Onset
- NF-NOS: Not otherwise specified

Q. Describe neurofibromatosis 1 (NF1).

A.

- Also known as Von Recklinghausen's neurofibromatosis as first described by Von Recklinghausen in 1882.
- It accounts for 90% of neurofibromatosis
- Incidence—approximately 1 in 3,000
- It is the commonest phakomatoses

Q. Which gene is involved in NF1?

A. *NF1* gene is located on chromosome 17q11.2 and encodes for protein neurofibromin (p stands for the short-petit arm of the chromosome and q stands for the long arm).

Q. Describe the pathogenesis of NF1.

A.
- *Neurofibromin* gene is a tumor suppressor gene.
- The neurofibromin protein shows significant regions of similarity to the GTPase-activating protein (GAP related protein) and is capable of down-regulating proto-oncogene RAS activity.
- RAS proto-oncogene when activated and turned to oncogene causes tumorogenesis.

Q. Describe the clinical features of NF1.

A.
- Cutaneous:
  - Café-au-lait macules (>90%)
    - Earliest skin lesion
    - Present at birth or appear in the first year
    - Sharply defined, light-brown macules that vary in size from 0.5 to 5 cm
    - The macules increase in size and number during the first decade
    - Number is not indicative of clinical severity, but it is important for diagnosis
  - Axillary and/or inguinal freckling (~80%)
    - Also known as Crowe's Sign
    - Yesudian sign—freckling over palms
  - Neurofibromas (60–90%)
    - CNFs are skin-colored to pink, tan or brown, polypoid or pedunculated nodules, soft/slightly rubbery and range from a few mm to several cm in diameter.
    - May be cutaneous or subcutaneous.
    - Buttonhole sign—upon applying pressure to the neurofibroma, it completely goes inside the skin and reappears on releasing the pressure.
    - Usually asymptomatic but sometimes becomes pruritic also.
    - Appear as early as 4–5 years of age but increase in number during puberty with acceleration in pregnancy.
  - Plexiform neurofibroma (25%) (plexiform—weblike)
    - Common along branches of trigeminal and cervical nerves, congenital in origin but become apparent at birth.

    - Large, diffuse elongated lesion with bag-of worms feel.
    - +/- overlying hyperpigmentation and hypertrichosis.
    - Elephantiasis neurofibromatosa-overgrowth of the subcutaneous tissue and of the skin pendulous and wrinkled.
    - Complication—may involve internal organs especially spinal cord deformity (dumb bell shaped neurofibromatosis). Involvement of nerves leads to neurological deficit. Can undergo sarcomatous change.
- Ocular:
  - Lisch nodules (90%)
    - Pigmented iris hamartomas appear as dome shaped yellow-brown papules on surface of iris on slit-lamp examination and rarely may be visible to naked eye also.
    - Asymptomatic.
    - Do not occur in segmental or NF2
  - Hypertelorism (25%)
  - Glaucoma
- Oral lesions:
  - Papillomatous tumors of palate, buccal mucous membrane, tongue and lips.
  - Macroglossia, usually asymmetrical.
- Scalp:
  - Cutis verticis gyrata (vertical longitudinal thickening of skin of scalp).
- Skeletal:
  - Cranial
    - Macrocephaly (20–50%)
    - Sphenoid wing dysplasia (<5%)
  - Spinal
    - Scoliosis (5–10%)
    - Spina bifida
  - Limbs (congenital)
    - Dysplasia of long bones; most commonly tibia (14%)
    - Pseudoarthrosis (2%)
    - Thinning of long bone cortex
    - Local bony overgrowth
    - Absent patellae
- Tumors:
  - Optic glioma (10–15%) +/- precocious puberty
  - Malignant peripheral nerve sheath tumor (3–15%)
  - Pheochromocytoma (1%)

- Juvenile myelomonocytic leukemia (especially in patients with concomitant juvenile xanthogranuloma)
- Astrocytoma, ependymoma, schwannoma
- Rhabdomyosarcoma, especially genitourinary
- Duodenal carcinoid
- Somatostatinoma
- Parathyroid adenoma
- Wilms tumor
- Malignant melanoma

- Endocrine disturbances:
  - Precocious puberty
  - Gynecomastia
  - Acromegaly
  - Addison's disease
  - Cushing syndrome
  - Hyperparathyroidism
  - Pheochromocytoma
  - Retinoblastoma
- Neurological:
  - Unidentified bright object on MRI (50–75%) of unknown significance.
  - Learning difficulties (30–50%)
  - Seizures (~5%)
  - Mental retardation (severe, <5%)
  - Aqueductal stenosis and hydrocephalus (~2%)
- Cardiovascular:
  - Hypertension (~30%), mostly essential due to renal artery stenosis or pheochromocytoma
  - Pulmonic stenosis
  - Renal artery stenosis

Q. What are the diagnostic criteria for NF1?

A. • Suggested by National Institute of Health Consensus Development Conference, 1988

Two or more of the following must be present:

- Six or more Café-au-lait macules >5 mm in prepubertal individuals and >15 mm in postpubertal individuals and 5 or more CALM with size 5 mm or more in children (also called Crowe's law)
- Two or more neurofibromas of any type or one plexiform neurofibroma
- 'Freckling' in the axillary or inguinal regions

- Optic gliomas
- Two or more Lisch nodules (iris hamartomas)
- Osseous lesion, such as sphenoid wing dysplasia or thinning of long bone cortex, with or without pseudarthrosis
- First-degree relative (parent, sibling or offspring) with NF1 by the above criteria

Q. Which investigation to be carried out in NF1?

A.
- Diagnosis is mainly clinical
- Thorough clinical examination of patient and family members
- Slit lamp examination of eye
- Skeletal survey
- Neurological imaging—CT scan and MRI depending upon clinical features
- Prenatal screening

Q. What are differential diagnosis of Café-au-lait macule?

A.
- Normal individuals (10–20%)
- Noonan syndrome
- Ataxia telangiectasia
- Piebaldism
- LEOPARD Syndrome
- McCune–Albright syndrome
- Bloom's syndrome
- Fanconi's anemia
- Cowden's syndrome
- Tuberous sclerosis
- Watson syndrome
- MEN syndrome

Q. What is the course and prognosis of NF1?

A.
- Course—variable and unpredictable
- Psychological morbidity due to unsightly appearance
- Early onset, rapid progression before puberty and extensive involvement—poor prognosis.
- Enlargement and pain in individual lesion—hemorrhage or malignant transformation.
- Sarcomatous change in neurofibromas occur in 1.5–15% cases.
- Highly aggressive malignant peripheral nerve sheath tumor may occur. In women, screening to be done for breast carcinoma

Q. How will you manage NF1?

A.
- Treatment is mostly symptomatic. Café-au-lait can be masked by cosmetics

- Large disfiguring or rapidly progressive painful lesions—excision or carbon dioxide laser
- Pruritus—antihistaminics
- Orthopedic intervention
- Life long surveillance usually an annual assessment by neurologist, ophthalmologist, regular blood pressure monitoring
- Counselling

Q. Which antihistaminics are used in pruritus of NF?

A. Mast cell stabilizers.

Q. What is the other name for NF2?

A. Bilateral acoustic schwannoma.

Q. Which gene is involved in NF2?

A. Gene on chromosome 22q11, encodes for protein Neurofibromin 2 or Merlin or Schwanomin.

Q. Describe NF2.

A.
- Autosomal dominant inheritance
- Incidence 1 in 40,000
- Characterized by bilateral acoustic schwannoma
- Associated with other meningeal and glial tumors
- Vestibular lesions manifest in third decade of life
- Juvenile posterior subcapsular cataract
- Café-au-lait macule (fewer as in NF1) are seen
- Cutaneous neurofibroma are seen
- No Lisch nodules, MR, learning disability

Q. What are the diagnostic criteria for NF2?

A. Either of the two:

1. Bilateral eighth nerve masses as demonstrated on CT or MRI.
2. A first degree relative with NF2 and either U/L eighth nerve mass or two of the following: neurofibroma, meningioma, glioma, schwannoma, and juvenile posterior subcapsular opacity.

Q. Describe the clinical features of segmental NF.

A. Either cutaneous neurofibroma or café-au-lait macule present or both present in segmental distribution.

Q. If one parent is affected with neurofibromatosis then what is the chance of offspring being affected with neurofibromatosis?

A. As neurofibromatosis is transmitted as an autosomal dominant disorder, so if one parent is affected then there is 50% chance that the child will have neurofibromatosis.

Q. If parents do not have neurofibromatosis, then what is the incidence that the child will have neurofibromatosis?

A. • If both the parents are normal then incidence of child getting neurofibromatosis is equal to that in normal population, i.e., 1 in 3,000 for NF1 and 1 in 40,000 for NF2.

• It is due to sporadic mutation.

Q. Is it difficult for a women with neurofibromatosis to conceive?

A. Yes. This is because neurofibromatosis patients frequently have leiomyoma of uterus which makes it difficult for women with neurofibromatosis to conceive.

Q. New modalities in treatment of NF2.

A. • Stereotactic radiosurgery—stereotactic radiosurgery (the gamma knife) has in recent years come to the fore as a suggested alternative to microsurgical removal in the management of vestibular schwannomas.

• Advantages—avoidance of an operation, a short hospital stay and no period of convalescence.

• Disadvantage—very long period of follow-up, with repeated scanning, significant morbidity to the hearing, both immediately and over time, and to the facial and trigeminal nerves. Risk of hydrocephalus.

67 Nipple Eczema, Hand Eczema and Pompholyx

Q. Define dyshidrotic eczema.

A. This form of eczema is characterized by vesicle and bullae on palms and soles. When it involves palms it is called cheiropompholyx, and when it involves soles it is called podopompholyx.

Q. What is pompholyx?

A.
- Pompholyx or dyshidrotic eczema, account for 5–10% of hand eczema. There is a family history or a personal history of atopy. Direct allergens implicated are primin, isopropyl-paraphenylenediamine, benzisothiazolinone and dichromates, perfumes, fragrances, balsam ingredients.
- They cause palmar vesicles, appearing in crops on palms and sides of fingers. Vesicles are very itchy, deep seated and look like sago grains. They dry up and overlying skin peels off. Lymphangitis and cellulitis can occur. Rubbing can produce secondary eczematous changes. Nail changes can occur.
- Vesicles are seen over palms and soles. Nickel sulphate was the commonest allergen (14%) followed by potassium dichromate, nitrofurazone. Patch testing is positive for one or more allergens.

Q. What is the treatment of pompholyx?

A.
- Severe cases require soaks and compresses of potassium permanganate (1:8,000) or burrows solution 1%. A soothing lotion like calamine lotion is given. Blister fluid can be aspirated with syringe. Topical steroids are useful in subacute and chronic cases. Topical tacrolimus 0.1% ointment with mometasone furoate can be used.
- Systemic treatment—short course of steroids is used. Sedative antihistaminics are used. Low dose methotrexate (5 mg/week) and dapsone are given.
- Other therapy are—local photochemotherapy, intradermal botulinum toxin can be given. Tap water iontophoresis can be used.

Q. Describe nipple eczema.

A.
- Eczema of the breast affects the nipple, the areolae and may extend to surrounding skin.
- Rarely seen in men. Eczema of the nipple is the moist type with oozing and crusting. Painful fissuring is seen. Atopic dermatitis is a frequent cause.
- It can be the only manifestation of atopy. Other causes of nipple eczema are allergic contact dermatitis, jogger's dermatitis, or from ill-fitting brassieres with seams in women with asymmetrical large breast.

Q. What are the signs of Paget's disease in breast?

A. If eczema of nipple or areola has persisted for >3 months and unilateral, a biopsy is to be done, to rule out Paget's disease. Retraction of nipple is an ominous sign.

Q. Treatment of nipple eczema.

A.
- Oral antibiotics are preferred treatment for secondary bacterial infections.
- Analgesia may be required and breastfeeding is suspended for the period.
- Pumping and the silicon nipple shield are useful.
- Oral fluconazole 150 mg is effective in case of candidial infection.
- Topical gentian violet 0.5%, mupirocin 2%, betamethasone 0.1% ointment is effective.
- Lactating consultant or nurse may be helpful in managing these patients, since poor positioning during breast-feeding is the cofactor.

Q. What are the types of hand eczema?

A.
- Allergic contact dermatitis
- Irritant contact dermatitis
- Atopic hand eczema
- Vesicular or vesiculobullous
- Hyperkeratotic endogenous hand eczema

Q. Which is the strong risk for hand eczema?

A. Wet work (contact with liquid or gloves for >2 h/day or hand-washing >20 times/day) is a strong risk factor.

Q. What are the high risk occupations for hand eczema?

A. High risk occupations—bakers, hairdresser, dental surgeon, kitchen worker/cooks, butchers, healthcare workers, cleaners, doctor/dentist/veterinarians, and laboratory technicians.

Q. What are the allergens in hair dressing?
A. Glyceryl monothioglycolate, ammonium persulfate.

Q. What is the allergen in cement?
A. Chromate and cobalt.

Q. What is the systemic treatment of hand eczema?
A. Methotrexate, azathioprine and mycophenolate mofetil (1–1.5 g twice a day for adult), cyclosporine, oral retinoids, alitretinoin 30 mg/day.

Q. What are the barrier products used?
A. Foams containing dimethicone and glycerin.

Q. What is the topical treatment of hand eczema?
A.
- Moisturizing is the critical component.
- Application of protective moisturizing cream or ointment after each hand wash. Petroleum jelly is also used.
- Superpotent or potent topical steroids. Addition of 2.5% zinc sulfate to clobetasol enhances the efficacy of topical steroids. Soaks of tar bath oil or application of 20% liquor carbonis detergent or 2% crude coal tar in an ointment base.
- Phototherapy—high dose of UVA-1, soaks or cream PUVA and oral PUVA. Superficial Grenz ray radiotherapy, in dose of 200 cG are delivered at weekly interval for total 800–1,000 cG. Therapy is repeated after months. Total lifetime dose should not exceed 5,000 cG.

Q. Newer modalities for the treatment for pompholyx.
A. Alitretinoin or 9-cis retinoic acid. This treatment has been efficacious in double-blind randomized studies, leading to 75% improvement in patients with recalcitrant chronic hand eczemas, with an impressive 50% remission rate.

68 Nummular Eczema

Q. What are the other names for nummular eczema?

A. Discoid eczema, nummular dermatitis, microbial eczema, nummular dermatitis.

Q. What is the meaning of the word nummular?

A. Coin-shaped.

Q. Define nummular eczema.

A. It is a condition characterized by oozing papulovesicular lesions or erythematous, scaly, eczematous lesions which are coin shaped with a clear demarcated edge.

Q. Which are the most common sites to be affected?

A. Usually extensors of limbs.

Q. Epidemiology.

A.
- More common in older age group (above 50 years)
- Men are affected slightly more often and at later age than women

Q. Factors implicated in the etiology.

A. Xerotic skin, atopic diathesis, neurogenic contributors (like substance P and calcitonin gene related peptide positive nerve fibers), alcohol, allergic contact dermatitis (to rubber, nickel, fragrances, mercury), sensitization to certain substances and drugs (gold, dental amalgam, methyldopa).

Q. What are the clinical features?

A. Initially erythematous papules or vesicles which coalesce to form large round lesions. Later lesion starts oozing and crust is formed. In late stages, lesions become dry, scaly, less erythematous that may appear annular. Usually symmetrically distributed over extensors of limbs, occasionally trunk. Itching is the main complaint. Hyperpigmentation or lichenification of skin can occur due to constant scratching.

Q. What are the histopathological findings?

A.
- New lesions—spongiosis, intraepidermal vesicles, papillary edema, perivascular infiltrate.

- Old lesions—psoriasiform epidermal changes, focal spongiosis, Mixed infiltrate with few eosinophils, alternating ortho and parakeratosis

Q. What is the prognosis?

A. Chronic course, partial remission, relapses common, worsens in winters.

Q. How to diagnose?

A. Mainly clinical, patch testing

Q. Differential diagnosis.

A.
- Allergic contact dermatitis
- Irritant contact dermatitis
- Tinea corporis
- Polymorphous light eruption
- Psoriasis
- Atopic dermatitis
- Mycosis fungoides
- Autoeczematization
- Bowen's disease

Q. Treatment.

A.
- All causative agents should be removed
- Topical steroids
- Antihistaminics
- Antibiotics
- Topical emollients
- Oral steroids (40 mg/day)
- Hand eczema

Q. What are the morphological pattern of hand eczema?

A. Pompholyx, hyperkeratotic palmar eczema, ring eczema, fingertip eczema, housewife's eczema, apron eczema, discoid eczema, juvenile plantar dermatosis.

Q. Classification of hand eczema.

A.
- *Endogenous*:
  - Atopic dermatitis
  - Discoid eczema
  - Pompholyx
  - Palmoplantar pustulosis
  - Hyperkeratotic eczema
- *Exogenous*:
  - Irritant contact dermatitis

- Allergic contact dermatitis
- Dissemination from a focus
- Systemic allergen
- Infective dermatitis

Q. Write a note on housewife's eczema.

A.
- It is a chronic, cumulative irritant dermatitis caused by household contact with soap, soda, detergent, cleanser
- Friction, trauma, cold and heat play a part. Atopics are more vulnerable. It develops usually after marriage or childbirth
- It commonly occurs on palmar surface of fingers, interdigital spaces, palms, and dorsal aspects of fingers mostly knuckles coal tar ointments

Q. What is ring eczema?

A. This pattern of eczema affects young women. An itchy patch of eczema appears beneath the ring finger and spreads to adjacent fingers and the palmar area. Very rarely radioactive gold in the ring may cause radiation dermatitis called "wedding ring dermatitis".

69 Other Deep Fungal Infections

Q. What is the causative agent of sporotrichosis?
A. *Sporothrix schenckii.*

Q. What do you mean by dimorphic fungi?
A. Fungi which is seen in yeast and mycelial forms.

Q. What is dematiaceous fungi?
A. The pigment producing fungi.

Q. Is there any seasonal variation in the incidence of sporotrichosis?
A. Highest in the first half of winter in which there is high humidity and temperature is between 16–22°C because these conditions favor saprophytic growth of *S. schenckii.*

Q. Why is history of occupation important?
A. After trauma, it is common in:
- Florists and gardeners (rose thorns)
- Forest tree workers
- Workers using straw as packing material
- Mine workers (decaying vegetable matter, e.g. timber with soil as a source)

Q. Predisposing factors.
A.
- Trauma—thorn/splinter/insect bite
- Adult males by view of occupation
- Walking barefoot (farmers)
- Alcoholics (systemic sporotrichosis)

Q. What are the clinical features of systemic sporotrichosis?
A.
- Ulcerated nodules on body/mucous membrane lesions and visceral lesions (bones/joints/lungs/meninges).
- Generally not painful
- Additional lesions appear weeks later typically developing as dermal and subcutaneous nodules and ulcers along the path of lymphatic drainage
- This is well known as "SPOROTRICOID" pattern.

Q. Which animal can transmit sporotrichosis?
A. Cat has been reported to transmit sporotrichosis.

Q. Portal of entry in systemic sporotrichosis.
A. Lung.

Q. What is the incubation period?
A. 8–30 days.

Q. Mode of spread.
A.
- Localized to subcutaneous tissue
- Spreads via subcutaneous lymphatics
- Disseminates in blood stream

Q. What are asteroid bodies? In which conditions are they seen?
A. They are small cigar shaped or oval yeasts surrounded by thick radiate eosinophilic substance and are seen in:
- Sporotrichosis
- Sarcoidosis
- Tuberculosis

Q. What are the two reasons suggested to be the cause of asteroid bodies?
A.
- Trapped collagen bundles
- Some components of cytoskeleton, predominantly vimentin intermediate filaments.

Q. Types of sporotrichosis.
A.
- Cutaneous
- Fixed
- Lymphangitic (most common type is localized lymphatic starting as pustule/nodule)
- Atypical (mycetoma like or cellulitic forms)
- Systemic

Q. What are the clinical types of fixed sporotrichosis?
A.
- Acneiform
- Nodular
- Ulcerated
- Verrucous
- Infiltrated plaques (high immunity) or red scaly patches.

Q. Why do some get lymphangitic and some fixed form of sporotrichosis?
A. Depends on host immune response and changes in temperature sensitivity of the organisms.

Q. Which mycobacterial infection closely resembles lymphangitic sporotrichosis?
A. *Mycobacterium marinum* causing fish tank granuloma.

Q. Describe the colonies.

A.
- Leathery moist, initially white later black due to production of conidia and partly due to addition of thiamine to media.
- Microscopy—slender hyphae bear small oval/pyriform conidia and conidiophores arising at right angles from the hyphae. Cigar shaped or oval yeasts on brain heart infusion agar incubated with sheeps blood at 37°C.

Q. How do you treat?

A.
- Itraconazole 100–200 mg daily
- Terbinafine 250 mg/day
- Potassium iodide 5 drops initially increasing to 4–6 mL of SSKI three times a day for 3–4 weeks after clinical cure.
- IV amphotericin B
- Local heat application (also in chromoblastomycosis)

Q. What are the agents causing chromoblastomycosis?

A. *Phialophora verrucosa, Fonsecaea pedrosoi, Fonsecaea compacta, Cladophialophora carrionii.*

Q. Why is it common in rural communities?

A. Walking barefoot predisposes to trauma (splinter of wood) especially in adult male agricultural workers (the organism is seen in wood and soil) and these conditions are prevalent in rural areas.

Q. Other names.

A. Verrucous dermatitis/chromomycosis.

Q. What are muriform or sclerotic cells or Medlar bodies (Copper penny bodies)?

A. Within giant cells, group of fungal cells which are chestnut or golden brown in color divided in several planes of division by thick septa (deeply pigmented and thick walled).

Q. What are the clinical features?

A. It starts as a warty papule leading to a verrucous hypertrophic plaque, ulcereration, Psoriasiform lesions.

Q. In which deep fungal infections can koebnerization be seen?

A. Chromoblastomycosis.

Q. What are the complications?

A.
- Secondary infection—itching/pain
- Elephantiasis (secondary infection by lymphatic stasis)
- Squamous cell carcinoma
- Brain abscess (hematogenous spread)

Q. How do you differentiate it from blastomycosis?

A. By the absence of sharp border containing minute abscesses and also absence of pulmonary lesions.

Q. What are the differential diagnosis of verrucous hyperkeratotic plaques?

A.
- Verruca vulgaris
- Tuberculosis verrucosa cutis
- Chromoblastomycosis
- Leishmaniasis
- Syphilis
- Verrucous discoid lupus erythematosus
- Verrucous hemangioma
- Inflammatory verrucous epidermal nevus

Q. Culture characteristics.

A. Dark gray/green to black and velvety or dawny with a black obverse.

Q. Treatment.

A.
- Itraconazole 100–200 mg daily
- Terbinafine 250 mg daily
- Flucytosine with amphotericin B
- Better with *Cladophialophora carrionii*
- Cryotherapy/local heat

Q. What is the indication of surgical excision?

A. Very small lesions and in these it should be combined with chemotherapy (larger lesions, if excised may lead to development of satellite lesions).

Q. What is Welsh regimen and Damle's regimen?

A. Welsch regimen:
- Intensive phase—it consists of amikacin sulphate 15 mg/kg twice daily (IM) in 2 divided doses + tablet cotrimoxazole double strength (DS) twice a days given for 3 weeks
- Maintenance phase—continue cotrimoxazole DS for 2 weeks after the last cycle.

Modified Welsh regimen:
- Intensive phase—it consists of amikacin sulphate 15 mg/kg twice daily (IM) in 2 divided doses + tablet cotrimoxazole DS twice a days given for 3 weeks + add rifampicin 10 mg/kg/day.
- Maintenance phase—continue cotrimoxazole DS for 2 weeks after the last cycle + tablet rifampicin 10 mg/kg/day.

Damle's regimen:
- It consists of addition of rifampicin to amikacin sulphate and cotrimoxazole combination.
- Itraconazole 100–200 mg daily

70 Parapsoriasis

Q. Define parapsoriasis.

A. It is a chronic, lymphoproliferative, asymptomatic, erythematous and scaly dermatosis, that includes, small plaque parapsoriasis (SPP) and large plaque parapsoriasis (LPP), acute and chronic variants of pityriasis lichenoides and lymphomatoid papulosis with significant overlap and progression to MF.

Q. What is differential diagnosis (DD) of parapsoriasis?

A.
- Mycosis fungoides (MF)
- Psoriasis
- Pityriasis rosea (PR)
- PR-like drug eruptions
- Dry nummular dermatitis
- Secondary syphilis
- MF-like drug eruptions
- Autoimmune connective tissue diseases

Q. Who defined parapsoriasis?

A. Brocq in 1902.

Q. Classify parapsoriasis.

A.
- Small plaque parapsoriasis
- Large plaque parapsoriasis
- Pityriasis lichenoides:
  - Pityriasis lichenoides chronica (PLC) (Juliusberg)
  - Pityriasis lichenoides et varioliformis acuta (synonyms PLEVA, Mucha-Habermann)

Q. Clinical features of small plaque.

A.
- It is chronic asymptomatic condition
- Persistent small scaly plaques on trunk
- Peak age being 40–50 years
- It can affect all races with the male female ratio being 3:1
- It consists of round or oval erythematous patches 2–6 cm in diameter
- Slight scaling with digitate appearance
- Poikiloderma
- The long axis of digitate lesion has 10–20 cm forming fingernail appearance.

Q. What is digitate dermatosis?

A. Small plaque parapsoriasis with typical finger print patches on the trunk which are >5 cm and follows the lines of cleavage of the skin and gives an image of a hug leaving a print. When lesion has yellowish hue, it is called xanthodermic perstans.

Q. What is the DD of poikiloderma?

A.
- Large plaque parapsoriasis
- Dermatomyositis
- Lupus erythematosus
- Chronic radiation dermatosis
- Bloom's syndrome
- Rothmund–Thompson syndrome
- Dyskeratosis congenita
- Xeroderma pigmentosum

Q. What are the various alternative names for parapsoriasis?

A.
- Chronic superficial scaly dermatitis.
- Persistent superficial dermatitis
- Xantho-erythroderma

Q. What are the other names of LPP?

A.
- Atrophic parapsoriasis
- Poikilodermatous parapsoriasis
- Poikiloderma vasculare atrophicans

Q. What are the clinical features of LPP?

A.
- It is a chronic condition characterized by presence of fixed large atrophic erythematous plaque mostly on trunk and sometimes limb.
- Ill-defined irregular persistent yellow orange erythematous to brown macules or plaques.
- Epidermal atrophy.
- Lesions are larger than 6 cm.
- Later they develop mottled hyperpigmentation and telangiectasias.
- Lesions are present on nonsun exposed parts also.

Q. What is parapsoriasis variegata?

A. Brownish red scaly papules arranged in a net or zebra-like pattern on trunk or extremities.

Q. What are alternative names?

A.
- Parapsoriasis lichenoids of Brocq
- Retiform parapsoriasis

Q. What is clonal dermatitis?

A. It is a term which includes a variety of lymphocyte-rich dermatosis often characterized by clonal T-lymphocyte proliferation which include presentation like primary erythroderma, nonspecific chronic spongiotic dermatitis, follicular mucinosis and large plaque parapsoriasis and pagetoid reticulosis. It may progress to MF.

Q. Explain the histopathology of parapsoriasis.

A. Small plaque epidermis shows:
- Hyperkeratosis
- Focal parakeratosis (focal scale crust)
- Mild spongiosis

The dermis shows:
- Perivascular lymphohistiocytosis
- CD4+ T cells

Q. Explain the treatment of parapsoriasis.

A.
- Topical emollients
- Tacrolimus 0.1%
- Coal tar
- Bexarotene
- Mechlorethamine
- Steroids
- Antihistaminics
- UVB therapy
- PUVA

Q. What is pityriasis lichenoides?

A.
- Idiopathic acquired dermatosis of unknown etiology
- Acute form is known as PLEVA

Q. Who discovered pityriasis lichenoids?

A.
- PLEVA: Jadassohn and Nieser 1894
- PLC: Juliusburg 1899

Q. Other name of PLEVA.

A. Mucha-Habermann disease.

Q. Epidemology of PLEVA.

A. • Young adults
- Male > female
- PLC > PLEVA

Q. What is the etiology?

A. Infections:
- Toxoplasma
- Cytomegalovirus
- Parvovirus
- Adenovirus
- Epstein–Barr virus
- Streptococci
- Staphylococci

Q. PLC synonyms.

A. • Chronic guttate parapsoriasis
- Dermatitis psoriasiform nodularis
- Parapsoriasis chronica

Q. What are the clinical features of PLEVA?

A. • Acute eruption associated with low grade fever, headache, malaise, arthralgia
- Eruptions begin as crops of erythematous macule → edematous papules → Central vesiculation
- Itching and burning sensation present
- Lesions present over the trunk, flexures
- Spares the face, palms, soles, scalps, mucous membrane
- Heals with varioliform scars, hypo and hyperpigmentation
- Polymorphous lesions are present

Q. DD of varioliform scars.

A. • PLEVA
- Varicella
- Hydroa vacciniforme
- Papulonecrotic tuberculides
- Disseminated pustular lesions
- Atrophic maculosa varioliformis cutis.

Q. What are the DD of PLEVA?

A. • Varicella
- Pyoderma gangrenosum
- Leukocytoclastic vasculitis

- Lymphomatoid papulosis
- Gianotti-Crosti syndrome
- Arthropod bite, sting, infestations
- Erythema multiforme, dermatitis herpetiformis, follicilitis
- Secondary syphilis

Q. Explain the histopathology of PLEVA.

A.
- Epidermal necrosis with hemorrhage and dense perivascular infiltrate in superficial and deep dermis.
- Lymphocytic vasculitis
- Vacuolar interface dermatitis.

Q. DD of PLC.

A.
- Guttate psoriasis
- Pityriasis rosea
- Lichen planus
- Secondary syphilis
- Small plaque parapsoriasis
- Drug eruption

Q. What are the clinical features of PLC?

A.
- It is the more common form of PL.
- Characteristically it shows a pleomorphic eruption.
- Asymptomatic lesions
- Red-brown colored oval round lichenoid papules 3–10 mm with centrally adherent mica like scales
- Scales detached with shiny brown pigmented surface.
- Site—trunk, proximal extremities; spares palms and soles.
- Heals with hyperpigmentation or hypopigmentation.
- Scarring is unusual.

Q. Explain the histopathology of PLC.

A.
- Compact parakeratosis
- Exocytosis of lymphocytes causing pseudo munro abcesses.
- Dermis shows lymphohistocytic perivascular infiltrate.
- Dermal edema.
- Vacuolar interface dermatitis.

Q. What is febrile ulceronecrotic Mucha-Habermann disease (FUMHD)?

A.
- It is a febrile ulcerative acute ulceronecrotic form of PLEVA.
- Sudden onset of diffuse purpuric papules with necrotic centres.

- Development of large necrotic ulcers associated with high fever malaise arthralgia.
- Gastrointestinal tract (GIT) and central nervous system (CNS) manifestations along with pneumonitis
- Lymphadenopathy
- Myocarditis
- Oral mucosa may be involved
- Pruritus and pain is present
- Ulcer may get secondarily infected which heals with atrophic scar

Q. Explain the treatment of PL.

A.
- Oral erythromycin 2 g/day
- Tetracycline 2 g/day
- Oral antihistaminics
- Oral corticosteroids

71 Palmoplantar Keratoderma

Q. Define palmoplantar keratoderma (PPK) (tylosis).

A. It is defined as heterogeneous group of disorders characterized by hyperkeratosis of palms and soles.

Q. Classify hereditary PPK.

A.
- Diffuse:
  - Nontransgrediens (confined to the palms and soles only)
    - Vorners
    - Unna-Thost
  - Transgrediens (extending onto the dorsum of palms and soles)
    - Camisa syndrome
    - Vohwinkel's syndrome
    - Greither's syndrome
    - Huriez syndrome
    - Mal de meleda
    - Olmsted syndrome
    - Papillon-Lefèvre syndrome
- Focal:
  - Focal PPK with oral leukokeratosis
  - Striate PPK
  - Howel-Evans syndrome
  - Richner-Hanhart disease
  - Pachyonychia congenita
  - Carvajal syndrome
- Punctate:
  - Punctate keratoderma of palm and soles
  - Punctate keratoderma of palmar crease, marginal papular acrokeratoderma

Q. What is nontransgrediens keratoderma?

A. *Types*:
- Vorner syndrome (epidermolytic)
- Unna-Thost (nonepidermolytic)

Clinical features:
- Thick yellowish hyperkeratosis involving the entire palms and soles with sharp erythematous cut off borders

- Isolated keratotic lesions on dorsum of hands, feet, knees, and elbows.
- Dirty appearance in epidermolytic PPK
- Waxy in nonepidermolytic PPK

Q. Treatment of nontransgrediens PPK.

A.
- About 6% salicyclic acid
- About 50% propylene glycol under occlusion
- Lactic acid-urea combination
- Oral retinoid therapy

Type	*Inheritance*	*Mutation*	*Clinical features*
Focal palmoplantar keratoderma (PPK) with oral leukokeratosis	AD	K16	Oral cavity and nail involved
Striate Howel–Evans	AD	Dsg1	Linear striate PPK, oral leukokeratosis, associated with malignancy
Richner–Hanhart	AR	*TAT* gene	Painful PPK, mental retardation
Paronychia congenita	AD	K16,17	Subungual hyperkeratosis of nail

Q. What is Mal de Meleda?

A. Synonyms—keratoderma palmoplantar transgrediens
- Autosomal recessive
- Named after Croatian islands Meleda from where first patients were described.
- Caused by mutation in *ARS* gene which encodes SLURP-1 (secreted by -6/PAR related protein)

Q. Clinical features of Mal de Meleda.

A.
- Starts in early childhood as erythema of palms and soles, followed by appearance of diffuse, waxy, ivory-yellow hyperkeratosis, extend on to dorsum (transgredience)
- Well-circumscribed psoriasis like plaques or lichenoid patches may be present on elbow and knees.

Q. How can you differentiate the above type from other PPK?

A.
- Hyperhidrosis
- Maceration
- Malodor
- Digital constriction
- Nail changes
- All present in Mal de Meleda

Q. What are the histopathological findings of Mal de Meleda?

A.
- Hyperkeratosis
- Acanthosis
- Pseudospongiosis
- Perivascular lymphohistiocytic infiltrate

Q. What is the treatment of Mal de Meleda?

A. Oral retinoids.

Q. What is progressive keratoderma?

A.
- Synonyms:
    - Greither's disease
    - Acral keratoderma of Sybert
    - Transgrediens et progrediens PPK
- Atopic dermatitis
- Mutations in gene encoding keratin 1 are responsible

Q. What are the clinical features of progressive keratoderma?

A.
- Onset in late child hood, symmetrical, glove and stocking distribution of PPK.
- Diffuse PPK extends onto dorsal aspects of hands and feet, knees and elbows with characteristic involvement of tendo achilles.
- Hyperhidrosis is common
- An early onset and a more severe form of pseudoainhum formation and auto-amputation of digits may occur.

Q. What is Vohwinkel's syndrome?

A. It's a cicatrizing keratoderma with hearing impairment.
- AD trait
- Honeycomb-like PPK, pseudoainhum of digits and stellate keratoses of knuckles and other extensor surfaces.
- Mutations in gene encoding connexin 26 which is found in cochlea as well as palmoplantar epidermis.
- Warty lesions on extensor surface and knuckles coalesce with spiky projections giving pathognomic starfish appearance on knuckles.
- Sensorineural hearing loss present.

Q. Histopathological findings in Vohwinkel's syndrome.

A.
- Hyperkeratosis
- Acanthosis, thickened granular cell layer with retained nuclei in stratum corneum.

Q. Causes of acquired PPK.

A.
- Menopause (keratoderma climactericum)
- Hypothyroidism
- Acanthosis nigricans
- Psoriasis
- Pityriasis rubra pilaris
- Tinea manuum/pedis
- Darier's disease
- Lichen planus
- Associated with esophageal carcinoma (Howel-Evans syndrome)

Q. Newer modalities of treatment.

A.
- Based on recent studies, topical sirolimus treatment was proven to be effective in treatment of painful plantar keratoderma in pachyonychia congenita using topical sirolimus.
- To avoid systemic toxicities, 1% sirolimus ointment was compounded to be used twice daily on both feet. The patients used an average of 2.5–4.5 mg sirolimus daily for about 4 months. There was significant improvement of pain within 4 weeks. Two months after treatment initiation, the thickness and size of the callus was markedly reduced.

72 Paronychia

Q. Why is this paronychia?

A. There is a localized swelling on the lateral nail fold with redness, edema, pain and occasionally purulent discharge with no change in the nail plate.

Q. Define paronychia.

A. Paronychia is the term used for inflammation of nail folds, and presents with painful periungual erythema and sometimes with purulence.

Q. What are the types of paronychia?

A. Acute and chronic.

Q. Which organisms cause paronychia?

A.
- Acute paronychia: Caused by bacteria such as *Staphylococcus, Streptococcus, Escherichia coli*
- Chronic paronychia: Due to *Candida* species, *Scytalidium* species, syphilis, tuberculosis, leprosy

Q. What are the clinical features of acute paronychia?

A.
- Usually bacterial in origin.
- May develop from a simple injury.
- Localized swelling on the lateral nail fold with redness, edema, pain and occasionally purulent discharge.
- May subside on its own.
- If it spreads it may cause nail deformity by affecting the matrix

Q. What are the predisposing factors for acute paronychia?

A. Bacterial infection due thumb sucking in children.

Q. What are the predisposing factors for chronic paronychia?

A.
- Exposure to wet activities such as in housewives, nurses, exposure to irritants, excessive manicuring, finger sucking.
- Chemical damage

Q. What is chronic paronychia?

A.
- Infection maybe mixed (fungal and bacterial—Gram negative bacilli)
- Nail dystrophy is seen.

- Course is prolonged
- Eczematization and subungual abscess formation may complicate the condition.

Q. How do you treat acute paronychia?

A.
- A quick and easy method to relieve pain and hasten healing is to stab the purulent area with number 11 scalpel blade and discharge the pus.
- Antibiotics and soaks should then be instituted.

Q. How do you treat chronic paronychia?

A.
- Avoidance of all causative and aggravating factors
- Long term systemic antibiotics and topical antibacterials or antifungal therapy

Q. Differential diagnosis of paronychia.

A.
- Herpetic whitlow
- Hallopeau's acrodermatitis
- Hypoparathyroidism
- Celiac disease
- Acrodermatitis enteropathica
- Reactive arthritis
- Acrokeratosis paraneoplastica
- Retinoid therapy
- Pemphigus
- Myremecious wart
- Cellulitis
- Felon
- Onychomycosis
- Nail psoriasis
- Squamous cell carcinoma

73 Parry–Romberg Syndrome

Q. What is seen in Parry–Romberg syndrome (PRS)?

A. Progressive hemifacial atrophy, epilepsy, exophthalmos, alopecia, enophthalmos, the deviation of mouth and nose to the affected side, and unilateral exposition of teeth, when lips are involved.

Q. What do you see in PRS when lower extremities are involved?

A.
- Associated spina bifida
- Faulty limb development
- Hemiatrophy
- Flexion contractures

Q. Which is the only type of PRS showing spontaneous resolution?

A. Childhood type with involvement of extremities.

Q. Why are roentgenograms done?

A. To detect melorheostosis as dense cortical hyperostosis.

Q. What remains the mainstay of treatment?

A. Physical therapy of involved limbs to prevent contractures and frozen joints.

74 Pearly Penile Papules–Hirsute Penis

Q. Why is it a case of pearly penile papules (PPP)?

A.
- They are pearly white dome-shaped papules present circumferentially on the coronal margin and sulcus of glans penis.
- Seen more in uncircumcised males.

Q. What else can it be?

A.
- Condyloma acuminatum
- Papillomas
- Hypertrophic sebaceous glands.

Q. How will you manage a case of PPP?

A.
- No treatment is necessary.
- If patient wants treatment, then laser ablation or shave excision can be done.

Q. What will you see on histology of PPP?

A.
- There is dermal proliferation of fibroblasts in a collagenous stroma with increased dilated blood vessels.
- Elastic fibers are decreased in number.

Q. What are the other cutaneous angiofibromas?

A.
- Adenoma sebaceum
- Fibrous papules of nose
- MEN type 1
- Segmental angiofibroma of tuberous sclerosis (TS)
- Cellular angiofibroma of vulva in older women
- Birt–Hogg–Dubé syndrome

75 Pediculosis

Q. What are the clinical features of pediculosis?

A.
- Itching
- On examination—nits and live lice
- Lymph node swelling

Q. What is the differential diagnosis of pediculosis capitis?

A.
- Pityriasis sicca (dandruff)
- Hair spray remnants
- Concretions
- Piedra
- Monilethrix/Pseudomonilethrix
- Scalp impetigo
- Peripilar keratin casts
- Insect bite
- Eczema
- Psoriasis
- Pseudonits

Q. What is pediculosis? What are the types?

A. Pediculosis is an infestation of lice, of any part of the body. It is caused by sucking lice of the order phthiraptera and suborder anoplura. There are three types of lice which form the ectoparasite fauna of man:
- Pediculosis humanus var capitis (head louse)
- Pediculosis humanus var corporis (body louse)
- Phthirus pubis (pubic louse)

Q. What is the life cycle of lice?

A. The life cycle of the head louse has three stages: Egg, nymph, and adult.

Q. What is the mode of transmission of head louse?

A. Close personal contact and sharing of headgear is the chief mode of transmission among susceptible contacts. They move from one infested hair to another with the help of claws on their legs.

Q. What are the differentiating points between head louse and body louse?

A. Head louse is relatively smaller (2.5–3 mm) in size compared to body louse (2.8–3.5 mm). It is darker or blackish in color whereas the body louse is grey or brownish in color. Also, the segments of antennae in head louse are smaller as compared to body louse. On an average, the female head louse lays 100 eggs during its 30 day lifetime, whereas a female body louse lays around 300 eggs.

Q. What are pseudonits?
A. Retained internal root sheath on the hair shaft.

Q. What are the diseases transmitted by head louse?
A. None.

Q. What are the disease transmitted by body louse?
A.
- Epidemic typhus caused by *Rickettsia prowazekii*
- Relapsing fever caused by *Borrelia recurrentis*
- Trench fever caused by *Bartonella quintana*

Q. What are the various treatment modalities of pediculosis capitis?
A. Treatment:
- General measures:
  - Fomite/environmental control
  - Avoid contact with contaminated items such as hats, hairbrushes, clothing, towel, combs, etc.
  - Bedding, clothing should be washed and dried
  - Combing wet hair with the fine toothed bug buster comb. It should be repeated every 4 days for 2 weeks
  - Robi comb—battery powered device with which dry hair with lice can be combed
  - Isopropyl myristate and cyclomethicone
  - Coconut and ylang-ylang spray—asphyxiate the lice
  - Others—devices that deliver hot air to hair
  - Simple shaving
  - Plant derived essential hair oils—lavender, tea-tree oil, and neem
  - Head louse repellents containing piperonol
  - Plant derived essential oils (citronella)
- Topical application:
  - 0.5% malathion-left on hair for 12 hours and washed off. It has a doubtful ovicidal action but kills adult and larva. Therefore, to be applied second time, 10–14 days later
  - Gamma-benzene hexachloride (lindane) 1%—short contact period even for 5 minutes is effective
  - 10% crotamiton—safer, but less effective and has to be left for >24 hours
  - Pyrethrins and carbaryl
  - 1% permethrin

- Systemic treatment:
  - Ivermectin:
    - 200 μg/kg
    - Two doses at 10 days interval required.
    - Not in children <15 kg

      (Ivermectin is an anthelmintic drug, structurally similar to the macrolide antibiotics without antibacterial activity, which is derived from *Streptomyces avermitilis*. Ivermectin binds to glutamate-gated chloride channels with high affinity and specificity, which occur in invertebrate nerve and muscle cells, causing an increase in the permeability of the cell membrane to chloride ions of the nerve or muscle cell. This results in hyperpolarization, leading to flaccid paralysis culminating in the death of the parasite.)
  - Cotrimoxazole:
    - Kills symbiotic bacteria living in lice
    - Controls pyoderma

      (When cotrimoxazole is administered to infested individual, drug reaches the circulation of lice during blood meal as a result, gut flora of *Pediculus* is killed, and thereby depriving the lice of essential vitamins. Death results from vitamin B deficiency. Cotrimoxazole is not approved for treatment of head lice.)
  - Albendazole:
    - 400 mg stat or repeated over 3 days
    - Repeat dose of 400 mg suggested at 7–10 days interval

      (Albendazole is a broad-spectrum antiparasitic, used worldwide for treatment of various helminthic and protozoal infections. It has manifold action against the parasite, chiefly—inhibition of mitochondrial function, uncoupling of oxidative phosphorylation and inhibition of glucose transport pathway, ultimately leading to adenosine triphosphate depletion and cell death)
  - Levamisole:
    - 3.5 mg/kg for 10 days
    - For children weighing 10–19 kg, 50 mg daily
    - For children weighing 20–39 kg, 100 mg daily

      (Levamisole is an acetylcholine nicotinic receptor agonist, which is rapidly and almost completely absorbed from the gastrointestinal tract. Due to its agonistic action on acetylcholine receptor, there is tonic paralysis of the ectoparasite and killing. Levamisole also interferes with the carbohydrate metabolism of the parasite by inhibition of enzyme fumarate hydratase).

Q. What are the newer treatment modalities of pediculosis capitis?

A. New treatment modalities:

- Cetaphil cleanser (Nuvo method)
  - Soak the scalp with cleanser
  - Remove excess by combing
  - Hair dryer to totally dry it
  - Wash out >8 hours later
  - Repeat the process weekly × 3 weeks
- 2010—Ulesfia
  - Benzyl alcohol 5% plus mineral oil
  - Dose by length of hair
  - 2 doses (day 1 and day 7)
  - 91% cure rate at day 8; age > 6 months
- 2011—Natroba
  - Benzyl alcohol 5% and 0.9% spinosad
  - 10 minutes application upto twice/week
  - 84–87% cure rate at 40 days post therapy
  - Age >4 years
- 2012—Sklice
  - Ivermectin 0.5% lotion
  - Single 10 minutes application
  - 71.4–76.4% cure rate
  - No nit combing required
  - A/E—conjunctivitis, burning sensation
  - Age >6 months
  - New, expensive, but just one application

Q. What is vagabond disease? What is its treatment?

A. Vagabond disease is the other name for pediculosis corporis. It is usually seen in homeless people who are wandering about or the nomads. It is characterized by parallel scratch marks and hyperpigmentation especially of upper back.

- Treatment:
  - Laundering of clothes especially underclothes and bedding at high temperature.
  - Use of hot iron with special attention to seams of clothing destroys the lice and nits. Scrub bath is advised for the patient and change of clothing. Dusting of the garment with gamma benzene hexachloride or malathion can also be done.

Q. What is macula cerulae?

A. Macula cerulae are blue-gray macules on the upper thigh and lower abdomen which is probably produced by altered blood pigment or as reaction to louse saliva.

Q. What is the treatment for phthiriasis palpebrarum?

A. Treatment consists of:

- Petrolatum applied thickly twice a day for two weeks. This interferes with respiratory function of the louse by blocking the spiracles.
- Freshly prepared 20% flourescin eye drops to the lid margins.
- Two drops of ivermectin 200 μg/kg at an interval of 10 days is also effective.
- Topical pilocarpine and physostigmine

Q. What is called as permethrin/pediculosis resistance?

A.
- Resistance can be developed by two mechanisms—either by genetic mutation or enzymatically by inhibition of oxidases in the lice.
- To overcome the enzymatic resistance, cotreatment with synergist piperonyl butoxide (3:1) and longer duration of treatment is done.

Q. Difference between live and dead lice.

A.
- Live knit—brown or yellow or white, oval in shape, attached at an acute angle, adherently to the hair shaft.
- Dead nit—clear or white, flat surface, attached at obtuse angle

Q. Deterrence and prevention.

A. To prevent head lice reinfestation, all household members and contacts of a patient should be examined and treated at the same time if infested. Bedmates should also ideally be treated even if they do not show evidence of infestation. Washing combs, brushes, and other fomites may reduce reinfestation.

76 Perioral Dermatitis

Q. What is perioral dermatitis?

A. It is a common acneiform eruption almost exclusively seen in women aged 20–30 years. It is characterized by erythema, scaling and follicular papules that occur around the mouth, nose, and less frequently on the eyelids.

Q. What is the etiology?

A.
- Fluorinated steroids
- Sunlight, heat
- Allergic dermatitis
- *Demodex folliculorum*
- *Candida*, fusiform
- *Helicobacter pylori*
- Cosmetics
- Oral contraceptive pill
- Hormones
- Fluorinated toothpaste
- Rosacea

Q. What is the differential diagnosis?

A.
- Rosacea
- Acne
- Seborrheic dermatitis
- Contact dermatitis
- Lupus miliaris disseminatus faciei
- Herpes simplex
- Factitious dermatitis
- Polymorphic light eruption
- Impetigo

Q. Treatment of perioral dermatitis.

A.
- Avoidance of fluorinated compounds
- 1% hydrocortisone
- Topical clindamycin and erythromycin
- Topical metronidazole 0.75%–1%

- Oral tetracycline for 6–8 weeks
  - Benzoyl peroxide
  - Erythromycin/Clindamycin
  - Tacrolimus
  - Tretinoin
- Oral medications
  - Tetracycline
  - Doxycycline
  - Macrolides erythromycin, clindamycin
  - Metronidazole
  - Isotretinoin
- Prevention—sunscreens, avoidance of cosmetics, and triggers.

77 Phrynoderma

Q. Meaning of the word phrynoderma.

A. • Phryno = toad-like, derma = skin
- Phrynoderma can now be considered as nonspecific finding in multivitamin deficiencies.

Q. Etiology.

A. • Mainly due to deficiency of vitamin A.
- Also due to deficiencies of vitamin B-complex, vitamin E, vitamin C, essential fatty acids
- Protein-energy malnutrition and general malnutrition state.

Q. Causes of vitamin A deficiency.

A. • Decreased intake
- Malabsorption
- Recent attack of measles

Q. Classical lesions.

A. Multiple, discrete, skin colored to pigmented, keratotic, follicular papules with central intrafollicular keratotic plug which projects as a horny spine which leaves a pit when expressed.

Q. Sites affected.

A. • Extensor aspects of extremities, especially over knees and elbows
- Sometimes anterior aspect of thighs.

Q. Grade various eye symptoms due to vitamin A deficiency.

A. • XN—night blindness
- X1A—conjunctival xerosis
- X1B—bitot spots
- X2—corneal xerosis
- X3—keratomalacia and corneal ulcerations
- XS—corneal scar
- XF—xerophthalmic fundus

Q. Other features of vitamin A deficiency.

A. Other than skin and eye manifestations, patient is prone to develop recurrent respiratory tract infections.

Q. Diagnosis.

A.
- Clinical.
- Serum vitamin A levels < 20 μg/dL

Q. Histopathology.

A.
- Hyperkeratosis
- Dilated follicular orifices with keratin plug
- Sebaceous gland atrophy

Q. Daily allowance of vitamin A.

A.
- Children—3,000 IU
- Adult female—4,000 IU
- Adult male—5,000 IU
- Pregnant female—6,000 IU

Q. Treatment.

A. Regimen-1
- Skin + eye involvement:
  - Injection vitamin A on day 0, 1, 14
  - <6 months—50,000 IU/dose
  - 6–12 months—100,000 IU/dose
  - >1 year—200,000 IU/dose

Regimen-2:
- Skin moderate-to-severe involvement:
  - Injection vitamin A on day 0, 3, 7
  - 100,000 IU/dose.

Regimen-3:
- Skin mild involvement:
  - Vitamin A capsule 50,000 IU/day till symptoms subside

Q. Symptoms of hypervitaminosis A.

A.
- Dry, scaly skin with desquamation
- Peeling of palms and soles
- Follicular hyperkeratosis
- Cheilitis-fissuring of the lips and mouth
- Raised intracranial pressure
- Alopecia
- Blurring of vision, pseudotumor cerebri
- Headache, arthralgia, myalgia, premature closure of epiphysis and spontaneous bone fracture, cortical hyperostosis

Q. Any teratogenic effect.

A. Yes, cranio-facial syndrome.

Q. Any precautions while giving vitamin A.

A. Never given with oral retinoids because of risk of pseudotumor cerebri.

Q. Phrynoderma is associated with conditions.

A.
- Intestinal malabsorption
- Anorexia nervosa
- Patient who had bariatric surgeries
- Small bowel bypass surgery
- Chronic alcohol intake
- Pancreatic insufficiency
- Inflammatory bowel disease
- Gallbladder disease

Q. Differential diagnosis of phrynoderma.

A.
- Keratosis pilaris
- Lichen spinulosus
- Follicular eczema
- Follicular lichen planus
- Follicular syphilis
- Pityriasis rubra pilaris
- Lichen scrofulosorum
- Darier disease

78 Piebaldism

Q. What is piebaldism?

A. It is an uncommon congenital autosomal dominant, stable patterned leukoderma characterized by frontal, median or paramedian depigmented patch with a white forelock. Also, macules with scattered hyperpigmented islets can be seen.

Q. What is the cause of piebaldism?

A. Mutation in *KIT* gene on chromosome 14 is the cause.

Q. What is the prevalence of piebaldism?

A.
- It affects one in 20,000.
- It affects males and females equally.

Q. Describe the clinical feature of piebaldism.

A.
- The classical feature is a white forelock or a white triangular elongated or diamond shaped macule on forehead since birth. The middle of eyebrows and eyelashes may be white. White patches can also be seen on abdominal wall and the anterior chest, often extending dorsally on to the back, mid thigh to calf and occasionally lower part of the neck and face, mid-upper arm to wrist, while other areas remain normally pigmented.
- Another characteristic feature is the presence of islets of hyperpigmented macules in leukodermic patches and on normally colored skin.

Q. Describe the pathology of piebaldism.

A.
- Absence of melanocytes and melanin in hair bulbs and white patches of depigmented areas.
- Negative dihydroxyphenylalanine (DOPA) reaction in depigmented skin.
- In the hyperpigmented macules, melanoytes are normal in number but with abundant melanosomes.
- The fault is mainly in differentiation, migration and survival of melanoblasts.

Q. How will you diagnose a case of piebaldism?

A.
- Congenital onset
- Typical pattern of depigmented macules.

- Presence of islets of hyperpigmented macules within the depigmented and normal skin
- Autosomal dominant inheritance pattern.

Q. What is Wolffe's syndrome?

A. Piebaldism with deafness but without other features of Waardenburg's syndrome is known as Wolffe's syndrome.

Q. What is the treatment for piebaldism?

A.
- Photoprotective measures.
- Skin grafting from normal melanotic areas to amelanotic sites.

Q. What are the newer treatment in piebaldism?

A. Recently, transplant of autologous melanocytes obtained through the culture of melanocytes or of melanocytes and keratinocytes has been described as a safe and effective treatment for patients with piebaldism.

79 Pigmented Purpuric Dermatosis

Q. What is the definition?

A. Pigmented purpuric dermatosis (PPD) are a group of benign asymptomatic disorders characterized by petechiae, pigmentation, and occasionally telangiectasia on the lower extremities.

Q. What is the etiology?

A. Following factors have been implicated:

- Contact with allergens (textile dyes, rubber, cobalt, benzoyl peroxide, and lidocaine 2.5% + prilocaine 2.5%).
- Drugs
- Venous stasis/acroangiodermatitis
- Venous incompetence
- Step aerobics
- Rheumatoid arthritis/diabetes mellitus
- Hodgkin's disease
- Hepatitis B, C
- Purpuric mycosis fungoides (MF)

Q. Which drugs have been implicated in etiology?

A. Following drugs:

- Nonsteroidal anti-inflammatory drugs (NSAIDs)
- Diuretics
- Glipizide

Q. What are the clinical features?

A. Multiple, well-defined, erythematous to hyperpigmented macules, few of them coalescing together to form larger patches, are present most commonly over lower limbs.

Q. What are the clinical variants?

A.

- Schamberg's disease
- Majocchi's disease (purpura annularis telangiectoides)
- Pigmented purpuric lichenoid dermatosis of Gougerot and Blum
- Eczematoid-like purpura of Doucas and Kapetanakis
- Lichen aureus
- Itching PPD (disseminated pruruginous angiodermatitis)

- Granulomatous PPD
- Segmental PPD
- PPD/MF overlap

Q. Which is the most common variant?
A. Schamberg's disease (cayenne pepper spots).

Q. What is the differential diagnosis?
A.
- Contact dermatitis
- Cutaneous necrotising vaculitis
- Stasis dermatitis and purpura
- Angioma serpingnosa
- Kaposi sarcoma (Gougerot–Blum)
- Mycosis fungoides

Q. What is the histopathological findings?
A.
- Epidermis normal.
- Vasculitis in upper dermis.
- Extravasation of red blood cells (RBCs).
- Presence of hemosiderin.

Q. Dermoscopy findings.
A. Coppery background with more clear red dots and globules.

Q. What is the treatment?
A.
- Topical steroids
- Pentoxifylline
- Ascorbic acid
- Psoralen plus ultraviolet A (PUVA) therapy
- Cyclosporine

80 Pityriasis Alba

Q. Why is this pityriasis alba?

A.
- Lesions are scaly hypopigmented macules on face with no loss of sensation or hair.
- There may be H/O waxing in winter and improvement in summer.
- Wood's lamp examination shows no accentuation or fluorescence.

Q. What are the differential diagnosis?

A.
- Early vitiligo
- Pityriasis versicolor
- Leprosy
- Postinflammatory hypopigmentation
- Hypopigmented mycosis fungoides
- Progressive macular hypomelanosis
    - Associated with atopic dermatitis (minor criterion for its diagnosis).

Q. What is the histopathology?

A.
- Follicular plugging
- Follicular spongiosis
- Atrophic sebaceous gland in early stages
- Chronic dermatitis in later stage.

Q. What is the meaning of pityriasis alba?

A.
- Pityriasis—bran-like
- Alba—white

Q. What are the clinical features?

A.
- It is the most common condition in children.
- These are asymptomatic ill-defined hypopigmented slightly scaly macules present primarily over face; though arms, neck and trunk may be rarely involved.
- In early stages, the lesion may be erythematous and show minimal scaling.
- It resolves spontaneously but may recur in subsequent years.

Q. What is progressive macular hypomelanosis?

A. It is characterized by ill-defined, nummular, nonscaly hypopigmented spots on the trunk, often confluent in and around the midline, and rarely extending to the proximal extremities and neck/head region.

Q. What is the treatment for pityriasis alba?

A.
- An emollient may be advised.
- If mild signs of inflammation are present, a mild topical steroid may be used for short period.
- Tacrolimus ointment 0.03% and pimecrolimus cream 1% may hasten resolution.

Q. What are the stages of evolution of pityriasis alba?

A.
- Slightly scaly pink patch or plaque with a just palpable papular surface.
- Hypopigmented patch or plaque with fine surface scale.
- Then postinflammatory hypopigmented macule without scale.
- Resolution.

81 Pityriasis Rosea

Q. What is pityriasis rosea (PR)?

A. It is an acute, self-limiting, papulosquamous disorder with characteristic skin rash and clinical course, mainly involving children and young adults.

Q. Define a classical primary lesion?

A.
- Primary lesion is known as a "herald patch" or "mother patch."
- Erythematous, well-defined, round to oval, 2–10 collarette of cm in diameter, with collarette of scales.
- Sites—chest, back, neck, abdomen.

Q. Describe a classical secondary rash?

A.
- Appears 5–15 days following mother patch.
- Comes in crops for a few week.
- Discrete, oval, erythematous scaly plaques of 0.5–1.5 cm diameter.
- Fine, dry collarette of scales.
- Lesions distributed in a Christmas tree pattern.
- Hanging curtain sign present.

Q. What are the differential diagnosis?

A.
- Secondary syphilis, drug rash, pityriasiform Seborrheic dermatitis
- Guttate psoriasis
- Pityriasis lichenoides chronica
- Pityriasis alba
- Tinea circinata

Q. What is the derivation of the word?

A.
- Pityriasis = scale (latin)
- Rosea = red (greek)
- Also called as Gilbert's disease

Q. What is the etiology?

A. Two main factors:
- Viral—human herpes virus 6 (HHV6), HHV7
- Drugs—angiotensin-converting enzyme (ACE) inhibitors, nonsteroidal anti-inflammatory drugs (NSAIDs), gold, D-pencillamine, beta-blockers
- Vaccinations: Bacillus Calmette-Guérin (BCG), H1N1, hepatitis B

Q. Reasons to support viral etiology?

A. Following facts support viral etiology:

- Case clustering in families
- History of upper respiratory tract infection
- Gap of few days between primary lesion and widespread rash
- Recurrence is rare
- Cephalo-caudal distribution of rash
- HHV-7 in lesional skin
- Children (mainly affected)

Q. What are the drugs causing PR like eruption?

A. Barbiturates, propylthiouracil, captopril, clonidine, arsenic, bismuth, gold, metronidazole, BCG vaccine, imatinib, mesylate, interferon, ketotifen, methoxypropane, tripelennamine hydrochloride, ergotamine, lisinopril, acyclovir, lithium, adalimumab.

Q. What is the histopathology?

A. Following features are observed:

- Tea-pot lid sign—focal angulated patchy parakeratosis
- Unna's sign—eczematous pattern
- Sabouraud's sign—extravasation of red blood cells (RBCs) in the papillary dermis and partly into the epidermis
- Lowenbach sign—absence or decrease of granular cell layer
- Coat-sleeve pattern inflammatory infiltrate
- Spongiosis
- Mild acanthosis
- Exocytosis

Q. Chus-diagnostic criteria for PR?

A.

- Essential—discrete circular/oval lesions
    - Collarate of scales
    - Just scaling
- Optional—distribution (swimming trunk)
    - Herald patch
- Exclusion—most lesions on palms and soles
    - Lesions are vesicular.
    - Lymphadenopathy or venereal disease research laboratory (VDRL) positive

Q. What is the age group and seasonal variation?

A.

- Between 10–35 years, peak in 20s.
- More common in winters and spring

Q. Distribution of lesions?

- Christmas tree pattern on trunk.
- In adults, mainly on trunk.
- In children, face may be involved.

Q. Types of PR.

A.
- Classical
- Inverse
- Linear
- Atypical
- Papular
- Urticarial
- Purpuric
- Lichenoid
- Vesico-bullous
- Mucosal
- Giant PR
- Large localized flexural lesions (vidal PR)

Q. What is the prognosis?

A.
- Self limiting.
- Mostly heals with hypopigmentation
- Recurrences are 5%

Q. What is the treatment?

A.
- Erythromycin (500 mg 4 times/day for 5 days)
- Roxithromycin (150 mg 2 times/day × 7 days)
- Acyclovir (800 mg 5 times/day for 7 days)
- Emollients
- Calamine
- Topical steroids
- Sun exposure
- Ultraviolet B phototherapy
- Psoralen plus ultraviolet A (PUVA) therapy
- Oral steroids

82 Pityriasis Rubra Pilaris

Q. Describe a classical skin lesion?

A.
- Multiple, small, pale to pink, keratotic, scaly, follicular papules coalescing together to form large plaques.
- Reddish-orange erythema is seen.

Q. What is the synonym?

A. Devergie's disease.

Q. What are the etiological factors?

A.
- Disorders of vitamin A metabolism
- Underlying immunological abnormality
- Preceding febrile illness and infections
- Bacterial superantigens
- Rarely hypogammaglobulinemias

Q. Describe other clinical features?

A.
- Diffuse salmon-colored erythema and scaling over scalp
- Horny follicular papules on back of fingers (nutmeg grater feel)
- Sometimes erythroderma (islands of normal skin within the affected areas)
- Yellowish hyperkeratosis of the palms and soles [pityriasis rubra pilaris (PRP) sandal]
- Hyperkeratotic papules on knees and elbows
- Nails—thick, brittle, dull, rough, subungual hyperkeratosis, splinter hemorrhage
- Rarely oral mucosa may be involved (diffuse ground glass appearance)

Q. Name the classification system used for classifying PRP.

A. Griffith's classification as follows:

- *Type I*: Classical adult type
- *Type-II*: Atypical adult type
- *Type-III*: Classical juvenile type
- *Type-IV*: Circumscribed juvenile type
- *Type-V*: Atypical juvenile type
- *Type-VI*: HIV associated PRP (added later on)

Q. What are the differential diagnosis?

A. Following conditions should be kept in mind:

- Psoriasis
- Erythrokeratodermas
- Follicular ichthyosis
- Lichen scrofulosorum
- Other follicular keratosis

Q. What is the histopathological findings?

A.
- Checker-board pattern of vertical and horizontal alternating ortho and parakeratosis
- Shouldering parakeratosis at the sides of hair follicle
- Hypergranulosis
- Thick suprapapillary plates
- Follicular plugging
- Broad rete ridges
- Narrow dermal papillae
- Sparse inflammatory infiltrate

Q. What is the treatment?

A. Following drugs have been tried:

- Keratolytics
- Emollients
- Topical steroids
- Isotretinoin (0.5–2 mg/kg/day)
- Acetretin (0.4 mg/kg/day)
- Vitamin A (50,000 IU thrice daily)
- TNF-α inhibitors
    - One of the few causes of erythroderma for which systemic steroids do not work.

83 Porokeratosis

Q. What is the morphology of porokeratosis?

A. It presents as a hyperkeratotic papule or plaque, with an annular appearance due to thread like elevated border that expands centrifugally.

Q. What are the differential diagnosis of porokeratosis?

A.
- Pityriasis rosea
- Dermatophyte infection
- Hansen's disease
- Annular lichen planus (LP)
- Sarcoidosis
- Syphilis
- Basal cell carcinoma (BCC)
- Granuloma annulare
- Basal cell epithelioma
- Actinic keratosis
- Inflammatory linear verrucous epidermal nevus (ILVEN)
- Incontinentia pigmenti (stage 2)
- Linear LP
- Verruca vulgaris
- Porokeratotic eccrine ostial and dermal duct nevus

Q. Types of porokeratosis?

A.
- Porokeratosis of mibelli
- Punctate porokeratosis
- Linear porokeratosis
- Disseminated superficial porokeratosis
- Disseminated superficial actinic porokeratosis (DSAP)
- Porokeratosis Palmaris et plantaris disseminata (PPPD)
- Porokeratosis ptychotropica
- Giant porokeratosis
- Porokeratosis eccrine postal dermal duct nevus

Q. What is the epidemiology of porokeratosis?

A.
- Autosomal dominant inherited disorder
- Porokeratosis of mibelli affects boys more than girls except DSAP
- PPPD is more common in males

- DSAP is more common in Caucasians and rare in blacks
- Linear porokeratosis has been reported in monozygotic twins

Q. What is the pathology of porokeratosis?

A.
- Cornoid lamella is the sine qua non for histological diagnosis.
- Thin column of tightly packed parakeratotic cells extending from an invagination of the epidermis through the adjacent statum corneum often protruding above the surface of the adjacent skin, under the lamella. Granular layer is absent or thinned, dyskeratotic, and pyknotic kerationocytes with perinuclear edema in the spinous layer beneath the lamella are seen. Dermal lymphocytic infiltrate is seen.

Q. What is the treatment of porokeratosis?

A.
- Unsatisfactory
- Topical retinoids, 5-fluorouracil (5-FU), imiquimod
- Cryotherapy, CO_2 laser local excision have been tried
- In widespread lesions, oral acitretin may be tried

Q. What is the dermoscopy of porokeratosis?

A. Dots and globules in the border (white tract structures) which corresponds to cornoid lamella.

84 Prurigo Nodularis

Q. What are the clinical features?

A. Multiple, well-defined, dry, scaly, warty, lichenified, hyperpigmented, excoriated, firm nodules varying in size from 1–3 cm. Mostly seen on extensor aspect of limbs.

Q. What are the differential diagnosis?

A.
- Hypertrophic lichen planus
- Insect bite reactions
- Benign epidermal tumors
- Pemphigoid nodularis
- Perforating disorders (e.g., acquired perforating dermatosis)
- Multiple keratoacanthomas
- Granular cell tumors
- Pruriginous epidermolysis bullosa
- Nodular scabies (few lesions)

Q. What is prurigo nodularis also known as?

A. Hyde's prurigo.

Q. What is the etiology?

A.
- Idiopathic
- Emotional stress
- Xerosis
- Atopy
- Systemic diseases like hyperthyroidism, hepatic or renal dysfunction, lymphoma and iron deficiency
- Insect bite (20%)

Q. Describe the clinical features?

A.
- Pruritus with lesions that are hard, dome-shaped papules or nodules with central scale-crust
- Variable color ranging from erythematous to brown to skin-colored
- In longstanding disease, lesions may be verrucous, lichenified or fissured surface
- Multiple excoriations, postinflammatory hyperpigmentation and superficial scarring

- Patients may present with a few or hundreds of lesions, usually in a symmetric distribution, with a predominance on the extensor surfaces of the limbs

Q. What is "butterfly sign"?

A. Sparing of the mid upper back from the lesions is referred to as the 'butterfly' sign.

Q. What are the associated internal diseases?

A. It can be associated with:

- Metabolic disorders like uremia, hepatic dysfunction
- Malignancies like Hodgkin's disease
- HIV infection
- Gluten-sensitive enteropathy

Q. Incidence?

A.

- Most common in 20–60 years.
- Rare in children.
- Equally seen in both sexes.

Q. Describe the histopathology?

A.

- Focal hyperkeratosis and acanthosis.
- Papillomatosis and irregular proliferation of the epidermis
- The dermis may show a nonspecific inflammatory infiltrate.
- Neural hyperplasia (variable degree).

Q. How will you investigate a case of prurigo nodularis?

A.

- Complete blood cell count
- Liver function tests
- Serum creatinine
- Thyroid function tests.
- Chest radiograph and abdominal CT scan (suspicion of lymphoma)

Q. How will you treat a case of prurigo nodularis?

A.

- General measures:
  - To reduce excoriation
  - Cutting the nails very short
  - Wearing gloves at night
  - Occlusion of the involved regions of skin with bandages, dressings or steroid impregnated tape.
- Topical therapy:
  - Emollients
  - Superpotent topical steroid under occlusion
  - Topical capsaicin (0.025–0.3%)

- Tacrolimus, calcipotriol, and calcitriol
- Topical antipruritic and moisturizing agents containing menthol and phenol or anesthetics, such as pramoxine.

- Intralesional steroid and cryotherapy
- Systemic therapy
    - Antihistaminics
    - Cyclosporine (3.0–4.5 mg/kg/day)
    - Thalidomide (100–300 mg daily)
    - Phototherapy
    - Azathioprine
    - Naltrexone
    - Antidepressants
    - Anxiolytics
- Psoralen plus ultraviolet A (PUVA)

85 Pseudoxanthoma Elasticum

Q. Why is it pseudoxanthoma elasticum (PXE)?

A.
- Asymptomatic, small, skin-colored to yellowish papules arranged in a reticular fashion over soft lax wrinkled skin giving characteristic cobblestone/chicken neck/Moroccan leather appearance on the neck, axillae, groin.
- Occasionally similar lesions are present over mucous membranes.
- Many individuals have oblique mental (chin) creases.

Q. What is the other name?

A. Gronblad-Strandberg syndrome.

Q. What is pseudoxanthoma elasticum?

A. It is an inherited autosomal recessive disorder characterized by generalized fragmentation and calcification of elastic fibers in various tissues and clinically involving skin, eyes and cardiovascular system.

Q. What is the genetic defect?

A.
- Gene coding for ABCC6, on chromosome 16 is defective.
- Absence of normal ABCC6 protein results in calcification of elastic fibers.

Q. What is the age of onset?

A.
- Age of onset is 13–15 years
- More in women

Q. What are the differential diagnosis?

A.
- Buschke-Ollendorff syndrome
- Juvenile elastoma
- Other dermatochalasis like cutis laxa, Ehlers-Danlos syndrome, granulomatous slack skin.

Q. Which all systems are affected?

A. Following systems are affected:
- Skin
- Eyes
- Cardiovascular
- Others

Q. What are the ocular manifestations?

A. *In retina*:

- Angioid streaks
- Leopard spotting
- Fibrovascular ingrowths in the retina lead to retinal hemorrhages, retinal detachment and visual loss.

In macula:

- String of pearls appearance (best visible on fluorescein angiography)

Q. Other causes of angioid streaks?

A. Remember the mnemonic "**PEPSI**"

P – Pseudoxanthoma elasticum
E – Ehlers–Danlos syndrome
P – Paget's disease of bone
S – Sickle cell anemia
I – Idiopathic other conditions like atherosclerosis, acromegaly, diabetes mellitus, hemochromatosis, lead poisoning, aging, NF, SWS.

Angioid streaks are due to breaks in the Bruch's membrane of the retina.

Q. What are the cardiovascular manifestations?

A.

- Intermittent claudication
- Diminished peripheral pulses
- Angina pectoris
- Myocardial infarction
- Mitral valve prolapse
- Hypertension
- Brain hemorrhage
- Seizures

Q. What are the other manifestations?

A.

- Recurrent abortions
- Gastrointestinal hemorrhage
- Pulmonary involvement
- Urinary involvement

Q. What are the other associations?

A.

- Osteoectasia
- Osteitis deformans (Paget's disease)
- Sickle cell anemia
- Beta thalassemia
- Tumoral calcinosis

Q. What are the causes of death in PXE?

A.
- Cerebral hemorrhage
- Coronary occlusion
- Massive hemorrhage in the gut

Q. What are the histopathological findings?

A.
- In mid and lower dermis elastic fibers are fragmented, clumped, degenerated, swollen and calcified
- Appear dark blue on hematoxylin and eosin (H&E) staining.
- Special stains like van Gieson and von Kossa can be used.

Q. What is the diagnostic criteria?

A.
- Major criteria:
  - Flexural yellow cobblestone lesions
  - Characteristic histopathologic features in lesional skin, using elastic and calcium stains
  - Angioid streaks in retina
- Minor criteria:
  - Characteristic histologic changes in nonlesional skin
  - Family history of PXE in first-degree relatives.

Q. What is the treatment?

A. Early diagnosis and appropriate treatment to prevent complications
- Genetic advice
- Avoid any activity that causes a sudden increase in blood pressure or injury to eyes
- Mainstay is surgical correction of lax skin.
- Laser photocoagulation helpful in preventing further retinal hemorrhage
- Other systemic manifestations should be treated promptly.
- Restriction of dietary calcium may help.
- Recently antiangiogenic drugs like Bevacizumab and Ranibizumab have been used
- Intraocular vascular endothelial growth factor (VEGF) inhibitors, such as bevacizumab for CNV

86 Pyoderma Faciale

Q. What is pyoderma faciale?

A. It is a facial disorder that consists of an intense reddish or cyanotic erythema, combined with superficial and deep abscesses, cystic lesions and sometimes sinus tracts.

Q. How is it differentiated from acne?

A. Absence of comedones, rapid onset, fulminating course.

Q. How do you treat pyoderma faciale?

A. Prednisolone 40–60 mg daily tapered over 3–4 weeks. Isotretinoin should be used in conjunction with the prednisolone in a dose of 1 mg/kg/day continued for 4–6 months.

87 Pyogenic Granuloma

Q. What is pyogenic granuloma?

A. Pyogenic granuloma is a benign vascular tumor of skin or mucous membranes characterized by rapid growth and friable surface.

Q. Other name for pyogenic granuloma?

A. Lobular capillary hemangioma.

Q. Pyogenic granuloma is seen commonly in?

A.
- Most commonly seen in infants and children.
- It can also be seen in adults particularly pregnant women.

Q. What are the clinical features?

A. It is a solitary, red, rapidly growing papule or nodule with a subtle collarette of scale [other causes collarette of scaling: Pityriasis rosea (PR), staphylococcal furuncle].

Q. What are the common sites?

A. Cheeks, forehead but virtually any body site.

Q. What are the differential diagnosis?

A.
- Bacillary angiomatosis
- Epithelioid hemangioma
- Kaposi's sarcoma
- Peripheral fibroma
- Infantile hemangioma
- Peripheral giant cell granuloma

Q. What are the histopathological findings?

A. Pyogenic granuloma is an exophytic often ulcerative lesion characterized by lobulated proliferation of capillary sized vessels in a loose and edematous stroma with an epidermal collarette formed at the margins in form of rete ridges.

Q. What is the treatment?

A.
- Simple curettage with electrocautery
- Excision
- LASER surgery with carbon dioxide and pulsed dye
- Cryotherapy
- Imiquimod cream 5%
- Timolol gel 0.5% and other topical (or oral) beta-blockers
- Intralesional steroid injection

88 Reticulate Acropigmentation of Kitamura

Q. What is acropigmentation of Kitamura?

A. Characterized by hyperpigmented, atrophic, angulated macules which initially appear over dorsum of hands, later on involving the whole extremities, rarely affecting the face.

Q. What are other clinical features?

A. Palmar pits are characteristic.

Q. What is the histopathology findings?

A. Epidermal atrophy and increased basal melanocytes.

Q. What is the relation with HP?

A. Many cases show histopathologic overlap, considered by some as varied presentations of same entity.

Q. What are the differential diagnosis?

A.
- Dowling-Degos disease
- Acropigmentation of Dohi

Q. What is the treatment?

A.
- Azelaic acid, a tyrosinase inhibitor has been shown to be a potential treatment option.
- Erbium-doped yttrium aluminium garnet (Er:YAG), an ablative laser that emits light at 2,940 nanometers for skin resurfacing and pigmentary disorders, is another therapeutic.

89 Rosacea

Q. Define rosacea?

A. Rosacea is characterized by a persistent erythema of the convex surfaces of the face, nose most frequently affected followed by brow and chin.

Q. What are the types of rosacea?

A.
- Erythemato-telangiectatic
- Papulopustular
- Phymatous
- Ocular
- Granulomatous

Q. What are the various stimuli for rosacea?

A.
- Emotional stress
- Hot drinks
- Alcohol
- Spicy foods
- Exercise
- Cold or hot weather/bath/shower

Q. What is the etiology?

A.
- Abnormal vasomotor response to thermal and other stimuli
- Chronic solar damage
- Chronic vasodilation, edema and compromise of lymphatic drainage and lead to telangiectasia and fibrosis.

Q. What are the eye changes in rosacea?

A.
- Blepharitis, recurrent chalazion, conjunctivitis, keratitis, iritis, episcleritis.
- Abnormal Schirmer test in 40% patients.

Q. What are the types of phymatous rosacea?

A.
- Rhinophyma
- Gnathophyma (with central chin typically involved)
- Otophyma (usually affects the lower half of the helices and lobes of the ears)
- Metophyma (cushion-like, firm swelling of central forehead)
- Blepharophyma (swelling of the eyelids)

Q. What is rhinophyma?

A. It is a subtype of glandular rosacea. Hypertrophic, hyperemic, large nodular masses are centered over the distal half of the nose.

Q. What is the histopathology of rosacea?

A. Pilosebaceous hyperplasia with fibrosis, inflammation and telangiectasia.

Q. What is Haber syndrome?

A. Rosacea-like facial lesions and multiple verrucous lesions on the non-sun exposed areas.

Q. What are the differential diagnosis of rosacea?

A.
- Polycythemia vera
- Carcinoid syndrome
- Mastocytosis
- Lupus erythematosus
- Dermatomyositis
- MCTD

Q. What is the treatment for rosacea?

A.
- Control of inflammation
- Topical application of adrenergic agonists, such as brimonidine or oxymetazoline may help to diminish the erythema
- Topical metronidazole
- Sodium sulfacetamide-sulfur
- Azelaic acid
- CO_2 laser therapy, electrosurgery, or surgical excision (in phymatous rosacea)
- Lavage of eyelid margins with dilute "baby" shampoo using cotton swabs combined with an oily tear replacement (in mild ocular rosacea)

90 Scabies

Q. Define scabies?

A. Scabies is a disease caused by itch mite called *Sarcoptes scabiei* var hominis characterized by intense itching which is mostly worse at night.

Q. What are the clinical features of scabies?

A.
- Itching is predominant symptom, which is worse at night
- In early stages, itching confined to areas of predisposition, but as disease progress due to delayed hypersensitivity response, patient may present with generalized itching.
- Scabies involves web of fingers, flexor aspect of wrists, elbows, anterior axillary folds, umbilicus and periumbilical region, genitalia, upper thighs, knees, ankles. In females, nipple and areola are involved
- The lower part of buttocks and natal cleft are common sites. In adults, scalp, face, palms and soles are spared but this areas are involved in infants and children
- The burrow is the primary lesion. It is a serpentine, threadlike, grayish or dark line. The open end is marked by papule or papulovesicles. The mite may be seen as a whitish dot at closed end. Lesions are often excoriated, eczematized.

Q. What are differential diagnosis of scabies?

A. *Infancy*:
- Atopic dermatitis
- Prurigo mitis
- Bacterial infection
- Acropustulosis of infancy

Adults:
- Contact dermatitis
- Dermatitis herpetiformis
- Insect bites
- Pruritus related to HIV disease

Elderly:
- Asteatotic eczema
- Pruritus related to systemic causes

Q. What is epidemiology of scabies?

A. • Affects all races
- Epidemics occur every 30 years according to studies with smaller epidemics occurring every 7 years (the other 7 years itch is marriage!)
- Mostly a disease of children
- Highest in age group below 5 years
- Decreasing prevalence with age
- No preponderance in either sex

Q. What conditions are favorable for transmission of scabies?

A. • High humidity and low temperature favors survival of scabies mite and high temperature and low humidity leads to death of the mite
- Transfer of young fertilized female mites is necessary for establishing infection of new host
- Prolonged intimate, personal contact within household is significant factor in transmission of scabies
- Overcrowding with regard to sleeping space
- Indirect spread by clothing, bedding or other fomites is uncommon

Q. What is the morphology of *Sarcoptes scabiei*?

A. • *Sarcoptes scabiei* var hominis is the causative agent of human scabies
- *Sarcoptes scabiei* are whitish hemispherical mites
- Female is 0.4×0.3 mm, with four pair of legs
- In females, front two pairs end in suckers and hind two pairs in long trailing bristles
- Male is smaller about 0.2×0.15 mm and its fourth pair also end in suckers
- Body of both male and females end in transverse corrugation with spines and bristles on dorsal surface

Q. What is lifecycle of *Sarcoptes scabiei*?

A. • Copulation—in a small burrow excavated by a female
- After copulation, the fertile female enlarges the burrow and begins laying eggs. Burrows are not confined to stratum corneum, but are inclined downward into epidermis
- Gradual penetration appears to occur as a result of production of a lytic secretion by mite
- The burrow is lengthened by approximately 2–3 mm daily. Eggs are deposited behind in the burrow

- About 40–50 eggs are laid at each time during a lifespan of 4–6 weeks, during which time she does not leave the burrow
- Six-legged larvae emerge from the eggs after 3–4 days and escape the burrow
- The larvae then dig short burrows (moulting pockets) in which they transform into nymphs
- After further moults, adult males and females develop

Q. What are the pathological features of scabies?

A.
- A patchy to diffuse infiltrate with prominent eosinophils as well as lymphocytes and histiocytes are noted in the reticular dermis. A transected scabies mite may occasionally be seen within the epidermis.
- Pink "pigtail"—like structures attached to the stratum corneum, which represent fragments of the adult mite exoskeleton, can serve as a clue.

Q. How is immune system related to scabies?

A.
- In scabies, cell mediated immune response is more important than humoral response
- The mite population is more in the early asymptomatic phase of infestation. Once symptomatic, their number reduces dramatically, as the mites are removed mechanically by scratching and the immune response causes an outpouring of fluid that makes stratum corneum in hospitable for mite
- In reinfestation, symptoms are earlier, mites are fewer in number and disappear spontaneously.
- Rash and pruritis are limited to site of infestation.
- Immunosuppressed patients are more prone for severe type of scabies with unlimited production of mites. Delayed hypersensitivity response help to contain infestation.

Q. What are different types of scabies?

A.
- Classical scabies:
  - Itching which worsens at night
  - Burrows can be present as wavy thread-like, grayish lines, which open as papule or vesicle
  - In severe cases, deep seated nodules are seen
- Scabies in clean:
  - Moderate itching with few scattered wheals and papules
  - Distribution limited to sites of predisposition
  - Minute papules with gritty feeling in between web spaces may be present
  - Genital and gluteal regions should be checked to see for the typical lesion

- Scabies in babies:
  - Classical lesions of scabies are replaced by excoriations, crusting, pyoderma
  - Vesicles are a prominent feature which may lead to blister formation
  - Recurrent attack of vesicles and pustules of hands and feet area a common feature
  - The duration is usually less than 2 months and the mite population is low because of severe inflammatory reaction as a result of scabies and pyoderma
- Nodular scabies:
  - Persistent nodules occur mainly over the elbows, anterior axillary folds, genitalia and gluteal region
  - Firm, dull, red nodules may persist for weeks, months or for a year
- Crusted scabies:
  - Hyperkeratotic, scaly, crusted lesions with large number of mites in them
  - In addition to classical sites of involvement, lesions are seen on face, scalp, palms, soles and neck
  - The helix of the ear is commonly involved
  - The nails are dystrophic and discolored with subungual hyperkeratosis
  - Poor personal hygiene, defective cell mediated and humoral immunity may predispose to crusted scabies
  - The disease is frequently associated with malnutrition, lepromatous leprosy, tuberculosis, Down's syndrome, diabetes mellitus, acute renal failure, pemphigus vulgaris, etc.
- Scabies incognito:
  - Scabies treated with topical or systemic corticosteroids present with unusual clinical manifestations, involving atypical sites
  - While corticosteroids reduce the itching and the inflammatory lesion, the mite population increases
  - Mites are easily demonstrable from scraping of lesion
- Animal transmitted scabies:
  - It is acquired from animals like dogs, horses, etc.
  - The distribution pattern is different
  - The lesions are most common on forearm, lower chest, abdomen, thighs and areas exposed to mite by the person carrying the affected animal

- The interdigital webs and genitalia are spared and burrow absent
- Short incubation period
- The disease frequently goes undiagnosed
- The dog may show patchy alopecia with scaling involving mainly the head, ears and intertriginous folds, characteristic mousy odor (the disease is called as sarcoptic mange because the dog actually gnaws at its own skin; mange = eating).

Q. What are the complications of scabies?

A.
- Secondary pyodermas presenting as impetigo, ecthyma, cellulitis, lymphangitis, furunculosis
- Acute glomerulonephritis
- Pediatric acute glomerulonephritis is also reported in some cases

Q. How will you diagnose scabies?

A. The five cardinal features in scabies are:
1. The presence of burrow specially on web-spaces and penis
2. The characteristic distribution pattern of lesion
3. The presence of history of similar illness in other members of household or other contacts
4. Intense pruritis, which tend to worsen at night
5. Demonstration of burrow, with the help of scalpel, slice of entire burrow, especially the blind end. This is placed on a slide. Addition of xylol or 20% potassium hydroxide helps to clear cellular debris. Examination under low microscope reveals the mite, ova or fecal pellets.

Q. What is the differential diagnosis of scabies?

A.
- Atopic dermatitis
- Allergic contact dermatitis
- Autosensitization ("id" reaction)
- Nummular dermatitis
- Arthropod bites
- Pyoderma
- Dermatitis herpetiformis
- Bullous pemphigoid

Q. What is the treatment of scabies?

A. Patient's education:
- All persons in the household, whether itching or nonitching should be treated.

- Even after effective treatment the itching may persist for up to 2 weeks
- The clothes should be disinfected.
- Woolen blankets, etc., should be kept locked inside the cupboard, as the mites die off if they do not come in contact with humans for 3–5 days.

Medical therapy:

- Apply 5% permethrin. These creams are applied from the neck down, left on overnight, then washed off. This application is usually repeated in 7 days. Permethrin is approved for use in people 2 months of age and older.
- An alternative treatment is 1 ounce of a 1% lotion or 30 g of cream of lindane, applied from the neck down and washed off after approximately 8 hours
- Ivermectin, an oral medication, is an antiparasitic medication that has also been shown to be an effective scabicide, at a dosage of 200 µg/kg body weight as a single dose, followed by a repeat dose 2 weeks later.
- Crotamiton lotion 10% and cream 10% is another drug that has been approved for the treatment of scabies in adults
- Sulfur in petrolatum 6% applied as a cream or ointment is one of the earliest known treatments for scabies. Sulfur is safe for use in pregnant women and infants
- Antihistamines can be useful in helping provide relief from itching

91 Sebaceous Hyperplasia

Q. Why is this sebaceous hyperplasia?

A. Multiple, yellowish, telangiectatic papules on the central or upper face.

Q. What are the differential diagnosis?

A.
- Rosacea
- Milia

Q. Describe sebaceous hyperplasia.

A. It does not represent a true neoplasm, but it represents benign enlargement of the sebaceous lobule around a follicular infundibulum.

Q. What are the clinical features of sebaceous hyperplasia?

A.
- It is relatively common and presents with one or more multiple, yellowish, telangiectatic papules usually on the central or upper face or sometimes on the trunk.
- The lesions display a central dent that corresponds to a central follicular infundibular ostium
- Beaded lines represent a unique expression of sebaceous hyperplasia in which a linear presence of papules is seen.
- The lesions are sometimes confused with basal cell carcinoma.

Q. What is the histopathology of sebaceous hyperplasia?

A.
- Thin rim of seboblastic cells surrounding the remainder of the gland, composed of mature sebocytes.
- The enlarged sebaceous lobules usually circumferentially surround a central infundibulum.

Q. What are the treatment options?

- Lesions can be removed by shave excision, light electrosurgical destruction, cryotherapy or laser ablation.
- Long-term topical retinoid may be helpful.
- Oral isotretinoin can be used in individuals with extensive disfiguring lesions.

92 Striae

Q. What are the synonyms?

A.
- Striae atrophicans
- Striae distensae
- Stretch marks

Q. What is the definition?

A. Striae are linear scars produced by stretching of skin leading to dermal damage.

Q. What is the etiology?

A. Occurs secondary to stress rupture of connective tissue network. This occurs in following conditions:
- Growth spur in adolescence
- Pregnancy
- In weight lifters/bodybuilders
- Cushing's disease

Also observed in HIV patients on indinavir therapy.

Q. What are the clinical features?

A.
- Striae rubra: Initial lesion, slightly raised, red to blue in color. Fade after some years.
- Striae alba: Atrophic linear scar like lesions.

Q. What are the sites affected?

A.
- Abdomen, thighs, shoulders, breasts
- During puberty, striae appears in areas where there is a rapid increase in the size.
- In girls - most common sites are thighs, hips, buttocks and breast

Q. Striae in Cushing's syndrome.

A. Larger, more widely distributed, involve flexors along with other regions.

Q. What are the histopathological findings?

A. Flattened epidermis, dermal edema, perivascular lymphocytic infiltrate, eosinophilic collagen bundles arranged parallel to surface. Thin, branched elastic fibers.

Q. What is the treatment?

A.
- Striae rubra can be treated with topical tretinoin and pulsed dye laser.
- Striae alba cannot be treated.
- Early Striae rubra treated with tretinoin 0.1%
- Other topical treatments including 0.05% tretinoin/20% glycolic acid and 10% L-ascorbic acid/20% glycolic acid, may also improve the appearance of stretch marks.

93 Superficial Fungal Infection

Q. What is a dermatophyte?

A. • Dermatophyte is a fungus that has developed the ability to live on keratin (hair, nails or skin scale) of animals. Dermatophytes are classified into three genera: *Microsporum, Trichophyton* and *Epidermophyton.*

- Those dermatophytes capable of reproducing sexually are members of the genus *Arthroderma* and *Nannizia*, of phylum *Ascomycota.*

Q. Dermatophyte classification?

A. Dermatophytes are classified as follows:

- Kingdom: Fungi
- Phylum: Ascomycota
- Order: Onygenales
- Genus: *Arthroderma, Nannizia*

Q. What are the predisposing factors?

A. Predisposing factors are underlying diseases such as diabetes mellitus, lymphomas, immunocompromised status, or Cushing's syndrome, which could produce severe, widespread, or recalcitrant dermatophytosis.

Q. What is the pathogenesis?

A. • Trauma, maceration, and increased hydration of skin make the inroad for pathogenic fungi.

- Once the infection is established in the stratum corneum, two factors are important in determining the size and duration of lesion. The growth rate of the organism and the epidermal turnover rate
- The fungal growth rate must either equal or exceed the epidermal turnover rate

Q. How are superficial fungal infections diagnosed?

A. Mostly by KOH mount (skin scraping + ½ drops of 10–20% KOH) hyphae of dermatophytes will be septate and demonstrate branching.

Q. Most commonly used culture medium.

A.
- Sabouraud's dextrose agar:
  - Nonselective culture medium consisting of peptone, dextrose agar and distilled water. Allows growth of bacteria and yeast.
- Mycosel/mycobiotic agar:
  - Selective growth medium consists of Sabouraud's + Cycloheximide (inhibits saprophytic fungi) and Chloramphenicol (inhibits bacteria) Dermatophyte and *Candida* grow on this.
- Dermatophyte test media:
  - Sabouraud's + Cycloheximide + Gentamicin + Chlortetracycline hydrochloride. Has a phenol red indicator. If dermatophytes are present, the color of media changes from yellow to red.

Q. Which dermatophyte causes the most fungal infections of the skin?

A. *Trichophyton rubrum.*

Tinea Barbae

Q. Why will you say this case is *T. barbae*?

A. Since the lesion is nodular and boggy like kerion and associated with seropurulent discharge and crusting. Seen mostly on the chin, neck, maxillary and submaxillary area. Perifollicular pustules are present. Heals with scarring and alopecia.

Q. Other names of *T. barbae*.

A. Also known as *Tinea Sycosis* and barber's itch.

Q. What the common types of *T. barbae*?

A.
- Inflammatory type (discussed above)
- Superficial/sycosiform type
  - Diffuse erythema with perifollicular papules and pustules
- Circinate/spreading type
  - Vesiculopustular lesions at periphery with central scaling.

Q. What are the differential diagnosis of *T. barbae*?

A. Sycosis barbae, acne, carbuncle, furuncle, herpes simplex.

Q. What are the atypical forms of *T. barbae*?

A.
- Granuloma annulare like/abscess like caused by *Microsporum canis*
- Verrucous granulomatous lesion caused by *Epidermophyton floccosum*

Q. Most common method of transmission of *T. barbae*?
A. Person to person by contaminated barbers razors.

Q. Treatment of *T. barbae*?
A.
- Oral
  - Griseofulvin—0.5–1 g/day × 2–4 weeks
  - Itraconazole—200–400 mg OD × 1 week
  - Terbinafine—250 mg OD × 2 weeks
  - Fluconazole—150–300 mg × 4–6 weeks
- Topical
  - Econazole
  - Miconazole
  - Fluconazole

  These creams applied BD for 4–6 weeks

Tinea Faciei

Q. Why will you say the above case is *T. faciei*?
A. The lesion begins as an erythematous scaly macule that extends peripherally and develops a raised border. Central area is hypopigmented/brown. It is associated with burning, itching and photosensitivity. Some cases show simple papular lesions and flat patches of erythema occur.

Q. What is *T. faciei*?
A. Dermatophyte infection that occurs on nonbearded areas of face. Commonly seen in women and prepubertal boys.

Q. What are the causative agents of *T. faciei*?
A. *T. mentagrophytes* and *T. rubrum.*

Q. Differential diagnosis of *T. faciei.*
A. Seborrhoeic dermatitis, atopic dermatitis, furuncle, carbuncle, irritant contact dermatitis, *P. alba*, Rosacea.

Q. What is the treatment?
A. Mostly topical treatment such as econazole, miconazole and ketoconazole cream. Applied BD for 4–6 weeks.

Tinea Cruris

Q. Why will you say the case is of *T. cruris*?
A. Annular plaque with well-marginated raised border composed of multiple, erythematous papulovesicles and a clear center. Common sites involved are genitocrural area and on medial aspect of upper thigh and usually bilaterally present. They coalesce and spread to buttock, lower back and abdomen. Itching present.

Q. What are the causative organisms?

A. The three most common causative organisms are *T. rubrum*, *T. mentagrophytes* and *M. canis*.

Q. What are the complications?

A.
- Lichenification
- Secondary bacterial infection
- Weeping, maceration and areas of Pustulation present.

Q. Differential diagnosis of *T. cruris*?

A. Candidiasis, *P. versicolor, erythrasma, intertrigo, psoriasis.*

Q. What is *T. cruris*?

A. Dermatophytic infection of groins. Also called Dhobi's itch/Jock itch.

Q. Why is *T. cruris* more common in males?

A. Because *T. pedis* (with which *T. cruris* is associated) is more prevalent in men, males perspire more, anatomical difference and clothing difference.

Q. Why is *T. cruris* more prevalent in obese persons?

A. Constant mechanical irritation of apposed surface, decreased aeration, increased sweating, difficulty in maintaining hygiene and inspecting area involved.

Q. What are the causative agents?

A. *T. rubrum, T. mentagrophytes*, and *E. floccosum.*

Q. Mode of transmission of *T. cruris*.

A. Direct contact or fomites.

Q. Treatment of *T. cruris*?

A. Oral:
- Fluconazole—150–300 mg once a week × 4 weeks
- Itraconazole—200–400 OD × 1 week
- Terbinafine—250 mg OD × 1 week
- Griseofulvin—500 mg OD × 2–4 weeks

Topical:
- Ketoconazole, econazole, terbinafine and ciclopirox cream.

Tinea Manuum

Q. Define *T. manuum*.

A. Defined as ringworm of palmar skin and with infections beginning under rings.

Q. What are the causative agents?
A. *T. rubrum* and *E. floccosum.*

Q. What are the predisposing factors for *T. manuum*?
A.
- Pre-existing foot infection
- Under rings
- Watches
- Bangles
- Poor circulation
- Tylosis
- Manual labor
- Hyperhidrosis
- Existing inflammatory dermatoses

Q. What are the types of *T. manuum*?
A. Noninflammatory squamous form:
- Hyperkeratosis of palms and fingers affecting skin
- Accentuation of flexural creases
- Hyperhidrosis present
- Nails involved

Inflammatory vesicular/dyshidrotic/eczematous form
- Vesicles occur in clusters mainly on palms though dorsal surface maybe affected. Lesions arranged in annular/segmental pattern.
- *T. mentagrophytes* is the usual causative organism in this case.

Q. What are the other clinical variants?
A.
- Crescentric, circumscribed vesicular patches
- Folliculopapular lesions
- Dorsal erythematous type

Q. What are the differential diagnosis of *T. manuum*?
A.
- Contact dermatitis
- Psoriasis
- Eczema
- Tylosis

Tinea Pedis

Q. Define *T. pedis.*
A. Dermatophyte infection of feet. Also called Athlete's foot.

Q. What is the etiology of *T. pedis*?
A.
- Hands and feet are a favorable environment for dermatophyte because of their lack of sebaceous glands that produce fungistatic lipids.

- Males > females
- Increased sweating washes off lipids that inhibit fungi
- Lateral toes affected particularly between 4–5th toes
- Hot, humid climate
- Occlusive shoes
- Immune deficiency condition

Q. What are the types?

A. Chronic intertriginous type:

- Commonest type
- Characterized by fissuring, scaling, maceration in interdigital or subdigital areas. Third and fourth toe webs are commonest sites of infection. Aggravating factor are warmth, humidity and hyperhidrosis.

Chronic papulosquamous type:

- Inflammation and a patchy/diffuse moccasin like scaling over soles
- Affected areas are soles, heels and sides of feet
- Multiple toenails involved
- One hand—2 feet presentation
- Seen in patients with atopic dermatitis

Vesicular/vesiculobullous type:

- *T. mentagrophytes var interdigitale, E. floccosum* are main causative agents of this type.
- Small vesicles/vesiculopustules seen near instep and on mid anterior plantar surface. Scaling present. Infection flares up in summer

Acute ulcerative variant:

- Maceration, weeping and ulceration present. White hyperkeratosis and pungent odor present. Complicated by secondary bacterial infection.

Q. What are the differential diagnosis of *T. pedis*?

A. Candidiasis, erythrasma, soft corn, pustular psoriasis, pompholyx.

Q. Write a note on athlete's foot?

A.
- Caused by bacteria and fungi.
- C/f are maceration, white hyperkeratosis and erosions with pain and pruritus.

Q. Why will you say the following case is of *T. incognito*?

A. Suppression of inflammation with change in morphology of lesion and decrease in associated symptoms. Raised margins are decreased, scaling lost and inflammation reduced. Due to chronic use of topical steroids, local side effects become obvious, i.e., concentric rings of erythema within atrophy and telangiectasia.

Tinea Incognito

Q. Define *T. incognito*.

A. Tinea modified by topical/systemic immunosuppressant treatment due to misdiagnosis or given for some co-existing dermatosis is known as *T. incognito*.

Q. Who first described *T. incognito*?

A. Ive and Marks, 1968.

Q. What is the recent cause of *T. incognito*?

A. Calcineurin inhibitors

Q. Why will you say this is a case of Majocchi's granuloma?

A. Because the patient complains of nonpruritic, solitary/multiple persistant papulopustules/plaques on the legs. Associated with onychomycosis/*T. pedis*

Q. Describe the types of Majocchi's granuloma.

A. Follicular type:

- Occurs secondary to trauma. Immunosuppression not associated. Common in young women who shave their legs repeatedly.

Subcutaneous nodular type:

- Immunocompromised state which maybe primary/drug induced. Develops on hair bearing area mostly on the scalp, face, forearm, hands and legs. Lesion begins as single/multiple well defined oval patch/scaly ones and evolve into perifollicular papulopustules and nodules.

Q. What are the differential diagnosis?

A. *T. incognito*, folliculitis, nodular scabies, kerion.

Q. How will you diagnose such a case?

A.
- Hematoxylin and Eosin (H&E)—Hyphal invasion in cornified keratinocytes of hair follicle which produces suppurative folliculitis with rupture of hair follicle and spillage of contents into dermis. Healing is with fibrosis.
- PAS—fungal hyphae in tissue surrounded by foreign body granulomatous reaction.

Tinea Corporis

Q. Why will you say this is a case of *T. corporis*?

A. • Typical lesion is annular/polycyclic. Borders are erythematous and vesicular/scaly but center is clear.
- Degree of inflammation varies depending on species of fungus, immune status and extent of follicular invasion. In inflammatory lesions-pustules/vesicles present
- In quieter lesions—scaling present
- Central skin may show PIH

Q. What are the differential diagnosis?

A. Pityriasis rosea, impetigo, nummular eczema, GA, psoriasis, seborrheic dermatitis, lichen planus, bacterial infection.

Q. Define *T. corporis*.

A. Dermatophytosis of glabrous skin with exclusion of palms, soles and groin.

Q. PDF.

A. Poor hygiene, poor nutrition, DM, leukemia

Q. Causative agents.

A. *T. rubrum, T. mentagrophytes, M. canis*

Q. What is *T. imbricata*?

A. Variant of *T. corporis* caused by *T. concentricum*. Limited to certain areas of far east, South Pacific and Central Americ. Synonym is Indian Tinea. Contracted in childhood and persist for lifetime. Lesions begin as squamous annular concentric plaques with erythema. Later they became lamellar as they have thick scales that adhere to one side giving appearance of tiles, fish scales, lace.

Q. Types of hair invasion in *T. capitis*.

A. • Endothrix—produced by fungi that invade the inside of hair shaft and are composed of fungal arthroconidia and hyphae.
- Causative agents—*T. tonsurans, T. violaceum, T. soudanese*
- Ectothrix—Produced by fungi that invade outside of hair shaft
- Favus—Invasion of hair by hyphae. Wood's lamp fluorescence is produced by:
    - *Trichophyton schoenleinii*
    - *Microsporum canis*
    - *Microsporum audouinii*
    - *Trichophyton distortum*
    - *Trichophyton ferrugineum*

- Nonfluorescent *T. capitis* caused by:
    - *Trichophyton tonsurans*
    - *Trichophyton violaceum*
    - *Trichophyton soudanense*

Q. What are the C/f of *T. capitis*?

A.
- Gray patch/noninflammatory: Lesions begin as small, erythematous papule surrounding hair shaft. Spreads centrifugally involving all hair in its path. Patches of hair loss, patches are circular in shape, show broken hair that are dull, gray and lustreless. Caused by *M. audouinii.*
- Kerion/inflammatory type: Due to *T. verrucosum/T. mentagrophytes.* Kerion is an inflamed boggy and tender swelling, i.e., studded with broken/unbroken hair, vesicles and pustules. Thick crusting with matting of adjacent hair. Secondary bacterial infection present. Heals with scarring.
- Black dot: Caused by endothrix organism. Hair shaft is brittle and breaks at level of scalp. Remnant of hair left behind in follicle appears as black dot. When hair loss occurs affected areas are multiple and polygonal.
- Favus: Yellow cup shaped crust composed of dense mat of mycelia and epithelial debris. Called scutulum due to shield shape. As infection progresses scutula enlarge and merge to form yellow crust. Odor present. Center of infected area is scarred and devoid of hair.

Q. What are the differential diagnosis?

A.
- Alopecia areata
- Trichotillomania
- Secondary syphilis
- Atopic dermatitis
- Seborrheic dermatitis
- Psoriasis

Q. Complications.

A. Secondary bacterial infection, cicatricial alopecia.

Q. What is the treatment?

A. Topical

- Ketoconazole

Oral

- Griseofulvin 20–25 mg/kg/day for 8 weeks
- Ketoconazole 200 mg OD for 4 weeks

- Itraconazole 5 mg/kg/day for 4–6 weeks
- Terbinafine 3–6 mg/kg/day for 4–8 weeks
- Fluconazole 3–6 mg/kg/day for 6 weeks

Q. What are the types of onychomycosis?

A.
- Distal and lateral subungual onychomycosis
- White superficial onychomycosis
- Proximal subungual onychomycosis
- Endonyx
- Total dystrophic
- 20 nail dystrophy

Q. Why will you say this is distal and lateral subungual onychomycosis?

A.
- Most common type
- Mostly caused by *T. rubrum*
- Toenails > Fingernails
- Starts by invasion of stratum corneum of hyponychium of distal/lateral nail bed. Subungual hyperkeratosis results from hyperproliferative reaction of nail bed response to infection. Splinter hemorrhages maybe seen due to mild inflammation compressing vessels.

Q. Why will you say it is white superficial onychomycosis?

A. Second most common type. There is invasion of dorsal surface of nail plate. Causative agent is *T. mentagrophytes*. Characterized by well circumscribed powdery white patches away from free edge of the nails. Ultimately whole surface of nail plate may be affected. Fingernails are not affected. Surface of nail is rough and friable.

Q. Why will you say it is proximal Subungual onychomycosis?

A. Least common variant of onychomycosis. Commonly caused by *T. rubrum*. First clinical sign is whitish to brownish area on proximal part of nail plate. The organisms invade the ventral surface of nail plate from proximal nail fold. This type is an early indicator of HIV and is associated with peripheral vascular compromise.

Q. What are the differential diagnosis?

A.
- Psoriasis
- Eczema
- Lichen planus
- Darier's disease

Tinea Nigra

Q. Why will you say this is a case of *T. nigra*?

A. Lesions are asymptomatic, macular, sharply defined, nonscaly patches. Most characteristic feature is the brown/black color which resembles $AgNO_3$ stain and which is due to accumulation of melanin like substance in fungus.

Q. Which are the most common sites affected?

A. Palms are most commonly affected but other parts of body such as soles, trunk, neck even penis maybe involved.

Q. What is the causative agent?

A. *Phaeoannellomyces werneckii.*

Q. What are the differential diagnosis?

A.
- Pityriasis versicolor
- PIH
- Addison's disease
- Syphilis
- Pinta
- Junctional nevi of palms
- Melanoma

Q. What is the treatment?

A.
- Topical antifungals
- Cotrimoxazole or econazole ointment
- Thiabendazole 10% suspension OD for 2 weeks
- Whitfield's ointment
- Topical retinoic acid, epidermal tape stripping and ciclopirox olamine
- Oral itraconazole and ketoconazole

Q. What are the investigations?

A.
- Scraped material shows branched thick septate hyphae.
- Culture on Sabouraud's dextrose agar and oatmeal agar.
- Growing colonies that are white/gray at 1st and later become more deeply pigmented and develop aerial hyphae.

Tinea Versicolor

Q. Why will you say this is a case of P. versicolor?

A. Usually the condition is asymptomatic. Chief lesion is macule that maybe hypopigmented/hyperpigmented and covered with branny scales. Upper trunk commonly involved but infection usually extends to upper arms, neck and abdomen.

Q. What are the differential diagnosis?

A.
- Vitiligo
- Pityriasis rosea
- Seborrheic dermatitis
- Secondary syphilis
- Hansen's
- *P. alba*

Q. What does pityriasis versicolor mean?

A. Pityriasis means bran like and versicolor means variegated color.

94 Tattoo

Q. What is the meaning of word "Tattoo"?

A. It comes from the Hawaiian word "Tatau" meaning rhythmic beat.

Q. What are the types of tattoos?

A. There are two types:

1. Decorative tattoos
2. Accidental tattoos: Pigmented particles may be introduced accidentally into the skin as in road traffic accidents, blast injuries, penetrating wounds, therapeutic or occupational hazards.

Examples: Therapeutic—iron salts, gentian violet, Collier's stripes.

Q. What are Collier's stripes?

A. Bluish gray angular or linear stripes at sites of abrasion in coal miners.

Q. What are the chemicals present in various inks and stains?

A.

Mercury	Red
Carbon	Black
Cinnabar and vegetable dyes	Red
Cadmium	Yellow
Cobalt	Light blue
Ochre and iron oxide	Brown
Chromium oxide	Green
Manganese	Purple

Q. What are the complications of tattoos?

A.

- Infections (bacterial infections like syphilis, leprosy, tuberculosis and atypical mycobacteria, viral infections like HIV, hepatitis B and deep fungal infection) and allergic reactions are the most common side effects of tattoos.
- Reactions are mostly in form of erythematous nodules and plaques.
- Lichenoid and eczematous reaction may also be seen.
- Photo-allergic reactions occurs in red or yellow tattoos containing cadmium sulphide.
- Tattoo granuloma

Q. Explain the histological findings of tattoo?

A. • In inflamed tattoo: Different patterns of inflammatory response including sarcoidal, foreign body granulomatous, lichenoid or pseudolymphomatous.

• In noninflamed tattoos: Dermis shows granules within macrophages and extracellularly, in the absence of an inflammatory infiltrate. Tattoo pigments appear black with hematoxylin and eosin (H&E) staining but sometimes red or yellow colors are apparent histologically.

Q. What are the skin diseases associated with tattoos?

A. Lichen planus, psoriasis and rarely lupus erythematosus can be seen in association with tattoos.

Q. What are the modalities for tattoo removal?

A. Lasers such as:

- Q-switched ruby
- Alexandrite
- Nd-YAG

The specific type of laser depends on the tattoo ink colors and the wavelengths to which they best respond.

Q. How will you manage an inflamed tattoo?

A. • Surgical excision is the treatment of choice.

• Topical steroids are generally found ineffective; but intralesional steroids can be tried.

• Laser treatment is contraindicated as there is a risk of systemic reaction following release of pigment in an already sensitized patient.

Q. Relationship between syphilis and tattoos.

A. Syphilis can be inoculated through tattoos (Syphilis d' emblee). Also in case of secondary syphilis, it is noted that the lesions spare a red tattoo since the red pigment is mercury and mercury is known to be active against treponemes.

95 Trichotillomania

Q. Why trichotillomania?

A. Patchy loss of hair in an easily accessible area, with hair broken a different length and no scaling or signs of inflammation.

Q. Trichotillomania is also known as.

A. Habitual hair pulling.

Q. What does trichotillomania mean?

A. Hallopeau in 1889 and is derived from the Greek '*thrix*' hair, '*tillein*' pull out and mania madness. Literally it means a morbid craving to pull out hair.

Q. In which age group is it more common?

A. Bimodal distribution.

- Children—More common in boys.
- Adolescent—More common in females.

Q. What are the diagnostic criteria for trichotillomania?

A. The revised DSM-IV diagnostic criteria for trichotillomania are:

- Recurrent pulling out of one's own hair resulting in hair loss
- An increasing sense of tension immediately before pulling out the hair or when attempting to resist the behavior.
- Pleasure, gratification or relief when pulling out the hair
- The disturbance is not better accounted for by another mental disorder
- The disturbance provokes clinically marked distress and/ or impairment in occupational, social or other areas of functioning

Q. Which body parts hair are involved in trichotillomania?

A. It involves scalp, eyebrows, eyelashes or pubic hair.

Q. What are the clinical features of trichotillomania?

A.
- Hair pulling and plucking is commonest from the scalp.
- Typically, the hairs are short, irregular, broken and distorted.
- The patterns of plucking activity are centrifugal from a single starting point or linear, in wave like activity.

- In extreme cases, the centrifugal pattern removes all hair except the most difficult to access (occiput). This shows as a '*tonsure pattern*' or '*Friar Tuck*' *distribution.*
- The eyelashes, eyebrows, facial and pubic hair may also be primarily affected.
- Plucking may be confined to a specific time and place, with ritualized manipulation of the pulled hairs prior to discarding.
- Some patients may practice trichophagia, the chewing and swallowing of the hair that has been pulled out, possibly leading to intestinal obstruction from trichobezoars.

Q. What are the differential diagnosis of trichotillomania?

A.
- Alopecia areata
- Tinea capitis

Q. What is trichobezoar?

A.
- Bezoars are ball-like aggregations of vegetable or fiber-like materials in the stomach and small intestine seen almost exclusively in girls and young women.
- Swallowed hair is retained within the folds of the gastric mucosa. Action of peristalsis stimulate the hair to become enmeshed into a ball. The hair ball may eventually completely fill the stomach. Hair ball is decomposed to a degree by gastric acidity and fermentation of fats and food in the interstices of the hair gives a putrid smell and significant halitosis.

Q. What are the complications of trichobezoar?

A.
- Halitosis
- Gastric erosions
- Intestinal bleeding, pancreatitis or obstructive symptoms, particularly if the hair bolus extends down the small intestine.

Q. What is the Rapunzel syndrome?

A. It is trichobezoar with a tail that extends at least to the jejunum producing gastrointestinal obstructive symptoms.

Q. What are the other "tricho" seen in trichotillomania?

A.
- Trichomalacia: The process of injured follicles forming soft twisted hair.
- Trichotemnomania: The patient cuts his/her hair with scissors.
- Trichoteiromania: Perpetual rubbing of hair leading to alopecia because of hair shaft breakage

Q. How will you investigate the case of trichotillomania?

A.
- Scalp biopsy
- Barium contrast (trichobezoar)

Q. What are the histological features?

A.
- Normal hair are seen amongst empty hair follicles in a non-inflamed dermis. Many of the empty hair follicles show evidence of changing into the catagen phase.
- Follicular plugging with keratin debris.
- The hair shafts are often broken or reduced to little dark bodies.
- Trichomalacia is seen as deep distortion and curling of the hair bulb.
- In severe damage there is intraepithelial and perifollicular damage.

Q. What is the treatment of trichotillomania?

A.
- Behavioral therapy
- Pharmacotherapy (tricyclic or SSRI antidepressants), N-acetyl cysteine
- For many adolescents and children, identification of stressful episodes with accompanying support and parent education. Teaching awareness and relaxation training can be done.

96 Tuberous Sclerosis

Q. Why is this tuberous sclerosis complex (TSC)?

A.
- Cutaneous angiofibroma (Adenoma sebaceum) 10 mm reddish pink, dome shaped papules, distributed symmetrical on nasolabial folds, cheeks, chin, eyelid, forehead, ears and scalp.
- Ash leaf spots: 1-3 cm lanceolate hypopigmented macules present on trunk or limb.
- Confetti like lesion—numerous 1-3 mm sized white spots symmetrically distributed on extremities.
- Fibrotic plaque/nodule. Skin colored, firm, large plaque or nodule present on forehead or cheek or scalp.
- Shagreen's patch—skin colored, raised, soft plaque with irregular thickening and multiple dimples at follicular opening stimulating orange peel appearance, vary from 1 cm to several inches surrounded by satellite lesion. It commonly occurs in lumbosacral region, but other areas like back of breast may be involved.
- Koenen tumors—smooth, skin colored, firm, periungual or subungual fibroma arising from nail folds.

Q. Define tuberous sclerosis complex.

A. Tuberous sclerosis complex is a multi system hamartomatous condition involving skin, eyes, CNS, CVS, lung, kidney and bones. It is also called Bourneville's disease or epiloia.

Q. What is epiloia?

A. Epi—epilepsy
Loi—low intelligence
A—adenoma sebaceum

Q. What is etiopathogenesis of tuberous sclerosis?

A.
- It is a genetic disorder following AD inheritance. It occurs due to mutation of two genes. TSC1 and TSC2 located on chromosome 9q34 and chromosome 16p13 respectively. Mutation may occur in TSC1 and TSC2.
- TSC1 and TSC2 encode for two protein hamartin and tuberin respectively. TSC1 is biologically similar to NF1 with tumor suppression activity.

- Loss of tuberin cause activation of Rap1 which is a GTPase activating protein in patient of TSC. Sporadic cases occur due to mutation in TSC2.

Q. What is ash leaf spot also known as?

A. Ash leaf spot is also known as Fitzpatrick macule or lanceolate macule.

Q. What are the different types of adenoma sebaceum?

A. Pringle type, Balzer type, Butterworth and Wilson type.

Q. What is the penetration of TSC?

A. High.

Q. Why is adenoma sebaceum a misnomer?

A. It is neither a adenoma nor does it arise from the sebaceous gland; it is an angiofibroma.

Q. What are the extracutaneous findings?

A. Systemic findings

- Ocular features:
  - Retinal hamartomatosis in 50% patients present as yellow gray streaks along blood vessels or elevated multinodular lesion resembling mulberries.
  - White pendulous tumors of palpebral conjunctiva
  - Glial hamartoma of optic disc
  - Retinal angioma
  - Colobomas
  - White spots on iris
- CNS features:
  - Sclerotic areas-subependymal nodules, tubers in cerebral cortex in region of gyri and wall of ventricles.
  - Subependymal giant cell astrocytoma
  - Seizures, mental retardation, obstructive hydrocephalus, behavioral disorders
- Cardiac lesion:
  - Rhabdomyomas occur in infancy in 50% patients
  - Asymptomatic
  - Second peak in puberty
  - Cardiac arrhythmias
- Renal lesions:
  - Involves 15% patients.
  - Most commonly angiomyolipoma, usually asymptomatic
  - Bilateral multiple renal cyst

  - Malignant angiomyolipoma
  - Renal cell carcinoma
- Pulmonary lesions:
  - It is rare
  - Multifocal, multinodular pneumocytes hyperplasia giving rise to recurrent spontaneous pneumothorax.
  - Pulmonary lymphangioleiomyoma gives rise to chylothorax.

Other systemic findings

- Colonic polyposis
- Cyst in liver
- Bony abnormalities

Q. What is diagnostic criteria of TSC?

A. Major features

- Facial angiofibroma or forehead plaque
- Nontraumatic periungal fibroma
- Hypomelanocytic macules >3
- Shagreen patch
- Retinal hamartomas
- Cortical tubers
- Subependymal nodules
- Subependymal giant cell astrocytoma
- Cardiac rhabdomyoma
- Lymphangiomatosis
- Renal angiomyolipoma

Minor features

- Dental enamel pits
- Hamartomatous rectal polyps
- Bone cyst
- Cerebral white matter migration lines
- Gingival fibroma
- Non renal hamartomas
- Retinal achromic patch
- Confetti skin lesion
- Multiple renal cyst
- Definite diagnosis: 2 major features or 1 major + 2 minor features
- Probable diagnosis: 1 major + 1 minor feature
- Possible diagnosis: Either 1 major or 2 or more minor features.

Q. What are investigations?

A. Fully manifested syndrome present with few problems in diagnosis.

- Difficulty in diagnosis arises in childhood when disease evolution is incomplete.
- In infancy and childhood, presenting features are seizure disorder, developmental delay, mental retardation, behavioral problem.
- Cutaneous lesion may be present at birth as ash-leaf spot, forehead plaque.
- In a child when other causes are ruled out, screening for TSC done by wood lamp examination of whole skin for ash leaf spots.
- Ophthalmic examination for retinal hamartomas
- CT/MRI scanning for brain
- Neonatal 2D echo for rhabdomyoma
- Fetal ECG
- In older patients, imaging of different organs.
- Calcification of skull seen in 50% cases.
- Detection of calcified periventricular nodules in CT/MRI brain
- Abdominal USG/CT helpful for detecting renal lesions.
- Other investigation—chest X-ray, ECG, X-ray of hand and feet for cystic lesion of phalanges and irregular thickening of cortex of metatarsal

Differential diagnosis

- Acne
- Trichoepithelioma
- Verruca
- Milia
- Xanthoma
  - Reddish hue of lesion is characteristic
  - Histopathology of the lesion reveals capillary dilation and dermal fibrosis and atrophy and downward displacement of sebaceous unit.
  - Ash leaf spots may be confused with vitiligo but can be confirmed histopathologically by presence of active melanocytes.

Q. What is course and prognosis of TSC?

A.
- Common causes of death are seizure and cranial disorder
- Life expectancy of severely affected patient is poor
- People without seizures may have normal intelligence and life span

Q. What is treatment of TSC?

A.
- Neurosurgical interventions are needed in presence of obstructive hydrocephalus.
- Microsurgical removal of brain neoplasm causes improvement in life expectancy and prognosis. Angiofibroma can be removed by pulse dye laser. Recently, Rapamycin/Sirolimus can induce regression of brain astrocytes. Two analogs of sirolimus including everolimus and prodrug temsirolimus have also been used.
- In patients with TSC associated with infantile spasm following

Formulations are used:
  - Vigabatrin (DOC)
  - Cannabidiol

97 Twenty Nail Dystrophy

Q. Who 1st described twenty nail dystrophy?

A. Hazelrigg and colleagues in 1977.

Q. What is twenty nail dystrophy?

A. Twenty-nail dystrophy is also known as 'trachyonychia'. It could be said that twenty-nail dystrophy is widespread trachyonychia involving all 20 nails. The condition is characterized by longitudinal ridging (alternating elevation and depression), pitting, loss of lustre, and roughening (similar to sandpaper) of the nail surface.

Q. What are the causes of twenty nail dystrophy?

A.
- Idiopathic
- Lichen planus
- Rarely psoriasis
- IgA deficiency
- Primary biliary cirrhosis
- Pemphigus (rare)

Q. What are the types of nail changes that occur?

A.
- Type 1: Whole nail gives appearance of having been sandpapered in longitudinal direction. Excessive ridging and roughness that makes nails lustreless.
- Type 2: Less severe, nail plate is shiny with myriad miniscule superficial punctate depression.
  Thinness, fragility, onychorrhexis, onychoschizia and distal clipping of nail plate may occur. Yellowish thickening of thumb and toe nails is seen.

Q. What is the HP findings?

A. Spongiotic inflammation with fairly dense mononuclear inflammatory infiltrate

Q. What treatment is available?

A. There is no specific treatment for twenty-nail dystrophy. It is a very difficult condition to treat and often results are unsatisfactory.

- Some treatments that have been tried include:
  - Systemic, topical and intralesional corticosteroids
  - Topical PUVA
  - Topical 5-fluorouracil
  - Oral biotin
  - Emollients

98 Urticaria

Q. What is urticaria?

A. Urticaria is characterized by very itchy weals (hives), with or without surrounding erythematous flares. The name urticaria is derived from the common European stinging nettle *Urtica dioica*. Urticaria can be acute or chronic, spontaneous or inducible.

Q. Causes of acute urticaria.

A. Common in children and young adults after allergy to food, drugs, insect bites, or acute viral infection.

Q. Causes of chronic urticaria.

A. Can be due to physical stimulus: Heat, pressure, vibration and cold or autoimmune basis.

Q. Name few mediators of causing vasodilation and increasing vascular permeability.

A. Histamine, prostaglandin D2, leukotriene C4 and D4, platelet activating factor, bradykinin.

Q. Causes of cholinergic urticaria.

A. Exercise, warm bath, showers, emotions are triggers, there is an increased efferent cholinergic output to skin leading to mast cell degranulation.

Q. Classification of urticaria.

A. If duration of symptoms less than 6 weeks then acute urticaria if more than 6 weeks then chronic urticaria.

- Acute urticaria: Mediated by B-lymphocyte produced IgE, and seen in patients with anaphylaxis, serum sickness, atopy, reactions to food, drugs. Food like, nuts, eggs, strawberries, tomatoes, chocolate, citrus. Infections—hepatitis B, *H. pylori*, parasitic infestation.
- Chronic urticaria: Causes—drugs, food additives, inhalants.
- Contact urticaria: Direct contact of chemical with skin, may be immunologic (drugs, cosmetics, natural latex rubber. Non-immunologic (stings, plants, chemicals.)

- Aquagenic urticaria: Water induced urticaria small papules resembling micropapular hives of cholinergic urticaria usually within minutes of exposure to water.
- Autoimmune urticaria: 30–40% of patients with idiopathic urticaria have clinically relevant functional autoantibodies, to high affinity IgE receptor on basophils and mast cells. Patients have chronic severe urticaria with highly symptomatic, with systemic complaints.
- Hereditary angioedema: Dominantly inherited disorder in which a normal serum inhibitor of the activated first components of complement of C1 esterase inhibitor is either deficient or nonfunctional.

Q. Describe lesions of urticaria.

A.
- Urticarial wheals are raised, erythematous, edematous plaques with sharply defined, serpiginous and polycyclic borders surrounded by erythematous halo.
- Diameter ranging from few mm to cm, individual lesions last upto 12 hours, if lesion lasting for more than 24 hours, then urticarial vasculitis should be a differential diagnosis.
- Angioedema—edematous plaques involving the face, not associated with pruritus but with pain or burning, the edema lasts up to 72 hours. Laryngeal edema is noted too.
- Cold urticaria—may be familial or acquired.
- Associated symptoms include fever, arthralgias, leukocytosis. Patients develop localized or generalized wheals or angioedema.
- Urticarial vasculitis—painful, burning urticarial papules/ plaques that last longer than 24 hours, postinflammatory hyperpigmentation or purpura may be noted. Evaluate for complement levels and systemic symptoms.

Q. What are the differential diagnosis of urticaria?

A.
- Allergic contact dermatitis
- Atopic dermatitis
- Urticarial vasculitis
- Drug eruptions
- Erythema multiforme
- Henoch-Schönlein purpura (IgA vasculitis)
- Mastocytosis
- Pityriasis rosea
- Scabies

Q. History and investigations in urticaria.

A.
- Medication history—aspirin, NSAID, COX-2 agents, ACE inhibitors, beta-blockers.
- Investigations—CBC, ESR, urine analysis, liver function test. Leukocytosis indicates chronic infection, total eosinophilic count may indicate cause as drugs, food, parasites, atopy. If suspicion of necrotizing vasculitis or collagen vascular disease. Autologous serum skin test (ASST) is a simple test for diagnosing autoimmune urticaria.

Q. How will we treat urticaria?

A.
- Traditional classic antihistamines exhibit sedation, anticholinergic properties and paradoxical excitation in children as side effects.
- An ideal antihistamine should have a quick onset of action and less side effects besides convenient dosage schedule.
- The new generation antihistamines fulfil these criteria and are the mainstay of treatment especially in chronic idiopathic urticaria.
  - Terfenadine—is as effective as chlorpheniramine and hydroxyzine but less sedative. Cardiac arrhythmias may result if given in excess dosage, i.e., >120 mg/day for adults.
  - Astemizole is very useful in chronic idiopathic urticaria and also in angioedema; and dermographism. The dose is 10 mg/day. A dose of 20 mg/day may cause ventricular arrhythmias.
  - Loratadine is intermediate between fast acting terfenadine and slower astemizole but less effective than cetirizine. The dose is 10 mg/day.
  - Cetirizine is compared more favorably with other nonsedating antihistamines. Dose of 10 mg/day has a more rapid and long-lasting effect when compared to terfenadine or loratadine.
  - Fexofenadine has been used in the treatment of chronic idiopathic urticaria at a dose of 180 mg/day. Notably Q-T interval prolongation occasionally seen with the parent compound, terfenadine, does not occur with fexofenadine.
  - Doxepin is an antidepressant and an antihistamine that blocks both H1 and H2 receptors and may be effective in refractory cases of urticaria in doses of 25–50 mg at bedtime or 10–25 mg 3–4 times a day.

Q. Can antihistamines be prescribed in pregnancy.

A. Antihistamines cross the placenta but are not teratogenic. They are better avoided in pregnancy and especially in the first trimester. Terfenadine is relatively safer in pregnancy. The ideal drug for chronic urticaria would need to have a broad spectrum of activities antagonizing not only histamine but also a range of other mediators such as neuropeptides, and possibly PAF and IL-1 as well.

Q. What are other lines of management?

A.
- In a limited number of patients, low-dose cyclosporine-A, can be effective.
- In resistant cases a brief course of systemic corticosteroid therapy may be necessary but the extended use of systemic corticosteroids should be avoided because of significant adverse effects.

Q. Can stress management be effective in treatment of urticaria?

A. As urticaria patients have significant psychological problems it is suggested that adjunctive treatment of urticaria should focus primarily on stress management training aimed at relieving anxiety and group therapy which focuses on an exploration of interpersonal issues. Doxepin hydrochloride, a tricyclic anti-depressant significantly suppresses histamine and codeine induced cutaneous weal response.

Q. Treatment of angioedema.

A. Adrenaline is used in the emergency treatment of nonhereditary angioedema involving larynx. It can be injected intramuscularly, subcutaneously or inhaled depending upon the severity of the reaction.

Q. Role of phototherapy in urticaria.

A. UVB or PUVA therapy may improve dermographism.

Q. How do we treat cold and solar urticaria?

A. Cold urticaria can be managed by repeated exposure to cold and inducing tolerance apart from H1 antagonists. Solar urticaria may be minimized by wearing appropriate clothing, avoidance of sunlight, or applying broad spectrum sun screens.

99 Xanthomas

Q. What is the definition of xanthomas?

A. Xanthoma is an uncommon skin manifestation of generalized or localized disturbance of lipid metabolism.

Q. Word is derived from?

A. Xanthoma = Yellow tumor (greek).

Q. What are the associated/underlying conditions?

A.
- Hyperlipoproteinemia
- Hypercholesterolemia
- Leprosy
- DM
- Xantho-erythrodermia
- Lipoid proteinosis
- Histiocytosis X
- Pancreatitis
- Biliary cirrhosis
- Multiple myeloma

Q. Types of xanthomas.

A. Following types:
- Eruptive xanthomas
- Plane xanthomas
- Xanthelasma palpebrarum
- Tuberous xanthomas
- Nodular xanthomas
- Tendinous xanthomas
- Generalized plane xanthomas
- Xanthoma disseminatum

Q. What are the characteristics of each type?

A.
- Eruptive xanthomas—Buttocks, thighs, flexors affected. Pin head sized, reddish brown or yellow papules. Sudden onset. Associated with mixed hypertriglyceridemia, DM
  D/D: syringomas, sarcoidosis
- Plane xanthomas—Flexors affected. Yellow or orange slightly elevated plaques. Yellow streaks in palmar crease (xanthoma striata Palmaris). Associated with lymphoma/leukemia.

- Xanthoma palpebrarum—Most common type. Around the eyes, over upper eyelids. Soft velvety, yellow - orange papules or plaques. Associated with familial hypercholesterolemia, hyperlipoproteinemias. Can be treated with lasers, chemical peals.
- Tuberous—Face, buttocks, extensors of limbs affected. Firm, yellow, indurated nodules. Associated with hypercholesterolemia, hyperthyroidism, biliary disease.
- Nodular—On pressure sites, ear lobes, neck. Multiple, yellow, dome shaped nodular lesions. Associated with biliary cirrhosis, biliary atresia.
  D/D: Granuloma annulare, leprosy, leishmaniasis
- Tendinous—Achilles tendon, dorsum of hand affected. Subcutaneous nodules attached to tendons. Associated with hypercholesterolemia, hyperlipoproteinemias.
- Generalized plane Xanthomas—Face, neck, chest affected. Yellow plane macules or plaques. Associated with myelomas, lymphomas. Xanthoma flexures, face, oral mucosa, disseminatum conjunctiva affected. Discrete, small, yellow - brown papules and nodules. Seen in normolipemic individuals.

Q. What are the histopathological findings?

A. Xanthoma cells/Foam cells present in dermis. Touton giant cells seen. Special stains like Scarlet red or Sudan black confirm presence of cholesterol laden cells in frozen sections.

Q. What are investigations advise?

A.
- CBC
- Blood sugars
- Thyroid profile
- Lipid profile
- Biopsy
- USG
- Serum amylase
- Serum electrophoresis

Q. What are the treatment options?

A. Dietary control, treatment of underlying disorders, lipid lowering agents (Probucol and Alirocumab) liquid nitrogen cryotherapy, pingyangmycin, radio frequency ablation, cauterization, surgical excision, chemical peels with TCA and lasers (CO_2, Q switched Nd-YAG, Argon laser, pulsed dye laser, potassium titanyl phosphate laser, diode laser)

100 Yellow Nail Syndrome

Q. Who first discovered the yellow nail syndrome?

A. Yellow nail syndrome (YNS), which was first described by Samman and White in 1964 and by Emerson in 1966.

Q. What is the YNS?

A. Uncommon disorder that is characterized by a classic triad of yellow dystrophic nails, lymphedema, and respiratory tract abnormalities.

Q. What is the criteria for diagnosis of this syndrome?

A. Need to fulfil two out of the three in the triad.

Q. What is the pathogenesis of YNS?

A. The specific etiology of YNS remains obscure; however, the pathogenesis is thought to reflect functional or anatomic defects in the lymphatic vasculature and flow. In a subset of YNS patients, lymphangiography demonstrated hypoplastic, deficient, or sclerotic lymphatic vessels. Such abnormal lymphatic ducts are hypothesized to result in reduced lymphatic drainage, which leads to peripheral edema, pleural effusions, and nail changes when affecting the nail bed.

Another subset of YNS patients had persistent hypoalbuminemia due to increased enteric loss of albumin, which suggested that increased microvascular permeability may contribute to pathogenesis of the syndrome.

Q. What are the nail changes seen?

A. Nail changes include slow growth (0.1–0.25 mm/week) (normal 0.5–2 mm/week), yellow and green discoloration, transverse and longitudinal over-curvature that results in a hyperconvex nail plate, swelling of periungual tissue, onycholysis, shedding, and loss of lunulae and cuticles, nail detachment. Affected nails are thickened and sclerotic. Erythema and edema of the proximal nail fold or chronic paronychia may be present.

Q. What are respiratory symptoms present?

A. Respiratory involvement may vary but most often manifests as chronic cough, sinusitis, bronchiectasis, and exudative pleural effusions.

Q. What are the respiratory abnormalities associated?

A. Pleural effusion, chronic sinusitis, bronchiectasis, chronic bronchitis, pulmonary tuberculosis (TB), and chronic obstructive pulmonary disease (COPD).

Q. What are the other systemic abnormalities associated with YNS?

A. Immunodeficiency syndromes and autoimmune diseases, such as thyroiditis, systemic lupus erythematosus, rheumatoid arthritis, and Guillain–Barré syndrome. Lymphoma and carcinoma of the breast, lung, larynx, endometrium, and gallbladder, mycosis fungoides, xanthogranulomatous pyelonephritis, nephrotic syndrome, D-penicillamine therapy, chronic graft-versus-host reaction.

Q. Treatment.

A. Topical and oral vitamin E, oral zinc supplementation, oral antifungals, and intralesional triamcinolone injections.

101 Xeroderma Pigmentosum

Q. What is xeroderma pigmentosum (XP)?

A. Xeroderma pigmentosum is a very rare skin disorder where a person is highly sensitive to sunlight, has premature skin ageing and is prone to developing skin cancers.

Q. What are the causes of XP?

A.
- Impaired nucleotide excision repair (NER) system.
- In addition to the genetic abnormality, the immunosuppressive effects of exposure to ultraviolet radiation (UV) contribute to the disease, for example by depleting Langerhans cells from the epidermis.

Q. Who gets XP?

A.
- Parents already with a child with XP have a 1 in 4 chance of having another child with XP.
- XP occurs worldwide and affects men and women of all races

Q. What are the stages of XP?

A. **Stage 1**

- The first stage occurs around 6 months after birth (skin appears normal at birth). Areas exposed to the sun such as the face show reddening of the skin with scaling and freckling. Irregular dark spots may also begin to appear.
- These skin changes progress to the neck and lower legs, and in severe cases, to the trunk. Over the winter months, these changes may diminish.

Stage 2

- Characterized by:
  - Poikiloderma
  - Skin atrophy
  - Telangiectasia
  - Mottled hyperpigmentation and hypopigmentation.

Stage 3

- The third stage is the development of actinic keratoses and skin cancers. These may occur as early as age 4–5 years and a mean of 8 years. They are more prevalent in sun-exposed areas such as the face.

- They include:
  - Basal cell carcinoma
  - Squamous cell carcinoma
  - Melanoma

Q. What is the mode of inheritance of XP?

A. Autosomal recessive disorder characterized by defective DNA thymine dimer excision repair, extreme sun sensitivity, freckling and skin cancer.

Q. What is the De Sanctis–Cacchione syndrome?

A. Xeroderma pigmentosum with mental deficiency, dwarfism and gonadal hyperplasia.

Q. In which group is De Sanctis–Cacchione syndrome common?

A. Complementation group D.

Q. Which group is spared of neurological symptoms?

A. Group C.

Q. At which age, are the skin cancers seen?

A. Below 10 years of age.

Q. Treatment of XP.

A.
- Family members and known carriers should undergo genetic counselling and avoid consanguineous marriage.
- Retinoids prevent appearance of new cancers
- Photoprotection
- Topical application of recombinant liposomal encapsulated
- T4 endonuclease
- V repairs
- UV induced
- Cyclobutane pyrimidine dimers

102 Molluscum Contagiosum

Q. Why is it a case of molluscum?

A.
- They are asymptomatic, discrete dome shaped, umbilicated waxy papules. Pseudokoebner's present. In children it is present over face, trunk, thighs. It is caused by direct contact. In adults genital lesions are seen due to sexual transmission.
- Most commonly seen in the skin folds (e.g., axillae, neck)

Q. What is the differential diagnoses of molluscum contagiosum?

A.
- Pyogenic granuloma
- Epithelioma
- Cutaneous cryptococcosis
- Keratoacanthoma
- Verrucae
- Condyloma accuminata
- Basal cell carcinoma
- Melanocytic nevi (especially spitz nevi)
- Papular granuloma annulare

Q. What is molluscum caused due to?

A. MCV 1–4. MCV 1 is the most common seen in the children MCV 2 most commonly seen in the adults who are immunocompromised.

Q. What will you see on histopathology?

A. Epithelial cells have large intracytoplasmic inclusion body (molluscum body) with the dilated follicle. Intracytoplasmic inclusion bodies (Henderson Peterson bodies).

Q. How will you treat molluscum contagiosum?

A.
- Curettage
- Cryotherapy
- Phenol
- Cantharidin 0.9%
- 40% silver nitrate paste
- 20% salicylic acid
- 10% potassium hydroxide
- 0.5% podophyllin
- 5% imiquimod cream on alternate nights
- 1% cidofovir ointment useful in HIV patients

Q. Is it necessary to treat molluscum contagiosum?
A. No, since it resolves in 9 months.

Q. Why do you get umbilicated central area lesion?
A. The bond between the keratinocytes is weakened due to the excessive intracytoplasmic molluscum bodies. This central part collapses due to certain extent and causes umbilication.

Q. What are the complications of molluscum?
A. Eyelid involvement can cause toxic conjunctivitis. Molluscum dermatitis patchy eczema develops around the lesions secondary bacterial infections like impetigo developed after scratching the lesion.

Q. What are the lesions in HIV patients?
A. Lesions may be present over the face and neck. The lesions are large, multiple. Atypical lesions resembling comedones, abscesses, furuncles, keratoacanthoma can be present.

Q. What are the diseases caused by pox-virus?
A. Molluscum contagiosum, monkey pox, small pox, cow pox.

Index

B

E

F

H

L

M

Q

R

S

U

V

W

X

Y

Z

DYP Survival Guide

For Post Graduate Dermatology Examinations

PART-2

DYP Survival Guide
For Post Graduate Dermatology Examinations
PART-2

Editors

Nitin Nadkarni MD DVD DDV
Professor, Department of Dermatology
Dr DY Patil Medical College and Research Centre
Nerul, Navi Mumbai, Maharashtra, India

Sharmila Patil MD DDV
Professor and Head, Department of Dermatology
Dr DY Patil Medical College and Research Centre
Nerul, Navi Mumbai, Maharashtra, India

Kiran Godse MD PhD FRCP (Glasgow)
Professor, Department of Dermatology
Dr DY Patil Medical College and Research Centre
Nerul, Navi Mumbai, Maharashtra, India

Assistant Editor

Aishwarya Rai MBBS
Senior Resident, Department of Dermatology
Dr DY Patil Medical College and Research Centre
Nerul, Navi Mumbai, Maharashtra, India

Foreword

Satish L Wadhwa MD DVD DDV FCPS

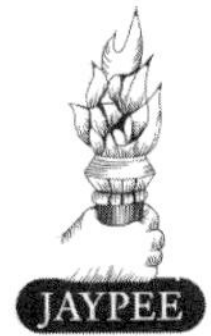

JAYPEE BROTHERS MEDICAL PUBLISHERS
The Health Sciences Publisher
New Delhi | London

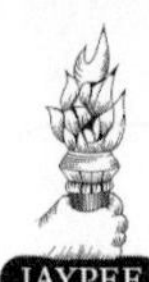

JAYPEE **Jaypee Brothers Medical Publishers (P) Ltd**

Headquarters

EMCA House, 23/23-B
Ansari Road, Daryaganj
New Delhi 110 002, India
Landline: +91-11-23272143, +91-11-23272703
+91-11-23282021, +91-11-23245672
e-mail: jaypee@jaypeebrothers.com

Corporate Office

4838/24, Ansari Road, Daryaganj
New Delhi 110 002, India
Phone: +91-11-43574357
Fax: +91-11-43574314
e-mail: jaypee@jaypeebrothers.com

Overseas Office

JP Medical Ltd.
83, Victoria Street, London
SW1H 0HW (UK)
Phone: +44-20 3170 8910
e-mail: info@jpmedpub.com

EU GPSR Authorised Representative

Logos Europe, 9 rue Nicolas Poussin
17000, La Rochelle, France
Phone: +33 (0) 6 67 93 73 78
e-mail: contact@logoseurope.eu

Website: www.jaypeebrothers.com
Website: www.jaypeedigital.com

Inquiries for bulk sales may be solicited at: jaypee@jaypeebrothers.com

DYP Survival Guide for Post Graduate Dermatology Examinations Part-2 / Nitin Nadkarni, Sharmila Patil, Kiran Godse

First Edition: 2014

Second Edition: 2023

Reprint : 2024, 2025, **2026**

ISBN: 978-93-5696-145-6

Printed at: Sterling Graphics Pvt. Ltd.

Contributors

Manjyot Gautam MD (Dermatology)
Professor, Department of Dermatology
Dr DY Patil Medical College and Research Centre
Nerul, Navi Mumbai, Maharashtra, India

Parag Chaudhari MD (Dermatology)
Assistant Professor, Department of Dermatology
Dr DY Patil Medical College and Research Centre
Nerul, Navi Mumbai, Maharashtra, India

Swagat Waghmare MD (Dermatology)
Assistant Professor, Department of Dermatology
Dr DY Patil Medical College and Research Centre
Nerul, Navi Mumbai, Maharashtra, India

Vedant Ghuse MD (Dermatology)
Assistant Professor, Department of Dermatology
Dr DY Patil Medical College and Research Centre
Nerul, Navi Mumbai, Maharashtra, India

Aswathy Radhakrishnan MD (Dermatology)
Assistant Professor, Department of Dermatology
Dr DY Patil Medical College and Research Centre
Nerul, Navi Mumbai, Maharashtra, India

Notice

Medical knowledge is a constantly changing science. Changes in treatment and drug therapy are essential as new research and clinical experiences enlighten our knowledge. The authors and publisher of this work have checked with sources which are believed to provide reliable and complete information in compliance with the standards, at the time of publication. Readers are encouraged to confirm with other sources the information that is provided in this work. As the possibility of human error exists and due to the ever-changing advances in medical sciences, neither the author nor the publisher or any other party involved in preparation or publication of this work assume any liability for any injury and/or damage to persons or property arising from this publication.

Foreword

It gives me great pleasure to introduce the second edition of *DYP Survival Guide for Post Graduate Dermatology Examinations*.

Success in exams is a matter of knowledge, hard work, presence of mind, and a proper attitude.

Ultimately, this requires not only hours and days of intense theoretical preparation but also practical presentation and rehearsals just as one would practice for a drama or a play.

I have the pleasure of knowing all the authors of this book personally. I have worked with Dr Nitin Nadkarni way back in 1984, when he was a lecturer in BYL Nair Hospital. Dr Kiran Godse has been my student in Nair for 3 years has proved to be hardworking and diligent. Dr Sharmila Patil has a very good name in Dermatology as Professor and Head of Dr DY Patil Hospital.

All these experienced teachers have come together and produced a book which gives a comprehensive approved to the practical examination at various levels in dermatology.

I am very sure this book will help in the understanding of the students of the various tips and tricks to succeed in the examination.

My best wishes to the authors and also to the readers of this book for a stress free and enjoyable exam experience.

Dr Satish L Wadhwa MD DVD DDV FCPS
Formerly Professor and Head
Department of Dermatology
Topiwala National Medical College and
BYL Nair Charitable Hospital
Professor of Dermatology
KJ Somaiya Medical College
Mumbai, Maharashtra, India

Preface to the Second Edition

Examinations are nothing but an ordeal, both for the students and (nowadays) for the examiners. It is a test of knowledge, competency, but above all, technique and temperament.

All of us have been candidates for examinations as well as examiners in our greater days. We have got (hopefully useful) experience which may help the unwary students to escape unscathed through the swampy fields of the viva and the practicals.

The aim of this book is to give advise on questions asked by examiners in tricky situations. We have divided the book into various sections including Long Cases, Short Cases, Spots and Viva. We have got feedback from various candidates who have emerged unscathed from the Post Graduate Examination in Dermatology.

In this book, we have tried to include recent information but omitted references for the sake of brevity. Some of these questions we have asked ourselves to the helpless candidates but we won't reveal which are our personal questions.

We gratefully acknowledge the help and cooperation by the Chancellor of the DY Patil Deemed-to-be-University Dr Vijay D Patil, as well as former Vice Chancellor of DY Patil University, Dr Shirish Patil, and our Dean Dr Rajiv Rao.

We would like to thank all the residents of our department who went through the proofs and also contributed to a few sections. We especially thank Bandhavi Muppalla, Aastha Menon, Edavally Sainath Reddy, Kazomi Shingala, Pooja Patel, Sahil Sethi, Jaisingh Solanki, Meghna Singh, Isheeta Manchandana and Sejal Kumar.

We would be remiss if we don't thank our own teachers, like Dr Satish L Wadhwa who wrote the Foreword, Dr Rui Fernandes and the doyens of Dermatology that are no more with us like Dr RG Valia and Dr VR Mehta. We are eternally grateful to all the teachers for have made us what we are today.

गुरु देवो भव!

We would also like to thank Torrent Pharmaceuticals and Jaypee Publishers for their help in distributing this book.

Nitin Nadkarni
Sharmila Patil
Kiran Godse

Preface to the First Edition

Examinations are a test, not only of knowledge and competence, but also of technique and temperament. Having (collectively) appeared for more than a dozen examinations, and having been examiners for a lot more, we are too aware of the foibles of examiners (including ourselves) and the follies of examinees. This book is a humble attempt to guide the unwary candidate through the pitfalls of dermatology postgraduate examinations at various levels (MD, DNB, DVD, FCPS, etc).

This book is intended for the examination-going candidate who is appearing (hopefully for the first and last time) for an important PG examination. We aim to give reliable advice on both simple and tricky questions asked by examiners in different clinical situations. We have divided the book into various sections, including long cases, short cases (and spots) as well as viva. We have collected common questions asked in the examinations, through "chatting up" our examiner friends, as well as quizzing candidates who have recently appeared for examinations (when their traumatic experiences are still fresh!). We have included lots of questions but have purposely omitted any references for the sake of brevity. Some of the questions (and the answers) reflect our own personal preferences and idiosyncrasies, but we think that is to be expected in a book of this nature.

We are extremely thankful to our teacher Dr Rui Fernandez, who went through the entire draft of this book and gave valuable suggestions, besides consenting to write the foreword. We gratefully acknowledge the help and cooperation given by the director of the Dr DY Patil Group of Hospitals, Mr Vijay D Patil as well as Dr Shirish Patil, dean of our hospital.

Lastly, we would like to thank the residents of our department, who helped with the nitty-gritty of preparing this book. Special mention must be made of Dr Aditya Mahajan and Dr Zubin Mandlewala, whose contribution to proofreading was invaluable. Many thanks to both of them.

Nitin Nadkarni
Sharmila Patil
Kiran Godse

Contents

1 Topical Agents

1.1. PRINCIPLES OF TOPICAL THERAPY

Q. Explain the pharmacokinetics of topical therapy.

A.
- In contrast to oral drugs, topical medications have a poor total systemic absorption and a very slow rate of absorption
- The stratum corneum plays the most significant role in limiting the percutaneous absorption of compounds
- After application of a topical agent, there is an initial lag phase, where the drug remains confined to the stratum corneum without being detectable in the blood stream
- Peak rates of absorption are reached up to 12–24 hours after application

Q. What are the factors affecting absorption of topical agents?

A.
- Drug factors:
    - Concentration of the drug used
    - Inherent potency of the drug
    - Drug diffusion coefficient—ability of the drug to penetrate all the layers of skin
    - Drug partition coefficient—ability of the drug to depart from the specific vehicle and enter the stratum corneum
    - Molecular size—smaller molecules lead to increased percutaneous absorption
    - Lipophilic drugs are better absorbed as compared to hydrophilic drugs
- Condition of the stratum corneum:
    - Diseased skin may have an altered stratum corneum (decreased, increased or absent) which must be taken into consideration while selecting the therapeutic agent and vehicle
    - Loss of barrier is seen in abraded or eczematized skin including conditions such as atopic dermatitis.
    - Hydration of the skin—hydration of skin prior to topical application increases absorption.

- Vehicle used for delivery:
  - Irritating vehicles such as solvents, surfactants, and alcohols can denature the cornified layer and increase penetration of the drug
  - Ointment is the best vehicle due to high lipid content while solutions are the weakest
- Site and total area of application—there are regional differences in drug penetration in different parts of the body, as follows (in decreasing order of absorption):
  - Mucous membrane > scrotum > eyelids > face > chest and back > arms and thighs > forearms and shins > dorsa of hands and feet > palmar and plantar skin > nails
  - Extensive body surface area involvement will lead to greater systemic absorption of the drug
- Age of patient:
  - Increased body surface area to body volume ratio in infants and children will cause enhanced systemic effects of topically applied drugs
  - In older patients although the stratum corneum is thin, low hydration and reduced hair follicles may impede absorption
- Occlusion:
  - Occlusion via air tight dressings or greasy ointment bases increases the hydration and temperature of the stratum corneum, limits rub off and wash off of the drug, and thus enhances drug penetration
  - However, occlusion may hasten the appearance of local adverse effects and may promote infections
- Frequency of application:
  - Frequency of application has little effect on absorption of the drug
  - Almost similar efficacy is observed with once daily as well as twice daily applications for many drugs such as topical corticosteroids
  - Nonspecific emollient and protective effects of drugs are enhanced by more frequent applications
- Compliance:
  - Compliance is a critical factor affecting efficacy of topical therapy
  - Low adherence to treatment regimens is seen in patients with extensive disease and disease on the face
- Rubbing/massaging—increases absorption by increasing surface area of application and improving cutaneous circulation.

- Micronization—reducing the particle size of the active ingredient increases the solubility of drug in its vehicle, thus enhancing penetration.

Q. What is a vehicle?

A.
- The term vehicle refers to all constituents of the formulation apart from the active pharmaceutical agent. Also referred to as the base
- It is the substance that brings the specific drug into skin contact
- An ideal vehicle is easy to apply and remove, nontoxic, nonirritant, nonallergic, homogenous, chemically stable, bacteriostatic, cosmetically acceptable and pharmacologically inert
- A vehicle can have one or more of three phases viz., powder (solid), liquid and greasy

Q. Name some monophasic vehicles.

A.
- Powders—inorganic (zinc oxide, bentonite) and organic (starch)
- Liquids—glycerol, glycerine, ether, etc.
- Greases—almond oil, lanolin, linseed oil, liquid paraffin, etc.

Q. What are biphasic vehicles?

A. Biphasic vehicles are made by combination of two monophasic vehicles. They include lotions, pastes, creams and liniments.

Biphasic vehicle	*Combination*	*Formulation*	*Example*
Shake lotion	Powder + liquid	Powder suspended in liquid	Calamine lotion
Drying pastes	Powder + liquid	Equal proportion of powder and liquid	Calamine paste
Greasy pastes	Powders + grease	Powders and greases in equal proportions	Lassar's paste
Liniments	Powders + greases	Powders in liquid greases	Calamine liniment
Creams	Liquids + greases	Mixtures of liquids and greases in presence of emulsifying agents	

Q. What are triphasic vehicles?

A. Triphasic vehicles are a mixture of greases, liquids and powders. Examples are cooling pastes and cream pastes.

Q. Define ointment.

A.
- Ointments are semi-solid vehicles composed of lipids
- They are greasy, occlusive, and do not require preservatives due to low water content
- They are used for smooth, nonhairy skin, and are avoided on hairy and intertriginous areas

Q. Define cream.

A.
- Creams are semi-solid emulsions containing both lipid and water
- They are suspensions, either of lipid droplets in water (oil in water type) or of water droplets in lipid (water in oil type)
- They are less greasy, nonocclusive
- They can be used for acute exudative inflammations and intertriginous areas

Q. Define paste.

A.
- Pastes are semi-solid preparations containing high concentrations of a finely powdered material
- Protective/fatty pastes are occlusive, protective, greasy and hydrating. Their stiffness permits accurate localization of the medication. They are difficult to apply and remove
- Drying/cooling pastes are mixtures of powder with liquid. They are nongreasy, water-miscible, and easy to apply and remove
- Pastes are useful for acute/subacute lesions with crusting and oozing and to absorb secretions

Q. Define lotion.

A.
- A lotion is a liquid formulation, generally a simple suspension or solution of a medication in water, alcohol, or other liquids
- They penetrate easily, leaving little residue
- They can be used for hairy areas

Q. What is a shake lotion?

A. An aqueous suspension of a powder such as calamine lotion, which requires shaking prior to each application is known as shake lotion.

Q. Define foam.

A. It is a liquid pressurized in an airtight can in which the active ingredient is combined with a hydrocarbon propellant (propane or butane). Easy to apply in hairy areas and is less drying. Can be used for sensitive scalp and sensitive skin.

Q. What are liniments?

A. Liniments are oily lotions. They may be oily substances suspended in aqueous medium (O/W) or aqueous solutions suspended in oily medium (W/O). They are less drying than lotions.

Q. What is a gel?

A.
- A gel is a semi-solid preparation containing high-molecular-weight polymers such as carboxy-poly-methylene or methyl-cellulose
- It is a semi-solid substance but liquefies on application to the skin leaving a thin transparent residue
- They are cosmetically acceptable preparations for use on the face
- They are nongreasy, least occlusive, and dry quickly
- They are preferred vehicles for acne, exudative inflammation, and hairy areas/scalp

Q. What are paints?

A. Paints are liquid preparations, either aqueous, hydroalcoholic, or alcoholic which are applied with a brush and generally evaporate.

Q. What are the advantages and disadvantages of different vehicles?

A.

	Ointments	*Creams*	*Gels*	*Lotions*
Composition	W/O emulsion	O/W emulsion	Semisolid emulsion in alcohol base	Powder in water (some with oil)
Relative potency	Strong	Moderate	Moderate	Low
Hydration/ drying	Hydrating	Some hydration	Drying	Drying
Stage of disease	Chronic	Acute/ Subacute	Acute/ Subacute	Acute
Sensitization	Very low	Significant	Significant	Significant
Irritation	Very low	Very low	Rather high	Moderate
Useful in	Nonfold areas	All areas	Oral, scalp	Scalp, folds
Avoid	Face, hands, groins	Sites with maceration	Fissures, macerated	Fissures, macerated
Patient preference	Often dislike greasiness	High acceptance	Variable	Variable

Q. What is a fingertip unit (FTU)?

A. A fingertip unit is the amount of ointment expressed from a tube with a 5 mm nozzle, applied from the distal skin crease to the tip of the index finger. It is a practical measure of amount of topical medication to be used.

One FTU = 0.5 g = 2% of body surface area (BSA).

Q. What is the rule of hand?

A. The "rule of hand" states that any area of the body of the size that can be covered by 4 adult hands can be treated by 1 g of ointment or 2 fingertip units.

One hand unit = 0.5 FTU = 1% BSA.

FTU guidelines for adults:

Anatomic area	*FTU required*	*Amount needed for twice daily regimen in grams*
Face and neck	2.5	2.5
Anterior and posterior trunk	7	7
Arm	3	3
Hand (both sides)	1	1
Leg	3	3
Foot	2	2

FTU guidelines for children:

Anatomic area	*FTU required/amount needed for twice daily regimen in grams*			
	3–6 months	*1–2 years*	*3–5 years*	*6–10 years*
Face and neck	1/1	1.5/1.5	1.5/1.5	2/2
Arm and hand	1/1	1.5/1.5	2/2	2.5/2.5
Leg and foot	1.5/1.5	2/2	3/3	4.5/4.5
Anterior trunk and posterior trunk	1/1	2/2	3/3	3.5/3.5
Buttocks	1.5/1.5	3/3	3.5/3.5	5/5

Q. What may be the local adverse reactions of topical agents?

A. Local reactions may be caused either by the active drug or the vehicle. Some of the examples include:

- Irritation
- Atrophy

- Comedogenicity
- Allergic contact dermatitis
- Contact urticaria
- Telangiectasias
- Contact purpura

The local adverse effects are usually minor and reversible.

Q. What are the systemic adverse effects of topical therapy?

A.
- Systemic adverse effects may be caused by the drug itself, its metabolites, or components of the vehicle
- Drugs absorbed topically bypass the hepatic first-pass effect
- When absorbed in high concentrations they may result in damage to the central nervous system (e.g., salicylic acid), kidneys and may even cause carcinogenicity and teratogenicity
- In rare instances, anaphylactic shock may be precipitated by topical drug application
- Young children are more susceptible to systemic adverse effects of topical medications

Q. Enumerate the various pregnancy categories of drugs.

A.
A: Completely safe in pregnancy (very few drugs, e.g., multivitamins, minerals and thyroid hormones)

B: No evidence of risk in pregnancy (e.g., penicillin group of antibiotics)

C: Risk cannot be ruled out (benefit > risk) (e.g., antileprosy drugs)

D: Positive evidence of risk (risk > benefit, e.g., tetracyclines and antimetabolites)

X: Absolutely contraindicated (e.g., thalidomide, retinoids)

1.2. TOPICAL ANTIBACTERIAL AGENTS

INTRODUCTION

- Aims of therapy:
  - Achieve high local drug concentration
  - Minimal systemic absorption—minimizes systemic adverse effects
- Classified as:
  - Antibiotic agents
  - Nonantibiotic agents

  Two broad categories:

  i. Drugs for wound care and minor topical bacterial infections

  ii. Drugs for acne and rosacea

Q. Discuss disinfectants and antiseptic.

A.
- Disinfectants—chemical agents primarily used on nonliving tissue to destroy bacteria as well as spores
- Antiseptics—chemical agents primarily used to destroy or decrease active bacterial population on intact skin
- Many times these terms are used synonymously
- These cannot be used on major wounds due to risk of systemic absorption, irritation and damage to cellular structures
- Can be used for hand hygiene for relatives and doctors to prevent hospital acquired infections
- *The various antiseptic agents are*:
    - Alcohol
    - Hydrogen peroxide
    - Chlorhexidine
    - Triclosan
    - Iodophor (Povidone iodine)
    - Sodium hypochlorite
    - Hexachlorophene

ALCOHOL

- Both ethyl and isopropyl alcohol can be used (60–95%)
- Denaturation of proteins
- Acts quickly but duration of action is limited. Action increased if combined with 4% chlorhexidine or povidone iodine

HYDROGEN PEROXIDE

- Kills bacteria by DNA damage due to formation of superoxide and hydroxyl radicals
- It also inactivates bacterial enzymes. However, it is not very bactericidal and may be actually detrimental to wound healing by damaging keratinocytes

CHLORHEXIDINE

- Kills bacteria by disrupting cytoplasmic membranes
- Extremely broad spectrum
- Acts slowly but long duration of action
- It has a major role in general skin cleansing, surgical site preparation and preoperative bathing

- It is superior to povidone iodine and useful in MRSA carriers
- Can be combined with isopropyl alcohol as a hand wash

TRICLOSAN

- It is a broad spectrum antimicrobial agent widely used in consumer products
- Kills bacteria by blockade of lipid synthesis
- Resistance to this product is emerging

IODOPHORS

- They are complexes of iodine with organic carrier compounds
- They act by destroying bacterial proteins and DNA through release of iodine
- The most common iodophor is povidone iodine which is a complex of iodine with polyvinyl pyrrolidine
- Acts rapidly but relatively short duration of action
- Broad spectrum, including MRSA and enterococci
- No significant resistance documented
- Adverse effects include—contact dermatitis and metabolic acidosis
- Contraindicated in pregnancy and thyroid disorders
- High concentration can impair wound healing

SODIUM HYPOCHLORITE

- Component of Dakin's solution
- Acts on cytoplasmic membranes
- Broad spectrum
- Used in pediatric patients with infected atopic dermatitis (added 1/2 cup per bath tub while bathing twice weekly)
- Also has anti-HIV effect

HEXACHLOROPHENE

- Bacteriostatic agent against gram positive bacteria
- Neurotoxic, hence, not used in infants

BACITRACIN

Introduction

Polypeptide antibiotic produced by Tracey I strain of Bacillus subtilis.

Mechanism of Action

Interferes with bacterial cell wall synthesis.

Indications

- Infections caused by gram positive (bactericidal) and few gram negative organisms
- Minor wounds and topical infections
- Bacitracin in combination with polymyxin B or neomycin reduces *S. aureus* contamination

Preparation

Bacitracin in creams and ointments—5 days application.

Adverse Effects

Localized itching and burning, allergic contact dermatitis; anaphylactic shock. May cross react with polymyxin.

Pregnancy Category: C

POLYMYXIN B

Introduction

Polymyxin B is a cationic decapeptide (isolated from aerobic gram positive rod Bacillus polymyxa), bactericidal against gram-negative bacteria.

Mechanism of Action

- Alters permeability of bacterial cytoplasmic membrane leading to leakage of ions and amino acids
- May neutralize endotoxins of bacteria

Indications

- 'Triple antibiotic' combination of neomycin, bacitracin, polymyxin B-for minor skin wounds
- Cutaneous infections caused by gram negative organisms mainly *Pseudomonas, Proteus* and *Serratia*. But ineffective against gram positive bacteria

Preparation

0.1–1% polymyxin cream.

Possible Side-effect

Contact dermatitis and acute renal failure reported.

Pregnancy Category: B

NEOMYCIN

Introduction

Bactericidal aminoglycoside produced by *Streptomyces fradiae*.

Mechanism of Action

It inhibits bacterial DNA polymerase; inhibits protein synthesis.

Indications

Minor wounds cutaneous infections; mixed infections of gram positive and gram negative bacteria.

Preparation

1% neomycin.

Adverse Effects

Ototoxicity, nephrotoxicity, deafness, very commonly ACD (allergic contact dermatitis) is seen. Sometimes also causes mast cell degranulation and histamine release.

Pregnancy Category: D

MUPIROCIN

Introduction

Mupirocin, which was previously known as pseudomonic acid, is a metabolite of *P. fluorescens*.

Mechanism of Action

- It inhibits bacterial RNA synthesis, protein synthesis and cell wall synthesis
- Excellent activity against *Staphylococcus aureus, Staphylococcus epidermidis, MRSA, Streptococcus pyogenes* and *β-hemolytic streptococci*. But noneffective against *Pseudomonas* and *Anaerobes*
- Binds to bacterial isoleucine—t-RNA synthetase. This prevents incorporation of isoleucine in the bacterial cell wall
- This mode of action is unique to mupirocin. Hence, no cross reaction to other antibiotics
- Resistance has been recently reported

Indications

- Impetigo
- Impetiginized eczema
- Folliculitis
- Burns

- Lacerations
- Leg ulcers
- Intranasally, perianally for elimination of staphylococci from chronic carriers

Preparation
2% cream, ointment.

Adverse Effects
Pain, burning, itching (due to vehicle base polyethylene glycol), ACD.

Pregnancy Category: B

RETAPAMULIN

Introduction
It is a semi-synthetic pleuromutilin derivative. Isolated from an edible mushroom.

Mechanism of Action

- Retapamulin is bacteriostatic and inhibits bacterial protein synthesis by targeting the 50s subunit of ribosome
- Acts at a site distant from other available drugs, hence, cross resistance is not yet a problem
- Effective against both MRSA and MSSA

Indications
Primary impetigo, secondary infected dermatitis, atopic dermatitis for bacterial decolonization.

Preparations
1% ointment—BD for 5 days.

Adverse Effects
Irritation, pruritus, paresthesia, pain at the site of application.

Pregnancy Category: B

SILVER SULFADIAZINE

Introduction
It is bactericidal against gram positive and gram negative bacteria.

Mechanism of Action

- Binds to bacterial DNA and inhibits its replication
- It is thought to combine the bactericidal activity of silver with the bacteriostatic activity of sulfadiazine

Indications

- Bactericidal against gram positive and gram negative bacteria including MRSA and *P. aeruginosa*
- Burns
- Higher concentrations of this drug also inhibit *Candida* and herpes zoster

Preparation

1% cream.

Adverse Effects

- Prolonged use in bullous disorders—renal insufficiency has been reported
- Transient neutropenia
- Argyria has occurred following extensive silver sulfadiazine application in patients with dystrophic epidermolysis bullosa

Pregnancy Category: B

FUSIDIC ACID

Introduction

Isolated from the mould fusidium. It has a ring structure similar to glucocorticoids. It has a reservoir effect in the stratum corneum.

Mechanism of Action

- Bactericidal against *S. aureus, Corynebacterium, Clostridium* and *Streptococci*
- It can penetrate both intact and damaged skin and also penetrate crusts and cellular debris
- Few reports of resistance

Preparation

2% cream, ointment.

Adverse Effects

Irritation, stinging and contact dermatitis.

Pregnancy Category: B

BENZOYL PEROXIDE

Introduction

- Broad spectrum bactericidal
- It is an antiacne agent for grade-I and grade-II acne vulgaris

Mechanism of Action

- Functions through its powerful oxidizing activity
- Inhibits triglyceride hydrolysis, thereby reducing inflammation
- Keratolytic and comedolytic activity
- Antibacterial action

Preparation

- Wash, lotion, cream, gel ranging from 2.5–20%
- BP is more effective on noninflamed areas and is superior to tretinoin for inflammatory lesions
- BP 4% gel reduces both inflammatory and noninflammatory lesions
- BP 5% and erythromycin 3% are more effective
- Formulations combining BP and topical retinoids have recently become available
- BP 5% gel for 12 weeks significantly reduces papules and pustules and is well tolerated

Adverse Effects

Irritant dermatitis with symptoms of dryness, irritation, burning, erythema and desquamation.

Pregnancy Category: C

Key Points

- Rapidly reduces bacterial count of *P. acnes*
- No bacterial resistance
- It can be combined with other antibacterials to prevent resistance

PROTEGRIN-1

Introduction

It is a naturally occurring, naturally available broad spectrum antibiotic identified in many organisms.

Mechanism of Action

- Binds to lipid component of bacterial cell membrane creating voltage dependent channels which rapidly lyse the bacteria
- It is broad spectrum and effective against MRSA also

PEXIGANAN

It is a peptide antibiotic with broad spectrum action and is rapidly bactericidal.

CLINDAMYCIN

Introduction

Synthetic derivative of antibacterial agent lincomycin, isolated from *Streptomyces* species.

Mechanism of Action

- Inhibits bacterial protein synthesis
- Bactericidal or bacteriostatic effect indications:
    - Acne vulgaris
    - It is effective against gram-positive cocci and anaerobic gram-positive and gram-negative organisms

Preparation

1% gel, 1% lotion, 1% solution.

Adverse Effects

Mild local reactions include itching, burning, excessive dryness, peeling, oily skin, stinging and erythema.

Pregnancy Category: B

ERYTHROMYCIN

Indications

Macrolide antibacterial agent—*Streptomyces erythraeus.*

Mechanism of Action

Bactericidal—inhibits bacterial protein synthesis.

Preparation

1–4% gel, cream and lotion.

Indications

Acne vulgaris.

Adverse Effects

Erythema, scaling, tenderness, burning, itching, dryness, oiliness.

Pregnancy Category: B

METRONIDAZOLE

Indications

It is a synthetic nitroimidazole antibacterial readily taken up by anaerobic organisms.

Mechanism of Action

- Uncertain. It is supposed to inhibit reactive oxygen species (ROS) which may have an immunomodulatory effect
- It results in DNA disruption and inhibition of nucleic acid synthesis
- It is minimally absorbed topically

Indications

- Papulopustular rosacea (alone or combined), seborrheic dermatitis, perioral dermatitis, acne vulgaris, cutaneous ulcers
- Treatment of toxicity caused by epidermal growth factor inhibitors. This often causes a papulopustular eruption resembling acne. For this metronidazole can be successfully used
- Odoriferous wounds associated with anaerobic infections
- Topical provocation testing to confirm the diagnosis of FDE or AGEP caused by systemic metronidazole

Adverse Effects

Rare, include dryness, itching, burning, stinging.

Preparations

0.75 % gel, 1% cream.

Pregnancy Category: B

AZELAIC ACID

Introduction

Saturated 9-carbon di-carboxylic acid.

Mechanism of Action

It interferes with neutrophilic functions through multiple mechanisms.

Indications

Acne vulgaris, rosacea, perioral dermatitis.

Adverse Effects

10% patient may develop itching, burning, scaling.

Pregnancy Category: B

DAPSONE

Introduction

Antimicrobial and anti-inflammatory agent.

Mechanism of Action

It interferes with neutrophilic functions through multiple mechanisms.

Indications
Acne vulagris (grade IV).

Preparation
5% gel.

Adverse Effects
Transient dryness, erythema, rash, sun burn.

Pregnancy Category: C

SODIUM SULFACETAMIDE

Introduction
Antibacterial and anti-inflammatory properties.

Mechanism of Action
It inhibits bacterial dihydropteroate.

Indications
Acne, rosacea.

Adverse Effects
- Mild-to-moderate dryness or transient pruritus
- It produces an orange-brown discoloration, which does not stain skin but stains clothes

Preparation
10% cream.

Pregnancy Category: C

1.3. TOPICAL ANTIFUNGAL AGENTS

INTRODUCTION

- First used during World War II
- Castellani's paint, Whitfield's ointment and gentian violet
- Irritating, staining and minimally effective
- Topical antifungals are considered 1st line therapy for uncomplicated superficial dermatomycoses due to high efficacy, low potential for systemic adverse effects

Q. Classify antifungal agents.

A. Antifungal agents can be classified as:
- Traditional or older antifungals:
  - Whitfield's ointment

  - Castellani's paint
  - Gentian violet
  - Undecylenic acid
  - Potassium permanganate
  - Selenium sulphide
  - Aluminium chloride
  - Zinc pyrithione

All these have nonspecific actions.

- Newer antifungal agents:
  - Polyenes
  - Azoles—imidazoles and triazoles
  - Allylamines/benzylamines
  - Morpholine—amorolfine
  - Miscellaneous—tolneftate, haloprogene, ciclopirox, iodochlorhydroxyquinoline

POLYENES

- Developed in late 1950's
- Multiple carbon atoms with conjugate double bonds

Nystatin

- First specific antifungal to be developed in 1949 by Hazen and Brown in New York state health laboratory—"nys"-tatin
- Polyene antibiotic produced by *S. nouseri* and *S. albidus*
- It is insoluble in water and not absorbed from intact skin, GIT or vagina
- MOA—increases cell membrane permeability by binding to ergosterol in susceptible species

Q. What are the indications for nystatin?

A. Nystatin is indicated in following conditions:

- Cutaneous or mucocutaneous mycotic infections caused by *Candida albicans*
- Not effective in dermatophytoses or *P. versicolor*

Q. What are the preparations available?

A. Available as cream, powder, ointment formulations for twice daily application and as a suspension and slowly dissolving pastille.

Q. What are the adverse effects of nystatin?

A. Adverse effects of nystatin are:

- Burning

- Pruritis
- Rash
- Eczema
- Pain on application

Q. Pregnancy category.
A. Category B.

AZOLES

Broader spectrum of activity.

Q. Classify azoles.
A. Azoles
- Imidazoles:
  - Topical: Clotrimazole, econazole, miconazole, oxyconazole
  - Systemic: Ketoconazole (topical also)
- Triazoles
- Systemic: Fluconazole (topical also), itraconazole, voriconazole, posaconazole

Q. What is the mechanism of action of azole?
A.
- Azoles act by inhibiting cytochrome P-450 dependent enzyme lanosterol 14-alpha demethylase which is an essential enzyme in ergosterol synthesis.
  - They are fungistatic at low concentration and fungicidal at high concentration.

Q. Name the azole antifungal agents.
A. The azole antifungal agents are:
- Miconazole
- Clotrimazole
- Ketoconazole
- Oxiconazole
- Econazole
- Sulconazole
- Sertaconazole

Miconazole

Penetrates the stratum corneum well and can be detected there up to 4 days after a single application.

Q. What are the indications of miconazole?

A. Miconazole is indicated in following conditions:
- Tinea pedis
- Tinea corporis
- Tinea cruris
- Tinea versicolor
- Cutaneous candidiasis
- Gram-positive bacteria—impetigo, erythrasma or ecthyma
- Twice daily application for all indications except tinea versicolor—once daily application
- A benzoyl peroxide and miconazole combination has also been studied in Rx of acne vulgaris

Q. What are the adverse effects of miconazole?

A. Adverse effects of miconazole are:
- Irritation
- Burning
- Maceration
- Allergic dermatitis at site of application

Q. Pregnancy category?

A. Category C.

Clotrimazole

Q. What are the indications for clotrimazole?

A. Clotrimazole is indicated in following conditions:
- Tinea pedis
- Tinea cruris
- Tinea corporis
- Tinea versicolor
- Cutaneous candidiasis
- Gram positive bacteria

Q. What are the various formulations available for clotrimazole?

A. The various formulations available for clotrimazole are:
- Available in cream, lotion, solution formulations for twice daily application
- Oropharyngeal candidiasis—troche—designed to slowly dissolve in mouth, administered 4–5 times daily for 2 weeks
- Intravaginal clotrimazole—once daily tablet insertion for 1–2 days

Q. What are the adverse effects of clotrimazole?

A. Similar to miconazole.

Ketoconazole

A.
- Synthesized in 1977
- Water soluble
- Broad spectrum antimycotic
- Not absorbed into systemic circulations, no detectable plasma levels

Q. What are the indications of ketoconazole?

A. Ketoconazole is indicated in following conditions:
- Tinea cruris
- Tinea corporis
- Tinea pedis
- Tinea versicolor
- Cutaneous candidiasis
- Seborrheic dermatitis (*Pityrosporum ovale*)

Q. What are the various formulations available for ketoconazole?

A. Ketoconazole is available as:
- 2% cream
- 2% shampoo
- 2% foam

Q. What are the adverse effects of ketoconazole?

A. Similar to miconazole.

Oxyconazole

First topical antifungal agent to be approved for once daily application.

Q. What are the indications for oxiconazole?

A. Oxiconazole is indicated for:
- Once daily application for Tinea pedis, including the hyperkeratotic plantar and interdigital subtypes
- Other superficial fungal infections
- 1% cream and 1% lotion (larger and hairy areas)

Q. What are the adverse effects of oxiconazole?

A. Similar to miconazole.

Econazole

Q. What are the indications of econazole?

A. Econazole is indicated in following conditions:
- Tinea pedis
- Tinea cruris

- Tinea corporis
- Tinea versicolor
- Cutaneous candidiasis
- Some gram-positive and gram-negative organisms—severe interdigital toe web infections

Sulconazole

- Has a sulfide bond in conjugate ring?
- Has modest antibacterial activity against gram-positive bacteria?

Q. What are the indications of sulconazole?
A. Similar to others.

Q. What are the adverse effects of sulconazole?
A. Similar to others.

Sertaconazole

- Most recent topical azole antifungal agent
- Lipophilic—greater reservoir effect in stratum corneum
- Binds to nonsterol cell membrane lipids, leading to altered membrane permeability and leakage of intracellular contents in susceptible microbes

Q. What are the uses of sertaconazole?
A. Sertaconazole is used in:
  - Sertaconazole nitrate 2% cream, gel, powder and solution formulations
  - Vaginal cream and intravaginal tablets—for single dose treatment of candidiasis
  - Tinea pedis—twice daily application for 4 weeks
  - Excellent activity against *Candida* species
  - Modest activity against gram-positive bacteria

Q. What are the adverse effects of sertaconazole?
A. Adverse effects of sertaconazole are: Rare cases of allergic contact dermatitis

ALLYLAMINES AND BENZYLAMINES

- New class of antifungal agents
- Broader spectrum
- Fungistatic + fungicidal

Action: Inhibition of squalene epoxide in ergosterol biosynthesis pathway.

Naftifine

- A synthetic allylamine antifungal
- High penetration power
- Concentration is high in the stratum corneum and hair follicle
- Its both fungicidal and fungistatic
- Available as 1% cream

Q. List the indications of naftifine.

A. Indications: Same as others

Q. What are the adverse effects of naftifine?

A. Naftifine is extremely well tolerated with <5% of patients experiencing adverse effects. They include:

- Mild burning/stinging
- Itching
- Erythema
- Irritation
- Rarely allergic reaction

Terbinafine

- It is a broad spectrum synthetic antimycotic agent
- Both fungistatic and fungicidal properties
- Probability of reinfection is less with use of this drug
- It is 10–100 times more potent as compared to naftifine
- On topical use 3–5% of terbinafine 1% cream is absorbed in systemic circulation

Q. What are the indications of terbinafine?

A. Same as others.

Q. What are the adverse effects of terbinafine?

A. Same as others.

Butenafine

- First and only benzylamine class of antifungal
- Fungicidal concentration in skin particularly in stratum corneum for atleast 72 hours after application leads to depot effect
- Available as 1% cream

Q. What are the indications of butenafine?

A.
- Same as others
- Not effective against *Candida*

Q. What are the adverse effects of butenafine?

A. Same as others.

OTHER AGENTS

Ciclopirox Olamine

- Acts by interfering with active membrane transport of essential macromolecular precursors, disrupting cell membrane integrity and inhibiting enzymes essential for respiratory processes
- Available as cream, gel, suspension, nail lacquer

Q. What are the indications of ciclopirox olamine?

A. Ciclopirox olamine is indicated in:
- FDA approved for Rx. of tinea corporis, tinea pedis, tinea versicolor and cutaneous candidiasis
- 1% shampoo formulation for seborrhea
- Demonstrates strong activity against gram +ve and gram -ve bacteria, and inherent anti-inflammatory property
- Ciclopirox nail lacquer 8%—potential to penetrate nail plate used for toenail onychomycosis. Daily use for 9–12 months

Q. What are the adverse effects of ciclopirox olamine?

A. Same as others.

Selenium Sulphide

- It is a liquid antiseborrheic, antifungal preparation for topical application
- 2.5% solution available only with prescription, 1% strength is available over-the-counter

Q. What are the indications of selenium sulfide?

A. Indications:
- Seborrheic dermatitis of scalp
- Tinea versicolor (short contact for 20 mins to be applied from head to toe excluding genital 5 days a week)
- Adjuvant to griseofulvin—tinea capitis

Q. What are the side effects of this agent?

A.
- Irritant contact dermatitis is very commonly seen
- Disagreeable odor
- Bleaching of ornaments
- Selenium is teratogenic in pregnancy

1.4. TOPICAL ANTIPARASITIC AGENTS

PERMETHRIN

Introduction

Permethrin is a synthetic pyrethroid derived from the pyrethrum flower *Chrysanthemum cinerariaefolium*. It has multiple uses for various arthropod infestations. Derivatives of pyrethroids have been originally used as insect repellants.

Q. What is its mechanism of action?

A. Permethrin acts on the arthropod cell membrane. It disables sodium transport across the cell membrane. This causes paralysis of the scabies mite. It is however, weakly ovicidal, since ova do not have fully developed central nervous system.

Q. What are its indications?

A.
- Scabies (FDA approved, treatment of choice in patients aged 2 months and older)
- Pediculosis capitis and Pthirus pubis
- *Demodex folliculitis*
- Other mite infestations—*Cheyletiella* mite infestation and rosacea-like demodicidosis

Q. What dose and formulations are available for this drug?

A
- 1% lotion
- 1%, 5% cream in a thixotropic vehicle (thixotropic, the medication is originally thick, but becomes less viscous over time when shaken)

Q. How is permethrin used in pediculosis?

A. For the treatment of head lice (1% lotion):
- Hair is shampooed, rinsed and dried. No conditioners should be used because it impairs the ability of permethrin to adhere to the hair shaft
- Shake the lotion and apply all over the scalp including the ears and the back of the neck
- Keep for 10 minutes, then properly rinse the hair and later dry the hair

Q. How can the knits be removed?

A. The knits are removed with fine-toothed metal comb. They can also be softened by treating with household vinegar (acetic acid) or formic acid.

Q. How is permethrin used in scabies?

A.
- Take a hot water scrub bath
- After drying the body, take one complete tube and apply all over from neck to toe (if face and scalp are involved, to apply to the affected area only)
- Wash the medication after 8–10 hours
- All family members living together should be treated simultaneously
- In case of infants and children, permethrin should be applied over face and scalp as these areas are frequently involved
- It is controversial whether clothing and linen should be washed because scabies mite cannot survive off the body for > 72 hours
- Most people recommend a second application after 7 days because the ova hatch within 7 days and also to kill any residual mites which have escaped the first application

Q. What is pregnancy category of the drug?

A. Category B.

Q. What are the adverse effects of this drug?

A. Adverse effects are rare, other than local reactions in the form of stinging, irritation, and tingling at times. Rarely, hypersensitivity reactions may occur if the patient is allergic to chrysanthemum or compositae family of plants.

Q. What are the other key features of this drug?

A.
- Systemic absorption of permethrin is minimal
- Resistance to permethrin has not been documented till date

GAMMA-BENZENE HEXACHLORIDE (LINDANE)

Introduction

- It is an organochlorine insecticide that inhibits neurotransmission, inducing respiratory and muscular paralysis in arthropods
- It is an ectoparasiticidal drug effective against lice, scabies and fleas

Q. What is the mechanism of action?

A. Lindane inhibits inositol in insect tissue. This affects neurotransmission thereby producing excitability, convulsions and ultimate death of the parasite.

Q. What are the indications?

A.
- Scabies
- Pediculosis capitis and pubis

Q. What are the contraindications?

A. GBH is to be avoided in:

- Patients with seizure disorders
- Children weighing <50 kg (<12 years)
- Patients with acutely inflamed raw skin
- Pregnant and lactating women
- Hypersensitivity

Q. What dose and instructions are given to the patient?

A.
- Available as a 1% cream or lotion
- Use the medication in adequate amounts, applied in a single overnight application over all parts of body from neck down
- It is washed off in morning with a bath
- Repeat application after 1 week (as it is not ovicidal)

Q. What are the adverse effects of this drug?

A. Effects on central nervous system:

- Seizures, excitability, agitation, delirium, tremors, dizziness, etc.
- Systemic absorption may lead to aplastic anemia

Q. What are the other key features of this drug?

A.
- Resistance of head lice to GBH has been reported
- Avoid contact with eyes and mucus membranes
- Avoid over exposure and frequent reapplications as it may lead to toxicity
- Avoid simultaneous application of oils and oily creams as they increase the systemic absorption of the drug
- Diazepam or barbiturates can be used to control CNS excitation and convulsions due to systemic toxicity of GBH

PRECIPITATED SULFUR

Introduction

Precipitated sulfur (6%) is a well tolerated drug, with no significant adverse reactions. It is a keratolytic, mild antiseptic and is parasiticidal.

Q. What is the mechanism of action?

A. Sulfur kills adult scabies mite by generation of sulfide radicals. However, it is not ovicidal.

Q. What are the indications?

A. It is considered by many to be the treatment of choice for scabies in pregnancy. It may also be used in infants less than 2 months (however, now a days permethrin is increasingly replacing sulfur for this indication).

Q. What dose and instructions given to the patient?

A. Sulfur ointment with 6% precipitated sulfur in petroleum jelly to be applied to the entire body at night for three consecutive nights.

Q. What are the contraindications?

A. Hypersensitivity.

Q. What are the other key features of this drug?

A. Sulfur "stinks, stings and stains".

CROTAMITON HYDROCHLORIDE

Introduction

Crotamiton has weak scabicidal activity along with an antipruritic effect. It is colorless or pale yellow oil used in the treatment of scabies.

Q. What is the mechanism of action?

A. Not known, but it is not ovicidal.

Q. What are the indications?

A.
- Scabies
- Pediculosis capitis
- Pruritus
- Nodular scabies
- As a follow-up treatment to other therapies

Q. What dose and instructions are given to the patient?

A.
- 10% cream or lotion
- It should be applied from the neck down twice daily for 5 consecutive days

Q. What is the pregnancy category of the drug?

A. Category C.

Q. What are the adverse effects of this drug?

A. Generally well tolerated. Its antipruritic effect is an added advantage. After application, irritation, redness and swelling may temporarily develop.

BENZYL BENZOATE (BB)

Introduction

It is derived from Balsam of Peru and has an acaricidal effect.

Q. What is the mechanism of action?

A. It is believed to be neurotoxic to the parasite, but not ovicidal.

Q. What are the indications?

A.
- Scabies
- Pediculosis

Q. What dose and instructions are given to the patient?

A. Overnight application of 25% emulsion lotion for adults or diluted 1:1 in children for three consecutive nights followed by a bath 24 hours after the last application.

Q. What are the adverse effects of this drug?

A. Pruritus, redness, swelling and allergic contact dermatitis.

Q. What are the other key features of this drug?

A.
- Inexpensive but not very effective
- Resistance reported
- Whole body immersion therapy (except head) was used as a mass treatment of scabies in communities where scabies was endemic. Patients were immersed in a tub containing 10% BB lotion and then were told to dry the skin and wear their usual clothing (Dr Rui Fernandez used this therapy).

TOPICAL IVERMECTIN

Introduction

Ivermectin is derived from fermentation of a soil dwelling fungus, Streptomyces avermitilis. Chemically, it is an avermectin. Ivermectin is effective orally for scabies. Topical application is controversial.

Q. What is its mechanism of action?

A. It is a neurotoxic drug. It increases synthesis of GABA (Gamma amino butyric acid), thereby blocking chloride channels. This causes tonic paralysis of the parasite.

Q. What are the indications?

A.
- Scabies
- Pediculosis
- Larva migrans
- Larva currens (Strongyloides)

Q. What dose and instructions are given to the patient?

A. 1% solution in propylene glycol applied twice with a one week interval is very effective in scabies.

Q. What are the relative contraindications?

A.
- In children <5 years or those who weigh <15 kg, and those who are breastfeeding
- In hepatic or renal disease

MALATHION

Malathion is an organophosphoric compound which has been used as an insecticide.

Q. What is the mechanism of action?

A. The active form is malaoxon. This irreversibly inhibits acetylcholinesterase enzyme of the parasite thereby resulting in neuromuscular paralysis. It is a potent ovicidal too.

Q. What are the indications?

A.
- Pediculosis capitis
- Scabies

Q. What dose and instructions are given to the patient?

A.
- Shampoo the hair and let it dry
- Applying 0.5% lotion and rinse with shampoo after 8–12 hours
- It is inflammable and patients should be warned about this
- In scabies, a 0.5% solution is applied for 24 hours and repeated after one week

Q. What is the pregnancy category of this drug?

A. Category B.

Q. What are the adverse effects of this drug?

A. Systemic toxicity has been reported only with oral ingestion (OP poisoning).

Q. What are the other key features of this drug?

A. Malathion has superior pediculicidal and ovicidal activity against naïve and permethrin-resistant lice. It has a residual effect for a few weeks due to slow bonding of the malathion to the sulfur atoms in the hair shaft.

THIABENDAZOLE

Introduction

Broad-spectrum anthelmintic agent.

Q. What is mechanism of action?

A. It inhibits helminth-specific fumarate reductase.

Q. What is indication?

A. Cutaneous larva migrans due to Ancylostoma braziliense.

Q. What dose and instructions are given to the patient?
A. 15% ointment in DMSO gel daily for 3–5 days.

Q. What is the method of application of topical thiabendazole in cutaneous larva migrans?
A. Thiabendazole topical suspension should be applied directly to the slowly advancing end of the larval burrow or tunnel in the skin.

Q. What is the pregnancy category of this drug?
A. Category C.

Q. What are the adverse effects of this drug?
A. Local irritation.

SPINOSAD (NATROBA)

Introduction

It excites the motor neurons of arthropods, resulting in muscle contraction, paralysis and death.

Q. What is its mechanism of action?
A. Exact mechanism not known, but spinosad causes disruption of the nicotinic cholinergic receptors.

Q. What is its indication?
A. Pediculosis capitis.

Q. What dose and instructions are given to the patient?
A. Apply to the scalp and hair and rinse after 10 minutes. Repeat after 1 week if necessary.

Q. What is the pregnancy category of this drug?
A. Category B.

Q. What are the adverse effects of this drug?
A.
- Erythema
- Skin irritation

MELALEUCA ALTERNIFOLIA (TEA TREE OIL)

Introduction

It is an Australian aboriginal traditional medication that has shown in vitro scabicidal activity. It is still under trial.

Q. What is the mechanism of action?
A. Not known.

Q. What are its indications?

A.
- Scabies
- Topical antiseptic
- Mild-to-moderate acne vulgaris
- Superficial fungal infections

Q. What are the adverse effects of this drug?

A.
- Generally well tolerated
- Contact sensitization occasionally reported

TETRAMETHYLTHIURAM MONOSULFIDE

Introduction

It is a pesticide as well as acaricide.

Q. What are its indications?

A. Fleas, lice and ticks.

Q. What dose and instructions are given to the patient?

A.
- Available as a 25% alcoholic solution. It should be diluted 2–3 times its volume by water to form an emulsion
- It should be applied once a day for 2–3 consecutive days
- It is also available as a toilet soap (5% concentration), mainly for prophylaxis

Q. What are the adverse effects of this drug?

A.
- Flushing, sweating and tachycardia have been reported when patients have taken alcohol before or after treatment (it is structurally similar to disulfiram—antabuse)
- Mild irritation

CARBARYL

It is an organophosphorus insecticide (1% aqueous and 0.5% alcoholic lotion) applied on the skin for 12 hours.

Q. Enumerate all possible antiscabetic agents with their concentrations.

A. 5% permethrin, 1% lindane, 6% precipitated sulfur, 10% crotamiton hydrochloride, 25% BB, ivermectin (topical 1% and oral 0.2 mg/kg), 0.5% malathion, 15% thiabendazole, spinosad, tea tree oil, 25% tetramethylthiuram monosulfide, carbaryl.

1.5. TOPICAL ANTIVIRAL AGENTS

CLASSIFICATION

- Viricidal—acyclovir, penciclovir, cidofovir, foscarnet, idoxuridine
- Immune enhancers—imiquimod, interferon
- Cytodestructive—bleomycin, podophyllin, trichloroacetic acid, cantharidine, salicylic acid, 5-Fluorouracil, sinecatechins

VIRICIDAL

Acyclovir

Acyclovir was first discovered in 1974 and the first formulation is the topical form.

Q. What is the chemical formulation of acyclovir?

A. Acycloguanosine.

Q. What is the mechanism of action of this drug?

A. Active moiety is acyclovir triphosphate which is potent inhibitor of viral DNA polymerase inhibiting DNA synthesis. It irreversibly incorporates into viral DNA chain causing DNA chain termination. However, the topical formulation does not achieve high intracellular concentration.

Q. What is the pregnancy category of this drug?

A. Pregnancy category B.

Q. What are the indications?

A.
- Genital HSV
- HSV labialis

Q. What are the adverse effects of the drug?

A.
- Burning, stinging, discomfort and mild pain at the site of application
- Less commonly—pruritus, erythema, edema or mucosal irritation when applied to genital lesion

Q. What are the contraindications of this drug?

A. Hypersensitive to drug, prodrug or any component.

Q. What are the doses and formulations available for this drug?

A.
- Initial genital HSV and HSV labialis: acyclovir 5% ointment 5 times daily for 7 days.

- Formulation—available as 5% ointment and cream form (A finger cot or rubber gloves have to be used while applying the medication to prevent autoinoculation or transmission to other persons).

Q. What are the key points of this drug?

A. Topical acyclovir is not found to be very effective in herpetic infection and hence cannot be used as a sole therapy for the treatment of the same.

Penciclovir

It is an acyclic purine nucleoside analogue of guanine.

Q. What is the mechanism of action of this drug?

A. Active moiety is penciclovir triphosphate which is inhibitor of viral DNA polymerase inhibiting DNA synthesis. It does not cause viral DNA chain termination so less potent than acyclovir.

Q. What is the pregnancy category of his drug?

A. Pregnancy category B.

Q. What are the indications?

A. HSV labialis in immunocompetent patients.

Q. What is the antiviral spectrum of this drug?

A. It is effective against HSV-1, HSV-2, HSV-3 and HSV-4 (EBV).

Q. What are the adverse effects of the drug?

A.
- Burning, stinging, discomfort and mild pain at the site of application
- Less commonly—headache, dysgeusia, decreased cutaneous sensations (particularly to touch and erythema)

Q. What are the contraindications of this drug?

A. Hypersensitivity to the drug, prodrug or any component.

Q. What are the doses and formulations available for this drug?

A.
- HSV labialis—penciclovir 1% cream 6 times daily for 4 days
- Formulation—available as penciclovir 1% cream
- Not available in India

Q. What are the key points of this drug?

A.
- It is less potent because it does not cause chain termination of viral DNA
- It has poor oral bioavailability
- Famciclovir is a prodrug of penciclovir

Cidofovir

It is an acyclic nucleotide that exhibits antiviral activity against a broad range of NA viruses.

It is a nucleoside analogue of deoxycytidine monophosphate.

Q. What is the mechanism of action of this drug?

A. Cidofovir phosphorylates to form cidofovir—diphosphate which is the active metabolite which inhibits viral DNA polymerase and thus prevents viral DNA synthesis.

Q. What is the pregnancy category of his drug?

A. Pregnancy category C.

Q. What are the indications?

A.
- Molluscum contagiosum
- Condyloma acuminata
- Verruca vulgaris
- Herpes simplex

Q. What are the adverse effects of the drug?

A. Application site pruritus, rash, pain, paresthesia and ulceration increased with increased concentration.

Q. What are the doses and formulations available for this drug?

A.
- Available in 1%, 3% or 5% gel form
- To be applied five times a week

Foscarnet

It is an antiviral agent and is a pyrophosphate analogue.

Q. What is the mechanism of action of this drug?

A. It directly inhibits DNA polymerase without activation by cellular or viral kinase.

Q. What are the indications?

A. Genital HSV which is resistant to acyclovir in immunocompetent/ immunocompromised patients.

Q. What are the doses and formulations available for this drug?

A.
- Genital HSV and acyclovir resistant vulvar HSV—foscarnet 1% cream applied 5 times weekly
- Available in 1%, 3% cream

IMMUNE ENHANCERS IMIQUIMOD

It is an immune response modifier that stimulates innate and adaptive immune pathway resulting in antiviral, antitumor and immunoregulatory properties.

It is a non-nucleoside heterocyclic amine.

Q. What is the mechanism of action of this drug?

A.
- Imiquimod induces cytokine production which indirectly produces interferon-gamma (IFN-γ) and enhancement of cell mediated immunity responsible for viral killing
- It is an activator of TLR-7
- It may also have indirect antiviral activity

Q. What is the pregnancy category of this drug?

A. Pregnancy category B.

Q. What are the indications?

A.
- FDA approved antiviral indication—external genital and perianal warts (response rate of 50% and relapse rate of 25% at 3 months)
- FDA approved nonviral indications:
  - Superficial small nonfacial BCC
  - Actinic keratoses
- Off-label dermatological uses:
  - Cutaneous wart
  - Molluscum contagiosum
  - Herpes simplex virus
  - Melanoma in situ
  - Keloid

Q. What are the adverse effects of the drug?

A.
- Cutaneous—erythema, ulceration, scaling, edema, pruritus, pain at the site of application
- Systemic—flu-like symptoms, fatigue, fever, headache, diarrhea, myalgia seen in 2% patients

Q. What are the contraindications of this drug?

A. Hypersensitivity to the drug, or any component.

Q. What are the doses and formulations available for this drug?

A.
- External genitalia and perianal wart—imiquimod 5% cream once a day on alternate days for 16 weeks
- Superficial small nonfacial BCC—imiquimod 5% cream once a day application for 5 days/week for 6–12 weeks

- Actinic keratoses—imiquimod 5% cream applied overnight, twice/week for 16 weeks
- Formulation available in 5% cream form

Interferon-α

Q. What is the pregnancy category of this drug?

A. Pregnancy category B.

Q. What are the indications?

A.
- FDA approved indication:
  - Malignant melanoma
  - Multiple condylomata acuminata in immunocompromised patients
  - Chronic granulomatous disease
- Off-label dermatological uses:
  - Verruca vulgaris
  - HSV infections
  - VZV infections
  - Keloid
  - BCC
  - Actinic keratoses
  - Squamous cell carcinoma
  - Kaposi's sarcoma

Q. What are the adverse effects of the drug?

A.
- Influenza like symptoms—fatigue, fever, headache, diarrhea, myalgia, arthralgia
- Fatal rhabdomyolysis and multiple organ failure
- Cardiovascular—significant hypotension, dysrhythmia, tachycardia
- Neurological and psychiatric effect—spastic diplegia, paresthesias, motor weakness, dizziness, confusion, dysarthria, short term memory loss
- Others—nausea, diarrhea, glomerulosclerosis

Q. What is the dosing of the drug?

A. Five million units intralesionally to be repeated once a week or once in two weeks depending on response.

Q. What are the drug interactions seen with interferon α?

A.
- Aminophylline—it decreases the clearance of aminophylline
- Zidovudine—along with this or other myelosuppressive agents may increase the risk of hematologic complication
- Interleukin-2—increased risk of renal failure

CYTODESTRUCTIVE DRUGS

Bleomycin

Introduction

It is a cytotoxic antibiotic derived from *Streptomyces verticillus*. Along with antiviral it has antitumor and antibacterial activity.

Q. What is the mechanism of action of this drug?

A. It binds to DNA in M and G2 phases of cell cycle leading to single strand break by removing purine and pyrimidine bases.

Q. What are the indications?

A.
- Resistant and difficult to treat verruca vulgaris specially around nails and plantar aspect
- Keloid

Q. What are the adverse effects of the drug?

A.
- Pain, erythema, swelling followed by blackened thrombotic eschar at the site of injection
- Uncommon—scarring, Raynaud's phenomenon, persistent nail dystrophy, flagellate hyperpigmentation, permanent loss of nail plate

Q. What are the doses and formulations available for this drug?

A.
- Verruca vulgaris and keloid—0.1 mL of 1 U/mL bleomycin in normal saline administered intralesionally every 2–3 weeks until resolution
- Formulation—Injection bleomycin 1% aqueous solution
- Storage—as it is rapidly deteriorated at room temperature, it is stored in glass at -22°C to maintain immunoreactivity for atleast 27 months

Podophyllin and Podofilox

It is a plant resin extracted from may apple plant (*Podophyllum peltatum/Podophyllum emodi*).

The most active and cytodestructive agent in podophyllin is podophyllotoxin.

Q. What is the mechanism of action of this drug?

A. It is an antimitotic agent which inhibits DNA synthesis in metaphase by binding reversibly to tubulin.

Q. What are the indications?

A.
- Condyloma acuminata
- Verruca vulgaris

Q. What are the adverse effects of the drug?

A. • Inflammation, burning, erythema and erosions
- Rarely it can cause peripheral neuropathy (podophyllin foot)
- Renal failure

Q. What is the pregnancy category of this drug?

A. • Podofilox is pregnancy category C
- Podophyllin is pregnancy category D

Q. What are the contraindications?

A. Should not be given in pregnant women as it causes birth defects, fetal death and still birth and CNS toxicity has been reported.

Q. What are the doses and formulations available for this drug?

A. • Podophyllotoxin (home application) 1% cream or 0.5% lotion available
- Podophyllin (office application) is 20% resin in tincture benzoin compound stored in amber colored bottle

Q. How to apply this drug?

A. • Podophyllotoxin to be applied twice daily for three consecutive days followed by a gap of 4 days, 4–6 such cycles are used
- The preputial skin is retracted and the area cleaned of smegma. The skin surrounding the wart is covered with petroleum jelly, the podophyllin is applied with a cotton tipped applicator carefully only over the lesion. Initially the patient is asked to wash with soap and water after 1 hour and this period is increased to 4 hours or even overnight
- Frequency of application is once a week. 6–8 weeks are usually required. Recurrence is fairly common

Q. Mention an important point about podophyllin.

A. After application of podophyllin, the epidermal cells become dyskeratotic and show abnormal mitotic figures resembling malignancy. Hence, if there is a suspicion of malignancy in a genital wart it has to be biopsied first and only later podophyllin should be applied.

Trichloroacetic Acid

It works through destruction of tissue by causing hydrolysis of cellular proteins, leading to inflammation and cell death.

Q. What are the indications?

A. • External genital warts
- Cervical HPV infection
- Nongenital warts

Q. What are the adverse effects of the drug?

A. Local pain and ulceration.

Q. What is the advantage of trichloroacetic acid (TCA) over podophyllin?

A. TCA can be used in treating genital warts in pregnant patient, minimal systemic side effects and no need for neutralization.

Q. What are the doses and formulations available for this drug?

A.
- Cervical HPV infection—60–80% TCA applied to entire cervix 1–4 application (revealed 81% clearance rate)
- External genital warts and nongenital warts—TCA applied over the lesion taking care that surrounding tissue does not come in contact and not destroyed. Adequate application is achieved when wart turns white. 4–6 application require for clearance

Salicylic Acid

It is a keratolytic agent that is a common component of over-the-counter medication for treatment of verruca vulgaris.

Q. What is the chemical formulation of salicylic acid?

A. It is a beta-hydroxy benzoic acid.

Q. What is the mechanism of action of this drug?

A.
- In lower concentration it softens the stratum corneum dissolving intracellular matrix and loosening connections between corneocytes
- In higher concentration it acts as keratolytic by exfoliating the virally infected keratinocytes and exposes cell to cellular immunity

Q. What are the indications?

A.
- Verruca vulgaris and calluses
- Ichthyosis
- Hyperkeratosis
- Keratoderma
- Other uses—scalp psoriasis, seborrheic dermatitis, acne, photoaging, chemical peels, dermatophyte infection

Q. What are the doses and formulations available for this drug?

A.
- Warts on hand and feet—lesion is initially soaked in warm water for 5 minutes and dead tissue removed with emery board or pumice stone. Then, salicylic acid containing medication is applied in concentrations ranging between 10 and 60%. Occlusion advised for enhancing penetration

- Formulation—available in 2-20% collodion based paints and gel, 10-50% liquid and plaster form
- Common formulation for treating warts is wart paint, which is as follows:
  Salicylic acid—16.7% + Lactic acid—16.7% + Flexible collodion-q.s. (it contains castor oil which is the only substance which can dissolve salicylic acid completely).

Q. What are the adverse effects of the drug?

A. Overuse, application over raw and inflamed area lead to "salicylism", i.e., systemic absorption leading to toxicity, which is more common in children.

Systemic toxicity

- GIT—nausea, vomiting
- Neurologic—confusion, dizziness, delirium, psychosis, stupor, death
- Metabolic—respiratory alkalosis, metabolic acidosis, hypoglycemia
- Miscellaneous—tinnitus, hyperventilation

Cantharidin

It is a vesiculating agent derived from "blister beetle" and is also known as Spanish fly. Formerly used as an aphrodisiac.

Q. What is the mechanism of action of this drug?

A. It interferes with mitochondria leading to epidermal cell death, acantholysis and blister formation with subsequent removal of wart.

Q. What are the indications?

A. Verruca vulgaris, molluscum contagiosum.

Q. What are the key points of this drug?

A.
- Cantharidin application is painless and non-scarring
- Applied after paring for warts and directly for molluscum
- Needs occlusion for 24 hours after application for warts
- Inadequate application results in annular or ring-like wart with flattening in center which is known as "doughnut wart"

Q. What is the formulation available of this drug?

A. 0.7% (not available in India).

5-fluorouracil

It is a cytotoxic agent with fluorinated pyrimidine analogue.

Q. What is the mechanism of action of this drug?

A. It inhibits DNA synthesis by blocking the function of thymidylate synthetase.

Q. What are the indications?

A.
- Actinic keratosis
- Resistant genital condyloma
- Verruca plana
- Verruca vulgaris
- Superficial BCC

Q. What are the adverse effects?

A. Hyperpigmentation, erythema, edema, erosive dermatitis, mucositis, ulceration.

Q. What is the pregnancy category of this drug?

A. Pregnancy category: X.

Q. What are the contraindications of this drug?

A. Hypersensitive or allergy to drug, or any component:
- Patient with known deficiency of DPD enzyme (dihydropyrimidine dehydrogenase) which is the key enzyme in 5-FU metabolic pathway
- Women who are or may become pregnant

Q. What are the doses and formulations available for this drug?

A.
- Resistant genital condyloma, verruca plana, verruca vulgaris—5% 5-FU once/week for 4–6 weeks
- Formulation—available as 0.5%, 1%, 5% cream and 1%, 2%, 5% solution form

Sinecatechin

It is a green tea polyphenol extract from *Camellia sinensis*.

Q. What are the key points of this drug?

A.
- Sinecatechin contain epigallocatechin gallate which protects cells from oxidative damage, induces apoptosis and inhibits telomerase activity
- Used in treatment of external genital and perianal warts
- Adverse effects include erythema, pruritus, ulceration, pain and edema
- Available in 10% and 15% ointment
- Not available in India currently

1.6. TOPICAL CALCINEURIN INHIBITORS

INTRODUCTION

Topical calcineurin inhibitors (TCI), namely tacrolimus and pimecrolimus, are nonsteroidal immunomodulator agents that modulate the immune responses of the skin.

Q. Topical calcineurin inhibitors are classified into which group of drugs?

A. Macrolactam (macrolides).

Q. Tacrolimus was formerly known as?

A. FK506.

Q. Which organism produces tacrolimus?

A. Soil bacterium *Streptomyces tsukubaensis.*

Q. What is pimecrolimus a derivative of?

A. It is a semisynthetic derivative of ascomycin which is a macrolactam isolated from the bacterium *Streptomyces hygroscopicus* var. ascomyceticus.

Q. Which drug does tacrolimus resemble in terms of structure and mechanism of action?

A. Cyclosporine (not suitable for topical application because its large molecular weight results in poor epidermal penetration).

Q. What is the neologism behind the nomenclature of tacrolimus?

A. T (*Streptomyces tsukubaensis* was found initially in Mount Tsukuba in Japan), *acrol* (macrolide), *imus* (immunosuppressive agent).

Q. What are the various mechanisms of action of topical calcineurin inhibitors?

A.
- Tacrolimus/pimecrolimus binds to FK506-binding protein (FKBP)

↓

Complex formed

↓

Complex interacts with Ca^+ binding protein—Calmodulin

↓

Calmodulin inhibition reduces calcineurin activity

↓

Calcineurin activity inhibition, inhibits the activity of NFAT

↓

NFAT inhibition reduces activity of IL-2

↓

IL-2 inhibition reduces activity of T cells

- Depletion of inflammatory dendritic epidermal cells in lesional skin of atopic dermatitis patients
- Dose-dependent decrease of histamine release from IgE-activated mast cells
- Blocks *Staphylococcus aureus* superantigen—induced T-cell proliferation in peripheral blood mononuclear cells in patients with atopic dermatitis

Q. What is the pregnancy category of topical calcineurin inhibitors?

A.
- *Tacrolimus*: Category C
- *Pimecrolimus*: Category C

Q. What preparations and formulations are topical calcineurin inhibitors available in?

A.
- *Tacrolimus*: 0.03% and 0.1% ointment
- *Pimecrolimus*: 1% cream

Q. What are the indications of topical calcineurin inhibitors?

A.
- FDA-approved: Atopic dermatitis
- Off-label:
  - Vitiligo (reduces TNF-α levels in the skin)
  - Psoriasis
  - Lichen planus (esp. oral LP)
  - *Pemphigus vulgaris*
  - *Bullous pemphigoid*
  - *Rosacea*
  - *Alopecia areata*
  - *Pyoderma gangrenosum*
  - Lichen sclerosus et atrophicus
  - Dermatomyositis
  - Graft-versus-host disease
  - Contact dermatitis
  - Hand dermatitis

Q. What are the adverse effects of topical calcineurin inhibitors?

A.
- Skin burning (minimized by refrigerating the tube at 4°C)
- Pruritus
- Increased susceptibility to infections (molluscum contagiosum, herpes simplex, warts, varicella zoster, fungal infections)

- Hyperesthesia
- Flu-like symptoms
- Possible photosensitizer

Q. What are the contraindications of topical calcineurin inhibitors?

A.
- Absolute—hypersensitivity to the medication
- Relative—children < 2 years of age (pimecrolimus can be used in children >6 months age) active skin infection (at site to be treated)

Q. Is there a risk of malignancy after chronic use of topical tacrolimus?

A.
- In certain clinical trials, few patients who were given topical tacrolimus for atopic dermatitis developed nonmelanoma skin cancer
- Few other clinical trials also demonstrate potentiality for development of non-Hodgkin's lymphoma and squamous cell carcinoma (SCC)

Q. Is there any specific warning with regards to topical calcineurin inhibitor use?

A. Yes, it is a "black box warning", which states that long term safety of topical calcineurin inhibitors has not been established. Although a causal relationship has not been established, rare cases of malignancy (e.g., skin and lymphoma) have been reported in patients treated with topical calcineurin inhibitors. Therefore, continuous, long-term use in any age group should be avoided, and application limited to areas of involvement with atopic dermatitis.

Q. What is "500 Dalton rule"?

A. The most commonly used topical applications have a molecular weight of <500 Daltons. According to this rule, no agent with molecular weight >500 Daltons penetrates the skin. Both tacrolimus and pimecrolimus have a molecular weight around 800 Daltons. Hence, these two drugs are a challenge to this rule.

Q. What is the advantage and disadvantage of TCIs vis-a-vis TCS?

A.
- TCS act rapidly, while TCIs take longer time to start their action
- The action of TCS is relatively short-lived, while that of TCIs is sustained
- Initial burning with TCIs is not seen with TCS
- Delayed local side effects seen with TCS are not seen with TCIs

Note: It is hence rational to start treatment in atopic dermatitis with TCI and TCS together and then wean off the TCS and further continue with TCI.

1.7. TOPICAL CORTICOSTEROIDS

INTRODUCTION

Topical corticosteroids were introduced into dermatologic therapy in 1952 by Sulzberger and Witten.

PHARMACOLOGY

1. Chemical characteristics and structural activity relationship:
   - All steroids are composed of a CPP ring (cyclopentano-perhydro-phenanthrene ring)
   - Hydrocortisone—3 hexane + 1 pentane ring
   - Substitution at key position can change its activity. For example, halogenation at 9-alpha position increases glucocorticoid activity. Removing hydrophilic chain at 16 or 17 position increases lipophilicity and thereby penetration.

Anti-inflammatory effects	*Immuno-suppressive*	*Antiproliferative and anthropogenic*	*Vaso-constrictive*
Induction of anti-inflammatory cytokines	Reduction of the number of Langerhans cells	Inhibition of interphase	Inhibition of the synthesis and production of nitric oxide
Inhibition of activator protein (AP-1) and nuclear factor kappa B (NFκB)	Decreasing Langerhans cell—dependent T-lymphocyte activation	Inhibition of keratinocytes and melanocytes	Prevention of degranulation of mast cells
Direct down regulation of pro-inflammatory cytokines	Indirect down regulation of pro-inflammatory cytokines	Causes hypoactive fibroblasts	Decrease in mast cells
Suppression of phospholipase A2 (PLA2) and Cyclooxygenase 2 (COX2) production	Superpotent TCS decrease in the number of cells expressing Langerhan's cell marker	–	–
Decrease in mast cell numbers and activity		–	–

2. Mechanism of action: Steroids bind to GCR in the cytoplasm and activates it. The steroid-GCR complex crosses the nuclear envelope to bind to DNA. This alters the regulation of genes and transcription of m-RNA molecules which produce the following actions.
3. Potency of TCS:
   - The term potency is used to describe the intensity of a TCS clinical effect.
   - American system classifies them into seven classes.
   - The most commonly used assay is the "Stoughton vasoconstrictor assay" to assess the potency of topical steroids.

*The classification of steroids is given on the next page.

Potency group	***Generic name***	***Formulation***
Class 1 (Superpotent)	Clobetasol propionate (0.05%)	Gel, ointment, cream, lotion, spray and shampoo
	Betamethasone dipropionate (0.05%)	Gel, ointment
	Diflorasone diacetate (0.05%)	Ointment
	• Fluocinonide cream (0.1%) • Flurandrenolide tape 4 mcg/ cm^2 • Halobetasol propionate (0.05%)	• Cream • Ointment, cream
Class 2 (High potent)	Amcinonide (0.1%)	Ointment
	Betamethasone dipropionate (0.05%)	Cream, lotion, gel, ointment
	Clobetasol propionate (Scalp application) (0.05%)	
	Desoximetasone	0.25% ointment and cream, 0.05% gel
	• Diflorasone diacetate (0.05%) • Fluocinonide (0.05%) • Halcinonide ointment (0.1%)	• Ointment and cream • Gel, ointment, cream, solution • Cream and solution
	Mometasone furoate (0.1%)	Ointment
	Triamcinolone acetonide (0.5%)	Ointment

Continued

Continued

Potency group	Generic name	Formulation
Class 3 (Medium-high potency)	• Amcinonide (0.1%) • Betamethasone dipropionate (0.05%) • Betamethasone valerate (0.1%)	• Cream, lotion • Cream, lotion • Ointment
	Fluticasone propionate (0.005%)	Ointment
	Triamcinolone acetonide (0.5%)	Ointment and cream
	Diflorasone diacetate (0.05%)	Cream
Class 4 (Medium potency)	Betamethasone valerate (0.12%)	Foam
	Desoximetasone (0.05%)	Cream
	Fluocinolone acetonide (0.025%)	Ointment
	Mometasone furoate (0.1%)	Cream and lotion
	Flurandrenolide acetonide (0.05%)	Ointment
	Hydrocortisone valerate (0.2%)	Ointment
	Triamcinolone acetonide	0.1% ointment and cream, 0.2% spray
Class 5 (Medium potency)	Betamethasone dipropionate (0.05%)	Lotion
	Betamethasone valerate (0.1%)	Cream and lotion
	Clocortolone pivalate (0.1%)	Cream
	Fluocinolone acetonide (0.025% and 0.01%)	Cream, oil and shampoo
	Fluticasone propionate (0.05%)	Cream and lotion
	Hydrocortisone butyrate (0.1%)	Ointment, cream and lotion
	Hydrocortisone valerate (0.2%)	Cream
	Triamcinolone acetonide (0.025% and 0.1%)	Ointment, lotion
Class 6 (Low potency)	Alclometasone dipropionate (0.05%)	Ointment and cream
	Triamcinolone acetonide (0.1%)	Cream

Continued

Continued

Potency group	Generic name	Formulation
	Desonide (0.05%)	Gel, ointment, cream, lotion, foam
	Fluocinolone acetonide (0.01%)	Cream, solutions
	Betamethasone valerate (0.1%)	Lotion
Class 7 (Low potency)	Topical with hydrocortisone, dexamethasone and prednisolone	

4. Vehicle:
   - The vehicle, or base, is the substance in which active ingredient is dispersed. The bases determine the rate in which the active ingredient is absorbed through skin.
   - They are available in ointments, creams, gels, lotions, solutions, etc.
5. Dose, frequency and duration of application:
   - The amount of cream required to cover a certain area can be calculated by remembering that 1 g of cream covers 100 cm^2 of skin. The entire skin surface of an average-sized adult is covered by 20–30 g of cream.
   - Tachyphylaxis refers to the decrease in responsiveness to a drug as a result of enzyme induction. It refers to acute tolerance to the vasoconstrictive action of topically applied corticosteroids. Recently, however tachyphylaxis is believed to be simply due to loss of compliance. Weekend or pulse therapy with topical steroid decreases the chances of tachyphylaxis.
6. Methods of application:
   - Simple application—creams and ointments should be applied in thin layers and slowly massaged into the site one to four times a day. It is not necessary to wash before each application. Continue treatment until the lesion is clear.
   - Hydration/occlusion—application to hydrated skin after bathing can increase absorption by 4–5 times. Occlusion (e.g., plastic wrap) increases absorption by up to 10 times. Short-term use of occlusion may be useful for severe lesions. If plastic occlusion is used, a maximum of 12 hours in a 24 hours period is recommended to reduce the potential problems of sweat retention, infection, and systemic side-effects.
7. Indications for use of topical steroids: The following chart enlists the indications of topical steroid. Very responsive disease generally

require low-medium potency topical steroid. For less responsive disease, high potency steroid, higher concentration and occlusion may be necessary.

Indications of TCS

Very responsive:

- Atopic dermatitis
- Seborrheic dermatitis
- Diaper dermatitis
- Lichen simplex chronicus
- Pruritus ani
- Late phase of allergic contact dermatitis
- Late phase of irritant contact dermatitis
- Nummular eczematous dermatitis
- Stasis dermatitis
- Psoriasis, especially of face and genitalia

Less responsive:

- Discoid lupus erythematosus
- Psoriasis of palms and soles
- Necrobiosis lipoidica diabeticorum
- Sarcoidosis
- Lichen straitus
- Pemphigus
- Familial benign chronic pemphigus
- Vitiligo
- Granuloma annulare

Least responsive (intralesional injection required):

- Keloid
- Hypertrophic scar
- Hypertrophic lichen planus
- Alopecia areata
- Acne cysts
- Prurigo nodularis
- Chondrodermatitis nodularis helicis

8. Adverse effects of topical steroid: Local adverse effects are far more prevalent than systemic reactions. A myriad of possible adverse effect of topical corticosteroids have been reported as shown in the table:

Local	***Systemic (if used for prolonged period over large areas or in children)***
Atrophic changes: • Steroid atrophy • Telangiectasia • Striae • Purpura • Stellate pseudoscars • Ulceration • Easy bruising • Topical steroid damaged facies (TSDF) or groin (TSDG) • Topical corticosteroid induced rosacea-like dermatitis (TCIRD)	*Endocrine*: Cushing disease, moon face, centripetal obesity, buffalo hump, striae distensae
Infections: • Masked microbial infections (tinea incognito) • Aggravation of cutaneous candidiasis, herpes or demodex • Reactivation of Kaposi sarcoma • Granuloma gluteal infantum	*Metabolic*: Glucose intolerance (hyperglycemia), osteopathy (fractures or aseptic necrosis), adrenocortical suppression, decreased growth rate
Ocular changes: • Ocular hypertension • Glaucoma • Cataract	*Electrolyte imbalance*: Edema, hypocalcemia, hypertension
Pharmacologic effects: • Steroid rebound • Steroid addiction • Tachyphylaxis	*Ocular*: Posterior subcapsular cataract, glaucoma
Miscellaneous: • Steroid acne • Perioral dermatitis • Steroid rosacea • Hypertrichosis • Hyperpigmentation • Hypopigmentation • Photosensitization • Rebound flare (psoriasis)	

Q. What is the procedure for performing Stoughton vasoconstrictor assay?

A.
- Prepare the test corticosteroid in 95% alcohol
- Apply it on volar surface of normal volunteer's forearm allow alcohol to evaporate
- Cover the test area with an occlusive dressing for 16 hours.
- Wash off the area
- Assess vasoconstriction 2 hours later on a blind basis by an experienced investigator using a multiple unit scale (0–3 or 0–4)
- Statistical analysis

Q. What are the allergens used as vehicles in TCS preparation which can cause allergic contact dermatitis?

A. Propylene glycol, sorbitan sesquioleate, formaldehyde-releasing preservatives, parabens, fragnance and lanolins. Most common—Propylene glycol and sorbitan sesquioleate.

Q. What are the most important factors in choosing the correct TCS preparation?

A. The following factors should be considered while choosing a TCS preparation:
- Disease responsiveness
- TCS potency
- Vehicle choice (potential for irritation, past allergic reaction)
- Price and cost-effectiveness considerations
- Proper amount to dispense
- Brand name versus generic products

Q. What is addiction/rebound syndrome with use of TCS?

A. Addiction/rebound syndrome is characterized by initial response with TCS, followed by lack of response after continued application, followed by a flare after TCS withdrawal. It most commonly occurs on facial, genital, perianal skin, with involvement on the face being most common.

Q. Give some examples of addiction or rebound syndrome.

A. Perioral dermatitis is a classical example. Others—acne, rosacea, infections (scabies incognito, tinea incognito, herpes incognito and impetigo incognito).

Q. What are the risk factors for developing local and systemic side-effects of TCS?

A.
- Systemic effects—young age, liver disease, renal disease, amount of TCS applied, potent of TCS, use of occlusion, lack of physicians supervision.
- Local—young age (infancy and childhood), potency of TCS (fluorination of steroid), use of occlusion, location (face, neck, axilla, groin, and upper inner thighs).

Q. Can TCS cause HPA axis suppression?

A. Yes, TCS can cause HPA axis suppression.

Q. What are the test for screening and monitoring HPA axis suppression?

A.
- Test of choice—8 AM plasma cortisol level
- For definitive diagnosis—Metyrapone test or insulin hypoglycemia test or ACTH stimulation test.

Q. What is tachyphylaxis?

A. Acute development of tolerance to the action of a drug after repeated doses.

Q. How will you prevent tachyphylaxis?

A. A proven regimen to prevent tachyphylaxis do not exists. Twice-daily application for 2 weeks on, then 1 week off, is recommended.

Q. Which classes of steroid are known to cause allergic contact dermatitis?

A.
- Nonfluorinated steroids. It is more in chronic diseases and when steroids are applied on the mucous membrane.
- There are four groups of steroid which do not cross react with each other:
  - Group A is hydrocortisone type
  - Group B is triamcinolone type
  - Group C is betamethasone type
  - Group D is hydrocortisone butyrate type

Q. What is the incidence of allergic contact dermatitis with use of TCS?

A. The incidence of allergic contact dermatitis to TCS is 0.5%.

1.8. DEMELANIZING AGENTS

Q. Classify demelanizing agents.

A.

Phenolic compounds	*Nonphenolic compounds*	*Combination formulas*
Hydroquinone	Azelaic acid	Kligman's formula
Monobenzyl ether of hydroquinone	Tretinoin	Pathak's formula
4-methoxyphenol	L-ascorbic acid	Webster's formula
4-isopropylcatechol	Kojic acid	–
N-acetyl-4-S-cystaminylphenol	N-acetylcysteine	–

HYDROQUINONE

Introduction

- Hydroquinone (HQ) benzene is a hydroxyphenolic compound which is used for hypermelanization
- It is also known as 1, 4-dihydroxybenzene

Q. What is the mechanism of action of hydroquinone?

A.
- Reduces melanocyte pigment production by inhibiting DOPA oxidase
- It breaks down, through auto-oxidation, melanin, tyrosinase and phenol oxidases into highly reactive oxygen radicals. These reactive substances prevent melanin production
- It inhibits the formation and melanization of melanosomes
- It also has a direct cytotoxic effect on melanocytes through reversible inhibition of DNA and RNA synthesis

Q. Pregnancy category of hydroquinone?

A. Category C.

Q. What are the indications of hydroquinone?

A.
- Melasma
- Postinflammatory pigmentation
- Periorbital hypermelanosis
- Freckles and lentigines

Q. What are the side effects of hydroquinone?

A.
- Burning, pruritus, irritation
- Allergic contact dermatitis

- Irritant contact dermatitis
- Hypersensitivity
- Exogenous ochronosis (late side effect seen with higher concentrations)
- Concerns have been raised about carcinogenic potential of high concentrations of HQ

Q. What is ochronosis?

A. It a long term side effect of high concentration of topical HQ which causes bluish-black discoloration of skin. The mechanism of HQ-induced ochronosis remains unknown. Histologically, the initial stages of ochronosis are characterized by the degeneration of collagen and elastic fibers. In later stages, ochronotic deposits (banana bodies) are seen, consisting of crescent-shaped, ochre colored fibers in the dermis.

Q. What is the formulation available for hydroquinone?

A. 2%, 4% and 6–8% cream.

Q. What is Kligman's regimen?

A. Kligman and Willis used a combination regimen of 5% HQ, 0.1% tretinoin, and 0.1% dexamethasone in a hydrophilic ointment and demonstrated an efficacy in the treatment of melasma, ephelides, and postinflammatory hyperpigmentation.

Q. What is modified Kligman's regimen?

A. It consists of 2% hydroquinone, 1% hydrocortisone and 0.05% tretinoin.

Q. What is the rationale for modified Kligman's regimen?

A.
- Hydroquinone is an effective depigmentary agent
- Tretinoin increases turn over rate of stratum corneum resulting in shedding of the pigment. It also increases the penetration of HQ
- Hydrocortisone reduces the inflammation caused by tretinoin and also decreases the activity of melanocytes
- Depigmentation occurs rapidly beginning within 3 weeks after twice-daily application of the formula and maximizing in 5–7 weeks

Q. What is Pathak's regimen?

A. *Pathak's formula*: 2% Hydroquinone, 0.05–0.1% Tretinoin in cream or ointment base. According to Pathak topical steroids may not be necessary, except in patients getting irritation to tretinoin.

Q. What is Westerhof formula?

A. • It is a combination of 4.7% N-acetyl cysteine (NAC), 2% HQ, and 0.1% triamcinolone acetonide

- The bleaching effect of NAC probably relates to the increase of intracellular glutathione that stimulates pheomelanin rather than eumelanin synthesis after binding with dopaquinone, clinically producing a lighter pigment

Q. What are the key points to be remembered while using hydroquinone?

A. • Exposure to sunlight causes repigmentation in patients of hydroquinone which may be prevented by broad spectrum sunscreen agents

- Arbutin is a derivative of hydroquinone. Many cosmetic companies use plant extracts such as bearberry that contain arbutin

AZELAIC ACID

Introduction

Azelaic acid is a naturally occurring, saturated 9-carbon dicarboxylic acid derived from Pityrosporum ovale, mainly used for acne vulgaris and hyperpigmentation of skin.

Q. What is the mechanism of action of azelaic acid?

A. • It is a weak reversible competitive inhibitor of the enzyme tyrosinase of melanin synthesis and is toxic to melanocytes. This molecule may have cytotoxic and antiproliferative effects on melanocytes, possibly by interfering with mitochondrial respiration and DNA synthesis in abnormal melanocytes

- Comedolytic, bacteriostatic and bactericidal against *P. acnes*
- Disruption of mitochondrial respiration and DNA synthesis
- Potential inhibitor of enzyme 5-alpha reductase that is responsible for androgenetic alopecia
- It decreases free radical formation

Q. Pregnancy category of azelaic acid?

A. Category B.

Q. What are its indications?

A. • Acne vulgaris (inflammatory and noninflammatory)

- Postinflammatory hyperpigmentation
- Melasma
- Rosacea

- Plaque psoriasis
- Solar freckles, senile freckles, lentigines, pigmentary seborrheic keratosis
- Periorbital dermatitis

Q. What are its side effects?

A. Burning, itching, scaling, allergic contact dermatitis.

Q. What are its formulations?

A. 10% and 20% cream and 15% gel.

Q. What are the benefits of azelaic acid over hydroquinone?

A. Unlike HQ, azelaic acid seems to target only abnormally hyperactive melanocytes, thus will not lighten skin with normally functioning melanocytes.

RETINOIC ACID

Introduction

Its generic name is all-trans-retinoic acid and was released in 1971.

Q. What is the mechanism of action of retinoic acid?

A.
- Comedolytic
- Increases the dispersion of melanin granules throughout the epidermis
- Gene transcription affects growth and differentiation of cells in the skin
- Normalizes follicular epithelial differentiation and keratinization

Q. What is its pregnancy category?

A. Category C.

Q. What are its indications?

A.
- US-FDA approved uses:
  - Acne vulgaris
  - Fine wrinkling
  - Mottled hyperpigmentation
  - Tactile roughness of facial skin
- Off-label uses:
  - Actinic keratosis
  - Hyperpigmentation (melasma, solar lentigines)
  - Hyperkeratotic disorder
  - Pretreatment of skin to augment wound healing
  - Early stretch marks or abdominal striae

Q. What are its adverse effects?

A. Irritation, erythema, peeling, temporary worsening of acne and photosensitivity.

Q. What are its contraindications?

A. Nursing, pregnancy, hypersensitivity, caution for eczematous skin, sunburn, hair depilatories or waxes.

Q. What are the key points to be remembered in retinoic acid?

A.
- It should be applied at night to prevent photosensitivity occurring due to thinning of stratum corneum and reduced melanin synthesis
- Sunscreens should be applied as retinoic acid is photo degradable
- It should not be applied near eye, nose or open wound and should be used for about 4 months to show visible effects

GLYCOLIC ACID

Introduction

It is an alpha-hydroxy acid or fruit acid that is found in sugarcane, sugar beets or ripened grapes.

Q. What is the mechanism of action of glycolic acid?

A.
- Facilitates progressive weakening of cohesion of the intercellular material of the stratum corneum, resulting in uniform exfoliation of its outermost layers
- Hydroscopic property promotes moisture retention by stimulating collagen and dermal glycosaminoglycans
- Possibly inhibits tyrosinase enzyme of melanin synthesis

Q. What is its pregnancy category?

A. Category B.

Q. What are its indications?

A.
- Pigmented acne scar
- Facial rejuvenation and wrinkles
- Facial hypermelanosis
- Postinflammatory hyperpigmentation
- Periorbital hypermelanosis
- Epidermal tumors and proliferations like actinic keratosis, dermatosis papulosa nigra, milia, seborrheic keratosis, verruca vulgaris
- Rhytides

Q. What are its contraindications?

A. Active infections, open wounds, prior hypersensitivities to peeling agents, prior radiation exposure, pre-existing inflammatory dermatosis such as atopic dermatitis, recent facial surgery.

Q. What are the side effects of glycolic acid?

A. Erythema, desquamation and postinflammatory hyperpigmentation.

Q. Combination therapy.

A. When used in combination with a modified Kligman-Willis formula (5% hydroquinone, 0.05% tretinoin, 1% hydrocortisone acetate), it was shown to decrease the MASI score by 79.9%, but the topical formula performed almost as well when used alone in this study, showing a 63.1% decrease in MASI score.

KOJIC ACID

Introduction

Kojic acid [5-hydroxy-2-(hydroxy methyl)-4-pyrone], a naturally occurring hydrophilic fungal derivative evolved from certain species of *Acetobacter, Aspergillus* and *Penicillium,* is used in the treatment of hyperpigmentation disorders. It was isolated from "Koji" or malted rice in Japan. It is a tyrosinase inhibitor in the fungus *Aspergillus oryzae.*

Q. What is the mechanism of action of kojic acid?

A.
- It inhibits tyrosinase enzyme by the chelation of copper ions and suppresses the tautomerization from dopachrome to 5,6-dihydroindole-2-carboxy acid
- Kojic acid and kojic acid esters also show antioxidant activity that enhances the depigmenting effect

Q. What is its formulation?

A. 0.75%–1%, 2%, 4% cream.

Q. What are its indications?

A. Melasma, postinflammatory hyperpigmentation, anti-aging.

Q. What are its side effects?

A. Burning and allergic contact dermatitis.

Q. What are the key points to be remembered?

A. It is a very unstable ingredient in cosmetic formulation and on exposure to sunlight or air, it loses its efficacy. Kojic dipalmitate is a more stable alternative.

Q. Combination formula.

A. Kojic acid is used in a 1–4% cream base, alone or in combination with tretinoin, hydroquinone, and/or a corticosteroid. It appears to act synergistically with glycolic acid.

MONOBENZYL ETHER OF HYDROQUINONE

Introduction

It is a derivative of hydroquinone. It is a known causative agent for occupational vitiligo mediating apoptotic melanocytic death. Monobenzyl ether of hydroquinone (MBEH) is a Food and Drug Administration approved drug used for depigmentation therapy of advanced vitiligo.

Q. What is its mechanism of action?

A. It has a similar mechanism of action to HQ on pigmented cells. MBEH is subjected to selective uptake by melanocytes and is metabolized into reactive free radicals that are capable of permanently destroying melanocytes and, hence, inducing permanent depigmentation. The process of depigmentation is long and may require 9–12 months of daily application to achieve total depigmentation.

Q. What are its indications?

A. It is used in generalized vitiligo with sparing of a few islands of normal skin. It induces permanent depigmentation of the spared normal skin to get uniformly depigmented skin which is cosmetically more acceptable.

Q. What are its contraindications?

A. It should not be used for other causes of hyperpigmentation as the hypo- or depigmentation induced by it may be permanent.

Q. What are its side effects?

A. Depigmentation of treated skin.

Q. What are the key points to be remembered?

A. While choosing the patient it is important to ensure that the vitiligo is stable and the patient understands that the effects will be irreversible.

NIACINAMIDE

Introduction

Niacinamide, also known as nicotinamide, is a water-soluble component of the vitamin B complex group.

Q. What is the mechanism of action of niacinamide?

A. Niacinamide inhibits melanin transfer to keratinocyte.

Q. What are the uses of niacinamide?

A.
- It reduces the appearance of hyperpigmented macules, fine lines and wrinkles, red blotchiness, skin sallowness, and increased skin elasticity
- In addition, niacinamide helps alleviate some of the symptoms of rosacea by increasing hydration, reducing transepidermal water loss, and improving the barrier function of the stratum corneum

OTHER DEMELANIZING AGENTS

Q. What is licorice extract?

A.
- Licorice extract derived from the root of Glycyrrhiza glabra, glabridin, has dual pigment modulating and anti-inflammatory properties
- Active ingredients are flavonoids, liquiritin and isoliquiritin
- Licorice extract inhibits tyrosinase, especially the rate-limiting first step of oxidation and leads to skin lightening primarily by dispersing melanin
- Licorice extract is considered a weak lightening agent and must be combined with other agents for optimal clinical results

Q. What is arbutin and deoxyarbutin?

A.
- Arbutin is a beta-D-glucopyranoside derivative of hydroquinone that is derived from uva-ursi folium (the bearberry plant) and can also be found in cranberry and blueberry leaves
- Its mechanism of action is inhibition of tyrosinase and 5,6-hydroxyindole-2-carboxylic acid (DHICA) polymerase and inhibition of melanosome maturation without associated melanocyte toxicity
- Higher concentrations may provide additional therapeutic benefit, but paradoxic darkening may occur
- Deoxyarbutin is a synthetically modified derivative of arbutin with enhanced pigment lightening properties

Q. What is aloesin?

A.
- It is a low molecular weight glycoprotein derived from the aloe vera plant
- It functions through the competitive inhibition of tyrosinase at the dihydroxy phenylalanine (DOPA) site
- Therapeutic application of aloesin is limited by its hydrophilic nature and inability to penetrate the skin

Q. What is Edelweiss complex?

A.
- Edelweiss complex is a new approach targeting skin discoloration. It relies on antisense oligonucleotides that block targeted gene transcription and modulate melanogenesis
- This technology offers unique specificity, biologic stability, and safety in whitening of all skin types

Q. What is the role of vitamin C in demelanization?

A.
- Numerous studies have confirmed the beneficial effects of systemic [oral and intravenous (IV) administration and topically applied ascorbic acid (vitamin C) in the treatment of melasma
- It decreases pigment by interacting with copper at the active site of tyrosinase and by reducing dopaquinone by blocking dihydrochinindol-2-carboxyl acid oxidation
- However, this molecule is rapidly oxidized, highly unstable, and does not work well alone; it is therefore usually combined with licorice extracts and soy to increase efficacy

Q. What is the role of soy as demelanizing agent?

A. Soybean trypsin inhibitor reversibly inhibits the protease-activated receptor-2 (PAR-2) pathway that is needed for melanosome transfer by keratinocyte phagocytosis of melanosomes.

MECHANISM OF ACTION OF DEMELANIZING AGENTS

Action	*Agent*
Tyrosinase inhibitors	• Hydroquinone • Kojic acid • Azelaic acid • Licorice • Arbutin
Stimulation of keratinocyte turnover	• Retinoids
Inhibition of melanin production	• Ascorbic acid • Glutathione
Reduction in melanosome transfer	• Retinoids • Soyabean trypsin inhibitors
Interaction with copper	• Kojic acid • Ascorbic acid
Inhibition of melanosome maturation	• Arbutin • Deoxyarbutin
Nonselective suppression of melanogenesis	• Indomethacin • Corticosteroids

1.9. MOISTURIZERS, EMOLLIENTS AND KERATOLYTIC AGENTS

DEFINITIONS

- Moisturizers are substances which hydrate the skin by preventing transepidermal water loss
- A related group of drugs is "humectants" which hydrate the skin by absorbing water from the atmosphere
- Another group is "emollients" which soften the skin (molle = butter)
- Natural moisturizing factor (NMF) is found within stratum corneum and constitutes 20–30% dry weight of this layer. It consists of 40% amino acids, sodium salt of pyrrolidine carbonic acid (PCA), lactate, urea, iron, sugar among other things. All these substances are water soluble and help to improve skin plasticity and barrier function
- Many of these substances are added to proprietary moisturizing medications
- The basic function of moisturizers is that it prevents the transepidermal water loss from a damaged skin barrier and it increases the softening of the skin and makes the skin smooth

Emollients are of the following types:

- Vegetable or animal fats
- Mineral greases
- Fatty acids
- Wax esters
- Vegetable waxes
- Phospholipids
- Cholesterol

The following are the common humectants:

- Glycerin
- Lactic acid
- Sodium lactate
- Sorbitol
- Gelatin
- Urea
- Propylene glycol
- Carboxylic acid
- Hyaluronic acid

EMOLLIENTS

Q. What are emollients?

A. Emollients soften and occlude the skin, helping it to be moist and preventing transepidermal water loss.

Q. How are they classified?

A. Emollients vary according to their oil to water ratio. In lotions lipid content is low and it is high in ointments (medium in creams). Emollients with high lipid contents are greasier and more sticky and they also make the skin more shiny.

- Soap substitutes
- Emollient bath additives
- Emollient creams and ointments

Q. What are the uses?

A. It is used in the following diseases:

- Atopic dermatitis
- Psoriasis
- Xerotic eczema and xerosis
- Erythroderma
- Pityriasis rosea
- Patch stage of mycosis fungoides
- Congenital and acquired ichthyosis
- Progressive symmetric erythrokeratoderma

Q. What are the adverse effects?

A. The adverse effects can include:

- Contact sensitivity
- Acneiform eruptions
- Occlusive miliaria
- Occlusion folliculitis

HUMECTANTS

Q. When should humectants not be applied?

A. In dry conditions as it will absorb the moisture from the skin and make the skin more dry.

KERATOLYTIC AGENTS

Q. What are keratolytic agents?

A. Keratolytic therapy is the treatment to remove warts and other lesions in epidermis produces excess skin. It causes the outer layer of the skin to thin and loosen. These are the agents which are used for the hyperkeratosis of the skin.

SALICYLIC ACID

Q. What is salicylic acid? What are the uses?

A. Salicylic acid is a monohydroxybenzoic acid and a beta hydroxyl acid and is the main keratolytic agent used in dermatology.

Main uses:

- Psoriasis and seborrheic dermatitis
- Tinea pedis
- Disorders associated with hyperkeratosis like corn, calluses, warts
- Acne vulgaris
- It can be combined with topical steroids to increase the penetration of the latter

Preparations:

- Ointment (6%, 12%)
- Lotion/Paint (16.7%)
- As a corn cap (40%)

Q. What is the mechanism of action?

A. It acts as a "keratolytic" agent by reducing the adhesion between keratinocytes and by dissolving the intercellular cementing substances. However, in concentrations below 3% it has a "keratoplastic" action, i.e., it increases the formation of stratum corneum.

LACTIC ACID

It is an alpha hydroxyl acid which is used as a humectant and keratolytic agent.

Q. What is the mechanism of action?

A. It causes the intercellular breakdown of the substances known as desmogleins. It absorbs moisture from the environment into the skin. It has a synergistic action with salicylic acid.

Q. What are the uses and availability of lactic acid?

A. Use is indicated in disorders associated with hyperkeratosis and dryness. It is available in concentration of 6–24% it is also available as ammonium lactate.

UREA

Urea is a potent keratolytic emollient and has properties of an exfoliating agent and humectant.

Q. What is the mechanism of action?

A. It dissolves the intercellular matrix of keratinocytes promoting desquamation of scaly skin, eventually resulting in softening of the hyperkeratotic areas. In nails, urea causes softening and eventually debridement of the nail plate.

Q. What are the indications?

A. Urea cream is indicated for removal of hyperkeratotic skin and promotion of normal skin formation. This is particularly true where healing is inhibited by local skin factors.

- In different concentrations, it can be used in different conditions.
  - 10–12%:
    - Keratosis pilaris
    - Phrynoderma
    - Palmoplantar keratoderma
  - 40%:
    - Callosities and corns
    - Chemical avulsion of the nails under occlusion
    - Urea can also be combined with topical corticosteroids to increase the penetration of the drug.

Q. What are the preparations?

A. It is available as a combined preparation of urea, propylene glycol, lactic acid and liquid paraffin.

Q. What are the side effects of urea cream?

A. Mild skin irritation, temporary burning sensation, stinging sensation, itching.

1.10. TOPICAL RETINOIDS

INTRODUCTION AND HISTORY

- A retinoid is defined as a substance that binds to retinoic acid receptors and is a vitamin A derivative
- The first topical retinoid, all-trans-retinoic acid, was developed by Dr Albert Kligman (USA) and thus was marketed for the treatment of acne vulgaris
- Retinoids have diverse functions throughout the body—this includes regulation of cell proliferation and differentiation immune function, tumor suppression, vision and growth of bone tissue.

Q. Describe the nomenclature of retinoids.

A. Vitamin A is a 20-carbon molecule with a cyclohexenyl ring. This is called as "all-trans-retinol" (naturally occurring retinoid). Oxidation of the end group results in "all-trans-retinaldehyde" while further oxidation results in "all-trans-retinoic acid = tretinoin".

Q. Classify retinoids.

A.
- First generation:
  - Retinol
  - Retinal
  - Tretinoin
  - Alitretinoin (natural retinoid)
- Second generation:
  - Etretinate
  - Acitretin
- Third generation:
  - Adapalene (synthetic)
  - Tazarotene (synthetic)
  - Bexarotene (synthetic)

Q. Which are the specific nuclear receptors to which topical retinoids bind?

A.
- Retinoic acid receptors (RAR-α, β, γ):
  - Tretinoin—all three equally bound
  - Adapalene—β, γ (strong affinity)
  - Tazarotenic acid (active metabolite of tazarotene)—preferentially to β and γ
  - Alitretinoin—all three equally bound
  - Bexarotene—no specific binding to RARs
- Retinoid X receptors (RXR-α, β, γ):
  - Bexarotene—all three equally bound
  - Alitretinoin—RAR > RXR

Q. How are the various retinoids metabolized?

A.
- Tretinoin—no conversion required as it is an active metabolite of all-trans-retinol
- Adapalene—active without metabolic transformation
- Tazarotene—rapidly metabolized (<20 minutes) to tazarotenic acid
- Bexarotene—unknown
- Alitretinoin—no conversion

Q. Where does distribution of majority of the retinoids take place?

A. Keratinocytes.

Q. What is the mechanism of action, resultant therapeutic effects, pregnancy category, concentration and formulation, indications, adverse effects, contraindications, and drug interactions of the various retinoids?

A.

TRETINOIN

Mechanism of action

Normalizes follicular epithelial differentiation and keratinization.

Therapeutic effects

- Comedolytic
- Reduces hyperpigmentation, wrinkling and roughness of facial skin

Pregnancy category

Category C.

Concentration and formulation

- 0.025, 0.05, 0.1% cream
- 0.01, 0.025% gel

Indications

- FDA-approved:
    - Acne vulgaris grade 1 and 2
    - Fine wrinkling and photo aging
    - Mottled hyperpigmentation
    - Tactile roughness of skin

Off-label

- Pigmentary disorders:
    - Melasma
    - Priming along with hydroquinone prior to peels

Viral disorders

- Viral warts
- Molluscum contagiosum

Photodermatoses

- Actinic keratosis
- Solar lentigines

Others

- Lichen amyloidosis
- Porokeratosis
- Pityriasis rubra pilaris
- Darier's disease

Adverse effects

- Irritation
- Erythema
- Dryness
- Desquamation
- Temporary worsening of acne

Contraindications

- Eczematous skin
- Sunburn
- Electrolysis
- Hair depilatories
- Waxing
- Nursing
- Pregnancy
- Netherton's syndrome

Drug interactions

- Photosensitizers (tetracyclines, thiazides, fluoroquinolones)
- Skin irritants (certain cosmetics)

ADAPALENE

MOA

- Normalizes follicular epithelial differentiation and keratinization
- Suppression of PMN chemotaxis
- IL-1,6,8 and TNF-α production

Therapeutic effects

Comedolytic.

Pregnancy category

Category C.

Concentration and formulation

- 0.1% cream
- 0.1% gel

Indications

- FDA-approved—acne vulgaris grade 1 and 2
- OFF label—as with tretinoin

Adverse effects

As with tretinoin.

Contraindications
- Pregnancy
- Hypersensitivity to adapalene or the vehicle.

Drug interactions
- Topical sulfur, salicylic acid, resorcinol
- Agents with high concentration of alcohol

TAZAROTENE

MOA
- Tazarotene is a prodrug which is rapidly hydrolyzed in tissues to its active metabolite, tazarotenic acid
- Affects expression of genes that modulate epidermal cell differentiation, proliferation, and inflammation, leading to normalization of keratinocyte differentiation and a reduction in cellular hyperproliferation and inflammation
- Suppression of migration inhibition factor related protein-8 marker in psoriasis, thereby reducing inflammation

Therapeutic effects
Same as tretinoin.

Pregnancy category
Category X.

Concentration and formulation
- 0.05, 0.1% cream
- 0.05, 0.1% gel

Indications
- FDA-approved:
  - Acne vulgaris
  - Psoriasis with <20% BSA involvement (specially palmoplantar and nail)
  - Off-label-cutaneous T-cell lymphoma

Adverse effects
- Irritation-induced exacerbation of psoriasis
- Erythema
- Desquamation

Contraindications
- Pregnancy (absolute)
- Koebnerizing psoriasis
- Eczematous skin

- Sunburn
- Hypersensitivity to tazarotene or the vehicle

Drug interactions

- Photosensitizers
- Medications with strong drying effect

BEXAROTENE

MOA:

- Binds to and activates RXR nuclear receptors resulting in the modulation of cellular differentiation, proliferation and apoptosis
- Activates PPARs through RXRs

Therapeutic effects

- Induces tumor regression
- Inhibits growth of tumor cells lines

Pregnancy category

Category X.

Concentration and formulation

1% gel.

Indications

- FDA-approved—cutaneous T-cell lymphoma (stage IA and IB)
- Off-label:
    - Psoriasis (specially palmoplantar and nail)
    - Alopecia areata
    - Hand dermatitis
    - Lymphomatoid papulosis

Adverse effects

- Irritation
- Erythema
- Pruritus

Contraindications

- Pregnancy
- Breastfeeding
- Hypersensitivity to the vehicle
- Drug interactions—agents containing DEET

Q. What time of the day should retinoids be preferably applied?

A. In the evening or at night because of the possibility of developing photosensitivity if applied during the day. It is also preferable to gradually increase the duration of retinoids application.

Q. What is retinoid dermatitis?

A. It is a retinoid-induced irritant contact dermatitis (ICD) characterized by erythema, scaling, dryness, burning and pruritus, which in turn, result in discontinuation of topical retinoid treatment. It is believed to occur within the first month of therapy and possibly results from epidermal hyperplasia.

Q. What are the precautions to be taken with use of retinoids?

A. Use of photoprotective (against UVA radiations) and moisturizing measures are advised.

Q. What are other indications of retinoids?

A.
- Lichen planus
- Rosacea
- Dysplastic nevi
- Oral leukoplakia
- Discoid lupus erythematosus
- Wound healing
- Keloid
- Confluent and reticulate papillomatosis of Gougerot and Carteaud
- Striae distensae

Q. What medications can be combined with retinoids in the treatment of acne?

A. Topical antibiotics, topical benzoyl peroxide. It is usually not advised that oral and topical retinoids be used concomitantly.

Q. What is microsphere technology?

A. Microsponges are biologically inert polymer particles that absorb, trap, or bind drugs or other chemical compounds. In the case of tretinoin and adapalene, irritation is concentration-dependent and is shown to be influenced by characteristics of the delivery system and formulation as well as the patients' skin type. This can be overcome by the use of microsphere technology that releases the active agent slowly over time. Topical microsponge delivery is associated with improved therapeutic outcomes and minimal irritation. The macroporous beads, which typically measure 10 to 25 μm in diameter, release active ingredient over time or in response to certain stimuli, such as change in pH, temperature, or physical manipulation when rubbed into the skin.

Q. Which topical retinoid causes most irritation?

A. Tazarotene.

Q. Which is preferred between adapalene and tretinoin in acne?

A. This apart from being a personal preference answer is that adapalene may be used more safely because though it is slightly less potent and it is much less irritant.

Q. Talk about topical isotretinoin.

A. More irritating, less effective and, hence, less popular.

1.11. SUNSCREENS

INTRODUCTION

Effective protection has to be taken against the harmful effects of UV radiation. This includes photoprotective strategies like staying in shade when possible, wearing dark colored closely woven clothing which covers majority of the skin surface, broad brim hats, sun protective lip balm, UV shielding goggles, and regular and judicious use of sunscreens.

Q. Discuss systemic photoprotective agents.

A. These would be more convenient compared to topical sunscreens. However, none have been studied extensively.

- The common ones are carotenoids (β-carotene, lycopene, lutein and zeaxanthin). Carotenoids have antioxidant activity and decreased reactive oxygen species (ROS). The second one would be retinoids like retinyl palmitate. These increase collagen production and epidermal thickness. They are also antioxidants
- Vitamin E in high doses can alter the human response to UVB while vitamin C is more effective topical
- Polypodium leucotomos (fern leaf extract) reduces UV induced epidermal proliferation
- Afamelanotide is a derivative of MSH and reduces UV induced DNA damage
- Polyphenols are naturally occurring plant products found in green tea with immunomodulatory, anti-inflammatory and anti-carcinogenic properties
- Similar properties are found in other plant extracts like silymarin, soya beans, senna and phytomelanin
- Micronutrients like selenium and nicotinamide are also associated with enhanced photo protection
- NSAIDs especially COX-2 inhibitors like celecoxib may reduce photocarcinogenesis

Q. Define sunscreen.

A. Sunscreens are chemical agents that shield the skin from the harmful effects of sunlight by either reflecting the sunlight or absorbing it. The first sunscreen was developed in US in 1928 and contained benzyl salicylate and benzyl cinnamate.

Q. Classify sunscreens.

A. Sunscreens are classified as:

- Physical (Inorganic)
- Chemical (Organic)
- Oral

Q. What are the indications of sunscreens in dermatology?

A.

- In patients not suffering from any skin disease, sunscreens can be used to prevent changes associated with long-term sun exposure namely, viz. wrinkling, yellowish discoloration, pigmentation, etc. (collectively called as "dermatoheliosis"). It can also be recommended for patients with type I or type II skin to reduce the risk of melanomas, actinic keratoses, and nonmelanoma skin cancers
- Diseases where sunlight plays a triggering factor, e.g., solar urticaria, actinic prurigo, actinic lichen planus, pellagra, photosensitive drug eruptions and polymorphous light eruption (PMLE)
- Diseases where sunlight plays an exacerbating factor, e.g., melasma, lupus erythematosus, dermatomyositis, pemphigus erythematosus, etc.
- Genetic diseases where exposure to sunlight is harmful, e.g., erythropoietic porphyria, erythropoietic protoporphyria, xeroderma pigmentosum, Bloom's syndrome, Cockayne's syndrome, Rothmund–Thomson syndrome
- Following therapy with photosensitizing molecules, e.g., following PUVA therapy for the treatment of vitiligo and psoriasis and following surgical procedures like peels, dermabrasion, LASER therapy

Q. What is the sun protection factor (SPF) of a sunscreen?

A. The sun protection factor (SPF) is one of the factors which measures the potency of a sunscreen. It is defined as the minimal erythema dose produced by a specific amount of the sunscreen applied on the skin (2 mg/cm^2). The MED is first measured with the sunscreen on (24 hours after irradiation) and also measured without the sunscreen.

$$SPF = \frac{\text{Minimal erythema dose of sunscreen protected skin}}{\text{Minimal erythema dose of unprotected skin}}$$

- It should be noted that SPF refers mainly to "UVB" light and not "UVA" light. There are no good criteria for measuring the latter. One of them is the "tanning protection index" (TPI) which is a measure of tanning produced without sunscreen compared to with sunscreen

Q. What is the substantivity of a sunscreen?

A. Substantivity of a sunscreen is defined as the ability of the sunscreen to stay on the skin in spite of potentially deleterious influences like water, sweating, itching, etc. Hence, sunscreens are often classified as "water-resistant" (where sunscreen is effective for maximum 40 minutes when the skin is in contact with water). Sunscreens can also be classified as "water proof" (when the sunscreen is effective for maximum 80 minutes).

Q. What are the common sunscreen components?

A. UVB blockers

- PABA (para amino benzoic acid), and PABA esters (octyl methyl PABA)
- Cinnamates—octyl methoxy cinnamate, cinoxate, octinoxate
- Salicylic acid derivatives—homosalate, octisalate
- Miscellaneous—octocrylene, ensulizole

UVA blockers

- Anthranilates—Methyl anthranilate
- Benzophenones—Avobenzone, oxybenzone
- Miscellaneous—Meradimate, ecamzule

Physical blockers

- Titanium oxide
- Zinc oxide
- Iron oxide
- Kaolin
- Calamine

Q. How to use sunscreens?

A.
- Select a sunscreen with SPF of atleast 15, with both UVA and UVB protection
- Apply the sunscreen atleast 20 minutes before the anticipated sunlight exposure
- Reapply every 2–3 hours when in sunlight

- Sunscreen should be applied generously using at least 2 mg/cm^2 overall exposed areas
- For exquisitely sun-sensitive patients (type I and type II skin), sunscreen application is even recommended indoors since fluorescent lights do emit UV
- Even in small children, sunscreens are recommended when outdoors but it is better to use physical sun-protective measures
- Water-resistant sunscreens should be preferably used for beach and outdoor activities associated with perspiration

Q. What are the contraindications of sunscreen?

A.
- Known sensitivity to any active sunscreen ingredient or vehicle ingredient
- Infants <6 months of age

Q. What are the side effects of sunscreens?

A.
- Allergic contact reactions
- Contact urticaria
- Photocontact reactions (esp. PABA)
- Acneiform eruptions (esp. comedones)
- Irritant contact dermatitis
- Photosensitivity (esp. PABA)
- There are theoretical concerns about development of vitamin D deficiency, which in turn could induce internal malignancies like prostate
- Sunscreens can cause paradoxical pigmentation due to excessive sun exposure because the patient can get a false sense of security. Also some sunscreens can cause photoallergic contact dermatitis

Q. What are the various Fitzpatrick skin types?

A. Various sun reactive skin types are:
- *Type 1*: Always burns, never tans
- *Type 2*: Always burns, tans minimally
- *Type 3*: Burns moderately, tans gradually
- *Type 4*: Rarely burns, tans darkly
- *Type 5*: Never burns, tans darkly black
- *Type 6*: Hyperpigmented (black)

Note: The most common Indian skin types are type 4 or type 5.

Q. Factors limiting regular sunscreen use?

A.
- Aggravation or appearance of acne with the use of sunscreen
- High cost of products

- Use of sunscreen with 2 hourly applications is cumbersome and difficult to maintain
- Stickiness and increased perspiration after use
- Many patients complain of increased tanning after regular sunscreen use. This maybe because of complacence after using sunscreen which actually leads to increased sunlight exposure as well as may be related to contact or photocontact dermatitis associated with sunscreen use
- Physical sunscreens often give a white appearance on the skin which is unsightly

Q. What is the risk of skin cancers?

A. Risk of skin cancers is definitely reduced with regular sunscreen use. Obviously this is more pertinent in people with fair skin who live in tropical climates, e.g., Australia and southern area of USA.

1.12. TOPICAL VITAMIN D3 DERIVATIVES

Q. What is vitamin D3?

A. Active form of vitamin D is vitamin D3 (1,25 dihydroxychole-calciferol).

Q. Which analogs for D3 are available for clinical use?

A.
- Calcipotriene (0.005%)—available as cream, ointment, solution
- Calcitriol (0.0003%)—available as ointment only
- Tacalcitol (0.002%, 0.004%)—available as ointment only
- Maxacalcitol (not available in India)

	Calcipotriol/ Calcipotriene	*Calcitriol*	*Tacalcitol*
Concentration (mcg/g)	50	3	2,4
Formulation	Cream, ointment, solution	Ointment	Ointment
Frequency	BID	BID	BID, OD
Maximum weekly amount	100 g	210 g	70 g
Side-effects: • Hypercalcemia		Maximum	
• Irritancy	Maximum		
Potency	Maximum		

Q. What is the mechanism of action of vitamin D3 analogs?

A.
- It acts through vitamin D receptor (VDR) to regulate cell growth, differentiation and immune function
- It inhibits the proliferation of keratinocytes and modulates epidermal differentiation
- It inhibits production of interleukin-2 and interleukin-6
- It blocks transcription of interferon gamma, granulocyte-macrophage colony-stimulating factor and messenger ribonucleic acid
- It inhibits activity of cytotoxic T cells and natural killer cells

Q. What cells in the skin have receptors for vitamin D3 analogs?

A. Keratinocytes, Langerhans' cells, melanocytes, fibroblasts and endothelial cells.

Q. What are the indications of vitamin D3 analogs?

A.
- *FDA approved*: Psoriasis
- *Off label uses*:
    - Disorders of keratinization (ichthyosis, epidermolytic hyperkeratosis)
    - Autoimmune disorders (morphea, vitiligo)
    - Cutaneous T cell lymphoma
    - Miscellaneous: Acanthosis nigricans, lichen sclerosus et atrophicus, confluent and reticulate papillomatosis, disseminated superficial actinic porokeratosis, erythema annulare centrifugum, ILVEN, lichen amyloidosis, Pityriasis rubra pilaris, prurigo nodularis, seborrheic dermatitis

Q. What is the pregnancy prescribing status?

A. Category C.

Q. What are the adverse effects?

A.
- Hypercalcemia
- Irritation
- Photosensitivity
- Allergic contact dermatitis

Q. What are the contraindications?

A.
- Should not be used in conditions causing hyperglycemia (e.g., patient on thiazide diuretics)
- Involvement requiring more than the maximally recommended quantity, e.g., 100 g/week of calcipotriol
- Abnormality in bone or calcium metabolism
- Renal insufficiency

- Allergy to the vitamin D3 analog or constituents of the preparation
- Pregnancy, lactation

Q. What is the effect of UVA light on calcipotriol?

A. UVA causes degradation of calcipotriol thereby reducing its efficacy.

Q. What are the combination regimens in which calcipotriol can be used?

A. The combinations are:

- Calcipotriol with topical steroids. One useful combination is for calcipotriol to be used for the weekdays and topical steroids on weekends
- Calcipotriol and salicylic acid. Salicylic acid will remove the scale and increase penetration of other drugs. However, it inactivates calcipotriol. Hence, salicylic acid and calcipotriol should be applied at different times of the day
- Calcipotriol with ultraviolet light. Calcipotriol can act as a sunscreen and is also deactivated by UV light. Hence, calcipotriol should be applied after the UV light has been given
- Calcipotriol and acitretin. Oral acitretin thins the skin. Therefore, concomitant use of calcipotriol can cause irritation. Emollients should be used along with calcipotriol
- Calcipotriol and methotrexate can be safely used

Q. Any unusual precautions to be taken for calcipotriol.

A. Calcipotriol should be kept away from dogs. Even a small quantity is fatal if ingested.

2 Systemic Agents

2.1. SYSTEMIC ANTIBACTERIAL AGENTS

EVOLUTION OF ANTIBIOTICS

- 1930s—sulfonamides
- 1940s—penicillins
- 1950s—macrolides and tetracyclines
- Early 1960s—ampicillin
- Late 1960s—aminoglycosides
- 1970s—cephalosporins
- 1980s—second and third generation cephalosporins
- Late 1980s—quinolones, carbapenems and monobactams
- Early 1990s—new β-lactam antibiotics
- Mid 1990s—fourth generation cephalosporins

PENICILLIN

- *Older generation penicillins* are inactivated by β-lactamase—penicillin V and penicillin G
- β-lactamase-resistant dicloxacillin, oxacillin
- Extension of antimicrobial spectrum of penicillins like ampicillin and amoxicillin which are the *second generation penicillins*
- Third generation extended spectrum penicillins such as carbenicillin
- Fourth generation penicillins such as piperacillin

Q. What is the mechanism of action of penicillin?
A. Interference with bacterial cell wall synthesis.

Q. What are the pharmacokinetics of penicillin?
A. Penicillins are vulnerable to gastric acid degradation and hence GI absorption is optimized by administration 1 hour before or after meal. All β-lactams are excreted renally.

Q. What are the various indications of penicillin?
A.
- SSTI's such as impetigo, cellulitis, etc., caused by susceptible bacteria
- Rare: Erysipeloid, anthrax, cutaneous diphtheria, Lyme disease, Vincent's angina

- Sexually transmitted diseases: Syphilis, gonorrhea (used in the past)
- Empirical use: Pityriasis rubra pilaris, systemic sclerosis

Q. What are the adverse effects of penicillin?

A. The adverse effects are as follows:

- Hypersensitivity reactions: The most severe being anaphylaxis. All penicillins can cross react with each other and sometimes with cephalosporins too
- Rare side effects: Hematologic, gastrointestinal (GI), etc.

Q. What are the drug interactions of penicillin?

A. Probenecid prolongs renal excretion of penicillins. While penicillins alter the coagulant effects of warfarin.

Q. What is this pregnancy category?

A. Category B.

Q. Which are the currently available penicillins?

A.
- Natural: Penicillin G, penicillin V
- Aminopenicillin: Ampicillin, amoxicillin
- Penicillinase resistant: Oxacillin, cloxacillin, dicloxacillin
- Carboxypenicillin: Ticarcillin (IM, IV)
- Combinations with β-lactamase inhibitors: Amoxicillin-clavulanic acid, ampicillin-sulbactam (IV)
- Uridopenicillin: Piperacillin (IM, IV)

CEPHALOSPORINS

Introduction

They were developed in the 1950s from a fungus *Cephalosporium acremonium*. It consists of a β-lactam ring attached to a dihydrothiazine ring, which confers resistance to β-lactamase. They inhibit a series of enzymes called as penicillin binding proteins which are important for synthesis of the cell wall.

Q. How do we classify cephalosporins?

A.

First generation		
Cephalexin	Sensitive against methicillin-susceptible *Staphylococcus aureus* (MSSA), *Streptococcus*, *Klebsiella* and *Proteus*	250–500 mg qid; 25–50 mg/kg/day in divided doses in children

Continued

Continued

Cefadroxil	Same as above, but longer half-life	250–500 mg bd; 30 mg/kg/day in divided doses in children
Second generation		
Cefaclor	Slightly increased activity against *Haemophilus influenzae* and *Moraxella*	250–500 mg tid; 20–40 mg/kg/day in three divided doses in children
Cefuroxime axetil	Increased stability against *Neisseria gonorrhoeae* and *H. influenzae*	250–500 mg bd; 20 mg/kg/day in divided doses in children
Third generation		
Cefixime	Effective against *N. gonorrhoeae* and streptococci, but poor activity against staphylococci	400 mg single dose for *N. gonorrhoeae*, 8 mg/kg/day in pediatric population
Cefpodoxime	Increased activity against *Staphylococcus aureus*, otherwise same as cefixime	100–400 mg bd; 10 mg/kg/day in two divided doses in children
Fourth generation		
Cefepime	Broad spectrum, highly resistant to most β-lactamases, good gram-positive and gram-negative coverage	1–2 g bd IV or IM
Fifth generation		
Ceftaroline, ceftobiprole	Methicillin-resistant *Staphylococcus aureus* (MRSA) coverage for skin and soft tissues	400–600 mg IV 12 hourly

Q. What are the pharmacokinetics of these group of drugs?

A. Cefaclor, cefadroxil, cephalexin and cephradine are best absorbed on an empty stomach while, conversely bioavailability of cefuroxime axetil is increased when taken with food. First and second generation cephalosporins are excreted by kidneys, while, cefoperazone and ceftriaxone undergo hepatic metabolism and excretion.

Note:

- *First generation*: Most active against staph and streptococci, but inactive against Methicillin-resistant *Staphylococcus aureus* (MRSA)

- *Second generation*: Decreased gram-positive activity but increased gram-negative activity
- *Third generation*: Increased gram-negative activity but less consistent activity against gram-positive organisms
- *Fourth generation*: Broad spectrum against both gram positive and gram negative

Q. What are the indications of cephalosporins in dermatology?

A. Dermatological indications:

- Skin and soft tissue infections (SSTIs):
    - Especially deeper and more severe ones such as cellulitis, erysipelas, and necrotizing fasciitis.
- Rare indications:
    - Lyme disease
- Sexually transmitted diseases (STDs):
    - Gonorrhea (cefixime), syphilis (ceftriaxone); third generation cephalosporins have been used against *Pseudomonas*

Q. What are the adverse effects of cephalosporins?

A.
- GI toxicities
- Hypersensitivity reactions (cross reactions with penicillins in 5% cases)
- Local reactions with parenteral preparations
- Hematological reactions like hemolytic anemia

Q. What are the drug interactions of cephalosporins?

A.
- Disulfiram-like reactions with alcohol, due to the N-methylthiotetrazole (NMTT) ring
- Prolonged prothrombin time
- Increased nephrotoxicity when combined with aminoglycosides

Q. What is the pregnancy category of cephalosporins?

A. Category B.

β-LACTAM AND β-LACTAMASES INHIBITOR COMBINATIONS

Q. Enumerate the mechanism of action of β-lactamase inhibitors.

A. β-lactamase enzyme is produced by many bacteria. It irreversibly hydrolyses the amide bond of the β-lactam ring, rendering the antibiotic inactive. β-lactamase production is mediated by chromosomal or plasmid genes, and is readily transferable. In the past few years, agents have been developed which are more resistant to β-lactams, e.g., penicillinase resistant penicillins, third generation cephalosporins, and carbapenems. Recently, β-lactamase inhibitors have been produced which inactivate plasmid mediated β-lactamases. These agents can be combined with various types of penicillins. These agents are clavulanic acid, sulbactam and tazobactam. These do not have antibacterial activity by themselves.

Q. Enumerate the clinical uses of β-lactamase inhibitors.

A.
- SSTI's caused by polymicrobial infections
- Animal or human bites infected—amoxicillin and clavulanic acid is recommended
- Ticarcillin/clavulanic acid and piperacillin/tazobactam are used for diabetic foot ulcers and infected pressure ulcers and burn wounds

Q. What are the drug interactions?

A.
- Probenecid: Increases the levels of β-lactams as well as sulbactam
- Allopurinol: Increases risk of ampicillin induced eruptions.

Q. What are the adverse effects of β-lactamase inhibitors?

A.
- GI complaints
- Hypersensitivity reactions
- Prolonged bleeding time
- Positive Coombs test
- Thrombocytopenia
- Pain at site of injection

CARBAPENEMS AND MONOBACTAMS

Carbapenems

- Imipenem (combined with cilastatin to reduce its nephrotoxicity), meropenem and ertapenem are available
- Most broad spectrum antibiotics available with activity against MRSA, pseudomonas
- Only given parenterally
- Used for severe SSTI's, decubitus ulcers, diabetic ulcers
- Toxicity causes increased risk of seizures (1–3%). Other side effects are similar to penicillin

Monobactam

- Aztreonam is only monobactam available
- Used in gram negative cutaneous infections like post operative wounds, ulcers, burns, ecthyma gangrenosum and anaerobic infections
- Adverse effects: Local reaction at site of injection, GI side effects
- Patients allergic to penicillin can be safely given aztreonam

VANCOMYCIN

Glycopeptide Antibiotic

Q. What is the mechanism of action of vancomycin?

A. It inhibits cell wall synthesis in gram-positive bacteria. However it is not effective against gram-negative bacteria since the latter have a different mechanism of cell wall synthesis. Vancomycin is pregnancy category C. It is used in treatment of staphylococcal infections that are resistant to several conventional antibiotics such as those caused by MRSA and methicillin resistant coagulase negative streptococci

Q. What are the indications of vancomycin?

A.
- Treatment of SSTI caused by MRSA and methicillin resistant coagulase negative staphylococci
- Treatment of hospital acquired MRSA
- Pseudomembranous enterocolitis caused by *Clostridium difficile*

Q. What are the adverse effects of vancomycin?

A.
- Red man syndrome and shock secondary to histamine release due to rapid transfusion of vancomycin
- Toxic epidermal necrolysis
- Linear IgA bullous dermatosis
- Dose related hearing loss in patients with renal failure
- Nephrotoxicity
- Fever
- Thrombocytopenia
- Phlebitis at infusion site

Q. What is the dosage?

A. 1 g IV bid, in a slow infusion.

Q. What are drug interactions of vancomycin?

A.
- Concurrent administration of vancomycin with aminoglycosides increases the risk of nephrotoxicity
- Vancomycin enhances the activity of nondepolarizing muscle relaxants

MACROLIDES (ERYTHROMYCIN, AZITHROMYCIN AND CLARITHROMYCIN)

They were isolated in 1952 from *Streptomyces erythreus*. They contain a macrocyclic lactone ring.

Q. What is the mechanism of action of macrolides?

A. They are bacteriostatic antibiotics which bind reversibly to the large 50S subunit of the bacterial ribosome, inhibiting RNA dependent protein synthesis.

Q. What are the indications of macrolides in dermatology?

A. Dermatological indications:

- Several types of SSTI's including pyodermas, abscesses, infected wounds, infected ulcers, erysipelas
- Rare diseases like Lyme disease, anthrax, cat-scratch disease, toxoplasmosis, atypical mycobacteria
- STDs like syphilis (3rd choice), gonorrhea (azithromycin), chancroid, donovanosis
- Leprosy (clarithromycin)
- For certain skin diseases with infectious component like acne vulgaris, rosacea and perioral dermatitis

Q. What are the differences between various macrolides?

A.
- Erythromycin has severe GI side effects, low oral absorption, short half-life and limited efficacy against gram-negative pathogens
- Azithromycin on the contrary has a long half-life and post-antibiotic effect. It is more effective against gram-negative pathogens and also against atypical mycobacteria. It is also effective in syphilis
- Roxithromycin is better absorbed orally and also effective against gram-negative pathogens
- Clarithromycin is effective against gonorrhea and *M. leprae*. It is also effective against atypical mycobacteria

Q. What are the adverse effects of macrolides?

A. Following are the adverse effects of macrolides:

- GI effects like nausea, abdominal pain, diarrhea
- QT prolongation and torsades de pointes with erythromycin in combination with ketoconazole, terfenadine or astemizole
- Azithromycin is associated with irreversible deafness, angioedema, photosensitivity, hypersensitivity and contact dermatitis
- Cholestatic hepatitis

Q. Should macrolides be used in lactating mothers and infants?

A. Macrolides are excreted in milk and therefore infant exposure can cause increased risk of hypertrophic pyloric stenosis and cardiovascular malformations.

Q. What are the drug indications of macrolides?

A. Erythromycin and to a lesser extent clarithromycin inhibit the metabolism and prolong the clearance of drugs like anticonvulsants, statins, theophylline and some antihistaminics.

FLUOROQUINOLONES

The first fluoroquinolone (FQ) introduced was nalidixic acid.

Food and Drug Administration (FDA) approved oral fluoroquinolones:

- Ciprofloxacin (500 mg bd)
- Gemifloxacin (320 mg od)
- Levofloxacin (500 mg od)
- Moxifloxacin (400 mg od)
- Sparfloxacin (200 mg od)
- Norfloxacin (400 mg bd)
- Ofloxacin (400 mg bd)

Q. What is the mechanism of action of fluoroquinolones?

A. The primary mechanism of action involves inhibition of DNA gyrase (topoisomerase II). This is the enzyme which introduces negative supercoiling of the bacterial DNA. Inhibition of this enzyme results in interference with DNA replication.

Q. What are the indications of fluoroquinolones in dermatology?

A. Following are the indications for fluoroquinolones:

- SSTI caused by multi-resistant gram-negative bacteria such as folliculitis, abscess, cellulitis, infected ulcers and wound infections
- Especially useful for gram-negative acne, gram-negative interdigital infections, diabetic foot ulcers, pseudomonas infections and decubitus ulcers
- Also effective against MRSA
- Ofloxacin, pefloxacin, sparfloxacin, moxifloxacin and gatifloxacin are used in leprosy. Gatifloxacin is banned due to the risk of hypoglycemia

Q. What are the adverse effects of fluoroquiolones?

A.
- GI symptoms like nausea, vomiting, diarrhea
- CNS adverse effects such as headache, dizziness, agitation, sleep disturbances, seizures, psychotic reactions, hallucinations
- Use in children can cause tendon rupture or cartilage formation alteration
- Hypersensitivity

- Photosensitivity reactions (spar > lome > pe > cipro > nor > oflox). Hence, evening doses may be preferred
- Congenital anomalies are associated with FQ when used in pregnancy
- Pefloxacin can cause blue-black pigmentation

Q. What are the drug interactions of fluoroquinolones?

A.
- Absorption reduced by antacids, sucralfate and iron salts
- Drug concentrations of theophylline (seizure potential) and warfarin are increased
- Increased risk of nephrotoxicity when given with cyclosporine
- Increased risk of cardiotoxicity with amiodarone

TETRACYCLINE, DOXYCYCLINE, MINOCYCLINE

Q. What is the mechanism of action of tetracyclines (TCN)?

A.
- TCN's are bacteriostatic and inhibit bacterial protein synthesis by binding to the 30s subunit of the bacterial ribosome
- TCN's also exhibit wide variety of direct and indirect anti-inflammatory properties

Q. What are the antibacterial properties of TCN?

A.
- TCN's exhibit activity against gram-positive and gram-negative bacteria as well as *Mycoplasma*, *Chlamydia*, and *Rickettsia* species, Spirochetes and some parasites
- Minocycline and doxycycline are more active against *S. aureus* as compared to TCN's

Q. What is the mechanism of resistance against TCN?

A. Two major TCN resistance mechanisms acquired by bacteria are:

1. Ribosomal protection
2. Drug efflux

Q. What are the types of TCN?

A.

Name	Dosage	Comments
Short acting:		
Tetracycline Oxytetracycline	250–500 mg 6 hourly	To be taken on an empty stomach, food and antacids decrease absorption, can cause esophagitis if swallowed dry

Continued

Continued

Name	***Dosage***	***Comments***
Intermediate acting:		
Demeclocycline	150–300 mg 12 hourly	High risk of photosensitivity, rarely diabetes insipidus
Long acting:		
Doxycycline	100 mg 12 hourly	Can be given with food and milk, safe in renal failure
Minocycline	200 mg stat, followed by 100 mg 12 hourly	Most active against *S. aureus*, risk of lupus, hepatitis, and pneumonitis is significant

Q. What are the indications of TCN?

A. FDA approved:

- Acne vulgaris:
  - Inhibits propionibacterium species, which metabolize lipids into FFA's which are irritant. *Propionibacterium acnes* is also proinflammatory, activating complement pathway and neutrophils. TCN's themselves may have an anti-inflammatory effect and hence can often be used in subtherapeutic doses (though this may promote bacterial resistance)
  - Doxycycline and minocycline are often preferred because of less frequent dosage and absorption with food
  - Minocycline has got a lipophilic action and gets stored in the fatty tissue to exert a more prolonged effect
- Rosacea:
  - Treatment of papulopustular rosacea with oral TCN's reduces inflammatory lesions, perilesional erythema, symptoms like stinging, burning, pruritus.
  - FDA approved: a minimal dose of 40 mg doxycycline od in rosacea

Non-FDA approved:

- Immunobullous dermatoses:
  - TCN's have been used in combination with nicotinamide for treatment of bullous pemphigoid, linear IgA bullous dermatosis, pemphigus vulgaris, pemphigus foliaceus, benign familial pemphigus, cicatricial pemphigoid, dermatitis herpetiformis
- Granulomatous dermatoses such as cutaneous sarcoidosis, Melkersson–Rosenthal syndrome, confluent and reticular papillomatosis, prurigo pigmentosa, oral lichen planus, acne keloidalis, pyoderma gangrenosum

- Aphthous stomatitis
- Community acquired MRSA infections
- Rickettsial disease, Vibrio-vulnificus infections
- Spirochete infections—syphilis, Lyme disease
- Less common sexually transmitted diseases like lympho granuloma venereum caused by *Chlamydia trachomatis*
- Atypical mycobacterial infections
- Leprosy (minocycline)

Q. What are the adverse effects of tetracyline?

A.
- GI effects, pancreatitis, hepatotoxicity, severe phototoxic reactions, may aggravate renal disease, brown discoloration of teeth and depressed bone growth in children. Hence, it is contraindicated in children <9 years
- Blue-black pigmentation with minocycline
- Lupus and hepatitis are fairly common with minocycline
- Superinfection like Candidal vaginitis are common

Q. What are the drug interactions of tetracyclines?

A. The drug interactions are as following:
- TCN's reduce the effectiveness of oral contraceptive (OC) pills
- There is augmented risk of benign intracranial hypertension caused by concurrent use of TCN's and oral retinoids
- Increased effect of oral anticoagulants

RIFAMYCIN

Q. What is the origin of the name rifamycin?

A. The rifamycins were isolated from *Nocardia mediterranei* in France. It was named riffi after a popular French movie (Le Riffi).

Q. Discuss the mechanism of action of rifamycin?

A. Rifamycins are bactericidal for both intra and extracellular organisms. They inhibit RNA synthesis by interacting directly with DNA dependant RNA polymerase. Thus, RNA transcription and subsequent protein translation is prevented.

Q. What is the difference between rifamycin and rifampicin?

A. Rifamycin is a natural antibiotic while rifampicin is a semi-synthetic derivative of rifamycin.

Q. What are the clinical uses of rifamycin?

A. The dermatological indications of rifamycin are as follows:
- Cutaneous TB along with isoniazid, pyrazinamide, ethambutol
- Atypical mycobacterial infections
- Hansen's disease

- Prevention and treatment of disseminated atypical mycobacterial infection
- *Bartonella* infections caused by *Bartonella henselae,* i.e., cat scratch disease, bacillary angiomatosis, peliosis, hepatitis, neuro-retinitis or Parinaud's oculoglandular syndrome
- Methicillin-susceptible *Staphylococcus aureus* (MSSA), methicillin-resistant *Staphylococcus aureus* (MRSA) infections: It is especially effective when combined with anti-staphylococcal antibiotics to prevent recurrent furunculosis
- Other infections and related diseases such as cutaneous leishmaniasis, rhinoscleroma, aspergillosis, brucellosis, tularemia, gonorrhea and chlamydial infection
- Pruritus associated with biliary cirrhosis
- Role in psoriasis: Rifampicin can reduce bacterial carriage and hence the concentration of superantigens which are important in the pathogenesis of psoriasis
- Rifampicin paste has been used in the treatment of molluscum contagiosum (not evidence based)

Q. What is the pregnancy category of rifampicin?

A. Category C.

TRIMETHOPRIM AND SULFAMETHOXAZOLE (TMS)

It is fixed ratio combination of 1 part trimethoprim with 5 parts of sulphamethoxazole.

Q. What is its mechanism of action?

A. Trimethoprim inhibits the conversion of para-aminobenzoic acid (PABA) to folic acid in the bacterial nucleus while sulphomethoxazole inhibits the conversion of folic to folinic acid (tetrahydrofolic acid). Because of this action, bacterial nucleic acid synthesis is impaired.

Q. What are the clinical uses of trimethoprim and sulfamethoxazole?

A.
- It is not used as a first line agent in most diseases. It is used in treatment of nocardiosis, actinomycotic mycetoma, and *Aeromonas* infection
- It is a treatment option for donovanosis, cat-scratch disease and melioidosis. It can be used in pyodermas, chancroid and LGV where other drugs fail or are contra indicated. It can also be used in acne vulgaris in TCN-resistant patients
- It can be used in gram-negative folliculitis.

Q. What are the adverse effects?

A. GI effects, hypersensitivity reactions, hematological toxicity and CNS effects. Also, renal stones have been reported.

Q. What is the pregnancy category of this drug?

A. Category C.

Q. What are the drug interactions of this drug?

A. Prolongation of prothrombin time when given concomitantly with warfarin and causes increased toxicity when given with methotrexate (MTX).

LINCOSAMIDES

Clindamycin

Q. What is the mechanism of action of clindamycin?

A. It binds to the 50s ribosomal subunit and then inhibits protein synthesis by blocking transpeptidation.

Q. What are the clinical uses of clindamycin?

A.
- SSTI's caused by staphylococci, cellulitis, folliculitis, furunculosis, carbuncles, impetigo, ecthyma, hidradenitis suppurativa, diabetic foot
- Deep soft tissue infection like streptococcal myositis and necrotizing fasciitis
- Acne vulgaris (mainly topical)

Q. What are the adverse effects of clindamycin?

A.
- Antibiotic associated pseudomembranous colitis (0.1–10% risk). Probably the risk is exaggerated because cephalosporin and ampicillin have a similar risk
- Bone marrow suppression and renal impairment
- Maculopapular or urticarial eruptions
- Rarely Stevens-Johnson syndrome (SJS) type reactions with polyarthritis

Q. What is its pregnacy category?

A. Category B.

Q. What are the drug interactions?

A. Clindamycin enhances the neuromuscular property of tubocurare and pancuronium.

Q. What is the dosage of clindamycin?

A.
- 50–300 mg twice daily.
- While conditions like hidradenitis suppurativa require 300 mg thrice daily

LINEZOLID

Q. What is the mechanism of action?

A. It binds to the 23s portion of the 50s ribosomal subunit.

Q. What is the spectrum of linezolid?

A. It has a wide spectrum of activity against resistant strains of MRSA, vancomycin-intermediate, resistant strains of staphylococci, penicillin resistant *Streptococcus pneumoniae* and vancomycin-resistant enterococci.

Q. What are its indications?

A.
- Skin infections due to *Staphylococcus* or *Streptococcus*
- SSTI's caused by *S. aureus*
- Community acquired MRSA in patients who have failed while on oral doxycycline, minocycline or vancomycin

Q. What are the adverse effects of these drugs?

A.
- Elevation in serum transaminases and creatinine
- Myelosuppression including anemia, leukopenia, pancytopenia
- Peripheral neuropathy with prolonged use
- Serotonin syndrome characterized by cognitive dysfunction, hyperpyrexia, hyperreflexia and incoordination

2.2. ANTILEPROSY DRUGS

Q. Elaborate about the history of treatment of leprosy.

A.
- Until 1940, the only known treatment was Chaulmoogra oil (*Hydnocarpus* oil), which was of limited efficacy
- It was given orally and intradermally, and was associated with severe side effects such as fever, nausea, local reactions. A better formulation of the oil was made by addition of camphor and resorcin
- In the 1950s, dapsone pills became the treatment of choice but in the late 1970s, reports showed widespread resistance against dapsone
- In 1980, the first multidrug therapy (MDT) was introduced in Malta, consisting of isoniazid, prothionamide, and dapsone (Isoprodian) combined with rifampicin
- In 1981, the WHO Expert Committee first recommended MDT for leprosy, combining dapsone, rifampicin, and clofazimine. This was not based on any field trials but only on theoretical grounds
- In the 2000s, concepts of fixed drug therapy, Uniform-MDT, and Accompanied-MDT were introduced

Q. Describe WHO recommended multidrug therapy (MDT) for leprosy.

A.

Type of leprosy	*Supervized therapy (once monthly)*	*Unsupervized therapy (daily)*	*Duration*
Multibacillary (MB) leprosy	Rifampicin (R) 600 mg Clofazimine (C) 300 mg	Clofazimine 50 mg Dapsone (D) 100 mg	12 months (to be completed in maximum 18 months)
Paucibacillary (PB) leprosy	Rifampicin 600 mg Clofazimine (C) 300 mg	Dapsone 100 mg Clofazimine 50 mg	6 months (to be completed in maximum 9 months)

DAPSONE (4, 4′-DIAMINODIPHENYL SULFONE) (DDS)

Introduction

Dapsone was synthesized by Fromm and Wittmann in Germany, in 1908. It is a sulfa drug.

Q. What is the mechanism of action of dapsone?

A.
- Dapsone is bacteriostatic and weakly bactericidal against *M. leprae*
- The mechanism of action of dapsone is similar to that of sulphonamides, i.e., by interference in folic acid synthesis through competition with para-aminobenzoic acid (PABA) for the enzyme dihydropteroate synthase
- It may also have an inhibitory effect on neutrophils
- Dapsone has also got an immunomodulatory effect

Q. Describe the pharmacology and metabolism of dapsone.

A.
- Following oral administration, the drug is almost completely absorbed from the gut and peak levels are reached within 4–6 hours
- Half-life is about 24 hours
- The metabolism of dapsone is primarily by two methods: (i) acetylation and (ii) hydroxylation
- Hydroxylation leads to formation of the metabolite dapsone hydroxylamine which is thought to be responsible for the hematologic adverse effects of dapsone
- Variability in acetylator status is not clinically relevant

Q. What is the pregnancy prescribing status of dapsone?

A.
- Dapsone is a pregnancy category C drug
- Hemolysis may occur in nursing infants of mothers taking dapsone
- It may cause kernicterus if given in the last trimester
- But treatment with dapsone during pregnancy may kill viable bacilli in breast milk, and thus may be advantageous

Q. What are the indications to prescribe dapsone? Name some uses of dapsone other than in treatment of leprosy.

A.

FDA approved indications:

- Leprosy
- Dermatitis herpetiformis

Other dermatologic indications (consistent efficacy):

- Linear IgA dermatosis
- Bullous systemic lupus erythematosus
- Erythema elevatum diutinum

Other dermatologic uses (variable efficacy):

- Autoimmune bullous dermatoses:
  - Bullous pemphigoid
  - Pemphigus vulgaris/foliaceus
  - Cicatricial pemphigoid
  - Subcorneal pustular dermatosis (IgA pemphigus)
- Vasculitis:
  - Cutaneous vasculitis (leukocytoclastic)
  - Urticarial vasculitis
- Neutrophilic dermatoses:
  - Acute febrile neutrophilic dermatoses (Sweet syndrome)
  - Pyoderma gangrenosum
  - Behçet's syndrome
- Infections:
  - Actinomycotic mycetoma
  - *Pneumocystis jiroveci* pneumonia in AIDS patients
- Other dermatoses:
  - Subacute cutaneous lupus erythematosus
  - Relapsing polychondritis
  - Granuloma annulare
  - Granuloma faciale
  - Rosacea (granulomatous)
  - Panniculitis
  - Pustular psoriasis
  - Nodulocystic acne

Q. Are there any contraindications to the use of dapsone?

A. Absolute contraindications:

- Prior hypersensitivity to dapsone (agranulocytosis and hypersensitivity syndrome)

Relative contraindications:

- G6PD deficiency
- Allergy to sulfonamides
- Significant liver or renal function impairment
- Significant cardiopulmonary disease
- Severe anemia
- Acute porphyria
- Preexisting peripheral neuropathy

Q. What is the dosage and suggested regimen of dapsone in leprosy?

A. The currently recommended dosage is 1–2 mg/kg daily as part of WHO prescribed MDT regimen, for a maximum period of 2 years. Usually, Dapsone is given 25 mg daily for patient aged <6 years, 50 mg daily for 6–14 years, and 100 mg for 14 years and above.

Q. What are the adverse effects due to dapsone?

A. Pharmacologic (dose-related) adverse effects:

Hemolytic anemia:

- Hemolytic anemia occurs in every patient on dapsone therapy
- Dapsone shortens the lifespan of RBCs from 120 days to 90 days
- Ageing RBCs are more susceptible to oxidative damage caused by N-hydroxy metabolites of dapsone (dapsone hydroxylamine)
- G6PD deficient individuals are more susceptible
- It is the most common adverse effect of dapsone therapy

Methemoglobinemia:

- Small amounts of methemoglobin can be seen even in individuals on low doses of dapsone
- Clinical effects relate to the patient's total hemoglobin and cardiopulmonary status
- Treatment: IV methylene blue 1–2 mg/kg, IV vitamin C, oral cimetidine 400 mg, oral vitamin E 800 IU

Nonpharmacologic (idiosyncratic) adverse effects:

Hematologic:

- Agranulocytosis
- Thrombocytopenia

Hepatic:

- Hepatitis (elevated transaminases)
- Infectious mononucleosis-like syndrome/dapsone hypersensitivity syndrome/"dapsone syndrome"/sulfone syndrome/"6 weeks syndrome"/drug reaction with eosinophilia and systemic symptoms (DRESS) syndrome/drug hypersensitivity syndrome (DHS):
    - Reports suggest that its frequency is on the increase since the introduction of MDT. The patient develops fever, maculopapular skin rash or exfoliative dermatitis, with lymphadenopathy and hepatitis, 3–12 weeks after starting dapsone. Peripheral eosinophilia is frequently seen. In almost half the patients, one or more manifestations may be missing (incomplete syndrome)
- Cholestatic jaundice (rare)

Cutaneous:

- Morbilliform rash
- Toxic epidermal necrolysis
- Fixed drug eruption
- Stevens–Johnson syndrome

Neurological:

- Woolly headache/light headedness (hence preferably taken at night)
- Dapsone psychosis
- Peripheral neuropathy (distal motor, reversible)

Gastrointestinal:

- Nausea
- Anorexia

Renal:

- Nephrotic syndrome

Q. Name some drug interactions of dapsone.

A.
- CYP3A4 enzyme inducers such as rifampicin and antiepileptics may reduce dapsone serum levels (loss of efficacy)
- Antacids and H_2 antihistamines may reduce gastrointestinal (GI) absorption of dapsone
- Probenecid decreases excretion of dapsone metabolites and increases toxicity
- Dihydrofolate reductase inhibitors (pyrimethamine, trimethoprim) increase hematologic risk of dapsone

Q. What are the monitoring guidelines during dapsone therapy?

A. Pre-therapy/baseline investigations:

- Complete blood count (CBC) with differential white blood cell (WBC) count
- Liver function tests
- Renal function tests
- G6PD levels
- Urinanalysis

During therapy:

- CBC with differential WBC count every week for 4 weeks, then monthly for next 3 months, then every 3–4 months
- Reticulocyte count as needed to assess response to hemolysis
- Renal and liver function tests every 3–4 months
- Methemoglobin levels when clinically indicated
- These monitoring guidelines are not practical in field treatment of leprosy and so for a leprosy case, these need not be mentioned

Q. Explain a spot test for evaluating compliance of dapsone therapy.

A. A drop of the patient's fresh urine is placed on a filter paper and Ehrlich's reagent is added. Development of a spot of orange color is seen when dapsone is present. This test is now rarely used.

Q. Explain tablet dodgers and clinic dodgers.

A. Clinic dodgers are those who don't come to the clinic for collecting drugs. Tablet dodgers are those who collect the drugs but don't take them. This can be detected by surprise visits to the house of the patient.

Q. What is the genetic basis of dapsone resistance?

A.
- Resistance occurs due to mutation of *folP* gene of *M. leprae*
- The main factors leading to development of resistance are the long practised dapsone monotherapy, poor compliance and suboptimal dosing
- Currently dapsone is recommended only as a component of MDT, to be given in a 50–100 mg daily dose, for as far as possible without interruption, up to completion of the regimen

RIFAMPICIN

Introduction

Rifampicin is a semisynthetic derivative of rifamycin B, originally derived from the organism *Streptomyces mediterranei*. Rees et al. first reported in 1970 that rifampicin had a rapid action in leprosy, the morphologic index (MI) reaching 0 in 5 weeks. It was found to be effective against dapsone-resistant bacilli as well.

Q. What is its mechanism of action?

A.
- Rifampicin is a highly potent bactericidal drug. It is the fastest acting antileprosy drug
- Its action is likely due to interference with mRNA synthesis by selective inhibition of bacterial DNA-dependent RNA polymerase
- Being lipophilic, it acts on both intracellular as well as extracellular organisms
- A single 600 mg dose of rifampicin kills 99.9% of nondormant *M. leprae*
- It has a postantibiotic effect which persists for a long time after taking it

Q. Describe the pharmacology of rifampicin.

A. Rifampicin should be given at least 30 minutes before food for complete absorption. With an oral dose of 600 mg, a peak serum level is reached within 2–3 hours, which is 40–50 times the minimal inhibitory concentration (MIC).

Q. How is rifampicin metabolized?

A. Rifampicin is rapidly metabolized and excreted into the bile. About 30% of total elimination may be urinary, which may cause orange-red discoloration of urine.

Q. Enumerate the indications of rifampicin.

A. FDA approved indications:
- Tuberculosis

Off-label uses:
- Leprosy (WHO approved use)
- Atypical mycobacterial infections
- *Anthrax*, brucellosis, *Legionella pneumophila* infections, *Bartonella* infections (cat-scratch disease, bacillary angiomatosis)
- Methicillin-susceptible *Staphylococcus aureus* (MSSA) and methicillin-resistant *Staphylococcus aureus* (MRSA) infections
- Cutaneous leishmaniasis, *rhinoscleroma, gonorrhea, mycetoma*

Q. What is the dosage of rifampicin?

A. Rifampicin is available as capsules of 150 and 300 mg. For leprosy, it is administered as a supervized monthly dose of 600 mg as part of the MDT regimen.

Q. What is the pregnancy prescribing status of rifampicin?

A. Rifampicin is a pregnancy category C drug. Given in last trimester, it may result in increased risk of bleeding in new born.

Q. What are the adverse effects caused by rifampicin?

A. Common adverse effects:

- Orange-red discoloration of body fluids and cutaneous discoloration at higher doses
- Central nervous system (CNS) symptoms: Headache, drowsiness, dizziness
- Gastrointestinal tract (GIT) symptoms: Epigastric distress, nausea, vomiting, diarrhea
- Hepatotoxicity

Uncommon adverse effects:

- Formation of rifampicin-dependant antibodies—causes cutaneous, gastrointestinal, and influenza-like syndromes. May also cause thrombocytopenia, hemolytic anemia and acute renal failure. This is often seen with intermittent rifampicin therapy (**RIPAS**—**r**espiratory, **i**nfluenza, **p**urpura, **a**bdominal pain and **s**hock)
- The "Flu syndrome" is characterized by episodes of fever and malaise which begin 1–2 hours after each treatment and last up to 8 hours, along with dyspnea and cough
- Stevens–Johnson syndrome (SJS) and toxic epidermal necrolysis (TEN)
- Urticaria

Q. What are the drug interactions with rifampicin?

A.
- Rifampicin is a potent inducer of multiple cytochrome P450 (CYP) isoforms including CYP3A4. It causes accelerated degradation of many drugs including steroids, oral contraceptives, oral hypoglycemics (sulfonylureas), warfarin, anticonvulsants, etc.
- Antacids increase absorption of rifampicin.
- Concomitant use with isoniazid increases risk of hepatotoxicity

Q. Explain the mechanism of rifampicin resistance.

A.
- Resistance to rifampicin in *M. leprae* has been shown to be due to mutations in the *rpoB* gene
- The pattern of resistance is of streptomycin type (single-step mutant type)

CLOFAZIMINE (LAMPRENE; B663)

Introduction

- Clofazimine is a red iminophenazine dye, initially developed for the treatment of tuberculosis. It has both antimicrobial and anti-inflammatory actions. It was first introduced in clinical trials by Dr Yawalkar

Q. Describe the mechanism of action of clofazimine.

A.
- Exact mechanism of action is not known. It possibly acts by blocking the template function of DNA
- It is bacteriostatic and mildly bactericidal against *M. leprae*
- It is inhibitory to multiplication of intracellular *M. leprae*. It also inhibits neutrophil motility

Q. Describe the pharmacology and metabolism of clofazimine.

A.
- Absorption from gut is 30–50%
- Large quantities of the drug accumulate in skin, subcutaneous fat, liver, lungs, adrenals, kidneys and GIT, causing discoloration of skin and organs
- Half-life is almost 2 months

Q. Name some indications of clofazimine.

A. **FDA approved indications:**
- Leprosy
- Erythema nodosum leprosum
- Other mycobacterial infections

Off-label uses:
- Pyoderma gangrenosum
- Pustular psoriasis, palmoplantar pustulosis, vitiligo, chronic discoid lupus erythematosus, acne fulminans, Oro-facial granulomatosis (Melkersson-Rosenthal Syndrome)

Q. What are the adverse effects of clofazimine?

A. **Cutaneous side-effects:**
- Red-brown pigmentation of skin and conjunctivae—initially "mauve" or "mahogany red" followed by "slate gray" or black. This occurs within 3 months of starting clofazimine therapy and may take up to 1 year to subside after stopping it. It is more prominent on the skin lesions and sun-exposed parts. It may give the patient an intoxicated look, which can cause non-compliance
- Dryness of skin and ichthyosis, which is more prominent on the skin lesions. This is due to impairment of lipid metabolism

Systemic side effects:
- Acute abdomen—nausea, vomiting, cramping, diarrhea
- Splenic infarction
- Eosinophilic enteritis
- Clofazimine deposition in the mesenteric lymph nodes
- Fatal enteropathy

Q. What is the pregnancy prescribing status of clofazimine?

A. • Pregnancy category C.
- No known teratogenic effects. The infant is born dark if clofazimine is given during pregnancy. However, this is temporary.

Q. What is the dosage of clofazimine?

A. Clofazimine is given in a daily dose of 50–100 mg. It is available as a 50 mg and 100 mg capsule.

OTHER DRUGS FOR TREATMENT OF LEPROSY: ETHIONAMIDE/PROTHIONAMIDE

Introduction

These drugs were used in patients who were unable to tolerate clofazimine as part of MDT. They are chemically related to isoniazid. Use of these drugs as monotherapy is not recommended.

Q. What is the mechanism of action of thionamides?

A. Powerful bactericidal effect against *M. leprae*. Exact mechanism of action is not known. Inhibition of mycolic acid and to some extent protein synthesis appears to be the mechanism. Effective in dapsone and rifampicin resistance.

Q. What are the side effects?

A. • Liver damage, gastric intolerance, nausea and vomiting
- GIT intolerance occurs in substantial proportion of patients
- Anorexia, salivation, and metallic taste
- Abdominal pain and diarrhea occur less commonly
- Less common—peripheral neuropathy, headache, depression, drowsiness, hypotension, visual disturbances, acne

THIACETAZONE

- It is a bactericidal antitubercular drug
- Was used for treatment in patients with coexistent leprosy and tuberculosis
- Now rarely used, due to severity of side effects (agranulocytosis, hepatotoxicity, severe drug rashes) and availability of safer drugs

Q. Name some newer drugs for the treatment of leprosy.

A. • Pefloxacin
- Sparfloxacin
- Moxifloxacin
- Gatifloxacin

- Minocycline (100 mg/day)
- Clarithromycin (500 mg/day)
- Rifabutin
- Rifapentine
- Cephaloridine
- Cephaloglycin
- Fusidic acid
- Cefoxitin

Q. What is ROM therapy for leprosy?

A.
- Single-dose ROM therapy (Rifampicin 600 mg, Ofloxacin 400 mg, and Minocycline 100 mg) was initially proposed for treatment of single skin lesion leprosy. However, it has been omitted as per recent WHO recommendations
- The reasons for its omission maybe that it is difficult to assess the number of lesions, especially in females. Also, ROM acts only on multiplying bacilli and all bacilli may not be multiplying at the time ROM is given, but may start multiplying later
- ROM therapy given in above doses every month is being evaluated for efficacy. Monthly ROM would be given for 6 months in PBL and 12 months in MBL. ROM-24 has also been given for MBL
- It is also being used as a substitute for the clofazimine component of MDT in patients not willing to accept clofazimine

Q. How would you treat a patient suffering from both leprosy and tuberculosis?

A. **Paucibacillary leprosy (PBL):**
- Intensive phase of antitubercular therapy (ATT): No new drug added
- Maintenance phase: Dapsone is added to ATT regimen

Multibacillary leprosy (MBL):
- Intensive phase: Dapsone and clofazimine are added
- Maintenance phase: Dapsone and clofazimine are added, and once daily rifampicin is stopped, monthly rifampicin is given

Q. What can be done in a PBL case if a patient is allergic to one of the two drugs?

A. In a truly paucibacillary (PB) case, patient can be continued on monthly rifampicin alone if he is allergic to dapsone. If he is allergic to rifampicin, however, it is better to add clofazimine to dapsone, since he may already be dapsone-resistant.

Q. What can be done in an MBL case, if patient is allergic to one of the three drugs?

A. If patient is allergic to dapsone, stop it and continue the other two drugs only. If patient is allergic to rifampicin, give minocycline plus ofloxacin for the first 3 months and then continue with either alone for the rest of the course, along with clofazimine and dapsone. If allergic to clofazimine, give minocycline or ofloxacin for the entire duration of MDT along with rifampicin or dapsone.

Q. Is MDT contraindicated in pregnancy and lactation?

A. No, it is not contraindicated and should not be stopped under any circumstances.

Q. What is "fixed drug therapy (FDT)"?

A. Giving MDT for PB patients for 6 months and for MB patients for 1 year, irrespective of initial smear status. However, some authorities recommend that if the initial smear is more than ++++, then therapy has to be given for 2 years.

Q. What is "uniform MDT"?

A. Giving D + R + C for 6 months to all patients, irrespective of whether they are PB or MB, is called uniform MDT; this simplifies the treatment for paramedical workers.

Q. What is "accompanied MDT"?

A. Normally, MDT is not given to anyone except the patient himself. However, for patients coming from remote or hilly areas, the MDT can be given for a few months at a time (or even the entire course), to a trustworthy person who can be relied upon to give the MDT to the patient.

Q. What is "field-modification" of MDT?

A. Here, the paramedical worker simply counts the number of lesions. If 5 or less, PB MDT is given, if >5 lesions, MB MDT is given.

Q. What are the minimum inhibitory concentrations (MICs) of antileprosy drugs?

A.

Drug	*MIC (µg/mL)*
Dapsone	0.003 (Dapsone produces blood level 500 × MIC, hence, a few doses skipped will not make much difference)
Rifampicin	0.3 (Rifampicin produces blood levels only 30 times MIC, hence even a single dose skipped can create Rifampicin resistance)

Continued

Continued

Drug	MIC (μg/mL)
Clofazimine	MIC unknown, since it gets distributed unequally in the tissues
Ethionamide/ Prothionamide	0.05 (A single dose produces levels 50 times MIC, so it is better not to interrupt the doses)
Minocycline/Ofloxacin/ Clarithromycin	Unknown

THALIDOMIDE (ALPHA-N-PHTHALIMIDO-GLUTARIMIDE)

History and Introduction

Thalidomide was first synthesized in West Germany by the company Chemie Grunenthal in 1954. It was promoted as an antiemetic, sedative, and hypnotic, and was in widespread use, including during the first trimester of pregnancy. In December 1961, an Australian obstetrician, William McBride, first reported the increased incidence of phocomelia in mothers taking thalidomide during the first trimester, in a letter to the Lancet journal. Following this, the drug was withdrawn from the market. However, it is estimated that atleast 12,000 newborn children were affected with thalidomide embryopathy before the drug was eventually withdrawn.

In 1965, Sheskin, an Israeli dermatologist, first reported the effects of thalidomide in treating erythema nodosum leprosum (ENL) in six leprosy patients. Since then there has been a growing interest in thalidomide as a possible immunomodulatory drug and its use in various diseases is being explored.

Q. Elaborate about the structure of thalidomide.

A. Chemically, it is an α-N-phthalimido-glutarimide consisting of a single central asymmetric carbon atom with a left phthalimide ring and a right glutarimide ring. The phthalimide ring is responsible for the teratogenic effects whereas the glutarimide ring, which is structurally similar to the one seen in other sedatives, mediates sedation. It is lipophilic and easily crosses the placenta.

Q. What is the mechanism of action of thalidomide?

A.
- Inhibits polymorphonuclear cell chemotaxis
- Decreases phagocytosis in PMN leukocytes and monocytes
- Inhibits lymphocyte proliferation, causing a significant reduction in CD4+ lymphocytes (correcting the CD4:CD8 imbalance occurring in ENL)

- It is a potent inhibitor of tumor necrosis factor alpha (TNF-α)
- Converts antigenic lymphocytic response from Th1 to Th2 type
- Exhibits a synergistic antitumoral effect with other antitumor drugs, though it is ineffective only by itself
- Also shown to inhibit replication of the HIV-1 virus
- Central depressant effect mediated by its glutarimide ring may be responsible for its antipruritic action seen in pruritic dermatoses

Q. Describe the pharmacokinetics of thalidomide.

A.
- Thalidomide is absorbed slowly after oral administration, peak levels reaching in 5 hours. It is not water-soluble and no parenteral forms are available
- Thalidomide is metabolized by non-enzymatic hydrolytic cleavage; the major route of elimination still remains undetermined
- As thalidomide is not metabolized by the CYP-450, it is unlikely to interact with the drugs metabolized by this enzyme

Q. What are the present day dermatological indications for use of thalidomide?

A. Very effective:
- Erythema nodosum leprosum
- Recurrent aphthous stomatitis of unknown etiology
- Behçet's syndrome
- Cutaneous lupus erythematosus
- Discoid lupus erythematosus
- Prurigo nodularis

Moderate/low/unproven efficacy:
- Actinic prurigo/Hutchinson's prurigo
- Recurrent erythema multiforme
- Chronic graft-versus-host disease (GVHD)
- Pyoderma gangrenosum
- Lichen planus (erosive)
- Sarcoidosis
- Langerhans cell histiocytosis
- Cachexia in TB

Use in HIV/AIDS: thalidomide has been used with success in management of AIDS patients with oral and genital aphthae (AIDS stomatitis) and coinfection with HIV, TB, and *Mycobacterium avium-intracellulare* (MAI). It has also been used for Kaposi's sarcoma in AIDS.

Q. What is the dosage of thalidomide?

A.
- Typical starting dose of thalidomide in dermatology is 200 mg/day taken at night. After clinical response, the dose is gradually tapered to a maintenance dose of 50–100 mg/day
- For treatment of ENL, thalidomide is given as 100 mg 3–4 times daily for 2 weeks, to be tapered off slowly over a couple of months, by reductions of 100 mg each month, to a maintenance dose of 50–100 mg daily. Every 6 months, effort should be made to discontinue therapy after gradual tapering of dose. The drug is restarted for another 6 months in case of recurrence of reaction
- In cases of recalcitrant aphthae, thalidomide is used in doses of 100 mg/day for 5–28 days
- In Behçet's disease, doses of 100–300 mg/day for a few days are used

Q. Discuss thalidomide embryopathy.

A. Teratogenicity is the most severe adverse effect of thalidomide, as seen during the thalidomide disaster in Europe in the 1960s. The deformities occur if the drug is taken between 20 and 40 days of gestation. The babies born with thalidomide embryopathy were known as "phocomelia" babies due to their resemblance to limbs of a seal.

The features of thalidomide embryopathy are:
- Limb deformities—amelia, phocomelia, bony hypoplasia, absence of bones
- External ear deformities—anotia, micropinna, absent auditory canal
- Eye deformities—enophthalmos, microphthalmos
- Neural tube abnormalities
- Rarely defects of internal organs
- Limb reduction in the upper limbs, and to a lesser extent in the lower limbs, is the most common abnormality followed by abnormalities of the eyes and ears
- During use of thalidomide in women of childbearing potential, it is necessary to perform two different pregnancy tests before starting therapy. It is mandatory to counsel the patient and use strict contraception with two different methods during the course of therapy, to be continued up to 1 month after stopping therapy. Pregnancy tests have to be repeated at monthly intervals, the last one being at 4 weeks after stopping therapy
- For male patients, use of condoms is advised during intercourse during therapy and for 1 month after stopping therapy

Q. What are the other adverse effects of thalidomide?

A. Apart from teratogenicity, the following are the other adverse effects observed with thalidomide:

- Neuropathy: It is a predominantly sensory, symmetric distal polyneuropathy. There is painful paresthesia of the hands and feet and numbness in a glove and stocking distribution. The reported incidence varies widely from 1–50% in various studies. It is unlikely to be a dose-related adverse effect
- Somnolence: This is a dose-dependent effect. Hence, bedtime administration of thalidomide is preferred
- Cutaneous adverse effects: Brittle finger nails, red palms, exfoliative and erythrodermic eruptions. Allergic vasculitis and pruritus may also occur. Severe reactions including TEN and erythema multiforme and erythroderma may occur requiring discontinuation of therapy
- Endocrine adverse effect: Myxedema, hyperglycemia, menstrual irregularities
- Constipation is a frequent side effect
- Others: Peripheral edema, increased thromboembolism, headache, nausea, leukopenia, sinus bradycardia, hypotension, etc., have been reported

2.3. SYSTEMIC STEROIDS

INTRODUCTION

Corticosteroids are anti-inflammatory and immunosuppressive agents. Cortisone was first described in 1935 by Kendall as compound E. The use of cortisone was first described in patients with rheumatoid arthritis in 1948 and in 1950. Hench and colleagues described the basic effects and toxicities of corticosteroids. In 1951, Sulzberger and associates described the use of cortisone in a variety of inflammatory dermatoses.

Q. What is the structure of corticosteroids?

A. Steroids are derived from cyclopentanoperhydrophenanthrene ring of cholesterol. The basic structure of all corticosteroids consist of three hexane rings and one pentane ring and this combined structure is known as the cyclopentanoperhydrophenanthrene nucleus. The rings are designated by the letters A, B, C, D and each carbon is numbered from 1 to 21. The designations "a" and "b" refer to the position of any added molecules. Manipulation of this basic structure can lead to production of different steroids, e.g., biologically active glucocorticoids have an 11-hydroxyl group.

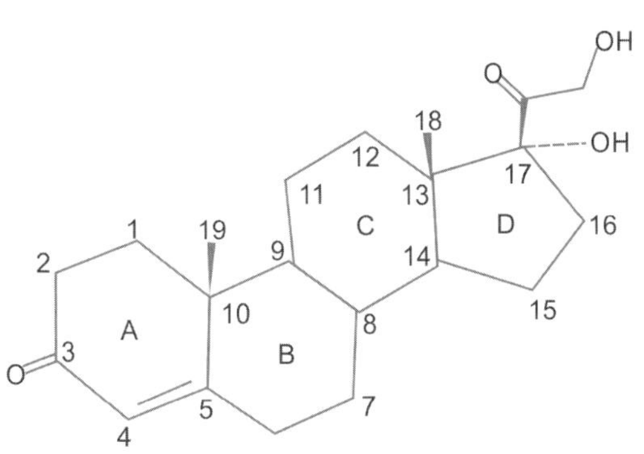

Structure of corticosteroids.

Q. Discuss the pharmacokinetics of glucocorticoids (GCS)?

A. Oral GCS are absorbed in the jejunum, absorption is delayed in the presence of food. In the plasma, they bind to a globulin called transcortin, as well as to albumin. The steroids which are free are the active steroids. Decreased serum proteins can lead to increased activity of steroids. Decreased renal function will also result in increased activity. Patients with hyperthyroidism show reduced effect of steroids, and hence the dose may have to be increased. GCS are distributed to all body tissues. Most GCS also have mineralocorticoid activity. Hydrocortisone has significant mineralocorticoid potency. Prednisolone has slight action, while methyl prednisolone has essentially no mineralocorticoid effects.

Q. What is the mechanism of action of corticosteroids?

A. Unbound corticosteroid enter the cells and exerts its effects by binding to the glucocorticoid receptor (GR). This complex is translocated to the nucleus and binds to the glucocorticoid responsive element of the steroid responsive genes. This binding essentially causes all the actions of steroids to occur.

Corticosteroids exert their anti-inflammatory and immunosuppressive effects through the following mechanisms:

- Inhibition of transcription factors (NF-κB and AP-1)
- Induction of eosinophil and lymphocyte apoptosis
- Phospholipase A_2 and cyclo-oxygenase 2 (COX-2) inhibition
- Decreased immunoglobulin synthesis by B cells and interleukin-2 (IL-2) production by T cells
- Depletion of Langerhans cells in the skin
- Lysosomal and cell membrane stabilization
- Inhibit degranulation of mast cells
- Vascular effects like angiogenesis, vasoconstriction and decreased permeability

- GCS inhibit tumor necrosis factor alpha (TNF-α), IL-1, IL-2, IL-8 and intercellular adhesion molecule (ICAM)
- GCS also produce neutrophilia, and a transient lymphopenia, eosinopenia and reduced destruction of RBCs

Q. What are the indications for use of systemic corticosteroids in dermatology?

A.

Short-term therapy (<3 weeks)	*Long-term therapy (>3 weeks)*
Contact dermatitis	Pemphigus (all types)
Photodermatitis	Pemphigoid
Drug reactions	Systemic lupus erythematosus
Severe urticaria and angioedema	Dermatomyositis
Atopic dermatitis	Mixed connective tissue diseases
Acute herpes zoster in elderly	Scleroderma (low dose)
Postherpetic neuralgia	Linear IgA bullous dermatosis
Leukocytoclastic vasculitis	Relapsing polychondritis
Acute widespread lichen planus	Epidermolysis bullosa acquisita
Erythroderma	Systemic sarcoidosis
Acute febrile neutrophilic dermatosis	Systemic vasculitis syndromes
Kerion	
Pyoderma gangrenosum	

Q. What are the contraindications of corticosteroids?

A. Absolute contraindications:

- Systemic fungal infections
- Herpes simplex keratitis
- Hypersensitivity

Relative contraindications:

- Cardiovascular: Hypertension, congestive heart failure (CHF)
- Central nervous system: Prior psychosis, severe depression
- Gastrointestinal: Active peptic ulcer disease, recent anastomosis
- Infections: Active TB (may give along with AKT), positive tuberculin test
- Metabolic: Diabetes mellitus
- Musculoskeletal: Osteoporosis
- Ocular: Cataracts, glaucoma
- Pregnancy

Human immunodeficiency virus (HIV) disease, even advanced HIV is not considered as a contraindication to short courses of systemic steroids. They are well tolerated and do not increase viral load or reduce CD4 count.

Q. What is the pregnancy prescribing status of corticosteroids?
A. Category C.

Q. How are corticosteroids metabolized and excreted?
A. Corticosteroids undergo reduction and conjugation in the liver to form relatively water soluble metabolites which are excreted by the kidneys.

Q. What are the equivalent doses and half-life of various corticosteroids?
A.

Corticosteroid	*Equivalent dose (mg)*	*Biologic half-life (hours)*
Cortisone	25	8–12
Hydrocortisone	20	8–12
Prednisone	05	24–36
Prednisolone	05	24–36
Methylprednisolone	04	24–36
Deflazacort	06	24–36
Triamcinolone	04	24–36
Dexamethasone	0.75	36–54
Betamethasone	0.75	36–54

Q. What are the various modes of delivering steroid therapy?
A. Options of therapy are:
- Short term oral therapy
- Long term oral therapy with tapering
- Intramuscular preparations (short and long acting)
- Intravenous delivery (daily or high dose pulses)

Q. Discuss short term oral therapy with corticosteroids.
A. This is therapy given for a duration of 3 weeks or less. The agent of choice is prednisolone or prednisone. Usually it is given in a single early morning dose, to avoid hypothalamic-pituitary-adrenal (HPA) axis suppression. The usual initial dose is 40–60 mg/day.

Q. Discuss long-term oral therapy.
A. It is therapy lasting for 4 weeks or longer, usually up to months or years. Prednisolone or methyl prednisolone are the best drugs for this because they allow the HPA axis to recover. It is always aimed to switch to alternate day therapy, because it allows the HPA axis to recover in the last 12 hours of the off-day of therapy.

Q. Discuss tapering of oral steroids.

A. The rate of steroid tapering depends on the nature of the disease, its severity, and the severity of side effects. Tapering of prednisolone can be accomplished by 20 mg decrease when the dose is greater than 60 mg/day, 10 mg reduction when the dosage is between 30–60 mg/day, and 5 mg reduction when the dosage is <30 mg/day. Once the physiological dose of about 5 mg/day is reached, the reduction should be in 1 mg decrements. Another method of decreasing is to convert from daily to alternate day therapy, once the prednisolone dose reaches 20–30 mg/day. The simplest method is to double the previous daily dose on the 'on' day and discontinue it on the 'off' day. Another way is to increase the 'on' day dose by 5 mg increments and decrease the 'off' day dose by 5 mg decrements.

Q. Discuss the advantages of alternate day therapy.

A. The following are the advantages of alternate day therapy:

- Recovery of HPA axis is faster
- Decreased risk of growth suppression, steroid myopathy and hypertension
- Decreases risk of opportunistic infections, electrolyte imbalances, and neuropsychiatric side effects
- However, two important side effects which are not minimized by alternate day therapy are osteoporosis and cataracts

Q. Discuss intramuscular (IM) and intravenous (IV) therapy.

A.

Drug	*Route*	*Concentration (mg/mL)*	*Duration of action*
Hydrocortisone sodium succinate	IM, IV	100–1000	4–6 hours
Dexamethasone phosphate	IM, IV	4	1–2 days
Betamethasone phosphate	IM	4	1–2 days
Triamcinolone acetonide	IM	40	21–25 days
Methylprednisolone acetate /succinate	IM–acetate IV–succinate	20–80	21–25 days

Q. What are the advantages and disadvantages of parenteral steroids over oral steroids?

A. Guaranteed compliance, and assured steady release of steroids through depot preparations. Also useful in patients with oral lesions who have difficulty in swallowing. The disadvantages of parenteral steroids are that it is nonphysiological, and there are risks of local problems like sterile abscesses at injection sites, or lipoatrophy (most common with triamcinolone). The other side effects are pain at site of injection, menstrual irregularities and purpura.

Q. Discuss pulse therapy with steroids.

A.
- Pulse therapy is therapy (usually parenteral) in a supra-pharmacological dose at regularly spaced intervals to treat a chronic and severe condition with the view of enhancing the therapeutic effect, increasing convenience of therapy, and reducing the side effects. Pulse therapy with steroids is usually given with either dexamethasone or methylprednisolone
- The dose of dexamethasone is 100 mg, while that of methyl prednisolone is 0.5–1 g. The medication is given as slow IV infusion in 5% dextrose over 2 hours on 3–5 consecutive days. It is often combined with 500 mg of cyclophosphamide on day 1, and 50 mg oral cyclophosphamide in the interval phase between pulses
- Pulse therapy in India was first used by Pasricha and Gupta for the treatment of Reiter's disease. However, it is today most commonly used for the treatment of pemphigus
- Other diseases responsive to pulse therapy are: Bullous pemphigoid, epidermolysis bullosa acquisita (EBA), systemic lupus erythematosus (SLE), pyoderma gangrenosum, systemic sclerosis, dermatomyositis, Behçet's syndrome, alopecia universalis

There are four phases of pulse therapy in pemphigus (Pasricha regimen):

1. DCP therapy at 28-day intervals with oral cyclophosphamide in the interval phase till all lesions heal (usually 6–9 months)
2. Same therapy as above continued for another 6–9 months after phase I
3. Only oral cyclophosphamide without IV dexamethasone for 9 months after phase II
4. Observation of the patient for 1 year without therapy

Q. Discuss the monitoring during pulse therapy.

A.
- Pulse, BP monitoring every 15 minutes for first hour, followed by every 30 minutes for rest of the time
- Pre-pulse investigations: Complete blood count (CBC), erythrocyte sedimentation rate (ESR), electrolytes, ECG, 2D echo, blood sugars, X-ray of chest, HIV, hepatitis B surface antigen, blood urea nitrogen (BUN)
- Post-pulse investigations: Electrolytes, RBS, BUN
- Intrapulse monitoring: CBC, LFT, RFT, sugars, urine routine analysis, X-ray of chest

Q. What are the side effects of pulse therapy?

A.
- Possible arrhythmias, and sudden death rarely if infusion is given too quickly. These are more common with methylprednisolone, due to acute hypokalemia. This may be prevented by infusion of potassium during therapy of methylprednisolone. This is not required with dexamethasone therapy, where hyperkalemia may occur
- Pulse therapy can increase the risk of osteoporosis and osteonecrosis, and also opportunistic infections due to its more potent immunomodulating effects

Q. Which patients have a higher risk for steroid toxicity?

A. Children, young adults and female patients are at a higher risk. Postmenopausal women are also at a higher risk. Patients with hypoalbuminemia, alcoholism, smokers and liver disease may get higher steroid toxicity. Patients with preexisting diseases like SLE, dermatomyositis, and rheumatoid arthritis (RA) may get more side-effects.

Q. What are the side effects of short-term glucocorticoid therapy?

A. Increased risk of infections, delayed wound healing, acneiform eruptions, GI side-effects, increased appetite, weight gain, fluid retention, muscle weakness, hyperglycemia, amenorrhea, mood changes.

Q. What are the side-effects of long term steroid therapy?

A.

System involved	*Specific side effects*
Gastrointestinal tract (GIT)	Nausea, vomiting, esophagitis, peptic ulcer disease and silent perforations, intestinal perforations, pancreatitis
Musculoskeletal	Myopathy, muscle atrophy, osteoporosis, avascular necrosis
Eye	Cataract (posterior subcapsular), glaucoma, hemorrhage, infections, exophthalmos
Metabolic	Growth retardation, hyperglycemia, hyperlipidemia, obesity, hypocalcemia, hypokalemic alkalosis
Gynecological/ obstetrics	Amenorrhea, menstrual irregularities (most with triamcinolone), fetal growth retardation (more with dexamethasone, less with prednisolone)
Hematological	Leukocytosis, neutrophilia, lymphopenia, eosinopenia, impaired fibroblast activity, immunosuppression and increased infections
Central nervous system (CNS)	Mood and personality changes, frank psychosis, seizures, pseudotumor cerebri, neuropathy

Q. What are the corticosteroid monitoring guidelines for long-term oral therapy?

A. Baseline

- Blood pressure, weight, height and weight on a growth curve in children
- Ophthalmoscopic examination of cataracts
- TB screening through tuberculin skin testing and chest X-ray
- Fasting glucose, triglycerides and potassium levels
- Dual energy X-ray absorptiometry (DEXA) scan in predisposed patients

Follow up: At 1 month, then every 3 months

- Blood pressure, weight, height and weight on a growth curve in children
- Ophthalmoscopic examination of cataracts and glaucoma every 6 months
- Thorough history to rule out adverse effects
- Fasting glucose, triglycerides and potassium levels every 3 months
- Near time of cessation of long-term therapy—morning cortisol levels
- DEXA scan repeated annually

Q. What are the drug interactions of corticosteroids?

A.
- Drugs that increase the serum levels and potential toxicity of corticosteroids:
  - Azole antifungal agents
  - Macrolide antibiotic agents
  - Sex steroids
- Drugs that decrease the serum levels or activity of corticosteroids:
  - Aminoglutethimide
  - Phenytoin, phenobarbital
  - Rifampin
  - Cholestyramine
  - Ephedrine
- Corticosteroids may increase the serum levels and potential toxicity of the following drugs:
  - Diuretics—potassium depleting
  - Immunosuppressants
  - Inotropic agents like digitalis
- Corticosteroids may decrease the serum levels or activity of following drugs:
  - Isoniazid
  - Insulin
  - Salicylates

- Other important variable interactions:
  - Anticoagulants; corticosteroids may increase or decrease warfarin activity
  - Xanthine bronchodilators; alterations in either theophylline or corticosteroid activity

Q. What are the cutaneous adverse effects from systemic corticosteroids?

A.
- Non-healing wounds, ulcers, striae, atrophy, telangiectasias
  - Steroid acne and steroid rosacea
  - Purpura including actinic purpura
  - Staphylococcal and herpes infections in particular
  - Telogen effluvium, hirsutism
  - Fat atrophy
  - Cushingoid features
  - Acanthosis nigricans
  - Rebound of poison ivy/oak, pustular psoriasis flare
  - Granuloma gluteale infantum (rare)

Q. What are the predictors of osteoporosis with steroids?

A. These are—postmenopausal females, history of high tobacco, alcohol or caffeine intake, calcium-poor or sodium-rich diet, prolonged immobilization, endocrine disorders like hyperthyroidism or hyperparathyroidism, and preexisting diseases like rheumatoid arthritis or renal failure.

Q. What are the ways to reduce steroid-induced osteoporosis?

A.
- Radiological screening for osteoporosis is an essential component. Plain X-ray is unreliable, because it is useful only when above 50% of the bone mass is lost. Hence, DEXA scan is used. It is sensitive, reproducible, involves low radiation exposure, and is quantifiable. DEXA scan is initially done on hip and lumbar spine and repeated annually at the same sites. The extent of osteoporosis is quantified by the 'T' score. A 'T' score of <2.5 signifies osteoporosis.
- The following measures are advised for patients on long-term GCS to reduce or prevent osteoporosis:
  - Tobacco avoidance
  - Restrict alcohol, caffeine
  - Weight-bearing exercises
  - Low sodium diet
  - Calcium (1.5 g) and vitamin D (800 IU) supplementation.
  - If urinary calcium is high, a thiazide diuretic can be added to decrease it.

- It is recommended that bisphosphonates may be started in high risk patients or if DEXA 'T' score 1–3. Alendronate 70 mg/week or Risedronate 35 mg/week, given early in the morning on empty stomach in the erect position. Bisphosphonates should be avoided during pregnancy. One rare but important side-effect is osteonecrosis of the jaw
- In patients in whom bisphosphonates are contraindicated, intranasal calcitonin may be given
- In patients who have failed to respond to bisphosphonates, teriparatide may be given which is a fragmented portion of human parathyroid hormone

Q. How can you differentiate between steroid myopathy and myositis?

A.

Steroid myopathy	*Myositis*
Weakness without myalgia	Weakness plus myalgia
Likely with high doses	Unlikely with high doses
Muscle tenderness absent	Muscle tenderness present
Normal creatine kinase (CK)	Elevated CK
Normal electromyography (EMG)	Abnormal EMG
Urine creatinine elevated but decreases on decreasing the dose	Urine creatinine elevated but increases with decreased dose
Muscle biopsy shows atrophy	Muscle biopsy shows myositis
Improves with decreased steroid dose	Worsens with decreased steroid dose

Q. Discuss osteonecrosis (avascular necrosis) occurring with steroid therapy.

A. It is believed to be secondary to intraosseous hypertension, leading to occlusion of terminal arterioles. Fat embolization is also believed to be important. It is more common in patients with alcoholism, cigarette smoking, fatty liver, hypertriglyceridemia, SLE, and post-renal transplant. Trauma is an inciting factor. The proximal femur is the most common site. Localized bone pain, initially during activity and later one even at rest is the usual symptom. MRI is the most sensitive and specific investigation. Early treatment is conservative (prevention of weight bearing) but more advanced cases may require core decompression, fibular grafting, or even arthroplasty.

Q. Discuss use of steroids in lupus erythematosus.

A. For cutaneous (discoid) lupus, only topical steroids are used, but systemic steroids can be used for widespread lesions. For subacute cutaneous lupus, steroids are used in conjunction with antimalarials. For lupus panniculitis it is often used as the first drug, while for bullous lupus, it is the second drug after dapsone. Steroids are the first line therapy for systemic lupus where they may be given alone or with immunosuppressive agents. Then, when psychosis develops in patients with SLE on glucocorticoids, it is often impossible to distinguish it from lupus psychosis. The only way is to reduce the dose. If the psychosis improves, it is likely to be steroid-induced psychosis.

Q. Discuss use of steroids in pemphigus.

A. Usually we start with 1–2 mg/kg/day of prednisolone, which is given for 1–3 months. After a good clinical response is seen, a very slow taper is recommended over the next one year, and after that the steroid can be stopped or given in an alternate day fashion. During this weaning process, cyclophosphamide, azathioprine, or mycophenolate mofetil can be added. Regular monitoring of anti-desmoglein antibody titers is recommended. Pulse therapy has been discussed above.

Q. Discuss steroids and psoriasis.

A. In general, systemic steroids should not be used for psoriasis. Though they cause immediate improvement, the patient slowly becomes refractory and the steroid dose has to be progressively increased. Moreover, taper of the steroids is often associated with a flare or even pustular psoriasis. However, steroids have been given in the past for arthropathic psoriasis, before better agents became available. They are still used in erythrodermic psoriasis where they may be lifesaving. As far as pustular psoriasis is concerned, impetigo herpetiformis, a variant occurring in pregnancy is treated with steroids, since acitretin, otherwise the drug of choice for pustular psoriasis, is contraindicated. Nowadays, cyclosporine is also used for this indication. Some dermatologists are still using systemic steroids for the treatment of "unstable" psoriasis where new lesions are rapidly forming. It is better to use cyclosporine in such a situation.

Q. Discuss the use of steroids in kerion.

A. Kerion often causes scarring alopecia, and this can be prevented by systemic steroids added to antifungals, at least in the initial phase. This may prevent scarring, and also dermatophytid reactions.

Q. Discuss the use of steroid in hemangiomas.

A. For life-threatening or functionally disruptive infantile hemangiomas, high dose systemic steroids are still important though oral and topical β-blockers are used routinely. Steroids prevent airway blockage, visual obstruction and ulcerations. The recommended dose is 2–3 mg/kg/day for atleast 8 weeks followed by tapering. Steroids play an important role in Kasabach–Merritt syndrome. With such a high dose, behavioral changes, irritability, and cushingoid appearance are common. Some doctors recommend prophylaxis for *Pneumocystis jirovecii* pneumonia (PJP) with cotrimoxazole.

Q. Discuss the use of steroid in herpes zoster.

A. Steroids limit the duration of acute neuralgia, but it is controversial whether it prevents postherpetic neuralgia. Many doctors give steroids with acyclovir in the treatment of herpes zoster in elderly patients or also in herpes zoster ophthalmicus. Dose is prednisolone 40–60 mg daily for 1–3 weeks with a rapid taper.

Q. Discuss the use of steroids in urticaria.

A. Steroids have to be used with antihistamines when there is angioedema with life threatening manifestations. However in acute urticaria itself, it may be used in severe situations in the dose of 1 mg/kg, for about 3–14 days. Its use in chronic urticaria is controversial because though effective, patients can become steroid dependent. Sometimes it is given in the same dose for 4–6 weeks. In autoimmune urticaria patients may not respond to steroids, and antimetabolites may have to be considered.

Q. Discuss the use of steroids in scleroderma.

A. Steroids along with methotrexate (MTX) or cyclophosphamide have been shown to be effective in rapidly spreading morphea, or in pansclerotic morphea. Steroids in the dose of 0.5–1 mg/kg of prednisolone are useful in systemic sclerosis to reduce the Rodnan skin score. However, high doses of steroids have been associated with malignant hypertension (scleroderma renal crisis) and should not be given. Pulse steroids have been used in systemic sclerosis with variable results. Steroids reduce the pulmonary complications of systemic sclerosis.

2.4. SYSTEMIC ANTIVIRAL DRUGS

Q. Discuss the historical development of antivirals.

A.
- The first antiviral developed was idoxuridine and Trifluorothymidine by William Prusoff who is often called as the father

of antiviral chemotherapy (*Note*: Paul Ehrlich is the father of antibacterial chemotherapy)

- In 1977, acyclovir was developed. The other agents later developed were famciclovir, penciclovir, ganciclovir and valacyclovir
- Valacyclovir is the prodrug of acyclovir, while famciclovir is the prodrug of penciclovir

Q. How do you classify antiviral drugs?

A.
- Antihuman herpes virus (anti-HHV) drugs:
  - Acyclovir, famciclovir, valacyclovir
- Anti-cytomegalovirus (anti-CMV) drugs:
  - Foscarnet, gancyclovir, cidofovir
- Antiretroviral drugs: (See later)

Q. List the available therapies for herpes virus infections.

A.
- Acyclovir
- Valacyclovir
- Famciclovir
- Penciclovir
- Ganciclovir/valganciclovir
- Cidofovir
- Fomivirsen
- Foscarnet

ACYCLOVIR

Introduction

Acyclovir is a synthetic purine nucleoside analog which is a derivative of acycloguanosine.

Q. What is the mechanism of action of this drug?

A. The active moiety is acyclovir triphosphate. It is a potent inhibitor of viral DNA polymerase thus inhibiting viral DNA synthesis. Acyclovir is first converted to acyclovir monophosphate by viral thymidine kinase, and then to acyclovir triphosphate in presence of cellular kinase. Viruses which are deficient in thymidine kinase will not respond to acyclovir (TK mutants).

Q. Describe the pharmacokinetics of acyclovir.

A. Oral acyclovir is incompletely absorbed from the GIT (about 20%). It is excreted by the kidney.

Q. What is the pregnancy category of this drug?

A. Pregnancy category B.

Q. What are its indications?

A. FDA approved:

- Herpes simplex infection—primary episode, recurrent episodes, suppressive therapy, in both immunocompetent and immunocompromized patients
- Varicella zoster infection—chicken pox, herpes zoster, in both immunocompetent and immunocompromized patients

Off-label indications:

- Recurrent herpes associated erythema multiforme
- Eczema herpeticum
- Herpetic whitlow
- Neonatal herpes

Q. What are the adverse effects of this drug?

A. Systemic:

- Hypersensitivity
- Headache, nausea, malaise
- Rash, sweating, hypotension, vomiting
- Reversible crystalluria-induced nephropathy due to intravenous acyclovir

Cutaneous:

- Morbilliform eruptions, Stevens-Johnson syndrome, urticaria, injection site reactions, angioedema
- In general incidence of side effects with acyclovir is very low.

Q. What are the contraindications of this drug?

A.
- Hypersensitivity to the drug, prodrug or any component.
- Dose adjustment required in patients with renal impairment, those taking any nephrotoxic medication.

Q. What are the doses and formulations available for this drug?

A. In immunocompetent patients:

- Primary herpes simplex virus (HSV) infection: 200 mg 5 times/day for 10 days
- Recurrent HSV infection: 200 mg 5 times/day for 5 days
- Chickenpox (in children): 20 mg/kg/dose times/day for 5 days
- Herpes zoster: 800 mg 5 times/day for 5 days

In immunocompromized patients:

- Primary HSV infection: 200–400 mg 5 times/day for 10 days
- Recurrent HSV infection: 400 mg TID/day for 7–10 days
- Chickenpox (children): 10 mg/kg IV 8 hourly for 7–10 days
- Herpes zoster: 800 mg 5 times/day for 5 days

Formulations:
- Tablets in dose of 200 mg, 400 mg, 800 mg available
- Injection 100 mL/vial containing 25 mg/mL acyclovir available
- 200 mg/5 mL banana flavored suspension

Q. What are its key points?

A.
- Sensitivity of acyclovir is more in HSV than varicella-zoster virus (VZV) so permit lower dose in HSV infection
- Duration and treatment in immunocompromized is longer and depends on clinical response
- Since acyclovir is excreted unchanged in urine, dose is to be reduced to 1/10th in case of renal failure
- All oral antivirals are supposed to be consumed with ample of water.

VALACYCLOVIR

Q. What is its chemical formulation?

A. L-valyl ester of acyclovir.

Q. What is its mechanism of action?

A. Valacyclovir is the prodrug of acyclovir. Mechanism of action is the same as acyclovir.

Q. What is its pregnancy category?

A. Pregnancy category B.

Q. What are its indications?

A.
- Initial and recurrent HSV genital infection
- Herpes zoster

Q. What are the adverse effect of this drug?

A. Hypersensitivity, headache, nausea and vomiting.

Q. What dose and formulations are available?

A.
- Primary HSV infection: 1,000 mg bd for 10 days
- Recurrent HSV infection: 500 mg bd for 5 days
- Prophylaxis for HSV infection: 1,000 mg od for 1–2 year
- Chickenpox: 1,000 mg tds for 5 days
- Herpes zoster: 1,000 mg tds for 5 days

Formulations:
- Formulations available in 500 mg and 1,000 mg tablet form

Q. What are the key points of this drug?

A.
- Valacyclovir has 45–50% oral bioavailability
- Convenient dosage schedule allows better compliance in patients
- Efficacy and safety profile not proven in immunocompromized patients

FAMCICLOVIR

Introduction

Famciclovir is a prodrug of penciclovir, an acyclic nucleoside.

Q. What is the mechanism of action of this drug?

A. Penciclovir is phosphorylated to pencyclovir triphosphate which inhibits viral DNA polymerase thereby inhibiting DNA synthesis.

Q. How is this drug metabolized?

A. Famciclovir is converted to penciclovir by deacetylation and oxidation in liver and intestine. Plasma half-life of penciclovir is 2 hours, and 60–70% drug is excreted in urine unchanged by glomerular filtration and tubular secretion.

Q. What is the pregnancy category of this drug?

A. Pregnancy category B.

Q. What are its indications?

A.
- Initial and recurrent HSV genital infection
- Herpes zoster

Q. What are the adverse effect of this drug?

A. Hypersensitivity, headache, nausea and vomiting.

Q. What dose and formulations are available for this drug?

A.
- Primary herpes simplex: 250 mg tds for 10 days
- Recurrent herpes simplex: 125 mg bid for 5 days
- Prophylaxis of HSV: 250 mg bd for 1–2 year
- Herpes zoster: 500 mg tds for 7 days
- Chickenpox: 500 mg tds for 5 days

Formulation:
- Available in tablet 125 mg, 250 mg and 500 mg

Q. What are the key points of this drug?

A. Famciclovir has a high oral bioavailability, more convenient dosage schedule, and may be preferred in immunocompromized patients. It has a doubtful role in preventing postherpetic neuralgia (PHN).

FOSCARNET

Introduction

It is a synthetic non-nucleoside analog. It is an analog of pyrophosphate.

Q. What is the mechanism of action of this drug?

A. It noncompetitively inhibits DNA polymerase by preventing the cleavage of pyrophosphate without the activation by cellular or viral kinase. It does not require phosphorylation for its antiviral activity and is therefore active against viruses that are resistant to acyclovir, famciclovir.

Q. What is pregnancy category of this drug?

A. Pregnancy category C.

Q. What are its indications?

A.
- Acyclovir resistant HSV infection
- Ganciclovir resistant CMV infection
- Treatment of CMV colitis
- Treatment of CMV retinitis in patients with AIDS

Q. What are the adverse effects of this drug?

A.
- Proteinuria
- Nephrogenic diabetes insipidus
- Increased creatinine level
- Hypokalemia, hypocalcemia, hypomagnesemia
- Headache, fatigue, fever, seizures
- Anemia, low white blood cell (WBC)
- In males, meatal irritation and ulceration (foscarnet ulcers), about 2 weeks after beginning of treatment

Q. Why is monitoring of the therapy required?

A.
- Use of foscarnet requires close monitoring of renal function especially at initial therapy due to its nephrotoxic effect and electrolyte abnormalities
- Renal function test and electrolytes should be checked frequently
- Saline hydration before administration and slow infusion of drug appear to reduce nephrotoxicity

Q. What dose and formulations are available for this drug?

A.
- 40 mg/kg 8 hourly for 10–42 days
- Available in injectable form

CIDOFOVIR

Introduction

Antiviral agent effective against cytomegalovirus (CMV).

Q. What is the mechanism of action of this drug?

A. Cidofovir is converted to cidofovir diphosphate by host cell enzymes. This acts as a competitive inhibitor of viral DNA polymerase and prevents transcription.

Q. What is the pregnancy category of this drug?

A. Pregnancy category C.

Q. What are its indications?

A.
- Treatment of CMV retinitis in patients with AIDS
- Treatment of resistant CMV infections
- Topical cidofovir is used for resistant molluscum contagiosum in immunocompromized patients (3% ointment has to be compounded)

Q. What are the adverse effects of this drug?

A.
- Renal tubular damage: Proteinuria, increased creatinine level, dose-dependent proximal tubular injury (Fanconi-like)
- Rash, nausea, alopecia, myalgia, fever

Q. What precautions has to be taken while starting this drug?

A. Intravenous hydration and oral probenecid appear to protect from nephrotoxicity.

Q. What dose and formulations are available for this drug?

A.
- Induction dose: 5 mg/kg IV once/week for 2 weeks
- Maintenance dose: 5 mg/kg IV every 2 weeks
- It has to be given in normal saline

GANCICLOVIR/VALGANCICLOVIR

Introduction

It is a deoxyguanosine analog. It accumulates in the virally infected cells and is phosphorylated by viral enzymes. This phosphorylated molecule competitively inhibits the incorporation of deoxyguanosine triphosphate into the viral DNA. Thus, DNA synthesis is inhibited.

Q. What are its indications?

A.
- It is approved for treatment and chronic suppression of CMV retinitis in AIDS patients

- Treatment of CMV pneumonia and CMV colitis in immunocompromized patients
- Prevention of CMV infections in renal transplant patients who are immunocompromized

Q. What dose and formulations are available for this drug?

A.
- Dose: 5 mg/kg bid given IV. May also be injected into the vitreous
- Oral valganciclovir can be used as a substitute for ganciclovir. Dose is 1 g 8 hourly orally, taken after food

Q. What are the adverse effects of this drug?

A. Side effects of both valganciclovir and ganciclovir are numerous and include myelosuppression, CNS toxicity and metabolic abnormalities.

FOMIVIRSEN

It is a phosphorothioate derivative. It acts through an antisense mechanism, to inhibit CMV replication. It is effective in cidofovir and ganciclovir resistant strains of CMV. It is given by intravitreal injection at the dose of 330 mg every two weeks. Adverse effects include iritis and glaucoma. The iritis can be treated by topical corticosteroids.

HELICASE–PRIMASE INHIBITORS

- This is a new class of drugs effective in resistant cases of herpes. There are two subtypes of this class, thiazole phenyls and thiazole ureas. Both these subtypes inhibit the helicase-primase complex, which is essential for DNA multiplication
- These drugs are effective in herpes virus but not against VZV and CMV

2.5. ANTIHISTAMINES

INTRODUCTION

Antihistamines are substances which antagonize the actions of histamine at the site of various receptors. They do so by acting as inverse agonists. The first clinically useful antihistamine was mepyramine. Its successor, diphenhydramine hydrochloride, was the first antihistamine formally introduced in North America in the late 1940s.

Q. Discuss histamine.

A. Histamine was first isolated by Sir Henry Dale in 1910. It is derived from L-histidine by the enzyme histidine decarboxylase. Histamine is an important mediator of immediate allergic reactions. It mediates its effects by binding to four receptor subtypes, H_1–H_4. Histamine is a very important neurotransmitter in the brain and hence inhibition of its action can cause drowsiness and sedation. Histamine is also a proinflammatory agent. Many antihistamines act by their anti-inflammatory properties in addition to their antihistaminic properties. This is particularly true of second generation antihistaminics, many of which inhibit eosinophil chemotaxis, inhibit leukotriene release and decrease intercellular adhesion molecule-1 (ICAM-1) expression.

Q. Classify antihistamines.

A.
- First generation antihistamines with their daily doses:
  - Ethanolamines—diphenhydramine (25–50 mg tid), clemastine (2 mg bid)
  - Alkylamines—chlorpheniramine (4–8 mg bid), brompheniramine (4–8 mg bid)
  - Ethylenediamines—pyrilamine and tripelennamine (4–8 mg bid)
  - Piperidines—cyproheptadine (4–8 mg bid), azatadine (1–2 mg tid)
  - Phenothiazines—promethazine (12.5–25 mg tid)
  - Piperazines—hydroxyzine (10–25 mg tid)
  - Antidepressants—doxepin hydrochloride (10–25 mg hs) (the most potent antihistamine)
- Second generation antihistamines (updosing is possible with many of these molecules up to 4 times their mentioned dose):
  - Piperazines-cetirizine (10 mg), levocetirizine (5 mg)
  - Piperidines-loratadine (10 mg), fexofenadine (180 mg), desloratadine (5 mg), mizolastine (10 mg), ebastine (10 mg), astemizole (not available)

Q. What is the mechanism of action of antihistamines?

A. H_1 and H_2 anithistamines are inverse agonists that down regulate the constitutively activated state of the corresponding receptors.

Q. What are the indications of anithistamines?

A.
- Allergic skin disorders—acute and chronic urticaria, angioedema, drug hypersensitivity, physical urticarias, chronic refractory urticaria
- Pruritus associated with skin lesions—scabies, lichen planus, atopic dermatitis, contact dermatitis, dermatitis herpetiformis, neurodermatitis
- Pruritus without skin lesions (antihistamines often not very useful)

- Mast cell stabilizing—mastocytosis
- Anti-inflammatory properties—bullous pemphigoid, type II lepra reaction

Q. Discuss first generation antihistamines.

A.
- H_1 antihistamines are inverse agonists that down-regulate the activated state of H_1 receptor. They do not bind significantly to H_2 (GI tract), H_3 receptors (pulmonary). They are relatively lipophilic and thus, cross the blood-brain barrier and bind to H_4 receptors in the brain, causing significant sedation. They reach plasma peak concentration in about 2 hours and are protein bound. They are metabolized via hepatic cytochrome P450 (CYP) system. In vitro these drugs decrease mediator release from mast cells and basophils
- Sometimes 1st generation antihistamines are used for anxiolytic effect (e.g., hydroxyzine)

Relative contraindications:
- Elderly individuals with cardiac problems
- Benign prostatic hyperplasia
- Chronic glaucoma
- Pregnancy and lactation
- Occupations requiring alertness and muscular coordination, e.g., drivers, heavy machinery operators, pilots, etc.

Adverse effects:
- Central nervous system—sedation, hyperexcitability (more common in children—paradoxical agitation), impaired cognitive function, increased appetite, blurred vision
- Gastrointestinal—dry mouth, constipation, epigastric discomfort, nausea, vomiting
- Genitourinary—dysuria, erectile dysfunction
- Cardiac—tachycardia, arrythmias
- Cutaneous (rare)—urticaria, maculopapular rash, fixed drug eruption, allergic contact dermatitis

Q. Write a note on second generation H_1 antihistamines.

A. They are inverse agonists of H_1 receptors. The most important feature is their high therapeutic index (ratio of minimum toxic dose and minimum therapeutic dose). They are poorly lipophilic and do not readily cross the blood-brain barrier. They have a highly selective action with little or no anticholinergic activity. Several nonsedating antihistamines have been developed—astemizole, terfenadine, loratadine, cetirizine, mizolastine, acrivastine, ebastine. The metabolite of loratadine (desloratadine) and the R-enantiomer (or L- isomer) of cetirizine (levocetirizine) and a derivative of terfenadine (fexofenadine) have also been introduced (so called 3rd generation antihistamines). Terfenadine and astemizole have been withdrawn from the market because of serious drug interactions involving QT interval prolongation, with resultant torsades de pointes. This is more common when they are given with drugs like erythromycin, cisapride and ketoconazole.

Q. Write a note on drug interactions of H_1 antihistamines.

A.
- Drugs that may increase serum levels of H_1 antihistamines and cause torsades de pointes with some of them:
  - Antibacterial/macrolides—erythromycin, clarithromycin
  - Azole antifungal agents—ketoconazole, and less commonly with itraconazole and fluconazole (doses 300 mg daily or higher)
  - HIV drugs/protease inhibitors—ritonavir, indinavir, saquinavir, nelfinavir
  - H_2 antihistamines—cimetidine
  - GI drugs—cisapride
- Drugs that may decrease serum levels and efficacy of several H_1 antihistamines by inducing the CYP3A4 system:
  - Antibacterial—rifamycin, rifabutin, rifapentine
  - Anticonvulsants—carbamazepine, phenobarbitone, phenytoin
- These drugs may lead to additive CNS depression along with sedating H_1 antihistamines:
  - Antidepressants—various tricyclics, nonselective reuptake inhibitors (venlafaxine)
  - Alcohol
  - Miscellaneous drugs—metoclopramide, thalidomide
  - Narcotics
  - Antipsychotic agents, barbiturates, central α_2 agonists, muscle relaxants
  - Sedatives—benzodiazepines, nonbenzodiazepines-zaleplon, zolpidem
- Other important interactions:
  - Monoamine oxidase inhibitors (MAOIs) like phenelzine, tranylcypromine, may intensify anticholinergic, sedative and other high-risk effects
  - Anticholinergic drugs such as darifenacin, solifenacin, disopyramide, doxazosin may increase the serum levels of low sedation H_1 antihistamines

Q. Discuss fexofenadine.

A. Fexofenadine is the pharmacologically active metabolite of prodrug terfenadine. Terfenadine undergoes hepatic metabolism via CYP3A4 system to its active metabolite fexofenadine. Fexofenadine is not metabolized by the liver and excreted unchanged. Only 20% is absorbed by the oral route. Elimination half-life is 11–15 hours. There is no evidence of cardiotoxicity with fexofenadine unlike with terfenadine. Therefore updosing of fexofenadine up to 720 mg/day (4 times the usual daily dose) is recommended for use in refractory urticaria.

Q. Discuss loratadine.

A. Loratadine is a piperidine tricyclic selective long acting, minimally sedating H_1 antihistamine. Its major metabolite is desloratadine. Its mean elimination half-life is 8–11 hours. It has negligible urinary excretion.

Q. Discuss cetrizine.

A. Cetirizine is the carboxylic acid metabolite of first generation H_1 antihsitamine hydroxyzine. It appears to have an inhibitory action on eosinophil accumulation and chemotaxis in various tissues. It is rapidly absorbed orally and its plasma half-life is 7 hours. Levocetirizine is the R-enantiomer of cetirizine and its major active metabolite.

Q. Write pediatric doses of antihistamines.

A. Some of the important doses are given below:

Generation	*Drugs*	*Dose*
1st	Diphenhydramine	1–5 mg/kg/day
1st	Hydroxyzine	2 mg/kg/day
2nd	Cetirizine	2–5 years: 2.5 mg od/bd 6–11 years: 5–10 mg/day >12 years: 10 mg/day
2nd	levocetirizine	>6 years: 5 mg/day
2nd	loratadine	2–12 years: 5 mg/day >12 years: 10 mg/day
2nd	Desloratadine	2–5 years: 1.25 mg/day 6–12 years: 2.5 mg/day >12 years: 5 mg/day
2nd	Fexofenadine	6–11 years: 30 mg bd >12 years: 60 mg bd

2.6. SYSTEMIC ANTIFUNGAL AGENTS

Treatment of superficial and deep dermatomycoses has improved considerably with the use and availability of modern antifungal agents.

Q. Classify systemic antifungal agents.

A. Systemic antifungal agents can be classified as:

- Allylamine—terbinafine.
- Azoles:
    - Imidazoles—ketoconazole
    - Triazoles:
        - 1st generation—fluconazole, itraconazole
        - 2nd generation—voriconazole, posaconazole, ravuconazole
- Antifungal antibiotics:
    - Heterocyclic benzofurans—griseofulvin obtained from mould *Penicillium griseofulvum*
    - Polyene antibiotics—amphotericin B

TERBINAFINE

It is an allylamine developed in 1974.

Pharmacokinetics:

- Skin—it is delivered to the stratum corneum by passive dermoepidermal diffusion, through sebum and migrating basal keratinocytes
- Nails—drug diffuses into the nail plate via nail bed and matrix
- Hair—drug is delivered to hair via the sebum or by hair matrix cells

Q. What is pregnancy category?

A. Pregnancy category B.

Q. What is the mechanism of action of terbinafine?

A. Mechanism of action—terbinafine causes fungal cell death by inhibiting squalene epoxidase, the main enzyme in sterol biosynthesis, resulting in ergosterol deficiency within fungal cell walls and accumulation of intracellular squalene. It has fungicidal activity against dermatophytes and some yeasts.

Q. What are the indications of terbinafine?

A. Indications are:

- **Superficial mycoses**

  FDA approved uses:
    - Onychomycosis caused by dermatophytes
    - Tinea capitis especially by species *Trichophyton tonsurans*

Off-label use (supported by significant clinical data):

- Onychomycosis causes by *Candida* species and non-dermatophyte molds.
- Tinea corporis/cruris
- Tinea pedis
- Majocchi's granuloma
- Tinea imbricata
- Pityriasis versicolor
- Seborrheic dermatitis

- **Deep or systemic fungal infections**

  Off-label uses (supported by significant clinical data):
  - Chromoblastomycosis
  - Aspergillosis
  - Cutaneous sporotrichosis
  - Black piedra

Q. What is the dosage of terbinafine?

A. Systemic dosage of terbinafine:

Dermatophytosis

- Adult—250 mg once daily for 2–4 weeks in tinea cruris, 6 weeks for tinea pedis, 4 weeks for tinea corporis and 6–12 weeks for nail infections
- Child—10–20 kg: 62.5 mg; 20–40 kg: 125 mg; >40 kg: 250 mg. Doses to be taken once daily. Treatment is usually given for 2 weeks for tinea capitis; 2–4 weeks for tinea cruris; 4 weeks for tinea corporis; 6 weeks in tinea pedis; 6–12 weeks for nail infections
- Terbinafine is also given as a pulse therapy for onychomycosis in the dose of 250 mg bd for 1 week/month for 3 consecutive months. This is however, not officially sanctioned by the FDA

Q. What are the contraindications for terbinafine?

A. Contraindications are:

- Hypersensitivity
- Active or chronic liver disease
- Lactation.

Q. What are the adverse effects of terbinafine?

A. Adverse effects are:

- Anorexia, nausea, abdominal pain, taste disturbances, diarrhea, rash, urticaria
- Potentially fatal—liver failure, Stevens-Johnson syndrome, neutropenia

ITRACONAZOLE

Q. What is pregnancy category?

A. Pregnancy category C.

Q. What is the mechanism of action of itraconazole?

A. Itraconazole decreases ergosterol biosynthesis by interfering with cytochrome P450 activity. This inhibits cell membrane function of susceptible fungi including *Microsporum* species, *Trichophyton* species, *Candida* species, *Cryptococcus neoformans, Histoplasma capsulatum, Blastomyces dermatitidis,* and *Paracoccidioides brasiliensis.* It is fungistatic. It also has antiprotozoal activity against *Leishmania major.*

Q. What are the indications for use of itraconazole?

A. Indications are:

- **Superficial mycoses**

  FDA approved uses:
  - Onychomycosis caused by dermatophytes
  - Oropharyngeal candidiasis (oral solution)
  - Esophageal candidiasis (oral solution)

  Off-label uses (supported by significant clinical data):
  - Onychomycosis caused by *Candida* species and non-dermatophyte molds
  - Tinea corporis/cruris
  - Tinea pedis
  - Majocchi's granuloma
  - Tinea imbricata
  - Pityriasis versicolor
  - Pityrosporum folliculitis
  - Seborrheic dermatitis
  - Chronic mucocutaneous candidiasis
  - Vaginal candidiasis
  - Cutaneous candidiasis
- **Deep or systemic fungal infections FDA approved uses:**
  - Blastomycosis
  - Histoplasmosis
  - Aspergillosis

  Off-label uses (supported by significant clinical data):
  - HIV-1 associated eosinophilic folliculitis

Q. What are the contraindications for itraconazole?

A. Contraindications are:

- Hypersensitivity to azole antifungals

- Pregnancy and lactation
- Hepatic disease
- IV: Creatinine clearance—<30 mL/min.

Q. What is the systemic dosage of itraconazole?

A. Systemic dosage of itraconazole for various infections are:

- Oral and esophageal candidiasis:
  - Oral liquid—200 mg daily in 1 or 2 divided doses held in the mouth for 20 s before swallowing
  - Double the dose in resistant infections
  - Capsule—100 mg daily for 15 days
- Prophylaxis of fungal infections in immunocompromised patients:
  - Adult: oral liquid—5 mg/kg daily in two divided doses.
- Vulvovaginal candidiasis:
  - Capsule—200 mg bid for 1 day
- Pityriasis versicolor:
  - Capsule—200 mg daily for 7 days
- Tinea cruris/corporis:
  - Capsule—100 mg daily for 15 days or 200 mg daily for 7 days
- Nail fungal infections:
  - Capsule—200 mg daily for 3 months. Alternatively, pulse therapy with 200 mg bid for 7 days, repeated once for fingernail infections and twice for toenail infections after drug-free intervals of 21-day
- Systemic fungal infections:
  - Capsule—100–200 mg once daily, increased to 200 mg bid for invasive or disseminated infections. For life-threatening infections: Loading dose of 200 mg tid for 3 days has been given
- Primary or secondary prophylaxis of infections in neutropenic or AIDS patients:
  - Capsule—200 mg daily increased to 200 mg bid, if necessary
- Tinea pedis:
  - Capsule—100 mg daily for 30 days or 200 mg bid for 7 days
- Tinea manuum:
  - Capsule—100 mg daily for 30 days or 200 mg bid for 7 days
- Intravenous:
  - Systemic fungal infections
  - 200 mg infused bid over 1 hour for 2 days. Maintenance—200 mg daily

Q. What are the adverse drug reactions of itraconazole?

A.
- Dyspepsia
- Abdominal pain
- Nausea, vomiting, diarrhea
- Menstrual disorders
- Constipation, rash, pruritus, urticaria
- Angioedema, anaphylaxis
- Increased liver enzyme values, jaundice, Stevens-Johnson syndrome, hypokalemia
- Potentially fatal—liver failure; heart failure; pulmonary edema; cardiovascular disease

FLUCONAZOLE

Q. What is pregnancy category?

A. Pregnancy category D.

Q. What is the mechanism of action of fluconazole?

A. Fluconazole decreases ergosterol synthesis by interfering with cytochrome P450 activity, thus inhibiting cell membrane formation of susceptible fungi including *Blastomyces dermatitidis, Candida* species, *Coccidioides immitis, Cryptococcus neoformans, Epidermophyton* species, *Histoplasma capsulatum, Microsporum* species, *Trichophyton* species, thus leading to cell death. It is a fungistatic agent.

Q. What are the indications of fluconazole?

A. Indications are:

- **Superficial mycoses**

  FDA approved uses:
  - Vaginal candidiasis
  - Oropharyngeal candidiasis
  - Esophageal candidiasis

  Off-label uses (supported by significant clinical data):
  - Onychomycosis caused by dermatophytes and *Candida* species.
  - Tinea corporis/cruris
  - Tinea pedis
  - Tinea capitis
  - Pityriasis versicolor
  - Chronic mucocutaneous candidiasis
  - Cutaneous candidiasis

- **Deep or systemic fungal infections**
  FDA approved uses:
  - Systemic *Candida* infection—prophylaxis (transplant patients receiving chemotherapy and/or radiation therapy)
  - Cryptococcal meningitis

  Off-label uses (supported by significant clinical data):
  - Lymphocutaneous and visceral fungal infections

Q. What are the contraindications for fluconazole?
A. Hypersensitivity.

Q. What is the systemic dosage of fluconazole?
A. Systemic dosage of fluconazole for various diseases are:

Superficial mucosal candidiasis:

Adult:
- Except genital candidiasis—50 mg daily, may increase to 100 mg daily, if needed. Recommended treatment duration
- 7–14 days (oropharyngeal candidiasis, except in severely immunocompromised patients)
- 14 days (atrophic oral candidiasis associated with dentures)
- 14–30 days (other mucosal candidiasis including esophagitis).

Child:
- >4 weeks: Loading dose—6 mg/kg followed by 3 mg/kg daily
- Renal impairment—normal initial doses; adjust subsequent doses based on CrCl. Patients on dialysis—single recommended dose after each session

Vaginal candidiasis
- 150 mg as a single dose

Candidal balanitis
- 150 mg as a single dose

Dermatophytosis/pityriasis versicolor/cutaneous candidiasis
- 50 mg daily for up to 6 weeks, or
- 150 mg/week for upto 6 weeks
- 400 mg single stat dose for pityriasis versicolor
- Renal impairment—normal initial doses; adjust subsequent doses based on CrCl. Patients on dialysis—single recommended dose after each session

If creatinine clearence is <50 and patient is not on dialysis the dose is reduced to 50% of recommended dose.

Systemic candidiasis

Adult:

- Initially, 400 mg followed by 200–400 mg daily. Maximum—800 mg daily in severe infections
- 6–8 weeks in cryptococcal meningitis
- To prevent relapse after a primary course of treatment for acute cryptococcal meningitis in AIDS patients: 100–200 mg daily, may also be given via intravenous (IV) admin

Child:

- >4 weeks: 6–12 mg/kg daily; Maximum—400 mg daily

Prophylaxis of fungal infections in immunocompromised patients:

- Adult: 50–400 mg daily. May also be given via IV infusion
- Child: 3–12 mg/kg daily

***Note*:**

- Renal impairment—normal initial doses; adjust subsequent doses based on creatinine clearance. Patients on dialysis—single recommended dose after each session

Creatinine clearance (mL/min)	Dosage recommendation
<50 and not receiving dialysis	Maintenance dose: 50% of the recommended doses

Q. What are the adverse drug effects of fluconazole?

A. Adverse drug effects are:

- Nausea, abdominal pain, vomiting, diarrhea, flatulence
- Elevated liver function values
- Headache
- Rash, exfoliative dermatitis
- Rarely, angioedema, anaphylactic reactions, and thrombocytopenia
- Potentially fatal—hepatotoxicity; rarely anaphylaxis; Stevens-Johnson syndrome

KETOCONAZOLE

Q. What is pregnancy category?

A. Pregnancy category C.

Q. What is the mechanism of action of ketoconazole?

A. Ketoconazole interferes with biosynthesis of triglycerides and phospholipids by blocking fungal cytochrome P450, thus altering cell membrane permeability in susceptible fungi. It also inhibits other fungal enzymes resulting in the accumulation of toxic concentrations of hydrogen peroxide. It is a fungistatic agent.

Q. What are the indications for ketoconazole?

A. Indications are:

- **Superficial mycoses:**
  FDA approved uses:
  - Tinea corporis/cruris (severe recalcitrant)
  - Tinea pedis (severe recalcitrant)
  - Tinea capitis (severe recalcitrant)
  - Chronic mucocutaneous candidiasis
  - Vaginal candidiasis
  - Cutaneous candidiasis

  Off-label uses (supported by significant clinical data):
  - Pityriasis versicolor
  - Seborrheic dermatitis
- **Deep or systemic fungal infections**
  FDA approved uses:
  - Chromoblastomycosis
  - Blastomycosis
  - Histoplasmosis
  - Coccidio and paracoccidioidomycosis

Q. What is the dosage of ketoconazole?

A. Dose of ketoconazole:

- Fungal infections—200 mg once daily, up to 400 mg once daily if needed. Usual duration—14 days and for at least 1 week after symptoms have cleared and cultures have become negative
- Chronic vaginal candidiasis—400 mg once daily for 5 days

Q. What are the contraindications of ketoconazole?

A. Contraindications are:

- Hypersensitivity
- Pre-existing liver disease
- Porphyria
- Concurrent use with cisapride, terfenadine or astemizole

Q. What are the adverse effects of ketoconazole?

A. Adverse effects are:

- Gastrointestinal (GI) disturbances, e.g., nausea and vomiting
- Rash, dermatitis, burning sensation, pruritus
- Headache, dizziness, somnolence, fever and chills

- Thrombocytopenia
- Gynecomastia, impotence
- Raised intracranial pressure, photophobia
- Transient elevations in liver function tests (LFTs)

Potentially fatal: Hepatotoxicity which may be silent or anicteric. There is a mortality of 1 in 10,000 with ketoconazole.

VORICONAZOLE

Q. What is the pregnancy category?
A. Pregnancy category D.

Q. What is the mechanism of action of voriconazole?
A. Voriconazole is a triazole antifungal agent which inhibits cytochrome P450-dependent enzymes thereby inhibiting ergosterol synthesis in fungal cell membranes. It has a broad spectrum of activity against all *Candida* species (including strains resistant to fluconazole), *Aspergillus* species, *Scedosporium* species, and *Fusarium* species.

Q. What are the indications of voriconazole?
A. Indications are:

- **Superficial mycoses**
  FDA approved uses:
  - Esophageal candidiasis
- **Deep or systemic fungal infections**
  FDA approved uses:
  - Aspergillosis
  - Systemic *Candida* infection (non-neutropenic and disseminated candidiasis)
  - *Scedosporium apiospermum* and *Fusarium* species. Infections (patients intolerant of or refractory to other therapy)

Q. What is the dose of voriconazole?
A. Dose of voriconazole:

- Candidemia; deep tissue *Candida* infections; invasive aspergillosis; scedosporiosis and fusariosis-
- Oral: >40 kg—400 mg 12 hourly for the first 24 hours. Maintenance—200 mg 12 hourly, up to 300 mg 12 hourly, if needed
- <40 kg—200 mg 12 hourly for the first 24 hour. Maintenance—100 mg 12 hourly, up to 150 mg 12 hourly, if needed
- IV-loading dose—6 mg/kg 12 hourly for the first 24 hour. Maintenance—4 mg/kg 12 hourly (3–4 mg/kg 12 hourly for

candidemia in non-neutropenic patients or patients intolerant of high doses)

- Maximum duration—6 month, maximum infusion rate—3 mg/kg/h over 1–2 hour

Q. What are the contraindications for voriconazole?

A. Contraindications are:

- Hypersensitivity
- Lactation.

Q. What are the adverse effects of voriconazole?

A. Adverse effects are:

- Transient and reversible visual disturbances
- Fever; headache; abdominal pain; chills
- Asthenia; back pains; chest pain; face edema
- Flu-like syndrome
- Hypotension; thrombophlebitis; phlebitis
- GI disturbances (e.g., nausea, vomiting, diarrhea); jaundice; cheilitis; cholestatic jaundice; gastroenteritis
- Blood dyscrasias; purpura; peripheral edema; facial edema
- Hypokalemia; hypoglycemia
- Dizziness; hallucinations; confusion; depression; anxiety; tremor; agitation; paresthesia
- Respiratory distress syndrome; sinusitis
- Rash; pruritus; photosensitivity; alopecia; exfoliative dermatitis
- Acute kidney failure; hematuria; infusion-related reactions.
- Increased LFT and serum creatinine; prolongation of QT interval

Potentially fatal: Stevens–Johnson syndrome, toxic epidermal necrolysis.

POSACONAZOLE

Q. What is pregnancy category?

A. Pregnancy category C.

Q. What is the mechanism of action of posaconazole?

A. Blocks the synthesis of ergosterol, a key component of the fungal cell membrane, through the inhibition of the enzyme lanosterol 14 alpha-demethylase and accumulation of methylated sterol precursors. Posaconazole has activity against *Candida* species, *Aspergillus* species, *Coccidioides immitis*, *Fonsecaea pedrosoi*, and some species of *Fusarium* and zygomycetes.

Q. What are the indications of posaconazole?

A. Indications are:

- **Superficial mycoses**
  FDA approved uses:
  - Onychomycosis caused by dermatophytes
  - Tinea corporis/cruris
  - Tinea pedis
  - Tinea capitis

  Off-label uses (supported by significant clinical data):
  - Tinea imbricata
- **Deep or systemic fungal infections**
  FDA approved uses:
  - Aspergillosis (prophylaxis-immunocompromised patients)
  - Systemic *Candida* infection (prophylaxis-immunocompromised patients)

Q. What is the dosage of posaconazole?

A. Dose of posaconazole:

Oral

- Prophylaxis of invasive fungal infections—200 mg 3 times/day
- Oropharyngeal candidiasis—loading: 100 mg twice daily on 1st day; maintenance: 100 mg once daily for 13 days
- For cases which are refractory to itraconazole and/or fluconazole—400 mg twice daily; treatment duration is based on patient's underlying disease and clinical response

Q. What are the contraindications of posaconazole?

A. Hypersensitivity. Coadministration with sirolimus, ergot alkaloids, CYP3A4 substrates (terfenadine, astemizole, cisapride, pimozide, halofantrine, or quinidine).

Q. What are the adverse effects of posaconazole?

A. Adverse effects are:

- Fever, headache, rigors, fatigue, edema
- Dizziness, weakness, blurred vision
- Diarrhea, nausea, vomiting, abdominal pain, constipation
- Anorexia, anemia
- Febrile neutropenia, thrombocytopenia
- Petechiae, thrombotic thrombocytopenic purpura
- Electrolyte imbalance
- Bacteremia, herpes simplex, cytomegalovirus infection
- Increased LFT's and bilirubin; increased serum creatinine; adrenal insufficiency.
- Potentially fatal—hypersensitivity reactions, Stevens-Johnson syndrome, QT-prolongation, hepatic failure, pulmonary embolus

GRISEOFULVIN

Griseofulvin is derived from *Penicillium griseofulvum.*

Q. What is pregnancy category?

A. Pregnancy category C.

Q. What is the mechanism of action of griseofulvin?

A. Griseofulvin is a fungistatic antibiotic that inhibits fungal cell division at metaphase and binds to human keratin making it resistant to fungal infections. It has activity against common dermatophytes including *Epidermophyton, Microsporum,* or *Trichophyton* species.

Q. What are the indications of griseofulvin?

A. Griseofulvin is indicated for:

- Dermatophyte infections of the skin, scalp, and nails
- Tinea infection of nails (6–9 months treatment due to poor keratin penetration of drug)
- Tinea imbricata

Q. What is the dose of griseofulvin?

A. Dermatophytosis

- Adult:
  - 0.5–1 g daily in single or divided doses for 2–8 weeks in hair and skin infections
  - Tinea corporis/cruris—250 mg bid until cure
  - Tinea pedis—1000 mg od or 500 mg bd daily for 4–8 weeks
  - 6 months in fingernail infections and 12 months or more for toenail infections
  - Tinea imbricata—500 mg bid for 4–6 weeks, may require concomitant topical therapy
- Child—10 mg/kg daily.

Q. What are the contraindications for griseofulvin?

A. Contraindications are:

- Severe liver disease
- Porphyria
- Monilial infection
- Systemic lupus erythematosus (SLE); pregnancy

Q. What are the adverse effects of griseofulvin?

A. Adverse effects are:

- Oral thrush
- GI distress, taste alteration
- Dizziness, confusion, headache (very common), depression, insomnia, fatigue

- Peripheral neuritis, photosensitivity
- Skin rashes, urticaria, erythema multiforme
- Leukopenia, proteinuria.
- Precipitation of acute intermittent porphyria
- *Potentially fatal*: hepatotoxicity; angioedema.

Comparison of itraconazole, fluconazole, and terbinafine

Properties	***Itraconazole***	***Fluconazole***	***Terbinafine***
Chemistry	Triazole	Bis-triazole	Allylamine
Lipophilicity	++	-	++
Mechanism of action	Inhibition of lanosterol demethylase	Inhibition of lanosterold-emethylase	Inhibition of squalene-epoxidase
CYP450 dependance	Yes	Yes	No
Effect on human sterol synthesis	Weak	Almost none	None
Resistance	Very rare	Rare	Very rare
Absorption	Requires acidic pH	Independent of pH and food	Independent of pH and food
Peak plasma concentration	At 5 hours	At 3 hours	At 2 hours
Plasma protein binding	>99%	12%	>98%
Metabolism in liver	Extensive	None	Extensive
Excretion	Urine + Feces	Urine	Urine + Feces
Diffusion to the skin	Through capillary vessels and sebum	Through capillary vessels and sweat	Through capillary vessels and sebum
Drug in the nails	Slow to appear but long persistence for 9 months	Rapid to appear but shorter persistence for 3–6 months	Rapid to appear but shorter persistence for 3–6 months

Potentially dangerous or life-threatening interactions with itraconazole:

- Patient taking any one of the following medications like lovastatin, simvastatin, triazolam, midazolam, and ergot alkaloids
- Arrhythmias can result if a patient is taking quinidine, dofetilide, cisapride and pimozide

ECHINOCANDINS

Q. Discuss the new class of antifungals called echinocandins.

A. The echinocandins are cyclic hexapeptides, which are systemically effective antifungals. They inhibit the synthesis of 1,3-β-d-glucan, a key component of the fungal cell wall. Caspofungin was the first echinocandin introduced, and recently anidulafungin and micafungin are also available.

Mechanism of action: By inhibiting glucan synthesis, they interfere with the structural integrity of the fungal cell wall. This causes osmotic destabilization and eventual cell lysis. Echinocandins also demask the glucan antigen thus enhancing immune recognition of the fungus by the body. As cell wall is not present in mammalian cells, interference of echinocandins with host metabolism is less.

Spectrum of action: *Candida* and *Aspergillus* species. They are ineffective against *Cryptococcus, Trichosporum, Fusarium,* and dematiaceous fungi species since all these lack glucan in the cell wall.

Pharmacokinetics: Only effective intravenously. Half life of anidulafungin is the longest (26 hours). It is metabolized independent of live enzymes while the other two are metabolized in livet.

Drug interactions: Caspofungin and micafungin interact with immune suppressants like cyclosporine and tacrolimus while anidulafungin has no significant interactions.

Side effects: Usually mild, histamine mediated immune reactions, skin rashes, liver dysfunction.

Doses: Treatment with anidulafungin and caspofungin starts with an initial loading dose of 200 or 70 mg, respectively, followed by a maintenance dose of 100 mg daily of anidulafungin or 50 mg daily of caspofungin. Micafungin is administered at 100 mg once per day.

Indications: Caspofungin and anidulafungin are licensed for the treatment of invasive *Candida* infections in adult patients.

Caspofungin is licensed for second-line treatment of invasive aspergillosis and empiric treatment of neutropenic patients with fever and suspected fungal infection. Micafungin is licensed for invasive candidiasis, esophageal candidiasis and prophylaxis of *Candida* infections in patients undergoing allogeneic blood stem-cell transplantation.

2.7. IMMUNOMODULATORS

AZATHIOPRINE

Q. Which is the parent drug of azathioprine?

A. 6-mercaptopurine (6-MP). An imidazole ring is attached to 6–MP to make azathioprine. Azathioprine seems to have a favorable therapeutic index over methotrexate, 5-fluorouracil and actinomycin-C. It is also substantially more affordable than agents like cyclosporine.

Q. What are the pros and cons of ordering baseline testing for thiopurine methyltransferase (TPMT) enzyme activity prior to initiating azathioprine therapy?

A. The pre-treatment TMPT enzyme testing may avoid catastrophic myelosuppression and guide proper dosing.

Q. Discuss metabolism of azathioprine.

A.

- Azathioprine is converted in the body by sulfhydryl compounds, to form 6-MP. This mercaptopurine molecule undergoes metabolism from three enzymes:
  - The catabolic enzyme thiopurine-S-methyltransferase (TPMT)
  - The catabolic enzyme xanthine oxidase
  - As a result of these enzyme activities, inactive metabolites are produced and decrease in their activity can increase toxicity
  - The anabolic enzyme hypoxanthine-guanine phosphoribosyltransferase (HPRT). HPRT produces active inosine monophosphate dehydrogenase and 6-thioguanine which are the most active metabolites
- These active metabolites disrupt the function of endogenous purines. This causes interference with the building blocks of DNA, RNA, and certain co-enzymes. Most cells have a salvage pathway and can resist this action to a certain extent. However, lymphocytes do not have such a pathway. Hence, they are peculiarly susceptible to azathioprine.

- Also, patients with Lesch-Nyhan syndrome have a mutated *HPRT* gene. Hence active metabolites are not produced. Hence patients with this syndrome do not respond well to azathioprine.
- The *TPMT* gene has got extremely variable activity. 0.3% patients have low TPMT activity and these individuals are likely to show toxicity with azathioprine. However, this mutation is very less common in India.

Q. What is the pregnancy category of azathioprine?

A. Pregnancy category D. It is not advised in lactating patients.

Q. What are the indications for azathioprine?

A. All dermatological indications of azathioprine are off-label.

- Immunobullous diseases—both pemphigus and pemphigoid respond to azathioprine. However, it has to be used in conjunction with steroids (steroid-sparing agent). It is more effective in pemphigoid compared to pemphigus
- Psoriasis—it is not so effective in the management of psoriasis. However, it can be used in severe cases where methotrexate produces side effects
- Eczematous diseases—azathioprine is extremely useful in disseminated eczematous eruptions
- Photodermatitis—it is useful in chronic actinic dermatitis (photosensitive eczema, persistent light reactions, and actinic reticuloid). It is extremely useful in severe polymorphous light eruptions and parthenium dermatitis where some people believe it is the drug of choice rather than steroids
- Miscellaneous—type II lepra reaction, Behçet's syndrome, cutaneous lupus, pityriasis rubra pilaris (PRP), erythema multiforme, vasculitis, scleroderma, dermatomyositis

Q. What are the pediatric uses?

A. Severe eczemas, systemic lupus erythematosus (SLE), dermatomyositis. However, it should be used only when other therapies fail. Treatment should not be continued for >6 months at a time.

Q. What are the drug interactions with azathioprine?

A. Azathioprine is absolutely contraindicated with allopurinol which is also a xanthine oxidase inhibitor. Concomitant use can result in severe hematologic toxicity. If both medications are absolutely essential, start azathioprine at 1/4th of the original dose. Azathioprine can also induce warfarin resistance, which can be manifest as severe bleeding after discontinuation of warfarin. Recurrent thrombosis has also been reported with this interaction.

Benzoic acid derivatives like sulfasalazine, increase active thiogunanine nucleotides and can cause hematologic side-effects. Prolonged use of cotrimoxazole with azathioprine can cause neutropenia.

Q. What are the absolute contraindications?

A.
- Pregnancy
- Hypersensitivity to azathioprine
- Active infections

Q. What are the relative contraindications?

A.
- Allopurinol use
- Prior use of alkylating agents

Q. What are the adverse effects?

A.
- Common side-effects:
  - Gastrointestinal (GI) side-effects like nausea, vomiting, and discomfort. If severe azathioprine has to be discontinued as this may be a part of hypersensitivity reaction
  - Bone marrow depression is a well-accepted concern, for which proper hematologic monitoring has to be done
  - Skin problems are more common with transplant patients, which may include alopecia, and fungal, bacterial and viral infections
- Uncommon side-effects—azathioprine hypersensitivity reaction can occur within the first four weeks and presents with GI symptoms, hypotension, and even death.

  Pancreatitis has been reported to occur as well as hepatic damage due to veno-occlusive disease.
- Malignancy potential—patients on higher and longer duration of azathioprine have been reported to have premalignant lesions followed by aggressive squamous cell carcinoma (SCC). This is more common in patients who are exposed to sunlight. There is also an increased risk of lymphomas. In dermatology patients, however, the doses used are lower and the risk of cancer is similar to other anti-metabolites.

Q. What is the dosage of azathioprine?

A. 2.5 mg/kg body weight in a patient with normal TPMT activity (14–20 U/mL)

In patients with low activity (<5 U), it should not be used while with intermediate activity (5–14 U) dose is 1 mg/kg body weight. Patients with high TPMT should be given 3 mg/kg body weight.

Q. What are the monitoring guidelines?

A. Baseline:

- Laboratory:
  - Pregnancy test
  - Complete blood count (CBC)
  - Serum lipid profile
  - Urine analysis
  - Tuberculin skin test
- Special test:
  - TPMT assay

Follow-up

- Laboratory (bi-weekly for first 2 months, every 2–3 months thereafter)
- CBC should be done bi-monthly
- Complete metabolic panel – monthly for first 2 months and then every 3 months
- Complete skin examination should be done once a year

CYCLOSPORINE

Q. What is cyclosporine derived from?

A. From a fungus *Tolypocladium inflatum* gams. It was initially developed as an anti-fungal agent. It was found to be extremely useful as an immunosuppressant in 1978. In 1979, it was found to be useful in psoriasis by chance (serendipity – other examples of serendipity in dermatology are methotrexate for psoriasis, minoxidil in male pattern baldness and thalidomide in lepra reactions). It was approved for the treatment of psoriasis in 1997.

Q. What is the structure of cyclosporine?

A. It is a neutral cyclic polypeptide composed of 11 amino acids.

Q. What is the mechanism of action?

A. Cyclosporine selectively acts on T-cells (helper > suppressor). Cyclosporine forms a complex with cyclophilin which is an intracellular immunophilin. This complex then inhibits the activity of calcineurin phosphatase which is normally involved in phosphorylation of nuclear factor of activated T-cells (NFAT). If phosphorylation of NFAT doesn't take place, transcription of certain genes required for full activation of the T-cell pathways doesn't occur. Consequently, T-cells are depleted. IL-2 seems to be the main cytokine required for this pathway which is targeted by cyclosporine. Cyclosporine also inhibits natural killer (NK) cells antigen presenting cells (APCs), keratinocytes and also down-regulates ICAM.

Q. Why is grapefruit juice avoided with cyclosporine?
A. Grapefruit increases levels of cyclosporine.

Q. What was cyclosporine used as initially when discovered?
A. It was used as an antifungal-antibiotic.

Q. What are the versions of cyclosporine?
A. It is available in two versions sandimmune and neoral.

Q. What are the differences between both the versions?
A. The original molecule, sandimmune, is less hydrophilic, while the newer version, neoral, has greater bioavailability and smaller variation in serum levels.

Q. What is the pregnancy category?
A. Pregnancy category C.

Q. What are the indications?
A. FDA approved

- Psoriasis

Non-FDA approved

- Atopic dermatitis
- Lichen planus
- Pemphigus
- Pemphigoid
- Epidermolysis bullosa acquisita
- Dermatomyositis
- Lupus erythematosus
- Scleroderma
- Behçet's disease
- Pyoderma gangrenosum
- Alopecia areata
- Granuloma annulare
- Sarcoidosis
- Pityriasis rubra pilaris
- Chronic actinic dermatitis
- Chronic urticaria, cold urticaria, solar urticaria

Q. What are the absolute contraindications?
A.
- Significantly decreased renal function
- Uncontrolled hypertension
- Serious infections

- Hypersensitivity to cyclosporin A (CsA) or any ingredients in formulation
- Previous history of malignancy except basal cell carcinoma (BCC)
- Previous high cumulative dose of psoralen plus ultraviolet A (PUVA) therapy

Q. What are the relative contraindications?

A.
- Age <18 years or >64 years
- Controlled hypertension
- Planning to receive a live attenuated vaccination
- On medications that interfere with cyclosporine metabolism or potentiate renal dysfunction
- Active infection or evidence of immunodeficiency
- Concomitantly receiving phototherapy, methotrexate, or other immunosuppressive agents
- Pregnancy or lactation
- Unreliable patients

Q. What are the specific indications for cyclosporine therapy in psoriasis?

A.
- Patients with severe flare ups
- Extensive psoriasis [> 20 % body surface area (BSA)]
- Psoriatic erythroderma
- Pustular psoriasis
- Psoriatic arthropathy
- Patients with severe or disabling psoriasis who cannot tolerate, have contraindications to, or have filled other systemic therapies.
- Patient with major life events (such as wedding) where substantial clearing is critically important

Q. What are the regimens of cyclosporine used in psoriasis?

A.
- Intermittent short-term therapy over 12–16 weeks (2.5–5 mg/kg body weight for 2–16 weeks)
- Rescue/bridging therapy along with acitretin–particularly useful in erythrodermic or pustular psoriasis. Here the initial dosage is higher (5 mg/kg body weight for 12–16 weeks)
- Long-term therapy (<5 mg/kg body weight for upto 1 year with gradual tapering)
- Combination with other drugs [3–4 mg/kg body weight combined with topical steroids, anthralin, vitamin D3 analogs, methotrexate (MTX), monomethyl fumarate (MMF), and fumaric acid esters]

- Rotational therapy (3–4 mg/kg body weight for 6–12 months, rotated with other modalities of therapy to avoid cumulative toxicity)

Cyclosporine is an effective modality for psoriatic arthropathy but can cause quick relapse.

Q. Drugs that increase the levels of cyclosporine.

A.
- Beta blockers
- Statins
- Oral contraceptive pills
- Diuretics
- Tetracyclines
- Ciprofloxacin

Q. Which are the drugs that decrease the levels of cyclosporine?

A.
- Rifampicin
- Isoniazid (INH)
- Anticonvulsants
- Terbinafine

Q. Which are the drugs which increase the renal toxicity of cyclosporine?

A.
- Nonsteroidal anti-inflammatory drugs (NSAIDs)
- Cotrimoxazole
- Methotrexate
- Aminoglycosides

Q. What are the common adverse effects?

A.
- Renal dysfunction
- Hypertension
- Tremors
- Headache
- Paresthesia, hyperesthesia
- Hypertrichosis
- Gingival hyperplasia
- Nausea, abdominal discomfort, diarrhea
- Myalgia, lethargy
- Arthralgia
- Hyperkalemia, hyperuricemia, hypomagnesemia, hyperlipidemia
- Reactivation of tuberculosis

Q. Discuss cyclosporine and renal dysfunction.

A. It is suggested that cyclosporine causes most of its side effects by interfering with mitochondrial ion channel regulation. Most cases of renal dysfunction are associated with prolonged therapy or higher doses. The changes in the kidney may be functional or structural. Functional impairment is usually in the short term. It is caused by vascular dysfunction [vasoconstriction of afferent blood vessels causing decreased glomerular filtration rate (GFR) and decreased creatinine clearance]. Tubular dysfunction causes decreased magnesium reabsorption, decreased bicarbonates and hyperkalemia. Endothelin-1 has been implicated in the vascular dysfunction. Structural impairment is usually due to chronic nephrotoxicity. It causes vasculopathy (arteriolar thrombus formation) and tubulopathy (necrosis in the proximal tubules). Tubulopathy is reversible whereas vasculopathy is potentially irreversible. The best predictor of permanent renal damage is a persistent increase in renal creatinine even 1 month after stopping therapy. Regular blood pressure monitoring and serum creatinine levels are mandatory when a patient is on cyclosporine especially with pre-existing or new onset hypertension, older age, obesity, concomitant nephrotoxic medications and pre-existing renal pathology.

Q. What are the monitoring guidelines?

A. Baseline

- Examination:
  - Complete history and physical examination
  - Two baseline blood pressures atleast a day apart
- Laboratory:
  - Baseline serum creatinine levels (two baseline serum creatinine levels atleast a day apart)
  - Blood urea nitrogen (BUN), urine analysis with microscopic examination
  - CBC and liver function test
  - Fasting lipid profile—triglycerides, cholesterol, high-density lipoprotein (HDL) cholesterol
  - Other laboratory test—magnesium, potassium, uric acid

Follow-up

- Examination:
  - Re-evaluate the patient every 2 weeks for 1–2 months, then every 4–6 weeks while on cyclosporine
  - Blood pressure checked at each visit
- Laboratory:
  - Laboratory surveillance every 2 weeks for the first 1–2 months, then monthly while on cyclosporine
  - Renal function—serum creatinine, BUN, urine analysis

- CBC and liver function tests
- Lipids—triglycerides, cholesterol

Q. What can be done if there is an elevation of serum creatinine?

A. If there is an elevation of at least 30% over the baseline values, the dose should be reduced by 1 mg/kg/day or by 25–50% for 4 weeks. Then the serum creatinine is repeated and if it does not improve then cyclosporine should be decreased by another 25–50%. If it still remains high then discontinue cyclosporine therapy till serum creatinine values normalize and then restart cautiously. If creatinine rises 30% over the baseline again then withdraw it permanently.

Q. What can be done if there is an elevation of blood pressure?

A. The percentage of patients with new onset of hypertension with cyclosporine therapy is 0–24%. It is more common in psoriasis compared to atopic dermatitis (metabolic syndrome). If the BP is higher than 140 mm Hg systolic or 90 mm Hg diastolic, observe the patient and repeat the BP after 2 weeks. If at this stage the BP is still high, reduce cyclosporine by 25–50%. Alternatively antihypertensive therapy can be given with calcium channel blockers of the dihydropyridine class (amlodipine or isradipine) since they have a vasodilating effect on the afferent arterioles. Verapamil and diltiazem interferes with cyclosporine levels, nifedipine potentiates gum hypertrophy caused by cyclosporine, while ACE inhibitors decrease GFR. Thiazide diuretics can cause increased nephrotoxicity while potassium sparing diuretics can potentiate hyperkalemia caused by cyclosporine. Hence only calcium channel blockers can be used as antihypertensives, though some studies have shown perindopril to be effective and safe.

Q. What is the method of sequential therapy involving cyclosporine and systemic therapies?

A. *With acitretin*:

- Acitretin is not ideal as a clearing agent, has a slow onset of action and adverse effects at high doses
- Cyclosporine seems to be a very good clearing agent but its merit for long term use as a maintenance agent is questionable
- Thus for patients with severe psoriasis, cyclosporine can be used first to induce clearance followed by acitretin for maintenance

With methotrexate: Combination therapy with cyclosporine and methotrexate has been proved safe in rheumatology patients and is FDA approved for rheumatoid arthritis.

With biologics: Sequential use of cyclosporine transitioning to adalimumab appears to be a very good option.

Q. What is the benefit of combination therapy of cyclosporine with retinoids?

A. It is not only efficacious but it may also protect against cutaneous malignancy.

Q. Why is cyclosporine more safe in pediatric age group?

A. Because risk of nephrotoxicity is less common.

Q. Discuss the use of cyclosporine in atopic dermatitis.

A. It is effective in refractory and generalized atopic dermatitis. In the induction phase, a higher dose is required (5 mg/kg/day) but later on the dose can be reduced by 1 mg/kg/day every 2 weeks. The lowest effective dose should be used. There is a rebound after stopping in a small number of patients, which was associated with a sudden increase in IgE levels and a shift to a Th2 response.

Q. Discuss the use of cyclosporine in chronic urticaria.

A. It may be used in chronic urticaria as an alternative to steroids or as a steroid sparing agent. It lowers the serum levels of cytokines IL-2, IL-5 and TNF-α. Two-thirds of patients treated with cyclosporine 3 mg/day achieved a short-term remission. In many of the others the dose of rescue medication (anti-histaminics) was reduced. Cyclosporine is also useful in Schnitzler's syndrome (urticaria, fever and gammopathy). The dose for urticaria suggested is 3 mg/kg/day in 2 divided doses for 6 weeks, 2 mg/kg/day for 3 weeks, and then 1 mg/kg/day for further 3 weeks.

Q. Discuss the use of cyclosporine in Lichen Planus.

A. There are no established guidelines for this indication, however, it may be effective in the initial phase of lichen planopilaris in a dose of 3 mg/kg/day. Topical cyclosporine has been used for the treatment of oral lichen planus. Cyclosporine is increasingly being used for the treatement of LP in children.

Q. Discuss role of cyclosporine in alopecia areata.

A. It is quite effective but withdrawal leads to significant relapse. It may be combined with methylprednisolone (IV pulse therapy). However, it is noted that there are patients who develop alopecia areata when on cyclosporine for organ transplants.

Q. Discuss use of cyclosporine in hidradenitis suppurativa (HS).

A. 4–5 mg/kg/day has been reported to be effective for healing of the sinuses and decreased pain. It can be combined with broad spectrum antibiotics and surgical excision.

Q. Discuss use of cyclosporine in scleroderma.

A. There is significant skin softening in upto 50% patients, and also resolution of digital ulcers in some. However, careful monitoring is required as cyclosporine can worsen renal disease or hypertension associated with scleroderma.

Q. Discuss topical cyclosporine.

A. Cyclopsorine is effective only on the mucosae because of good absorption, hence, used in oral LP. Intralesional cyclosporine has been tried for psoriasis and pyoderma gangrenosum, but is associated with severe pain.

METHOTREXATE

Introduction

The use of methotrexate (MTX) occurred by chance in 1951 when Gubner noted clearance of psoriatic skin lesions in cancer patients undergoing treatment with aminopterin. Aminopterin is less stable and more toxic and its derivative MTX also called as amethoptrein has replaced it.

Q. Discuss the pharmacokinetics of MTX.

A. There is significant variability in absorption with food probably decreasing absorption. Maximum blood levels occur 1–2 hours after absorption and 35–50% of the drug is bound to proteins.The drug is well distributed throughout the body except in the brain. The primary active metabolite is a polyglutamate derivative which has a long half-life.

Upto 50–90% of the drug is excreted in the urine within 24 hours. A minor degree of enterohepatic circulation occurs.

Q. What is the mechanism of action of MTX?

A. There are 2 types of action of MTX. The antiproliferative action (mediated by folate dependent pathway) and anti-inflammatory action [due to increase in 5-aminoimidazole-4-carboxamide ribonucleotide (AICAR) levels]. The folate dependent action involves enzymes like methionine synthetase (DNA methylation), thymidylate synthetase (pyrimidine synthesis) and transformylase (purine synthesis). Thus DNA multiplication is inhibited at multiple sites. The drug is active only in the S-phase of the cell cycle.

The anti-inflammatory action can be due to folate dependent pathways or folate independent pathways. The inhibition of polyamines is thought to be contributory when MTX is given in low doses. In higher doses the enzyme inhibited is AICAR transformylase. This leads to increased amount of AICAR. AICAR increases adenosine levels and adenosine is a potent anti-inflammatory compound which inhibits chemotaxis, cytokine factors including TNF-α and down regulates intercellular adhesion molecule (ICAM).

Q. What are the indications of MTX?

A.

Group of diseases	*Specific entities*
Papulosquamous	Psoriasis (FDA approved), PRP, PLEVA, PLC, Reiter's syndrome and widespread LP
Allergic	Chronic refractory urticaria
Dermatitis	Atopic dermatitis, actinic dermatitis and refractory pompholyx
Vesiculobullous	Pemphigus (all types), pemphigoid (all types)
Collagen vascular diseases	Morphea, dermatomyositis, cutaneous LE
Vasculitis	Leukocytoclastic, rheumatoid, Behçet's, PAN
Granulomatous	Cutaneous sarcoid and GA
Lymphoproliferative	Lymphomatoid papulosis, CD30+ lymphoma, MF and Sézary syndrome (FDA approved)

(FDA: Food and Drug Administration; GA: granuloma annulare; LE: lupus erythematosus; LP: lichen planus; MF: mycosis fungoides; PAN: polyarteritis nodosa; PLC: pityriasis lichenoides chronica; PLEVA: pityriasis lichenoides et varioliformis acuta; PRP: pityriasis rubra pilaris)

Mode of administration

Oral, intravenous, intramuscular, or subcutaneously.

Contraindications

Algorithm for initiating and monitoring MTX:

- Rule out absolute contraindications (pregnancy, significant anemia, leukopenia, thrombocytopenia)
- Evaluate for relative contraindications (renal and hepatic impairment, chronic infections or immunocompromised states, diabetes, obesity or heavy alcoholic consumption, significant drug interactions or recent vaccinations). If significant factors exist, consider alternative therapy
- Evaluate laboratory parameters at baseline (full blood count, renal and liver function tests, baseline liver biopsy may be considered in patients with hepatic risk factors, X-ray chest and pregnancy test). If these are abnormal, clinical re-evaluation is indicated
- Initiate therapy (some recommend a test dose of 2.5 mg of MTX)

- Monitor treatment with following parameters:
  - Hematologic surveillance—complete blood count (CBC) and platelets (PLT) count weekly for first 2 weeks, 2 weekly for next month, then monthly or 3 monthly depending on the clinical picture
  - Renal surveillance; renal function tests (RFTs) including glomerular filtration rate (GFR) every 3 months
  - Hepatic surveillance—liver function test like SGOT (serum glutamic-oxaloacetic transaminase), SGPT (serum glutamic-pyruvic transaminase), alkaline phosphatase and serum albumin every 4–8 weeks. More frequent if hepatic risk factors
  - Pregnancy surveillance—women of childbearing age and sexually active must take contraceptive measures

Both men and women wanting to have a child should be off MTX for at least 3 months before attempting to conceive.

Q. What are the risk factors for hepatic toxicity?

A. The risk factors are—obesity, moderate to heavy alcohol consumption, type 2 diabetes mellitus (T2DM), past history of chronic hepatitis, significant exposure to hepatotoxic drugs, persistent abnormal liver enzymes, and hyperlipidemia.

Q. Should liver biopsy be done in every patient on MTX?

A. Baseline liver biopsy is not indicated for every patient on MTX, however, patients with risk factors should be subjected to a liver biopsy, though not at the beginning of therapy as liver biopsy itself has complications. It may be done after a few weeks, once we are sure that the patient is going to be maintained on MTX.

Serial biopsies are recommended in psoriatics when the cumulative dose exceeds 1.5 g, but may not be recommended when the initial biopsy is normal, enzymes are normal, or when the weekly dose is <15 mg.

Q. Discuss procollagen III aminoterminal propeptide (PIIINP).

A. It is serum type III procollagen aminopeptide. It is a test for fibrinogenesis. A recent study showed that patients with normal PIIINP had a low risk of developing liver toxicity. However, in some other conditions causing fibrosis (e.g., systemic sclerosis and rheumatoid arthritis), PIIINP levels are falsely elevated.

Q. What are the drug interactions of MTX?

A.
- Increase in methotrexate serum levels—doxycycline, minocycline, tetracycline
- Decrease in methotrexate serum levels—ciprofloxacin, penicillin
- Decrease in serum levels of digoxin

- Dapsone, sulfonamides inhibit dihydropteroate synthase
- Trimethoprim inhibits dihydrofolate reductase

MYCOPHENOLATE MOFETIL

Mycophenolic acid was used for the treatment of psoriasis in the 1970s. However, it was associated with severe gastrointestinal (GI) side effects and concern for malignancies. It was therefore, withdrawn. In the 1990s, a prodrug of mycophenolic acid was developed called mycophenolate mofetil (MMF), and was approved for prevention of graft rejection. A few years later, it was used for several immune mediated skin conditions.

Q. What is MMF?

A. It is an immunosuppressant, prodrug of the antimetabolite of mycophenolic acid.

Q. What is the absorption and bioavailability?

A.
- Peak levels—12 hours
- Bioavailability—nearly 100%
- Protein binding—97% (to albumin)

Q. Which is the active metabolite?

A. Mycophenolic acid. It is metabolized in the liver to form mycophenolic acid glucuronide (MPAG) which is inactive but can be reconverted to MPA through enterohepatic circulation.

Q. What is the half life?

A. 16 hours.

Q. How is it excreted?

A. Over 90% excreted in urine.

Q. What is the mechanism of action?

A. Mycophenolate mofetil is hydrolyzed to its active metabolite mycophenolic acid, by plasma esterases. MPA inhibits inosine monophosphate dehydrogenase (IMPDH) and depletes guanosine nucleotides, which are required for purine synthesis. The IMPDH affected is the type 2 isoform which is present on lymphocytes. Thus, lymphocytes are more affected by MMF. Moreover, all other cells of the body (except T and B lymphocytes) have a salvage pathway by which guanosine nucleotides are synthesized. These two facts explain the selective nature of MMF for lymphocytes.

Q. What is the pregnancy category of this drug?

A. Category D.

Q. Compare azathioprine with MMF.

A.

Azathioprine	*Mycophenolate mofetil*
Inhibits purine synthesis	Inhibits purine synthesis
Targets several enzymes (XO and TPMT), hence less selective	Targets only one enzyme (IMPDH) hence, more selective
TPMT deficiency can cause severe side-effects	Not relevant
One of the metabolites 6-thioguanosine can cause mutagenesis and chromosomal breakage	Potentially less mutagenic

(IMPDH: inosine monophosphate dehydrogenase; TPMT: thiopurine-S-methyltranferase; XO: xanthine oxidase)

Q. What are the indications?

A. Dermatitis

- Psoriasis
- Atopic dermatitis
- Dyshidrotic eczema
- Chronic actinic dermatitis

Bullous dermatoses

- Pemphigus vulgaris
- Pemphigus foliaceus
- Bullous pemphigoid
- Paraneoplastic pemphigus

Autoimmune connective tissue disease

- Systemic lupus erythematosus
- Subacute cutaneous lupus erythematosus
- Chronic cutaneous lupus erythematosus
- Chilblain lupus erythematosus
- Diffuse systemic sclerosis
- Dermatomyositis

Vasculitis

- Wegener's granulomatosis
- Microscopic polyangiitis
- Churg-Strauss syndrome

Miscellaneous

- Pyoderma gangrenosum
- Cutaneous Crohn's disease

- Sarcoidosis
- Recalcitrant lichen planus
- Chronic urticaria

Q. What are the absolute contraindications?

A.
- Pregnancy (teratogenic)
- Drug allergy

Q. What are the relative contraindications?

A.
- Lactation
- Peptic ulcer disease
- Hepatic/Renal disease
- Azathioprine (concomitant administration increases risk of bone marrow suppression)
- Drugs that interfere with enterohepatic circulation (cholestyramine)

Q. What are the adverse effects?

A.
- Carcinogenicity—lymphoproliferative disorders
- Gastrointestinal—nausea, diarrhea, soft stools, anorexia, abdominal cramps, vomiting, anal tenderness
- Genitourinary—urgency, frequency, dysuria, burning, sterile pyuria
- Infectious—viral, bacterial, atypical mycobacteria, fungal
- Hematologic—neutropenia, anemia, thrombocytopenia, agranulocytosis
- Neurologic—weakness, fatigue, headache, tinnitus, insomnia
- Teratogenicity—first trimester loss, external ear/facial abnormalities, anomalies of distal limbs, heart, esophagus, and kidneys

Q. What are the doses and preparations available?

A.
- Preparations: 250 mg capsules, 500 mg tablets, and an oral solution 100 mg/mL
- *Dose*: 2–3 g divided doses twice daily

Q. What are the monitoring guidelines?

A. **Baseline**
- CBC with differential and platelet count
- Serum chemistry panel including serum creatinine
- Serum liver function tests
- Hepatitis B and C panel
- Purified protein derivative
- Serum or urine beta-human chorionic gonadotropin

Follow-up

Every 2–4 weeks following dose escalation and every 2–3 months once dose is stable:

- CBC with differential and platelet count
- Serum chemistry panel including serum creatinine
- Serum liver function tests

LEFLUNOMIDE

Leflunomide is an oral disease modifying antirheumatic drug (DMARD) approved by FDA in 1998 for treatment of rheumatoid arthritis.

Q. What is leflunomide?

A. It is a synthetic isoxazole derivative. It is a prodrug.

Q. What is the pregnancy category?

A. Pregnancy category X.

Q. What is the mechanism of action?

A. Competitively and reversibly inhibits pyrimidine synthesis by inhibiting the mitochondrial dihydroorotate dehydrogenase. This enzyme is critical in maintaining a sufficient pool of pyrimidines for proliferation of T and B cells.

Q. Pharmacology of leflunomide.

A.

Bioavailability (%)	80
Peak plasma time (h)	6–12
Protein bound (%)	>99
Half life (days)	15–18
Elimination	Feces—48%; urine—43%

Q. For how long is it detected in the blood?

A. For up to 2 years.

Q. What are the indications?

A.
- Psoriatic arthritis
- Psoriasis vulgaris (plaque type and pustular)
- Bullous autoimmune disorders (bullous pemphigoid)
- Wegener's granulomatosis
- Systemic vasculitis (Takayasu's arteritis)
- Rheumatoid arthritis
- Subacute cutaneous lupus erythematosus (SCLE)
- Sjögren's syndrome associated vasculitis

- Systemic sclerosis
- Atopic dermatitis
- Cutaneous sarcoidosis
- Synovitis-acne-pustulosis-hyperostosis-osteitis (SAPHO) syndrome
- Multicentric reticulohistiocytosis

Q. What are the contraindications to leflunomide?

A.
- Hepatic infections
- Heavy alcohol intake

Q. What are the adverse effects?

A. **Cutaneous**
- Reversible alopecia (most common)
- Oral ulcerations (common)
- Hypersensitivity syndrome
- Erythema multiforme
- Stevens-Johnson syndrome
- Toxic epidermal necrolysis
- Erythroderma
- Lichenoid drug eruption
- Alopecia areata
- SCLE (more seen in patients with rheumatoid arthritis)

Systemic
- Gastrointestinal disturbances (most common)
- Ankylosing spondylitis
- Hypertension
- Elevated transaminases

Q. What are the doses and preparations?

A. Tablets—10 and 20 mg.
- Dose—100 mg loading dose for 3 consecutive days, followed by 10–20 mg daily as maintenance therapy
- However, loading dose may precipitate GI intolerance, and may therefore, be omitted. In such cases, therapy is started with a 10 mg daily dose

2.8. ANTIRETROVIRAL THERAPY AND HAART

INTRODUCTION

The first antiretroviral (ARV) drug was introduced in 1986 (Zidovudine). ARV drugs are those that inhibit multiplication of human immune virus and the search for a cure of AIDS has led to extensive studies in different treatment modalities resulting in >20 Food and Drug Administration (FDA) approved antiretroviral drugs.

Q. Classify ARV drugs and state their pregnancy categories.

A.
- Nucleoside reverse transcriptase inhibitors (NRTIs)
    - Zidovudine (pregnancy category C)
    - Didanosine (pregnancy category B)
    - Zalcitabine (pregnancy category C)
    - Stavudine (pregnancy category C)
    - Lamivudine (pregnancy category C)
    - Abacavir (pregnancy category C)
    - Emtricitabine (pregnancy category B)
- Non-nucleoside reverse transcriptase inhibitors (NNRTIs)
    - Nevirapine (pregnancy category B)
    - Efavirenz (pregnancy category D)
    - Delavirdine (pregnancy category C)
    - Etravirine (pregnancy category B)
- Nucleotide reverse transcriptase inhibitors—tenofovir (pregnancy category B)
- Protease inhibitors (PIs)
    - Indinavir (pregnancy category C)
    - Ritonavir (pregnancy category B)
    - Saquinavir (pregnancy category B)
    - Nelfinavir (pregnancy category B)
    - Amprenavir (pregnancy category C)
    - Fosamprenavir (pregnancy category C)
    - Lopinavir (pregnancy category C)
    - Atazanavir (pregnancy category B)
    - Tipranavir (pregnancy category C)
    - Darunavir (pregnancy category C)
- Fusion inhibitors—enfuvirtide (pregnancy category B)
- Entry inhibitor/CCR5 coreceptor antagonist—maraviroc (pregnancy category B)
- Integrase inhibitor—raltegravir (pregnancy category C)
- Miscellaneous—hydroxyurea (pregnancy category D)

Q. What is the mechanism of action of NRTI's?

A. They inhibit RNA dependent DNA synthesis by inhibiting reverse transcriptase enzyme after phosphorylation by cellular enzymes.

Q. What are the indications of NRTI's?

A.
- As a part of highly active antiretroviral therapy (HAART) regimen of antiretroviral therapy
- In the prevention of perinatal transmission of HIV
- Combination therapy for postexposure prophylaxis

Q. What are the adverse effects of NRTI's?

A.
- Zidovudine—alopecia and nail pigmentation, myelosuppression (causing anemia), hepatotoxicity, lactic acidosis, myopathy, neurotoxicity, headache, myalgia
- Lamivudine—side effects mild and uncommon, rarely lactic acidosis and severe hepatomegaly, pancreatitis, peripheral neuropathy, splenomegaly reported
- Stavudine—lactic acidosis, hepatotoxicity with steatosis, peripheral neuropathy are relatively common. Pancreatitis, arthralgia, hypersensitivity, myalgia, anorexia, chills, fever, rash, asthenia, gastrointestinal (GI) disturbances, headache, insomnia

Note:
- Zidovudine cannot be given with didanosine as it may increase the chances of peripheral neuropathy. Zidovudine cannot be given with Stavudine as it causes in-vivo antagonism. Zidovudine decreases the transformation of Stavudine to its active form

Q. What is the mechanism of action of NNRTI's?

A. These drugs bind noncompetitively to the viral RNA dependent DNA polymerase altering its structure thereby inhibiting its function. Unlike NRTIs, these drugs do not require activation.

Q. What are the indications of NNRTI's?

A.
- As a part of HAART regimen of antiretroviral therapy
- As a single dose to prevent perinatal transmission
- Combination for postexposure prophylaxis

Q. What are the contraindications of NNRTI's?

A. Hypersensitivity, severe hepatitis, renal failure.

Q. What are the adverse effects of NNRTI's?

A.
- Nevirapine—Stevens-Johnson syndrome/toxic epidermal necrolysis (SJS/TEN), liver toxicity, fever, GI intolerance
- Delavirdine—liver failure, morbilliform eruption
- Efavirenz—SJS/erythema multiforme (EM), dizziness, insomnia, amnesia, cutaneous vasculitis
- Etravirine—SJS/TEN, EM, GI intolerance, fatigue, liver failure

Q. What is the mechanism of action of protease inhibitors?

A. These drugs block the protease enzyme involved in the final processing of viral proteins. This results in decreased assembly of new viruses from recently as well as chronically infected cells.

Q. What are the indications of protease inhibitors?

A. • As part of HAART especially in patients with high viral load
- Combination therapy for postexposure prophylaxis

Q. What are the adverse effects of protease inhibitors?

A. • Saquinavir—hyperglycemia, hyperlipidemia, lipodystrophy, GI intolerance
- Ritonavir—GI intolerance, paresthesia, dysgeusia
- Indinavir—hyperbilirubinemia, kidney stones, insomnia, sicca syndrome
- Nelfinavir—diarrhea in upto 30% of patients, asthenia, hypertension
- Amprenavir—morbilliform eruptions, SJS, perioral paresthesia, GI intolerance
- Atazanavir—fatigue, GI intolerance, jaundice

Q. What is postexposure prophylaxis for HIV?

A. • Basic regimen—zidovudine 300 mg + lamivudine 150 mg twice daily for 28 days
- Expanded regimen—zidovudine 300 mg twice daily + lamivudine 150 mg twice daily + nevirapine 200 mg twice daily/efavirenz 600 mg once daily/indinavir 800 mg thrice daily for 28 days

Q. What is pre-exposure prophylaxis?

A. It is used for prevention of HIV infection in men who have a documented negative HIV antibody test and desire to have sex with men. The patient initially has to be determined eligible for this therapy by testing for HIV antibodies, screening for hepatitis B and screening for other sexually transmitted diseases (STDs). The patient is prescribed 300 mg tenofovir + 200 mg emtricitabine daily given for 3 months at a time, but which can be renewed if periodic HIV testing confirms that the patient is negative. The patient is also advised about risk reduction and adherence counselling. The blood urea nitrogen (BUN) and serum creatinine have to be monitored.

Q. How to prevent perinatal transmission of HIV?

A. • Single dose of nevirapine 200 mg to the mother at the onset of labor and 3–4 mg/kg twice daily to the neonate within 72 hours of birth
- Zidovudine 100 mg five times a day after 14–34 weeks of pregnancy until the start of labor. During labor zidovudine 2 mg/kg intravenous (IV) over 1 hour followed by a continuous IV infusion of 1 mg/kg/h till clamping of the umbilical cord post delivery. The neonate should receive 2 mg/kg orally every

6 hours starting within 12 hours after birth and continuing through to 6 weeks of age

Q. What is HAART?

A. Highly active antiretroviral therapy is an aggressive treatment regimen used to suppress HIV viral replication and progression of the disease and it constitutes the combination of three or more different drugs. For example, two NRTI's and one PI or two NRTI's and one NNRTI and other such combinations.

Q. What are the advantages of HAART?

A.
- Reduces the chances of infections with common and opportunistic infections
- Improves CD4 counts and constitutional symptoms
- Reduces the chances of malignancies and their progression
- Reverses HIV-induced encephalopathy, diarrhea, thrombocytopenia, bone marrow suppression and adds to life expectancy

Q. What are the disadvantages of HAART?

A.
- Relatively expensive therapy
- Serious side effects, compliance to medications difficult, intolerance to drug
- Endpoint is not known

Q. What is IRIS or HAART attack?

A. Immune reconstitution inflammatory syndrome (IRIS) is an unusual inflammatory reaction to an opportunistic infection which occurs in late HIV (CD4 <200/μL) during the reconstitution of the immunity in the initial months of HAART. There is unmasking of dormant infections, pulmonary extrapulmonary tuberculosis or manifestations due to altered immunological reactivity like psoriasis or Reiter's disease. IRIS has to be differentiated from antiretroviral therapy (ART) failure by the finding of increasing CD4 counts and decreasing viral load.

Q. What is ART failure?

A. Antiretroviral therapy failure is suspected in the presence of decreasing CD4 counts and increasing viral load.

- Virologic failure—failure to achieve 70% reduction in plasma viral load after 1 month period
- Immunologic failure—there is a decrease in viral load but CD4 counts fail to rise despite ART
- Clinical failure—there is a decrease in viral load, increase in CD4 count in a patient on ART but without expected clinical improvement.

Q. What are the causes of ART failure?

A.
- Discontinuation of therapy due to socioeconomic reasons
- Intolerance to ARV medications
- Monotherapy and drug resistance

Q. What is the revised World Health Organization (WHO) clinical staging for HIV?

A.
- Primary HIV infection—asymptomatic or acute retroviral syndrome
- Clinical stage I—asymptomatic or persistent generalized lymphadenopathy
- Clinical stage II—moderate/unexplained weight loss, herpes zoster, recurrent oral ulcerations, angular cheilitis, recurrent respiratory tract infections, papular pruritic eruptions, seborrheic dermatitis, onychomycosis.
- Clinical stage III—can be subdivided into conditions where a presumptive diagnosis can be made on the basis of clinical signs alone, and conditions where confirmatory diagnostic testing is required. The first group includes severe weight loss, unexplained chronic diarrhea, unexplained persistent fever, oral candidiasis, oral hairy leukoplakia, recently diagnosed pulmonary tuberculosis (TB), severe presumed bacterial infections, and acute necrotizing stomatitis, gingivitis or periodontitis. The second group includes unexplained anemia, neutropenia or thrombocytopenia
- Clinical stage IV—can be subdivided into conditions where a presumptive diagnosis can be made on the basis of clinical signs alone, and conditions where confirmatory diagnostic testing is required. The first group includes HIV wasting syndrome, pneumocystis pneumonia, recurrent bacterial pneumonias, chronic herpes simplex infections, esophageal candidiasis, extrapulmonary TB, Kaposi's sarcoma, central nervous system (CNS) toxoplasmosis, and HIV encephalopathy. The second group includes extrapulmonary cryptococcosis, nontuberculous mycobacterial infections, progressive multifocal leukoencephalopathy, pulmonary candidiasis, isosporiasis, cytomegalovirus (CMV) infections, disseminated mycosis, lymphomas, invasive cervical carcinomas, and visceral leishmaniasis

Q. What are the WHO guidelines for starting a patient on ART?

A. If CD4 testing is available:
- WHO stage IV disease, irrespective of CD4 cell count

- WHO stage III disease with consideration of using CD4 cell counts <350/mm^3 to assist decision making
- WHO stage I OR II disease with CD4 cell count <200/mm^3

If CD4 testing unavailable:
- WHO stage IV disease, irrespective of total lymphocyte count
- WHO stage III disease, irrespective of total lymphocyte count
- WHO stage II disease, with a total lymphocyte count <1200/mm^3

Q. What are the ARV regimens?

A. First line ARV regimens in adults and adolescents
- Stavudine/Lamivudine/Nevirapine
- Zidovudine/Lamivudine/Nevirapine
- Stavudine/Lamivudine/Efavirenz
- Zidovudine/Lamivudine/Efavirenz
- Tenofovir/Efavirenz/Emtricitabine

Adult dosages
- Stavudine—20–40 mg bid
- Lamivudine—150 mg bid, 300 mg od
- Nevirapine—200 mg bid
- Zidovudine—300 mg bid, 200 mg tid
- Efavirenz—600 mg od
- Tenofovir—300 mg od
- Emtricitabine—200 mg od

ARV regimens for infants and children

First line regimen:
- Stavudine/Zidovudine + lamivudine + NNRTI: Nevirapine/ Efavirenz

Second line regimen:
- Abacavir + didanosine + PI: Lopinavir + ritonavir, or nelfinavir, or saquinavir if weight <25 kg

Pregnancy and women of childbearing age:
- Avoid efavirenz-based regimens
- First line regimen is stavudine/zidovudine + lamivudine + nevirapine

Q. What is status of HAART in patients coinfected with TB?

A. In HIV coinfection with TB, the drug of choice is efavirenz. Avoid nevirapine because it may increase the risk of hepatotoxicity and lowers rifampicin serum levels. Some people advise to change rifampicin to rifabutin. A cautious use of a ritonavir-boosted lopinavir-based regimen may also be used. Atazanovir may also be used. Moxifloxacin is a potential substitute for the rifamycins.

2.9. PSORALENS AND PHOTOTHERAPY

INTRODUCTION

- Phototherapy includes PUVA (Psoralens and ultraviolet A: 320–340 nm) and UVB
- PUVA can be topical PUVA and systemic PUVA
- Psoralens are naturally occurring or synthetic agents used for photosensitizing the skin and are widely used in dermatology for photochemotherapy
- First compounds used as psoralen were methoxsalen (obtained from seeds of *Ammi majus* plant) and trioxsalen (synthetic compound)
- Ultraviolet radiation (UVR) reaching the earth's surface can be divided into UVB (280–320 nm) and UVA (320–400 nm). UVA can be further subdivided into UVA I (340–400 nm or "far UVA") and UVA II (320–340 nm or "near UVA")
- UVB can be broadband UVB (BBUVB: 280–320 nm) and narrow-band UVB (NBUVB: 311-313 nm) and UVC <280 nm

Q. What are the types of phototherapy?

A.
- UVA
- UVB
- Targeted phototherapy—excimer light and excimer laser
- Photodynamic therapy
- Extracorporeal phototherapy

Q. What is the mechanism of action of psoralens?

A. Various mechanisms are:
- Suppression of DNA synthesis by formation of monoadducts and cross-links (oxygen independent) and production of free radicals (oxygen dependent)
- Selective immunosuppression (depletion of Langerhans'cells and apoptosis of CD4 lymphocytes)
- Selective cytotoxicity
- Stimulation of melanocytes

Q. What are the indications for phototherapy?

A.

FDA approved indications	*Off-label uses*
• Psoriasis • Vitiligo • Increasing tolerance to sunlight • Enhancing pigmentation	• Neoplastic disorders: o Mycosis fungoides o Histiocytosis X • Papulosquamous disorders: o Atopic dermatitis o Seborrheic dermatitis o Lichen planus o Pityriasis lichenoides o Parapsoriasis • Photosensitivity dermatoses: o PMLE o Erythropoietic protoporphyria o Solar urticaria o Chronic actinic dermatitis • Others: o Morphea o Linear scleroderma o Pruritus (idiopathic or aquagenic) o Chronic urticaria

Q. What are the types of PUVA?

A. Systemic PUVA

Drug	*Preparation*
8-methoxypsoralen (8-MOP)	10 mg tablets
5-methoxypsoralen (5-MOP) (better tolerated but not available in India)	
Trimethylpsoralen (trioxsalen/TMP)	Tablet 5 mg, 25 mg
Khellin	100 mg tablets

Topical PUVA

Drug	*Preparation and concentration*
8-MOP	1% solution (1:10 dilution with ethanol), 0.75% ointment (apply 15 min before exposure)
TMP	0.2% solution (apply 15 min before exposure)
Khellin	2% solution (apply 15 min before exposure)

Q. What is the pregnancy prescribing status?

A. Pregnancy category C (for psoralens). No confirmed data for khellin.

Q. What are the contraindications?

A.

Absolute	*Relative*
• Pemphigus and pemphigoid • Xeroderma pigmentosum • Lupus erythematosus • Lactation • Hypersensitivity to psoralen	• Pregnancy • Young age • Severe cardiac renal or liver disease • History of skin cancer or chronic photodamage • History or family history of melanoma • Prior exposure to ionizing radiation or arsenic • Photosensitivity or photosensitizing medications

Q. What are the side effects?

A.

Short-term side effects	*Long-term side effects*
• Due to methoxypsoralen ○ Gastrointestinal disturbances ○ Bronchoconstriction ○ Central nervous system disturbance ○ Drug fever ○ Exanthems ○ Hepatotoxicity	• Photoageing • Melanoma • Nonmelanoma skin cancer
• Phototoxic reactions ○ Symptomatic erythema (most common, 10% of cases) ○ Psoralen plus ultraviolet A (PUVA) itch ○ Photoonycholysis ○ Koebner's phenomenon ○ Friction blisters on hands and feet ○ Hypertrichosis ○ Phytophotodermatitis ○ Subacute phototoxicity	
• Others ○ Herpes simplex recurrences ○ Photosensitive eruptions	

Q. What are the principles of PUVA therapy?

A.
- Psoralen has to be taken with water 1 hour after food
- Exposure is either twice or thrice a week and not every day as PUVA induced erythema takes minimum 48 hours to subside

- Assess erythema due to previous exposure. Stop treatment if the patient complains of burning, tenderness, and blisters
- Eyes should be protected during PUVA therapy by wearing UV-blocking glasses. The whole day eyes are to be protected and sometimes even the second day. Face is protected by using sunscreen
- Genitals also need to be protected by genital shields, under-garment, jockstrap
- Increment of exposure dose should be done at every sitting, modified depending upon the clinical response and side effects
- The final dose that maintains the clearance is held constant and then gradually reduced
- Concurrent topical corticosteroid therapy is required for areas naturally shielded from exposure to UVA (like scalp, intertriginous areas)
- On nontreatment days, protect skin by avoiding sun exposure and by using sunscreens

Q. What is minimum erythema dose (MED)?

A.
- MED is the minimum dose of ultraviolet light that produces perceptible and well-defined erythema.
- MED testing is carried on covered sites
- Such as the buttocks and read 72 hours after light exposure. Ideally, MED should be determined before the initiation of PUVA therapy
- Phototherapy is started with 50% of MED dose

Q. What are the combination treatments utilizing PUVA photo-chemotherapy?

A.
- PUVA + retinoids (acitretin)- RePUVA
    - Acitretin 1 mg/kg, started 2 weeks prior to PUVA
    - Acitretin + PUVA until clearance
    - Stop acitretin and PUVA continued
- PUVA + methotrexate
    - Methotrexate 7.5 mg started 3 weeks prior to PUVA
    - Methotrexate + PUVA until clearance
    - Methotrexate stopped and PUVA is continued
- PUVA + UVB
    - PUVA + high dose broadband UVB (75% of MED with 20% increments)
    - Both treatments given at same time
    - Stop UVB when clear
- PUVA + topical tazarotene

Q. What are the combination treatments utilizing UVB photochemotherapy?

A.
- UVB + systemic retinoids
- UVB + saltwater bath
- UVB + topical tazarotene
- UVB + calcipotriol

Q. Which drugs should not be used concomitantly with phototherapy?

A.
- Calcipotriol—phototherapy degrades calcipotriol
- Salicylic acid—it has photoprotective properties which will reduce the efficacy of phototherapy

Q. What are the drug interactions in PUVA therapy?

A. The following agents should not be used with PUVA therapy.
- Phototoxic agents—doxycycline and fluoroquinolones (acute phototoxic erythema)
- Drugs that activate CYP450 enzymes—carbamazepine and phenytoin (enhance metabolism of methoxsalen)

Q. What is turban-PUVA?

A. Turban-PUVA therapy can be considered a useful method of administering a dilute psoralen solution containing 8-MOP selectively to the scalp. It is well-tolerated and is an efficient therapeutic alternative in the treatment of scalp psoriasis and alopecia totalis.

Q. What is soak PUVA therapy?

A.
- It can be used for palmoplantar psoriasis, palmoplantar pustulosis, and hand eczema
- Prepared by adding 0.5–1 mL of 0.75% 8-MOP solution in 2L of water
- Hands or feet are immersed in the solution for 30 minutes, then dried off and exposed to UVA
- Initial UVA dose, 5 J/cm^2
- UVA increments—0.5–1 J/cm^2
- Frequency—thrice weekly
- Dorsa of hands and feet require 50% of the dose for palms and soles

Q. What is PUVASOL therapy?

A. Exposure to natural sunlight (11 AM to 2 PM) 1–2 hours after taking psoralen tablets or 15–20 minutes after application of topical psoralens.

Q. What is balneotherapy?

A. Any bath followed by phototherapy is balneotherapy. For example—bath PUVA, dead sea therapy

Q. What is targeted phototherapy?

A. Ultraviolet exposure (NBUVB) limited only to affected areas (targeted).

Q. What are the advantages of targeted phototherapy?

A.
- Larger doses are delivered to the target sites
- Less incidence of phototoxicity in the surrounding normal skin
- Rapid results

Q. What are the difference between excimer laser and excimer lamp?

A. Although the excimer lamp and laser use the same wavelength, they are different devices with distinct radiation properties. Following are the differences between the two.

Properties	*Excimer laser*	*Excimer lamp*
Wavelength (nm)	308	308
Results	+++	+++
Energy	250 mW/cm^2	50 mW/cm^2
Spot size	4.9 cm^2	Upto 16 cm^2
Price	10×	1×
Weight	100 kg	1.5 kg
Optical energy	1,000 mW	800 mW
Mobility	Less	More
Long-term costs	Higher (10 times)	Lower
Protection of surrounding tissue	+++	+++

Q. What is high dose UVA1 therapy?

A. UVA 340–400 nm.

Q. What is blue light therapy?

A.
- Exposure to blue light in visible rays
- Used for noninflammatory acne vulgaris as it targets the organism *Propionibacterium acnes* (*P. acnes* produces porphyrins which is a natural photosensitizer)
- The wavelength is 450–495 nm

Q. What are the predictors of NBUVB phototherapy?

A. Good response

- Lesions on face
- Young patient
- Skin type III–IV
- Early initial response (during 1st month of treatment)

Poor response

- Lesions on the body
- Skin type I–II
- Late initial response (after 1st month of treatment)

Q. What are the monitoring guidelines for PUVA therapy?

A.

Baseline	*Follow-up*
• Cutaneous examinations for skin cancer, premalignant lesions and actinic damage • Ocular examination—examination of lens, cornea, and retina and assessment of the visual acuity • Laboratory—renal and liver function tests	• Cutaneous examination yearly for screening skin cancer • Ocular examination—yearly

Q. Discuss the American and the European protocols for PUVA.

A. In the American protocol, patient's skin type is determined, and patient is treated two to three times a week with an increase of 0.5–1 J/cm^2 gradually. In the European protocol, the minimum phototoxic dose (MPD) is determined and the patient is given more aggressive therapy 4 times/week.

Q. Compare UVA with UVB?

A.

UVA	*UVB*
It requires psoralens	It does not require psoralens
Contraindications; in children <12 years of age, elderly patients, during pregnancy and lactation and in patients with compromised hepatic and renal functions	It can be given in children, elderly patients, during pregnancy and lactation and in patients with compromised hepatic and renal functions
Response is earlier with UVA	Response sustained
Skin and eye protection against sunlight throughout the day	No eye protection required outside the chamber

Continued

Continued

UVA	*UVB*
Longer exposure time side effects of psoralens less expensive	• Shorter exposure time • No side effects associated with psoralens • More expensive
More carcinogenic	Less carcinogenic

Q. What is photodynamic therapy?

A. Photodynamic therapy (PDT) is a form of phototherapy. It uses a nontoxic photosensitizer which when exposed to appropriate wavelengths of light becomes toxic and causes a desired therapeutic effect. Thus the drug and the light are nontoxic but the combination is lethal to the target cells. The mechanisms of action are as follows.

- Generation of reactive oxygen species—they can be free radicals (type I PDT) or singlet oxygen species (type II PDT)
- Vascular injury which leads to platelet and neutrophil activation, causing vessel thrombosis
- Inflammatory response—cell membrane damage leads to release of various inflammatory mediators
- The photosensitizers used are aminolevulinic acid (ALA), methyl aminolevulinic (MAL) acid, porphymer sodium. All these are applied topically but rarely systemic therapy can also be given. The wavelengths used range from 635 to 1,200 nm. The wavelengths below 635 nm are absorbed by hemoglobin, while the higher ones are absorbed by water. The light sources could be coherent (lasers like Nd:YAG, argon, or gold vapour) or incoherent (halogen lamps and xenon lamps)

Q. What are the indications of PDT?

A. The indications could be classified into malignant and premalignant conditions or nonmalignant conditions. The former include actinic keratosis, Bowen's disease, epidermodysplasia verruciformis, basal cell carcinoma (BCC), squamous cell carcinoma (SCC), keratoacanthoma, kaposi's sarcoma, Gorlin's syndrome, cutaneous metastasis, mycosis fungoides, etc. The latter include acne vulgaris, psoriasis vulgaris, alopecia areata, cutaneous vascular malformations, hair removal, hirsutism, condyloma acuminata, and wound healing.

Q. What are the side effects of PDT?

A. Burning pain, stinging, and itching can occur at the site of irradiation. The lesion can become crusted and erythematous, and rarely blistering and ulceration can occur. Photophobia can occur and exacerbation of systemic lupus erythematosus (SLE), psoriasis, and melanoma have been reported. However, most people tolerate it very well.

Q. Can PDT be combined with other modalities?

A. Yes, it can be combined with surgical debulking or chemotherapy in the treatment of tumors.

2.10. SYSTEMIC ANTIPARASITIC AGENTS

IVERMECTIN

Introduction

Ivermectin is a semisynthetic anthelmintic derived from the fermentation products of *Streptomyces avermitilis*. It is the 22,23-dihydro derivative of avermectin B1 and is classified as a macrocyclic in the avermectin family.

Q. What is mechanism of action?

A. It has GABA-nergic action, blocks chloride channels leading to tonic paralysis of parasites.

Q. What are the indications?

A.
- Scabies
- Pediculosis
- Onchocerciasis
- Filariasis
- Larva currens
- Strongyloidiasis

Q. What dose and formulations are available for this drug?

A. 12 mg single dose to be repeated after 2 weeks, 200 µg/kg single dose in children.

Q. What is pregnancy category of the drug?

A. Category C.

Q. What are the adverse effects of this drug?

A.
- Systemic: Headache and giddiness
- Cutaneous: Local irritation with topical preparation

Q. What are the other key features of this drug?

A. Ivermectin has an advantage of single dosing in all the conditions for which it is used. Cure rates of 60–70% are observed with a single dose of ivermectin in scabies. An additional dose of ivermectin after 2 weeks improves cure rate.

ALBENDAZOLE

Introduction

Broad-spectrum anthelmintic is a congener of mebendazole. chemical name for albendazole is methyl 5-(propylthio)-2-benzimidazolecarbamate.

Q. What is mechanism of action?

A. It causes depletion of glycogen stores and blocks glucose uptake in the parasite. It binds to β-tubulin of susceptible worms and inhibits polymerization of the cells of the worm.

Q. What is indication?

A.
- Round worm/hookworm/trichuriasis
- *Enterobius vermicularis*
- Tapeworms/strongyloidiasis
- Neurocysticercosis
- Larva migrans/Larva currens

Q. What dose and formulations available for this drug?

A. 400 mg single dose, 10–14 mg/kg in children.

Q. What is pregnancy category of the drug?

A. Category C.

Q. What are the adverse effects of this drug?

A.
- Systemic: Well tolerated, GIT disturbances, diarrhea, headache and dizziness can occur. Less frequent reactions include hypersensitivity reactions presenting with rash, pruritus or urticaria.
- Cutaneous: Alopecia is reported.

Q. What are the other key features of this drug?

A.
- Inconsistent absorption
- Widespread distribution
- Good CSF penetration
- Less effective than mebendazole for trichuriasis

MEBENDAZOLE

Introduction

Broad-spectrum benzimidazole anthelmintic.

Q. What is mechanism of action?

A. It causes depletion of glycogen stores and blocks glucose uptake in the parasite. It binds to β-tubulin of susceptible worms and inhibits polymerization of the cells of the worm.

Q. What is indication?

A.
- Round worm/hookworm/trichuriasis
- *Enterobius vermicularis*
- Tapeworms
- *Trichinella spiralis*

Q. What dose and formulations available for this drug?

A.
- 200 mg bid/tid
- 100 mg chewable tablet
- 100 mg/5 mL suspension

Doses and duration is same for children above 2 years and adults. Half dose is required for children less than 2 years of age.

Q. What is pregnancy category of the drug?

A. Category C.

Q. What are the adverse effects of this drug?

A.
- Systemic: Well tolerated, GIT disturbances can occur
- Cutaneous: Allergic reaction, alopecia with high doses

Q. What are the other key features of this drug?

A. Minimal absorption; 75–90% of oral mebendazole passes in feces. Fatty food increases absorption. Complete clearance of the parasite from GI tract may take up to 3 days. More effective than albendazole for trichuriasis. Though used extensively for mass treatment, a 3-day dosage schedule is a potential drawback as far as compliance is concerned.

THIABENDAZOLE

Introduction

Broad-spectrum anthelmintic agent.

Q. What is mechanism of action?

A. It inhibits helminth-specific fumarate reductase.

Q. What are the indications for its use?

A.
- Cutaneous larva migrans (*Ancylostoma braziliense, Necator americanus*)
- Larva currens (*Strongyloides stercoralis*)
- Visceral larva migrans (*Toxocara canis*)
- Trichinosis
- Guinea worm infestation
- Scabies (topical)

Q. What dose and formulations available for this drug?

A.
- 1.5 g for two successive days, 25 mg/kg bid
- 500 mg chewable tab
- 500 mg/5 mL suspension

Q. What is pregnancy category of the drug?

A. Category C.

Q. What are the adverse effects of this drug?

A.
- Systemic: Nausea, vomiting, and diarrhea.
- Cutaneous: Local irritation with topical preparation.

Q. What are the other key features of this drug?

A.
- Thiabendazole tablet should be first chewed and then swallowed
- May increase plasma levels of theophylline

DIETHYLCARBAMAZINE (DEC)

Introduction

Diethylcarbamazine is an antifilarial agents.

Q. What is mechanism of action?

A. It modifies microfilariae so that they are engulfed by phagocytes but do not have direct microfilaricidal action.

Q. What is indication?

A.
- Filariasis
- Loiasis

Q. What dose and formulations available for this drug?

A.
- Filariasis: 6 mg/kg/day in three divided doses after meals for 2 weeks
- Loiasis: 50 mg tid on day 1 and 2,
  100 mg tid on day 3, and
  2 mg/kg tid from day 4–2,
  60 mL syrup 50 mg/5 mL

Q. What are the adverse effects of this drug?

A. Systemic: Nausea, vomiting, diarrhea, headache and giddiness.

Q. What are the other key features of this drug?

A.
- Adequate data not available for safety in pregnancy
- Advisable to defer use until delivery DEC has no effect on the adult parasite
- Brugian filariasis is more susceptible to treatment than bancroftian filariasis

Q. What is Mazzotti reaction?

A. Mazzotti reaction is a severe, potentially life-threatening allergic response that occurs within 7 days of treatment of microfilariasis with DEC. The reaction correlates with the intensity of infection. The clinical features consist of fever, urticaria, swollen and tender lymph nodes, tachycardia, hypotension, arthralgia, edema, and abdominal pain. It occurs due to liberation of microfilarial antigens on treatment.

ANTILEISHMANIAL AGENTS SODIUM STIBOGLUCONATE (SODIUM ANTIMONY GLUCONATE)

Introduction

It is a water-soluble pentavalent antimonial.

Q. What is mechanism of action?

A. It inhibits SH-dependent enzymes of the parasite and bioenergetics of the parasite is interfered. Blocks glycolic and fatty acid oxidation pathways.

Q. What are the indications?

A. Kala azar.

Q. What dose and formulations available for this drug?

A.
- 20 mg/kg (maximum: 850 mg) daily by IM (in the buttocks) or IV injection for:
  - 28 days for mucocutaneous and visceral disease
  - 20 days for cutaneous leishmaniasis
- Formulation: 100 mg/mL in 30 mL vial.

Q. What are the adverse effects of this drug?

A. Nausea, vomiting, metallic taste, cough, abdominal pain, pain and stiffness of injected muscle, sterile abscesses and liver and kidney damage.

Q. What are the other key features of this drug?

A. Drug of choice for kala azar.
- Rapidly absorbed from the site of IM injection. It is excreted unchanged in urine
- Liver and renal function tests should be done at the baseline and after 10 days of therapy
- Repeated doses are cumulative, increasing efficacy as well as risk of liver and renal toxicity

PENTAMIDINE

Introduction

Pentamidine isethionate is an antiprotozoal agent.

Q. What is mechanism of action?

A. Probably interacts with kinetoplast DNA or inhibits aerobic glycolysis.

Q. What is the indication of pentamidine in dermatology?

A. Used only as salvage therapy after antimonial failure.

Q. What dose and formulations available for this drug?

A.
- 4 mg/kg IM or slow IV injection on alternate days; total 12–15 injections.
- Dry powder in 300 mg vial.

Q. What is pregnancy category of the drug?

A. Category C.

Q. What are the adverse effects of this drug?

A.
- Acute reactions: Sharp fall in BP, palpitation, fainting, vomiting, rigor and fever (with IV injection, less frequent with IM).
- Others: Rashes, ECG changes, liver and kidney damage, rarely cardiac arrhythmias.

Q. What are the other key features of this drug?

A.
- Used only as salvage therapy after antimonial failure.
- It initially causes cytolysis of pancreatic β-cells—release of insulin, hypoglycemia and later permanent diabetes.

AMPHOTERICIN B

Introduction

Amphotericin is a broad-spectrum systemic antifungal drug and also used for disseminated and visceral leishmaniasis.

Q. What is mechanism of action?

A. Like fungi, *Leishmania* have a high percentage of ergosterol and hence are susceptible to amphotericin B.

Q. What are the indications?

A. Mucocutaneous and disseminated leishmaniasis.

Q. What dose and formulations available for this drug?

A. 0.5 mg/kg by slow intravenous infusion for leishmaniasis, total dose of 7–20 mg/kg is usually required.

Q. What is pregnancy category of the drug?

A. Category B.

Q. What are the other key features of this drug?

A.
- Reserved for patients not responding to both antimonial and pentamidine.
- Useful in mucocutaneous and disseminated leishmaniasis.

ALLOPURINOL

Introduction

It is a xanthine oxidase inhibitor, that has also been used in leishmaniasis.

Q. What is mechanism of action?

A. It inhibits protein synthesis. Purine salvage pathway in *Leishmania* metabolizes allopurinol into corresponding nucleotides, which are incorporated in RNA resulting in interference with protein synthesis.

Q. What is the indication?

A. Leishmaniasis.

Q. What dose and formulations available for this drug?

A. 4–12 mg/kg tid for 3–4 weeks.

Q. What is pregnancy category of the drug?

A. Category C.

2.11. ORAL RETINOIDS INTRODUCTION

INTRODUCTION

- The term retinoids includes all synthetic and natural compounds that have biological activity like that of vitamin A
- Isotretinoin was first synthesized in 1955 and got US FDA approval for treatment of acne in 1982
- Etretinate and acitretin were first synthesized in 1972, and etretinate got US FDA approval for treatment of psoriasis in 1986 but was phased out in 1998 and acitretin has been approved for the same use since then.

Q. How do you classify retinoids?

A.

Classification	*Chemical structure*	*Retinoid*
First generation	Monoaromatic	Isotretinoin, tretinoin
Second generation	Monoaromatic with replaced rings	Etretinate, acitretin
Third generation	Polyaromatic	Bexarotene, tazarotene, adapalene

Q. What is the mechanism of action of oral retinoids?

A. Retinoids bind to a specific retinoic acid response element (RARE) on some target genes. These are up regulated and transcription takes place. The proteins produced help in:

- Regulates cell growth, differentiation and morphogenesis of keratinocytes; i.e., normalizes keratinization.
- In contrast the anti-inflammatory action of oral retinoids are mediated by a down regulation of genes which do not contain RARE
- Retinoids also activate Toll-like receptors
- They also have an antikeratinizing and comedolytic effect
- Inhibition of carcinogenesis and tumorigenesis
- Immunomodulatory action

Q. What is the pregnancy category of oral retinoids?

A. Category X.

Q. What are the indications of oral retinoids?

A.

Drug	*FDA approved indication*
Isotretinoin	Nodulocystic and recalcitrant acne with scarring tendency
Acitretin	1. Generalized or localized pustular psoriasis 2. Combination therapy with phototherapy, cyclosporine or biologics
Bexarotene	Mycosis fungoides (resistant to at least one systemic therapy)

Other dermatologic uses are:

Group	*Specific disease*
Pilosebaceous disorders	Rosacea, perioral dermatitis, pyoderma faciale, scalp folliculitis, eosinophilic folliculitis, dissecting cellulitis, hidradenitis suppuritiva
Disorders of keratinization	Icthyosis, pityriasis rubra pilaris (PRP), keratoderma, Darier's disease, porokeratosis
Neoplastic processes	Basal cell carcinoma (BCC), advanced squamous cell carcinoma (SCC), keratoacanthoma, Bowen's disease, actinic keratosis, Langerhans cell histiocytosis
Miscellaneous	Lichen planus, lupus erythematosus, lichen sclerosus, sarcoidosis, granuloma annulare (GA), subcorneal pustular dermatosis

Q. What are the contraindications of oral retinoids?

A. Absolute contraindications:

- Pregnancy and lactation

Relative contraindications:

- Hyperlipidemia
- Children
- Diabetes mellitus
- Liver disease
- Raised intracranial pressure
- Suicidal ideation

Q. What are the side effects of oral retinoids?

A. Relatively common minor adverse side effects:

- Cutaneous—xerosis, palmoplantar desquamation, retinoid dermatitis, photosensitivity, pyogenic granulomas, *Staphylococcus aureus* infections
- Hair—telogen effluvium, abnormal hair texture, dryness
- Nails—fragility with nail softening, paronychia, onycholysis
- Ocular—dry eyes, blepharoconjunctivitis, photophobia
- Oral—cheilits, dry mouth, sore mouth and tongue
- Nasal—nasal mucosa dryness, decreased mucous secretion, epistaxis
- Musculoskeletal—arthralgia, myalgia, fatigue, muscle weakness, tendonitis
- Neurology—headache, mild depression
- Gastrointestinal—nausea, diarrhea, abdominal pain

Potentially serious adverse effects:

- Teratogenicity—retinoic acid embryopathy (facial, heart and bone defects), spontaneous abortions
- Ocular—reduced night vision (it is absolutely contraindicated in pilots), persistent dry eyes, *Staphylococcus aureus* infections
- Bone—diffuse interstitial skeletal hyperostosis (DISH), osteophyte formation, premature epiphyseal closure
- Lipids—hypercholesterolemia, hypertriglyceridemia
- Gastrointestinal—inflammatory bowel disease flare, pancreatitis
- Hepatic—transaminase elevations, toxic hepatitis
- Other endocrine effects—hypothyroidism
- Hematologic—leukopenia, agranulocytosis
- Neurologic—psuedotumor cerebri, depression (suicidal ideation)
- Muscle—myopathy

Q. What are the monitoring guidelines for oral retinoids?

A. Baseline:

- Careful history and physical examination
- Urine pregnancy test (FDA advises a serum pregnancy test also)
- Complete blood count (CBC)
- Liver function tests (LFT)
- Lipid profile

Follow up:

- Monthly for the first 3–6 months, then every 3 months:
- Clinical examination
- CBC
- LFT
- Urine pregnancy test
- X-ray of wrists ankles, or thoracic spine with long-term therapy to look for DISH syndrome
- Radiography of symptomatic joints with long-term therapy to look for DISH syndrome
- Complete ophthalmic examination if patient reports visual changes (optional)

Q. Why has acitretin replaced etretinate?

A. Etretinate is extremely long acting since it is lipophilic. Hence pregnancy cannot be allowed for 2 years after stopping it due its teratogenic potential. Acitretin is a metabolite of etretinate and has a shorter half-life. It was believed therefore that the interdiction period would be shortened. However, it is now known that acitretin gets reconverted to etretinate in the body especially in the presence of alcohol. Hence, the interdiction period for pregnancy is still 2 years in case of acitretin and its replacement of etretinate has not made any difference.

Q. How are oral retinoids metabolized and excreted?

A. Oral retinoids are metabolized by the hepatic cytochrome P450–3A4 system and are excreted in the bile and through the kidneys.

Q. What is the interaction of alcohol with retinoids?

A. Alcohol and retinoids are synergistically hepatotoxic. Moreover, alcohol increases conversion of acitretin to etretinate which is more embryotoxic. Hence, alcohol should be strictly avoided when on retinoids. Even cough syrups containing alcohol should be avoided.

Q. How does isotretinoin work in acne?

A.
- It inhibits sebum production by inhibiting sebaceous proliferation, differentiation, decreasing sebaceous gland size and skin dihydrotestosterone and down regulation of androgen receptors in skin
- Indirect antibacterial action due to reduction of follicular space and nutrient supply of *Propionibacterium acnes*
- Anti-inflammatory action by regulating Toll-like receptors

Q. How does acitretin work in psoriasis?

A. It helps in normalizing keratinization by causing growth differentiation. It also has an immunomodulatory action. It is especially useful in pustular and erythrodermic psoriasis. In plaque psoriasis it has to be combined with other modalities of therapy. It is not given in guttate psoriasis (since it is self-limited) while it is not effective in psoriatic arthropathy.

Q. What are the doses of retinoids?

A. Conventional dose of isotretinoin is 0.5–1 mg/kg/day for 16–20 weeks to a cumulative dose of 120–140 mg/kg. With this dose, there is very often a flare of acne after 3–6 weeks of treatment. This may be related to apoptosis of the sebaceous cells. Hence the recent trend is to use lower daily doses to reduce the incidence of adverse effects. It has also been noted that at low doses acne scarring is paradoxically less. A recent study has even shown as low a dose as 5 mg/day has been effective. The duration of treatment with this low dose has been increased to about 6 months for facial acne and 18 months for truncal acne.

Acitretin can be used either as monotherapy or combination therapy. The optimal dose range for monotherapy is 25–50 mg/day.

The improvement is very gradual and may take up to 3-6 months for response, very often there may be an initial flare after starting acitretin which may last for 1-2 months; higher doses will result in more side effects. Acitretin monotherapy is more preferred for pustular and erythrodermic types while combinations are preferred for plaque psoriasis if combination is given, it is better to start with an even lower dose of acitretin 10-25 mg/day.

Q. Discuss combination strategy in psoriasis.

A.

Group	***Specific disease***
Pilosebaceous disorders	Rosacea, perioral dermatitis, pyoderma faciale, scalp folliculitis, eosinophilic folliculitis, dissecting cellulitis, hidradenitis suppuritiva
Disorders of keratinization	Icthyosis, PRP, keratoderma, Darier's disease, porokeratosis
Neoplastic processes	Basal cell carcinomas, advanced SCC, keratoacanthoma, Bowen's disease, actinic keratoses, Langerhans cell histiocytosis
Miscellaneous	Lichen planus, lupus erythematosus, lichen sclerosus, sarcoidosis, GA, subcorneal pustular dermatosis

Q. Discuss various combinations of acitretin.

A. They are:

- Acitretin + PUVA: The patient is started on low dose acitretin for 10-14 days. PUVA is then added till lesions are clear. Maintenance therapy maybe continued with either acitretin or puva, this is called RE-PUVA therapy
- Acitretin + UVB: This is especially useful in difficult to treat areas like scalp, palms and soles
- Acitretin + methotrexate: Acitretin is started with a dose of 25-50 mg/day and if there is no response methotrexate is added in the dose of 15-25 mg/week. In this therapy there is a concern of hepatotoxicity
- Acitretin + cyclosporine: This therapy is called as sequential therapy where in cyclosporine is used as a clearing agent and acitretin as a maintaining agent. Transition between the drugs involves gradual tapering of cyclosporine while acitretin is maintained

Q. What are the precautions advised to the patients on oral retinoids?

A.
- Use of contact lenses should be avoided
- Alcohol intake should be avoided
- The patient should be advised strict contraception while on therapy and for 1 month after stopping therapy in case of isotretinoin and 2 years after stopping therapy in case of acitretin

Q. Discuss the adverse effects of acitretin in psoriasis.

A.

System	*Very frequent*	*Often*	*Infrequent*	*Rare*
Mucocutaneous	Cheilitis	Rhinitis	Epistaxis	Dry mouth
Cutaneous		Alopecia, peeling	Dry skin, onycholysis, itching	Paresthesia, paronychia, sticky skin
Eye	-	-	-	Dry eyes
Musculo-skeletal	-	-	-	Arthralgia, DISH
Central nervous system	-	-	-	Pseudotumor cerebri
Liver	-	-	-	Hepatitis
Pancreas	-	-	-	Pancreatitis due to triglyceridemia

Q. Discuss drug interactions of acitretin.

A.
- Tetracyclines and minocycline should not be used with acitretin due to the risk of photosensitivity and pseudotumor cerebri
- Alcohol increases conversion rate of acitretin to etretinate as well as increases hepatotoxicity
- Vitamin A can cause overdosing
- Caution is to be exercised with antidiabetic agents (alteration in blood glucose)
- Caution is to be exercised with steroids (pseudotumor cerebri and hyperlipidemia)
- Caution to be exercised with methotrexate (increased levels and hepatotoxicity)
- Acitretin interferes with contraceptive effect of progestin mini pills but not with the usual oral contraceptives
- Excessive UV exposure is to be avoided with acitretin as it can cause retinoid dermatitis

2.12. ANTIANDROGENS AND ANDROGEN INHIBITORS

Q. What are antiandrogens and androgen inhibitors?

A. "Antiandrogens" are agents that block androgen receptors while, "androgen inhibitors" block androgen synthesis.

Q. Name a few dermatological disorders due to androgen excess.

A.
- Acne vulgaris
- Androgenetic alopecia (AGA)—male pattern AGA, female pattern AGA
- Hirsutism
- Hidradenitis suppurativa

Q. Name a few antiandrogens and androgen inhibitors.

A. Antiandrogens (block or inhibit androgen receptor):
- Spironolactone
- Progesterone
- Cyproterone acetate
- Cimetidine

Androgen inhibitors (inhibit or block enzymes leading to DHT production, such as 5-α reductase):
- Finasteride
- Dutasteride
- Ketoconazole
- Progestin hormone agents
- Leuprolide
- Nafarelin
- Herbal products like saw palmetto, green tea, pygeum, stinging nettle, spearmint, etc.

Q. Write a note on spironolactone.

A.
- Spironolactone is an aldosterone antagonist. It inhibits androgen biosynthesis. It may be converted to other active metabolites via progesterone 17-hydroxylase. It reversibly inhibits adrenal and cytochrome P-450 enzymes resulting in decreased testosterone and DHT production. Bioavailability from oral administration is 90%. Food increases absorption of spironolactone. It is 98% protein bound and metabolized in the liver. Its primary metabolite is canrenone. Metabolites are excreted in bile and urine, peak levels arise after 2–4 hours with a plasma half-life of 12.5 hours. Doses range from 50 to 200 mg BID daily for 2–3 months.

- Indications—hirsutism, acne vulgaris, androgenetic alopecia, hidradenitis suppurativa
- Contraindications—renal insufficiency, anuria, hyperkalemia, pregnancy, abnormal uterine bleeding, family or personal history of estrogen—dependent malignancy
- Pregnancy category D
- Adverse effects—headache menstrual abnormalities, feminization of male fetus, hyperkalemia, agranulocytosis, estrogen-dependent malignancies
- Drug interactions—drugs which increase the risk of hyperkalemia like angiotensin converting enzyme inhibitors, aliskiren (a direct renin inhibitor), angiotensin II receptor blockers, aldosterone inhibitors
- Laboratory monitoring—monitoring of DHEA-S every 3–4 months is recommended for successful androgen suppression, complete suppression after 4–12 months of spironolactone therapy

Q. Discus drospirenone.

A. Drospirenone is a synthetic progestational compound and spironolactone analog with antimineralocorticoid activity. It has antiandrogenic activity but no estrogenic or glucocorticoid activity. Available as the following formulations—3 mg drospirenone and 0.02 ethinylestradiol and 3 mg drospirenone and 0.03 mg of ethinylestradiol.

Dermatological indications

- Acne vulgaris
- Female pattern alopecia
- Hirsutism

Contraindications

- Hepatic dysfunction
- Adrenal insufficiency
- Renal insufficiency

Q. Write a note on progesterone.

A. Progesterone can be given intramuscularly or orally. It shows good absorption via both the routes. Peak levels are reached in 1–2 hours with a half-life of 8–9 hours. It is metabolized in the liver to hydrophilic metabolites. It is excreted via renal and hepatobiliary route. Most commonly used oral formulation is medroxyprogesterone acetate. Also available as injectable and topical gels.

Indications in dermatology

It has been used as a topical agent for treating AGA in 2–5% concentrations.

Side effects

Menstrual irregularities, flare-up of acne.

Q. Write a note on finasteride.

A. Finasteride is a specific inhibitor of type II 5-α reductase. This enzyme catalyzes the conversion of testosterone to DHT. By inhibiting this enzyme, finasteride reduces the levels of DHT in the hair follicle. It does not directly bind to androgen receptors but has secondary effects on it via feedback mechanisms that affect androgen receptor levels like local suppression of DHT. Its half-life is 4–8 hours and is metabolized in the liver. Standard dose—1 mg od (for AGA) and 5 mg od for prostatic hyperplasia.

Indications

- Male pattern androgenetic alopecia (FDA-approved dermatological indication)
- Female pattern androgenetic alopecia
- Hirsutism
- Acne vulgaris
- Hidradenitis suppurativa

Contraindications

- Hypersensitivity to finasteride or any component of product
- Use in children
- Use in women of child bearing age
- Blood donation is contraindicated for atleast 6 months after the last dose of finasteride, to prevent blood donation to a pregnant female transfusion recipient, which may harm the male fetus
- Pregnancy category X

Adverse effects

- Loss of libido, erectile and ejaculatory dysfunction, gynecomastia
- Hypersensitivity reactions
- Severe myopathy
- Depression
- Decreases prostate specific antigen (PSA) and adjustment factors may be needed to determine whether the PSA is in the normal range. However, finasteride is also believed to reduce the risk of carcinoma prostate.
- Teratogenicity

Interactions

Nevirapine may reduce the levels and efficacy of finasteride.

Q. Discuss dutasteride.

A. Dutasteride is a very potent dual 5-α reductase inhibitor that inhibits both type I and type II isoenzymes. Peak levels are at 2–3 hours and the half-life is 4–8 weeks. Its bioavailability is 60% with a protein binding of 90%. It undergoes hepatic metabolism and is excreted in urine and feces.

Indications

- Male pattern androgenetic alopecia
- Female pattern androgenetic alopecia
- Frontal fibrosing alopecia (controversial)
- Hirsutism
- Acne vulgaris
- Hidradenitis suppurativa
- Benign prostatic hypertrophy

Dosage

Available as 500 μg soft capsules.

Drug interactions

Drugs that increase the serum levels of dutasteride are several CYP 3A4 enzyme inhibitors like azoles, macrolides, calcium channel blockers, and some anti-HIV drugs.

Precautions and contraindications

- Refer to finasteride
- Men on Dutasteride therapy should not donate blood for atleast 6 months after stopping therapy.

Q. Write a note on ketoconazole.

A.
- Ketoconazole causes inhibition of CYP-450 enzyme in the liver which reduces metabolism of estrogens and increases its levels. Hence, it has an antiandrogenic effect.
- Further discussion will be found in the chapter on antifungals.

Q. Write about the herbal remedies available for hair growth.

A. Herbal remedies available for hair growth that claim to have antiandrogenic properties against androgen receptors or androgen inhibiting activity against 5-α reductase enzymes include:

- Saw palmetto
- Green tea
- Pygeum
- Stinging nettle
- Spearmint herbal tea
- Lignans (phytoestrogens)
- Curcumin (found in turmeric)

- Caffeic acid
- Methanol extract of heartwood
- Alizarin

2.13. VITAMINS AND TRACE ELEMENTS

There are two types:

1. *Fat soluble vitamins which include*: Vitamins A, D, E, and K.
2. *Water soluble vitamins which include*: Vitamin B1 (thiamine), vitamin B2 (riboflavin), vitamin B3 (niacin or niacinamide), vitamin B4 (adenine), vitamin B5 (pantothenic acid), vitamin B6 (pyridoxine), vitamin B7 (biotin or vitamin H), vitamin B8 (inositol), vitamin B9 (folic acid), vitamin B10 (para-aminobenzoic acid), vitamin B11 (salicylic acid), vitamin B12 (cyanocobalamin), vitamin B13 (orotic acid) and vitamin C (ascorbic acid).

FAT SOLUBLE VITAMINS

Vitamin A

Q. What are the dietary sources of vitamin A?

A. *Animal sources*: Fish, meat
Vegetable sources: Green leafy vegetables, carrot

Q. What is the mechanism of action of vitamin A?

A. Maintaining the integrity of epithelial membranes, normalizing keratinization, antioxidant and anti-inflammatory effect, preventing tumorigenesis and carcinogenesis.

Q. What are the symptoms of vitamin A deficiency?

A. Nyctalopia (night blindness), Bitot's spots, phrynoderma, xerophthalmia, keratomalacia (appearing in this order).

Q. Is phrynoderma associated with any other deficiency?

A. Yes, possibly related to biotin or essential fatty acid deficiency (linoleic, linolenic, arachidonic acids), vitamin C and E.

Q. What are the uses?

A. Vitamin A has largely been replaced by retinoids. However, it is effective in vitamin A deficiency.

Q. What is the RDA of vitamin A?

A. 5,000 IU/day up to 6,000 IU/day in pregnancy.

Q. What is the dosage of vitamin A in phrynoderma?

A. 50,000 IU/day until lesions resolve (monitor for hypervitaminosis A).

Q. What are the drug interactions?

A. Vitamin A can interact with birth control pills, blood thinners such as warfarin, bexarotene, cholestyramine.

Q. What are the adverse effects?

A. This includes hypervitaminosis A if the consumption is > 200,000 IU for prolonged periods. Initial symptoms include lethargy, lassitude and headache, there is xerosis, erythematous, scaly and cracked skin. Hair loss and mucosal bleeding may follow.

Key point

Vitamin A is the only vitamin which can be teratogenic in high doses.

Vitamin D (Cholecalciferol)

Q. What are the sources of vitamin D?

A. Fatty fish (mackerel, tuna) and also food fortified with vitamin D. Most of our vitamin D is obtained through sunlight.

Q. What is its mechanism of action?

A. It stimulates the absorption of calcium from gastrointestinal tract and increases the rate of mineralization of the bones.

Q. What are the uses of vitamin D in dermatology?

A. Vitamin D can be used for the following conditions—topical therapy with vitamin D analogs is used in many skin diseases, for example, Psoriasis, vitiligo, morphea.

Q. What is the recommended daily allowance (RDA) of vitamin D?

A. 400 IU/day.

Vitamin E

Vitamin E is a fat soluble vitamin found in many foods including vegetable oils, cereals, meat, eggs. It has got antioxidant properties.

Q. What are its indications?

A. Vitamin E is empirically used in the following conditions:

- Periorbital darkening
- Lichen sclerosus et atrophicus
- Striae
- Epidermolysis bullosa
- Morphea

Q. What is the RDA of vitamin E?
A. 15 mg/day.

Vitamin K (Menadione)

Vitamin K is a fat soluble vitamin that the body needs for blood coagulation and in metabolic pathways in bone and other tissues.

Q. What are the indications?
A. Purpura, ecchymoses, hematoma secondary to vitamin K deficiency.

Q. What is the RDA of vitamin K?
A. 90 mcg/day.

Q. What are the adverse effects?
A. Intramuscular vitamin K can result in cutaneous necrosis (Nicolau syndrome or embolia cutis medicamentosa).

WATER SOLUBLE VITAMINS

Name	*RDA (mg/day)*	*Indications*	*Side-effects*
B1 (Thiamine)	1.1	Beri-beri disease	–
B2 (Riboflavin)	1.1	Oro-oculo-genital syndrome, naso-labial dyssebacia, lactic acidosis	–
B3 (Niacin)	20 (6.6 mg/1000 cal) dietary sources—fish, chicken, peanuts, mushroom	Pellagra, VBDs, hypertriglyceridemia, erythema elevatum diutinum	Flushing of the skin, hypotension, pruritus, headache
B5 (Pantothenic acid)	5 to 6	Burning feet syndrome, greying of hair	–
B6 (Pyridoxine)	1.3 to 1.7	Supplementation with INH to prevent neuropathy, homocystinuria, pellagroid dermatitis	Ataxia, hypoxia, and blistering

Continued

Continued

Name	RDA (mg/day)	Indications	Side-effects
B7 (Biotin)	0.1	Congenital biotin deficiency, telogen effluvium, uncombable hair syndrome	–
B9 (Folic acid)	0.4 to 0.6 dietary sources–beans, legumes, dark leafy vegetables fruits and nuts	Supplementation with MTX therapy, erythroderma, homocystinuria, aphthous ulcers	Drug interactions with NSAIDs increase requirement of folic acid
B12 (Cyano-cobalamin)	0.02	Canities, Addisonian pigmentation	Pruritus, hypersensitivity

Vitamin C (Ascorbic Acid)

It is an essential vitamin since it is not synthesized by the human body. It is an important antioxidant and free radical scavenger. It is a cofactor in protein and carbohydrate metabolism. Dietary sources—green vegetables, citrus fruits, tomato, guava, papaya.

Q. What are the indications?

A. It can be used in the following conditions:

- Scurvy—the first symptom reduced is the spongy and bleeding gums, later the purpuric lesions, and lastly the hair and skin lesions
- It is used both topically and systemically as a photoprotective agent
- It helps in wound healing
- Used empirically in pigmented purpuric dermatosis

Q. What is the RDA of vitamin C?

A. 75–90 mg/day.

Zinc

Zinc is an essential cofactor for many enzymatic reactions occurring in the body. Dietary sources—seafood, lamb, spinach, pumpkin.

Q. What is the mechanism of action?

A. It has an antioxidant, wound healing and lysosomal stabilizing action. It is a cofactor in enzymes like carbonic anhydrase.

Q. What are the adverse effects?

A. Intramuscular vitamin K can result in cutaneous necrosis (Nicolau syndrome or embolia cutis medicamentosa).

Q. What are its indications?

A.
- Zinc deficiency like acrodermatitis enteropathica and acquired zinc deficiency due to gastric and intestinal resections, and in conditions where total parenteral nutrition is required
- Chronic nonhealing ulcers
- Aphthous ulcers
- Recurrent erythema nodosum leprosum
- Acne vulgaris
- Hidradenitis suppuritiva
- Alopecia areata
- Nonspecific hair loss

Q. What are the adverse effects?

A. High dose exposures may lead to nausea, vomiting, diarrhea, abdominal pain, and dizziness.

Q. What is the RDA of zinc?

A. 15 mg of elemental zinc/day. Zinc is supplied as zinc sulphate or zinc gluconate containing 220 mg of salt which gives 22.5 mg of zinc/day.

Iron

Iron is a micronutrient which is an essential component of heme moiety of hemoglobin.

Q. What are the indications for iron therapy?

A. Following are the indications for iron therapy:
- Iron deficiency states
- Telogen effluvium
- Plummer—Vinson syndrome

Q. What are the adverse effects?

A. Nausea, vomiting, constipation, diarrhea and dark colored stools.

Q. Can you have decreased body iron with normal hemoglobin?

A. Yes. Hence, serum ferritin has to be done in doubtful situations.

Q. What is the RDA of iron?

A. 8 mg/day which is tripled during pregnancy.

Q. Which is the best iron salt?

A. There is none which is the best, but ferrous sulphate is cheap and easily absorbed.

Copper

Copper is an essential micronutrient which is a component of several enzymes, the most important of which is tyrosinase.

Q. What is its mechanism of action?
A. It helps in the post-translational modification of collagen.

Q. What are the indications?
A. It has been empirically used in vitiligo, nonspecific hair loss.

Q. What is the RDA of copper?
A. 0.9 mg/day.

Selenium

It is an important micronutrient as it plays an important role in many dermatological manifestations.

Q. What is its mechanism of action?
A. Selenium is an antioxidant.

Q. What are the indications?
A. As an antioxidant for photoprotection, topical selenium sulfide is used as a treatment for dandruff and pityriasis versicolor.

Q. What is the RDA of selenium?
A. 55 mcg/day.

Q. What are the adverse effects?
A. In high doses it causes alopecia, anonychia and xerosis of skin. It is also teratogenic in animals.

ESSENTIAL FATTY ACIDS

EFA contributes to the formation of the lamellar bodies by the stratum granulosum which form principle intercellular lipids in stratum granulosum.

Q. What is its mechanism of action?
A. It is an anti-inflammatory agent causing synthesis of n-3 type of fatty acid which replaces the n-6 type of fatty acids in the cell membrane. The latter are proinflammatory while the former are anti-inflammatory.

Q. Which are the essential fatty acids?
A. Linoleic acid, linolenic acid, and arachidonic acid. They are not synthesized by the human body, hence, they are called essential.

Q. What are the indications for the use of essential fatty acids?

A. Essential fatty acids can be useful for the following conditions:

- Phyrnoderma
- Psoriasis
- Atopic dermatitis
- Empirical use in acne

Q. What are its dosages?

A. 12 g eicosapentaenoic acid, daily for 6 weeks. Each 1 g capsule contains 170 mg Eicosapentaenoic acid (EPA) and 115 mg Docosahexaenoic acid (DHA).

2.14. ANTITUBERCULOUS DRUGS

Q. Classify antituberculosis drugs.

A. They are classified as first line drugs and second line drugs.

Drugs:

First line

- H-Isoniazid
- R-Rifampin/Rifampicin
- Z-Pyrazinamide
- E-Ethambutol
- S-Streptomycin drugs

Second line

- Tzn-Thiacetazone
- PAS-Para-aminosalicylic acid
- Etm-Ethionamide
- Cys-Cycloserine
- Kmc-Kanamycin
- Am-Amikacin second line newer drug
- Ciprofloxacin
- Ofloxacin
- Clarithromycin
- Azithromycin
- Rifabutin

Q. What are the therapeutic goals of AKT?

A. The therapeutic goals of AKT are as follows:

- Prevention or prophylaxis
- Cure of clinical disease
- Requirements:
    - Prolonged therapy

- ○ Combined therapy
- ○ Compliance
- ○ Prevention of development of drug resistance
- ○ Cures ideally, 95–100%

Q. Enumerate the various properties of *Mycobacterium tuberculosis.*

A. Properties of *Mycobacterium tuberculosis*:

- Cell wall has high lipid content
- Mycolic acid is a major component
- Slow growth
- Survive within phagocytes

ISONIAZID

- Primarily tuberculocidal
- Fast multiplying organisms are killed, quiescent ones are inhibited
- Act on extracellular and intracellular bacilli
- Cheapest antituberculosis drug

Q. What is the mechanism of action of isoniazid?

A. Inhibits mycolic acid synthesis which is an essential component of mycobacterial cell wall.

Q. What is the dose of isoniazid?

A. Adult dose:

- 300 mg/day PO
- 600 mg/dose PO in thrice weekly DOTS schedule

Pediatric dose:

- 5 mg/kg/day PO
- 10 mg/kg/dose PO in thrice weekly DOTS schedule

Q. Enumerate the adverse effects of isoniazid.

A. Peripheral neuritis—slow acetylators—paresthesia, numbness, mental disturbances, convulsions. It is due to interference with utilization of pyridoxine and its increased excretion in urine.

Pyridoxine can be used as 10 mg/day-prophylactic and 100 mg/day-for toxicity.

Hepatitis-older and alcoholics-dose related damage to liver cells. Reversible on stopping the drug.

Rash, fever, acneiform eruption, arthralgia, Stevens-Johnson syndrome, hypersensitivity, erythema multiforme, drug induced LE, pellagroid rash (interference with pyridoxine metabolism which is an essential coenzyme for niacin metabolism), toxic epidermal necrolysis.

RIFAMPICIN

- Semisynthetic derivative of rifamycin B
- Source—*Streptomyces mediterranei*
- Bactericidal
- As efficacious as INH
- Both extra and intracellular organisms are affected

Q. Enumerate the spectrum of rifampicin.

A.
- *M. tuberculosis*
- *M. leprae*
- *M. kansasii*
- *M. scrofulaceum*
- *M. avium intercellulare*
- *M. fortuitum*
- *Staphylococcus aureus*
- *N. meningitidis*

Q. Enumerate the mechanism of action of rifampicin.

A.
- Inhibits DNA dependent RNA polymerase
- Suppress initiation of chain formation in RNA synthesis

Q. What is the dose of rifampicin?

A.
- *Adult dose*: 600 mg/day if weight >35 kg, and 450 mg/day if weight <35 kg PO
- *Pediatric dose*: 10–20 mg/day PO

(dose remains the same in both groups for DOTS thrice weekly dosing schedule)

Q. Discuss the drug interactions of rifampicin.

A. It is a microsomal enzyme inducer.

Q. Discuss the adverse effects of rifampicin.

A. Refer to the chapter on antileprosy drugs.

Q. Enumerate the other uses of rifampicin.

A.
- Treatment of TB-10 mg/kg 600 mg
- 2nd/3rd line for MRSA, diphetheroids, legionella
- Leprosy
- Eradication of staphylococcal nasal carrier state in furunculosis
- Atypical mycobacteria infection
- Mycetoma (Damle's regimen)

PYRAZINAMIDE

- Weakly tuberculocidal
- Lethal to intracellular bacilli
- Helps shorten regimen and decreases relapse

Q. Discuss the mechanism of action of pyrazinamide.

A. An enzyme activates pyrazinamide to pyrazinoic acid which interacts with a different fatty acid synthetase causing inhibition of synthesis of mycolic acids.

Dose:

- *Adult dose*: 1500 mg/day
- *Pediatric dose*: 15–30 mg/kg/day

Dose remains the same in thrice weekly DOTS dosing schedule.

Q. Enumerate the adverse effects of pyrazinamide.

A. Hepatotoxicity, hyperuricemia, gout, arthralgia, flushing, rashes, fever, loss of diabetes control.

Q. Enumerate the drug interaction of pyrazinamide.

A. Concurrent administration with rifampicin has more risk of hepatotoxicity.

ETHAMBUTOL

- Tuberculostatic
- Fast multiplying organisms are affected
- Atypical mycobacteria
- Hasten sputum conversion and prevent development of resistance

Q. Discuss the mechanism of action of ethambutol.

A. Diffuses in the tubercle bacilli and impairs cell metabolism by inhibiting synthesis of one or more metabolites which causes cell death.

Dose:

- *Adult dose*: 800 mg/day or 15–25 mg/kg/day and 1200 mg/dose as part of DOTS thrice weekly dosing schedule.
- *Pediatric dose*: not recommended in children < 6 years of age (risk of optic neuritis which is difficult to diagnose in children).

Q. Enumerate adverse effects of ethambutol.

A. Dose related and duration dependent:

- Loss of visual acuity/red-green color vision
- Optic neuritis-field defects

- Nausea, rashes, fever, hyperuricemia, neurological changes-headache, dizziness, mental confusion, hallucination, tingling of fingers

STREPTOMYCIN

Introduction

- First clinically useful anti-TB drug
- Tuberculocidal
- Acts only on extracellular bacilli
- Penetrate TB cavities
- Does not cross CSF
- Resistance has increased-bacilli selectively multiply and stage a comeback after initial control

Q. Discuss the mechanism of action of streptomycin.

A. Binds to 30s causing inhibition of protein synthesis:

- Prevent polysome formation
- Promote disaggregation to monosome
- Cause misreading of codon

Dose:

- *Adult dose*: 15 mg/kg/day IM
- *Pediatric dose*: 20–40 mg/kg/day IM
- *DOTS regimen*: 0.75 mg/dose

Q. Enumerate the adverse effects of streptomycin.

A. Ototoxicity:

- Vertigo
- Rash
- Nephrotoxicity
- Fever

Q. What is the pregnancy category of this drug.

A. Pregnancy category D.

Q. What are the indications of streptomycin?

A.
- Life threatening TB
- Resistant TB
- In MAC and *M. kansasii* infection
- It is also used in mycetoma and was used in the past for treatment of chancroid with bubo formation, and also for treatment of donovanosis.

SECOND-LINE DRUGS

Thiacetazone

- Tuberculostatic drug
- Low efficacy
- Low cost
- Used as a substitute of PAS along with INH

Dose:

- *Adult dose*: 150 mg/day
- *Pediatric dose*: 2–3 mg/kg/day

Q. Enumerate the adverse effects of thiacetazone.

A.
- Hepatitis
- Exfoliative dermatitis
- Stevens Johnson syndrome and TEN
- BM depression
- Contraindicated in HIV patients

PARA-AMINO SALICYLIC ACID (PAS)

- Tuberculostatic drug
- PABA analog

Q. What is the mechanism of action?

A.
- Folate synthase inhibition
- Delays development of resistance-directly inhibit episomal resistance transfer
- Metabolism by acetylation

Dose:

- *Adult dose*: 12 g/day PO in 2 or 3 divided doses
- *Pediatric dose*: 150 mg/kg/day PO in 3 or 4 divided doses

Q. What are the adverse effects of PAS?

A.
- Anorexia
- Nausea
- Epigastric pain
- Rash, fever, malaise
- Goiter
- Liver dysfunction
- Blood dyscrasias
- Tuberculostatic drug

ETHIONAMIDE

Q. What is the mechanism of action?

A.
- Inhibits mycolic cell wall
- Acts on both extra and intracellular organisms
- Rapid resistance

Dose:
- *Adult dose*: 0.5–1 g/day PO in 2 or 3 divided doses
- *Pediatric dose*: 15–20 mg/kg/day PO in 3 or 4 divided doses

Q. What are the adverse effects?

A.
- Anorexia
- Nausea
- Vomiting
- Aches
- Pain
- Rash
- Optic neuritis

CYCLOSERINE

Introduction
- *Source*: *S. orchidaceus*
- Tuberculostatic drug

Q. What is the mechanism of action of cycloserine?

A.
- Analog of D-alanine
- Inhibits cell wall synthesis by inactivating enzyme which racemizes L alanine

Dose:
- *Adult dose*: 0.5 g/day per oral in divided doses
- *Pediatric dose*: 10–20 mg/kg/day

Q. Enumerate the adverse effects of cycloserine.

A. Sleepiness, headache, tremors, psychosis, convulsions.

KANAMYCIN, AMIKACIN, CAPREOMYCIN

- Reserve in rare cases-toxic
- Not combined among themselves or Streptomycin

Q. What is the mechanism of action of aminoglycosides?

A. Act by inhibiting bacterial synthesis. None penetrate the meninges.

Q. What are the adverse effects of aminoglycosides.

A.
- Ototoxicity—cochlear damage
- Neuromuscular blockade
- Nephrotoxicity

NEWER DRUGS

Quinolones

Ciprofloxacin, Moxifloxacin, Ofloxacin, Gatifloxacin, Sparfloxacin.

Q. Enumerate the spectrum of quinolones.
A. *M. tuberculosis, MAC, M. fortuitum.*

Q. What is the mechanism of action of quinolone?
A. Penetrate cell and kill mycobacteria lodged in macrophages.

Q. What is the indication of quinolones.
A. MDR TB.

MACROLIDES

Clarithromycin, Azithromycin
Used for Non TB mycobacteria like *MAC, M. fortuitum, M. kansasi, M. marinum.*

Clarithromycin

- Has low MIC value
- *Dose*: 500 mg BD

Azithromycin

- Has better tissue and intracellular levels
- *Dose*: 500 mg od

RIFABUTIN

- It is a weak enzyme inducer
- More active against MAC
- MAC prophylaxis—300 mg/day
- Used for treatment along with clarithromycin/azithromycin

Q. Enumerate the adverse effects of rifabutin.
A. GI intolerance, rash, granulocytopenia, myalgia, uveitis, substituted for rifampin in HIV patients.

Q. What are the regimens used for treatment of tuberculosis?

A. Under the latest RNTCP guidelines, the following regimens are used for treatment of all cases of pulmonary as well as extrapulmonary TB:

Category	*Cases included*	*PWB color*	*Intensive phase*	*Continuation phase*
I	All new, previously untreated cuses (including HIV-TB coinfection)	Red	$2H_3R_1Z_3E$	$4H_3R_3$
II	All previously treated cases (treatment for more than 1 month)	Blue	$2H_3R_1Z_3E_3S_3$ + $1H_3R_3E_3$*	$5H_3R_3E_3$

* Drug is given for 3 days in a week (alternate day dosing), the number at the left indicates number of months for which the drugs are to be given

(PWB: Patient-wise Box; H: Isoniazid; R: Rifampicin; Z: Pyrazinamide; E: Ethambutol; S: Streptomycin)

Q. What is DOTS?

A. DOTS (Directly Observed Treatment—Short Course) is the name given to the tuberculosis control strategy recommended by WHO. Under these programs, all doses of the intensive phase and at least the first dose of each week of the continuation phase are given under direct observation by a DOT provider.

Q. What is DOTS plus?

A. DOTS plus are DOTS programs with added components for MDR-TB diagnosis, management, and treatment.

Q. What is MDR and XDR TB?

A. An MDR-TB case is a TB patient, whose sputum is culture positive for *Mycobacterium tuberculosis* and is resistant in vitro to isoniazid and rifampicin with or without resistance to other antitubercular drugs.

An extensively drug resistant tuberculosis (XDR TB) case is an MDR-TB case whose *M. tuberculosis* isolate is resistant to at least isoniazid, rifampicin, a fluoroquinolone (ofloxacin, levofloxacin, or moxifloxacin) and a second-line injectable anti-TB drug (kanamycin, amikacin, or capreomycin).

Q. What is the treatment regimen for MDR-TB?

A. Intensive phase:

6–9 months of Kanamycin + Levofloxacin + Ethionamide + Cycloserine + Pyrazinamide + Ethambutol.

Continuation phase:
18 months of Levofloxacin + Ethionamide + Cycloserine + Ethambutol.

Q. What were the treatments for tuberculosis before anti TB treatment was introduced?

A. They were:

- Sanatorium treatment where patients were hospitalized and given rest, sunlight and plenty of high protein food
- Artificial pneumothorax and artificial pneumoperitoneum where the affected lung was collapsed and rested
- Injectable vitamin D in high doses which helps to resolve tuberculoid granulomas
- Phototherapy where high dose UVB was given in special chambers. This was especially used in cutaneous TB. It was introduced by Niels Finsen who won the Nobel Prize for this advance, and as yet, is the only dermatologist to be so honored.

2.15. BIOLOGICALS

Q. What is a biological (or 'biologic')?

A. A biological is a therapeutic or a diagnostic agent synthesized from the product of living organisms. It targets specific mediators of inflammation and is relatively selective. It is used in the treatment of many inflammatory and some neoplastic disorders.

Q. Classify biologicals.

A. Biologicals can be grouped according to the site of their therapeutic action.

- Cytokines as biological, e.g., IFN-α, GM-CSF
- Monoclonal antibodies against:
    - Cytokines, e.g., infliximab (anti-TNF)
    - Cell surface molecules, e.g., rituximab (anti-CD20)
    - IgE, e.g., omalizumab (anti-IgE)
    - Tumor antigens, e.g., cetuximab (anti-EGF receptor)
- Fusion proteins:
    - Soluble cytokine receptors, e.g., etanercept (anti-TNF)
    - Soluble cellular ligands, e.g., abatacept (CTLA-4)

Q. What is the difference between classical immunosuppressants and biological?

A. Classical immunosuppressants are low molecular weight compounds, while biological are high molecular weight proteins.

The former are metabolized in the body to reactive compounds, while the latter are not metabolized and act 'as is.' The former are given orally or parenterally, while the latter are parenteral only. The immune response with the former is mostly cellular, while with the latter, it is mostly humoral. Drug interactions are common with the former, while rare with the latter.

Q. What is a biosimilar?

A. A biosimilar is a biological product that is highly similar to an already approved product. It may have minor differences in its clinically inactive components. However, there are no clinically meaningful differences between the biosimilar and the approved biological product in terms of the safety, purity, and potency of the product. A major advantage of a biosimilar is that it is comparatively cheap.

Q. How is its nomenclature derived?

A. Monoclonal antibodies (mab), e.g., Adalimumab

- mo = mouse, u = human, xi = chimera, zu = humanized chimera
- lim = immune
- tu = miscellaneous tumor
- Receptor fusion protein (cept), e.g., alefacept
- Receptor antagonist (ra), e.g., anakinra

Q. Discuss the general adverse effects with biologicals.

A. These have been recently classified into types α, β, γ, δ and ε.

- Type α (overstimulation) is due to the cytokine storm caused because of biological therapy. These are dose—dependent reactions. For example, flu-like symptoms due to IFN.
- Type β (hypersensitivity) is due to nonhuman part of the biologic molecule. Thus, the patient can develop human antimurine antibodies (HAMA), human antichimeric antibodies (HACA) and rarely, even human antihuman antibodies (HAHA). These reactions may be dose-dependent or dose-independent and are in the form of urticaria, anaphylaxis or serum sickness.
- Type γ (immune deviation) is due to immunodeficiency caused by biological, e.g., TB after TNF inhibitors or autoimmunity (e.g., SLE with infliximab). It is dose-dependent.
- Type δ (cross-reactivity) is due to similarity with the target structures on which the biologic acts (e.g., acneiform eruption caused by cetuximab). It is dose-dependent.
- Type ε (nonimmunologic) due to an unknown mechanism. For example, retinopathy and depression caused by IFN-γ. It is dose-dependent.

Q. What are the acute reactions to biologicals?

A. These reactions occur within the first two days of the infusion but mostly within the first two hours. These can affect:

- *Skin*: Itch, flushing, exanthems, urticaria and angioedema
- *Eye*: Nose—itch, visual disturbances and rhinoconjunctivitis
- *GIT*: Nausea, cramps, vomiting, diarrhea
- *Respiratory*: Dyspnea, wheezing
- *Cardiovascular*: Chest pain, hypotension, incontinence, cardiac arrest
- *CNS*: Vertigo, dizziness, unconsciousness

Q. How to manage the aforementioned reactions?

A. The role of premedications with antihistaminics and steroids (parenteral) is controversial. However, some people give it to reduce the severity and frequency of the reaction. Once the reaction occurs, the infusion is stopped, legs are elevated, airway is secured and (except if the reaction is very mild) patient is given intramuscular epinephrine 0.5 mL 1:1000 solution. Normal saline is given IV, IV antihistaminics are given (e.g., pheniramine 2 mL) and IV steroid (hydrocortisone – 100 mg). Oxygen is also administered intranasally.

Q. Discuss TNF-α and its antagonists.

A. TNF-α is a proinflammatory cytokine. It is released by tissue-specific cells like keratinocytes and dendritic cells, as well as by circulating cells like macrophages and T-lymphocytes. It exists in membrane-bound and soluble (circulating) forms. It produces inflammation by activating nuclear factor (NF-κB), as well as by inducing IL-1, IL-2 and IL-6. It also upregulates adhesion molecules like ICAM and VCAM, promoting leucocyte migration. At present there are three main biologics which block the action of TNF-α, viz. etanercept, infliximab and adalimumab.

Q. What is etanercept?

A.
- Etanercept is a fusion protein consisting of the extracellular domain of the p75 TNF receptor and the Fc portion of human IgG1. It binds sTNF-α preventing its interaction with the receptor, and changes the cytokine pattern from type 1 to type 2.
- Etanercept is a fully human soluble TNF receptor fusion protein. It has two TNF type-2 receptors joined by the Fc part of IgG1.
- Etanercept binds primarily to soluble and less to membrane-bound TNF-α. It prevents TNF from binding to its receptor, thus, blocking the functions mentioned in the previous answer.
- It also binds to TNF-β. It does not however, fix complement, cause cytotoxicity, or promote apoptosis.

Q. What are the indications of etanercept?

A. FDA approved—it was the first TNF antagonist approved.

- Rheumatoid arthritis and juvenile RA
- Psoriatic arthropathy
- Ankylosing spondylitis
- Psoriasis (plaque type)

Off-label indications of etanercept

- Acute graft-versus-host disease (combined with methylprednisolone)
- Behçet disease
- Hidradenitis suppurativa
- Kawasaki disease
- Pemphigus vulgaris
- Pustular psoriasis
- Pyoderma gangrenosum
- Scleroderma/systemic sclerosis

Q. What are the absolute contraindications?

A. Active infection, tuberculosis, hypersensitivity, demyelinating diseases.

Q. What is the pregnancy category of etanercept?

A. Pregnancy category B (common to all TNF antagonists).

Q. What is its preparations and dose?

A. Available as injection 25/50 mg vial prefilled syringe with autoinjector. It is given as a subcutaneous self-administered injection. In psoriasis it is given as 50 mg twice weekly for 12 weeks followed by 50 mg once weekly. In RA, AS and psoriatic arthropathy it is given as 25 mg twice weekly.

Q. What are the side effects of etanercept?

A. It is generally well-tolerated, however injection site reactions are seen in up to 40% patients. Antietanercept antibodies develop in <10% patients and are not associated with decreased efficacy.

Q. What are the off-label indications of etanercept?

A. See later (given in common).

Q. What is infliximab?

A. It is a chimeric (human + mouse derived) IgG monoclonal antibody. It has human constant and murine variable sequences. It binds and neutralizes both soluble and membrane-bound TNF (unlike etanercept), but does not bind TNF-β (unlike etanercept). It fixes complement and induces cytotoxicity resulting in lysis of cells.

Q. What are indications of infliximab?

A. FDA approved—psoriasis and psoriatic arthritis, RA, Crohn's disease, ulcerative colitis and ankylosing spondylitis.

Q. What is the preparations and dose?

A. It is available as a 100 mg vial. It is given as a slow intravenous infusion in normal saline in a dose of 3–5 mg/kg at baseline, week 2, week 6 and repeated every 8 weeks thereafter.

The commonly followed protocol is of administering at 0, 2 and 6 weeks, and subsequently every 8 weeks for maintenance. No systemic accumulation of infliximab occurs upon continued repeated treatment.

Q. What are the precautions to be taken with infliximab?

A. As mentioned above.

Q. What are the side effects of infliximab?

A. In 10% cases infusion reactions can occur. Because infliximab is a dimeric antibody, patients can develop human antichimeric antibodies (HACA) in 15–50% cases. These are associated with decreased efficacy and higher infusion reactions.

Q. How to minimize HACA formation?

A. Concomitant immunosuppressive therapy, premedication with steroids and a 3-dose induction regimen as mentioned above followed by maintenance dosing.

Q. What is adalimumab?

A. It is a fully humanized monoclonal antibody (unlike infliximab). It is highly specific to TNF, binding both to soluble and membrane-bound forms. It also fixes complement and causes lysis of cells which express membrane-bound TNF. The chances of developing HACA are less with adalimumab because being fully humanized it is less immunogenic. However, its therapeutic effect is as good as infliximab.

Q. What are the preparations and dose of adalimumab?

A. It is available as injection form (40 mg/0.8 mL) and is given subcutaneously in a dose of 40 mg every week or alternate weeks.

Q. What are the side effects of adalimumab?

A. Most common are—infections (e.g., upper respiratory, sinusitis), injection site reactions, headache and rash. Antiadalimumab antibodies are found in only 12% patients and reduced to 1% if methotrexate is given simultaneously.

Q. What are the general problems with TNF antagonists?

A. They are:

- TB—the number of cases of TB are significantly higher and most of these represent reactivation of latent disease. Many patients also develop disseminated or atypical disease because TNF is required for proper granuloma formation and sequestration of mycobacterium. Hence, every patient on TNF antagonists should undergo X-ray chest and PPD to detect latent TB
- Deep fungal infections like histoplasmosis, aspergillosis, cryptococcosis have been reported especially after infliximab
- Lymphomas and other malignancies have been reported with infliximab and adalimumab
- Demyelinating diseases have been reported including multiple sclerosis
- Elevated liver enzyme levels are seen with infliximab and adalimumab
- New onset cardiac failure has been reported with infliximab and etanercept
- Autoimmune diseases can develop with infliximab

Note: The patient should change injection sites each time, atleast 1 inch away from the previous injection site, usually on the thighs, abdomen, or upper arms.

Q. What are the off-label indications of TNF antagonists?

A. They can be classified into:

- Granulomatous diseases, e.g., sarcoidosis, granuloma annulare, necrobiosis lipoidica, hidradenitis suppurativa (increasingly being used for this indication)
- Neutrophilic dermatoses, e.g., pyoderma gangrenosum, Sweet's syndrome, subcorneal pustular dermatosis, neutrophilic and granulomatous vasculitis
- Autoimmune blistering diseases, e.g., bullous pemphigoid, mucous membrane pemphigoid
- Autoimmune connective tissue diseases, e.g., lupus erythematosus (controversial), systemic sclerosis, dermatomyositis, Behçet's disease, GVHD
- Miscellaneous diseases, e.g., pityriasis rubra pilaris, multicentric reticulohistiocytosis, toxic epidermal necrolysis, erythema annulare centrifugum, Hailey-Hailey disease

Q. Why is efalizumab withdrawn from the market?

A. It is withdrawn due to various reports of progressive multifocal leukoencephalopathy (PML).

Q. What is rituximab?

A. It is a chimeric murine—human monoclonal antibody to CD20 which helps in depletion of B cells with CD20 receptors thus, reducing production of disease—causing antibodies.

Q. What is the mechanism of action of rituximab?

A. CD20 is a B cell specific antigen expressed on the surface of B lymphocytes but not on plasma cells or stem cells. Rituximab acts by three mechanisms, namely, inducing apoptosis, antibody dependent cytotoxicity and complement mediated lysis. Since plasma cells or stem cells are not affected, Ig levels do not fall dramatically and B gradually return to normal within 6 months of therapy.

Q. What are the indications of rituximab therapy?

A. FDA approved:

- Non-Hodgkin B cell lymphoma CD20+
- Chronic lymphocytic leukemia CD20+
- Rheumatoid arthritis
- Granulomatosis with polyangiitis
- Microscopic polyangiitis
- Pemphigus vulgaris

Off label:

- Vesiculobullous diseases:
  - Pemphigus vulgaris
  - Pemphigus foliaceus
  - Paraneoplastic pemphigus
  - Epidermolysis bullosa acquisita
  - Bullous pemphigoid
  - Mucus membrane pemphigoid
- Collagen vascular disorders:
  - Dermatomyositis
  - Scleroderma
  - Cutaneous lupus erythematosus
  - Graft-versus-host disease (GVHD)
- Vasculitides:
  - Wegener's granulomatosis (WG)
  - Microscopic polyangiitis
  - Cryoglobulinemic vasculitis
  - Churg-Strauss syndrome
- Miscellaneous:
  - Chronic urticaria—phase I and II trial
  - Cutaneous B-cell lymphoma

Q. What are the preparations of rituximab?

A. It is available in injection form at a concentration of 10 mg/mL in 10 mL or 50 mL vials.

Q. What are the various protocols available for rituximab therapy?

A.
- Lymphoma protocol—dose of 375 mg/m^2 is administered weekly for 4 weeks
- Rheumatoid arthritis protocol—two doses of 1 g administered at an interval of 15 days
- Other modifications:
  - Low dose rituximab—two doses of 500 mg given at a interval of 15 days
  - Combination therapy—IVIgG, dexamethasone pulse

Q. What are the contraindications of rituximab therapy?

A.
- Active infections or sepsis
- CHF
- Poorly controlled diabetes, immunosuppression
- Malignancy
- Renal impairment
- Asthma
- CNS demyelinating disease
- Blood dyscrasias
- Tuberculosis
- Pregnancy (relative)

Q. What are the adverse effects?

A.
- Opportunistic infections:
  - Pneumocystis pneumonia
  - Septic hip (12 weeks later)
  - Cytomegalovirus infection
  - Malignancy induction—SCC and Merkel cell carcinoma (possible)
  - Fatal hypersensitivity infusion with arrhythmias
  - SJS, TEN, vesiculobullous reaction

Q. What are investigations needed prior to start of rituximab therapy?

A.
- Routine investigations
- HCV, HbsAg, HIV
- Chest X-ray (PA)—repeat after 1st dose
- Mantoux test (if < 10 mm patient can be started with therapy)

- HRCT (when indicated)
- ECG, 2D - Echo
- TB Quantiferon test (controversial)

Q. What are premedications for rituximab therapy?

A. Inj. Pheniramine (Avil) 25 mg, Injection Hydrocortisone 100 mg, Inj. Ranitidine 50 mg IV, Tab. Paracetamol 500 mg stat.

Q. How to monitor a patient on rituximab therapy?

A. Monitor pulse, BP, O_2 saturation every 15 minutes. If no fever, rash or breathlessness, continue with the infusion of 500 mg in 500 mL NS for 5 hours. Monitor every 1/2 hourly.

Q. What are postmedication?

A.
- Tablet Cotrimoxazole DS once a day, Monday-Wednesday-Friday for 3–6 months.
- Tablet Acyclovir 400 mg twice daily for 6 weeks.

Q. What is omalizumab?

A. It is a IgG1 type of humanized monoclonal antibody which has 95% human and 5% murine fraction, the latter being active.

Q. What is the mechanism of action of omalizumab?

A. It binds to the Cε3 site of IgE which is very close to the binding site of high and low affinity IgE receptors. Omalizumab reduces the free IgE levels in plasma because it forms small complexes with IgE which are biologically inert and do not activate complement. It also blocks the binding of IgE to FCεR1 (high affinity IgE receptor) and prevents the release of histamine and other vasoactive amines. It also indirectly reduces the number of these receptors in the target cells. Moreover, it can act on other target cells like CD4 T-lymphocytes (increased activity) and B-lymphocytes (decreased activity).

Q. What are the preparations and dose of omalizumab?

A. It is available as prefilled syringes for subcutaneous injection of two doses—75 mg and 150 mg. The dose is between 75–375 mg at 2–4 weeks intervals. The most effective dose in urticaria is 300 mg once in 2–4 weeks.

Q. What are the indications of omalizumab?

A. **FDA approved:** Asthma

Off label: Chronic urticaria (including chronic autoimmune), atopic dermatitis, mastocytosis.

Q. What are the adverse effects of omalizumab?

A. The common adverse effects are:

- Local skin reactions, urticaria, headache, mild fever, upper abdominal pain.
- Rare—anaphylaxis (0.2%), syncope, serum sickness, thrombocytopenia, laryngeal edema, etc.

Q. How to manage the adverse effects of omalizumab?

A. The patient should be provided with self-injectable vials of epinephrine. The patient should be observed for up to 2 hours after each injection.

Q. Discuss alefacept.

A. Alefacept was the first biologic agent approved for the treatment of moderate-to-severe chronic plaque psoriasis.

Alefacept is a dimeric fusion protein. Its binding domain is derived from LFA-3. This ligand binds to CD2 on effector memory cells, thereby inhibiting their activation. It also induces apoptosis of CD8 cells. It was earlier approved for psoriasis in USA, but now is withdrawn voluntarily. The dose of alefacept is 15 mg weekly intramuscular for 12 weeks. Besides psoriasis, it has been used in lichen planus, alopecia areata, sarcoidosis and GVHD. It is contraindicated in patients with history of malignancies and low CD4 counts. A common side effect is flu-like symptoms and decline of CD4 counts. Some patients develop antibodies to alefacept.

Q. Discuss anakinra.

A. Anakinra is a human recombinant IL-1 receptor antagonist. It selectively binds to the receptor of IL-1 and inhibits its activity. IL-1 is believed to be the key to innate immunity, thus inflammation is inhibited.

Q. What are the indications of anakinra?

A. Anakinra is used in the treatment of hidradenitis suppurativa, urticarial rash in the CINCA (chronic infantile neurologic cutaneous and articular) syndrome. It is also used Schnitzler's syndrome and Muckle Wells syndrome. It has been used in metastatic melanoma also.

Q. What are the side effects of anakinra?

A. Injection site reactions, lichenoid drug eruptions, granulomatous drug eruptions, new-onset psoriasis, new-onset, melanoma, neutropenia.

Q. What is the dose and preparations of anakinra?

A. It is administered in a dose of 1–2 mg/kg (maximum 100 mg daily) by subcutaneous injection.

Q. What are the newer biologicals recently introduced?

A.
- Daclizumab—a humanized monoclonal antibody against CD25, which blocks T cells. It has been used in blistering diseases, psoriasis and erythrodermic leukemia.
- Basiliximab—it is a chimeric monoclonal antibody against CD25, which is used for similar indications as 'daclizumab.'
- Cetuximab—it is a chimeric monoclonal antibody which targets the EGF receptor. It is used in EGFR positive colorectal cancer. The dose is 400 mg/m^2 as the first dose and subsequent weekly doses are 250 mg/m^2. The most common side effect is the PRIDE syndrome (papulopustular acne and paronychia, regulatory disturbances of hair growth including trichomegaly, dryness of skin with EGFR receptor. It is used in dermatology for advanced cutaneous SCC. It may also be useful in other diseases like psoriasis and BCC.
- Abatacept—it is a fusion protein that appears to work by specifically inhibiting full activation of T cells by binding to CD80 and CD86, and blocking interaction with CD28. At present it is used for the treatment of rheumatoid arthritis.

2.16. CHLOROQUINE AND HYDROXYCHLOROQUINE

Chloroquine (CQ) and hydroxychloroquine (HCQ) are used as systemic photoprotective agents in dermatology.

Mechanism of Action

- Anti-inflammatory and immunomodulatory:
  - Stabilization of lysosomal membranes
  - Lymphocytes and macrophages—reduced chemotaxis and phagocytosis
  - Decrease in pro-inflammatory cytokines like IL-1, IL-2, IL-6, TNF
  - Decreased leukotrienes and bradykinin
- Photoprotective effect:
  - Bind to melanin
  - Antioxidant
  - Bind to porphyrin-facilitate their clearance
  - Solubilize and mobilize hepatic porphyrins and their clearance
- Lowers triglyceride level, cholesterol level, and glucose level

Q. What are the indication for antimalarials in dermatology?

A.
- Lupus erythematosus
- Photosensitive dermatoses
- Polymorphous light eruption (PMLE)
- Solar urticaria
- Pemphigus foliaceus
- Porphyria cutanea tarda
- Hydroa vacciniforme
- Rheumatoid arthritis
- Type I and II reaction in leprosy
- Dermatomyositis
- Sarcoidosis

Q. What is the dose of antimalarials in dermatology?

A.
- Chloroquine: 250–500 mg/day
- Hydroxychloroquine: 200–400 mg/day

Q. What is the bioavailability of the drug?

A.
- Chloroquine: 50%
- Hydroxychloroquine: 75%

Q. What is the ocular safety limit?

A.
- Chloroquine: 3.5 mg/kg/day for 6 months
- Hydroxychloroquine: 6.5 mg/kg/day for 6 months

Q. Which drug has better gastrointestinal (GI) tolerance?

A. Hydroxychloroquine.

Q. What are the modes of excretion?

A.
- Chloroquine—mainly in urine. Hence should not be given in renal failure patients
- Hydroxychloroquine—mainly in bile. Hence cannot be given in renal failure patients

Q. What are the side effects of antimalarials?

A. **Ocular**
- Reversible:
  - Corneal deposits
  - Loss of accommodation
  - Retinal field defects
  - Retinal pigmentation
- Irreversible:
  - Central scotoma
  - Bulls, eye retinopathy
  - Loss of vision
  - Generalized pigmented retinopathy

Cutaneous side effects

- Rashes
- Urticaria
- Lichenoid like drug eruptions
- Morbilliform rash
- Erythroderma
- Purpura
- Acute generalized exanthematous pustulosis (AGEP)
- Pigmentation of skin, hair, and nails
- Flareup of psoriasis

Gastrointestinal

- Nausea, vomiting, and diarrhea

Nervous system

- Irritability, nervousness, altered mood, psychosis, headache, vertigo, tinnitus,nystagmus, myopathy

Q. Describe the pigmentary changes due to antimalarials?

A.
- Pigmentary changes are due to chloroquine binding with melanin pigment in dermis
- Blue-black pretibial, facial and palatal pigmentation
- Bleaching of hair
- Pigmentary bands over nail

Q. How will you monitor guidelines for antimalarials?

A.
- Vision, perimetry, slit lamp examination fundoscopy—baseline every 6 months for 1 year then yearly
- Serum transaminases—at 1 month, 5 months, 6 months

Q. What is the duration of onset of action of CQ and HCQ?

A.
- Onset of action 2–8 weeks
- Adequate responses after 1–3 months

Q. What are the indications of antimalarials in lupus erythematosus?

A.
- Chronic cutaneous lupus erythematosus (CCLE) not responding to the other lines of treatment
- Subacute and acute lupus erythematosus (LE) with cutaneous lesions, photosensitivity and arthritis
- Prevention of flareup in systemic lupus erythematosus (SLE)

Q. How will you use antimalarials in porphyria cutanea tarda?

A.
- HCQ 100 mg thrice a week 1 month
- 200 mg thrice/week 1 month
- 200 mg thrice/week 6–18 months till uroporphyrin level falls below 100 mg/day

Q. What are the interactions of antimalarials?

A.
- CQ and HCQ should not be given together as the combination causes additive renal toxicity
- It increases digoxin and D-penicillamine level
- Decreased bioavailability of ampicillin
- Kolin and magnesium trisilicate decreased absorbtion

Q. What are the other indications of antimalarials in dermatology?

A.
- Pemphigus vulgaris
- Psoriatic arthritis
- Recurrent and persistent erythema nodosum
- Actinic lichen planus (LP)
- Rosacea

Q. Diffentiate between CQ and HCQ?

A.

	Chloroquine (CQ)	*Hydroxychloroquine (HCQ)*
Salt	Phosphate	Sulphate
Dose	250–500 mg/day	200–400 mg/day
Bioavailability	30%	75%
Ocular toxicity	More common	Less common
Gastrointestinal tolerance	Poor	Better
Excretion	Urine	Bile

Q. What are the other antimalarials used in dermatology?

A.
- Quinine
- Quinacrine

2.17. CRISABOROLE

Q. Mechanism of action of crisaborole.

A. Inhibition of phosphodiesterase 4 (PDE4) by crisaborole leads to elevated levels of cyclic adenosine monophosphate (cAMP). Increased intracellular levels of cAMP inhibit the NF-kB pathway and suppress the release of pro-inflammatory mediators such as TNF-α and various interleukins that play a causative role in psoriasis and atopic dermatitis (AD). Suppression of downstream effects in different cell types may explain the therapeutic role of crisaborole in immune-mediated skin diseases.

Q. Pregnancy category.

A. It belongs to pregnancy category B1. Adequate data about its use in pregnant women are not available.

Lactation

Information about secretion in human milk after topical application in breastfeeding is unknown. Breastfeeding mothers should avoid its application to the breast in order to prevent entry in the mouth of the newborn.

Concentration and formulation

2% crisaborole ointment.

Q. Indications.

A. Crisaborole is a first-in-class, nonsteroidal, topical anti-inflammatory, PDE inhibitor approved for the treatment of mild-to-moderate AD.

Q. Adverse interaction.

A.
- The most common side effect of crisaborole is application site pain, such as burning or stinging.
- Crisaborole may cause hypersensitivity reactions at the application site or at a distant site.
- These can be serious and may include hives (contact urticaria), itching, swelling, and erythema.
- If signs and symptoms of hypersensitivity occur, crisaborole should be discontinued immediately and appropriate therapy initiated.
- Crisaborole is contraindicated in patients with known hypersensitivity to crisaborole or any component of the formulation.

Q. Dosage and administration.

A.
- Crisaborole is for topical use only and not for ophthalmic, oral, or intravaginal use.
- It is applied as a thin layer over the affected area(s) twice daily.
- Inactive ingredients in the ointment include white petrolatum, propylene glycol, mono- and diglycerides, paraffin, butylated hydroxytoluene, and edetate calcium disodium.

2.18. APREMILAST

Introduction

It is a PDE4 inhibitor which is a small molecule drug. Their small size allows them to be readily absorbed into the bloodstream after oral or topical administration and subsequently reach many different tissues in the body. At the target cell, unlike larger biologic drugs, these molecules can also easily penetrate the cell membrane to interact with intracellular proteins.

Q. What is the mechanism of action?

In inflammatory cells, cAMP is converted to adenosine monophosphate (AMP) via PDE4. Increased level of AMP lead to release of proinflammatory cytokines, such as TNF-α, IL-23 and IL-17 and decreased expression of anti-inflammatory cytokines, such as IL-10. Apremilast inhibits the action of PDE4, which increases levels of cAMP, decreases levels of AMP and which translates to a more anti-inflammatory downstream cytokine profile (increased anti-inflammatory cytokines and decreased proinflammatory cytokines.

Q. Indications.

A. US food and Drug Administration—approved indications

- Psoriasis
- Psoriatic arthritis

Off-label dermatologic uses

- Neutrophilic dermatoses
- Behçet disease
- Synovitis-acne-pustulosis-hyperostosis-osteitis (SAPHO) syndrome
- Autoimmune connective tissue diseases
- Discoid lupus erythematosus
- Papulosquamous dermatoses
- Lichen planus pityriasis rubra pilaris
- Pigmentary disorders
- Vitiligo

Q. Pharmacokinetics.

A.
- Apremilast is metabolized in the liver, primarily by cytochrome P450 (CYP)3A4.
- The apremilast half-life is approximately 6–9 hours, necessitating apremilast as twice daily dosing.
- The drug is excreted primarily through the urine, but a small portion is excreted through the feces.

Q. Contraindications.

A. Hypersensitivity to apremilast or components formulation.

Q. Adverse effects.

A.
- Gastrointestinal—severe nausea, vomiting, diarrhea reported, especially first few weeks of therapy. May cause weight loss; monitor regularly
- Psychiatric—use with caution in patients with prior depression, suicidal ideation/behavior
- Renal—caution with creatinine clearance <30 mL/min

Q. Pregnancy.

A.
- Traditional US Food and Drug Administration rating—category C
- Newer rating—moderate-to-high risk

Q. Interactions.

A.
- Relatively high-risk drug interactions
- Anticonvulsants—phenytoin, carbamazepine, others
- Rifamycins—rifampin, rifabutin
- BRAF inhibitors—dabrafenib
- Lower—risk drug interactions
- Biologics
- Tocilizumab

2.19. JAK INHIBITORS

- Full form
  - JAK-STAT—Janus kinase and signal transducer and activation of transcription
- Mechanism of action
  - JAK-STAT pathway is utilized by cytokines, which include ILs, IFNs and certain other molecules which help transmit signals from cell membrane to nucleus.
    - Cytokines bind to specific JAK receptors and stimulates JAK proteins leading to → dimerization and autophosphorylation.
    - Recruitment of STAT proteins followed by phosphorylation.
    - These are translocated into the nucleus where they induce the transcription of target genes.
    - The result is proliferation and differentiation of cells of innate and acquired immunity.
  - JAK family of kinases include four proteins—JAK1, JAK2, JAK3, TYK2
  - STAT family includes seven proteins—STAT1, STAT2, STAT3, STAT4, STAT5a, STAT5b, STAT6
- MoA–AD
  - AD is a predominantly Th2 disease. The key cytokines (IL-4, IL-5, IL-13, IL-17, IL-22, IL-23, IL-31, IL-33, and IFN-γ) play a central role in AD pathogenesis, and JAK, STAT and spleen tyrosine kinase (SYK) pathways are involved in signaling these cytokines. In AD, the use of JAK inhibitors block both IL-4 and IL-13 in acute phase and IFN-γ in chronic phase.

- MoA–AA
  - AA occurs as a result of breech in the immune privilege of anagen hair follicles. It is mediated by MHC-II suppression and shutdown of pro-inflammatory mechanisms including action of APCs, mast cells, and NK cells. Disruption in these mechanisms lead to collapse of immune privilege and progression of AA. Immune mechanisms in AA is mediated by CD8+ T cells via IL-15 within follicular epithelial cells and mediated through JAK pathway. JAK inhibitors prevent the release of cytokines along with IFN-γ and IL-15.
- MoA–vitamin
  - Depigmentation in vitiligo is mediated by IFN-γ and CXCL10. JAK inhibitors downregulates CXCL10 expression by inhibiting IFN-γ and therefore, resulting in repigmentation.
- MoA–psoriasis
  - The inflammatory response in psoriasis is driven by T cells and mediated by multiple cytokines such as TNF, IL-17 and IL-23. These pro-inflammatory cytokines bind to cytokine receptors leading to activation of intracellular signalling mediated by JAKs, formation of dimers/heterodimers with subsequent autophosphorylation and STAT activation which then translocates to cell nucleus regulating gene transcription.
  - JAK inhibitors inhibits signal pathway and gene transcription, reducing inflammation.
- Generations of JAK-I
  - 1st generation - Tofacitinib - JAK1/3
  - Ruxolitinib - JAK1/2
  - Baricitinib -JAK1/2
  - Oclacitinib - JAK1
  - 2nd generation - selective JAK inhibitors
  - Upadacitinib - JAK 1
  - Filgotinib - JAK1
  - Abrocitinib - JAK1
  - Beprocitinib - TY2
  - Ritlecitinib - JAK3
- FDA approved JAK-I/diseases
  - Tofacitinib—RA, PsA
  - Baricitinib—AA (approved by US-FDA)
  - Ruxolitinib—myelofibrosis, PCV
  - Upadacitinib—RA, AD
  - Filgotinib—RA

- Indications of JAK-I—FDA approved and off label
    - FDA approved - PsA, RA, UC
    - Off-label-
    - A/I ds—psoriasis, AA, vitiligo, DMS, LE, LPP
    - Dermatitis—AD
    - Photodermatitis—chronic actinic dermatitis
    - Miscellaneous—EM, hypereosinophilic syndrome
- Contraindications
    - Chronic kidney disease—GFR <30 mL/min/1.73m^2
    - Pancytopenia
    - Underlying malignancy
- Monitoring guidelines/pre-
    - Lab investigation
        - Complete blood count—watch for neutropenia/anemia
        - Lipid profile
        - Blood sugar levels
        - Creatinine/Glomerular filtration rate
        - Liver profile
        - R/o latent TB—Chest X-ray, Mantoux, QuantiFERON Gold
        - Pregnancy test—women of reproductive age group
        - Hepatitis B/Hepatitis C panel
        - HIV testing

    CBC, liver function tests and lipid profile—repeat at 4–8 weeks after treatment initiation and then at every 3 months
    - Clinical evaluation prior to starting Rx:
        - Active infections—herpes zoster vaccine/herpes simplex virus
        - Interstitial lung disease/diverticulitis
        - Renal/liver pathology history
        - H/O malignancy
- Pregnancy category C
- ADR
    - Risk of upper respiratory tract infection (URTI), urinary tract infection (UTI)
    - Varicella-zoster virus (VZV) reactivation
    - Latent tuberculosis (TB) reactivation
    - Impaired response to vaccination
    - Thrombocytopenic purpura, anemia
    - Diarrhea, fatigue, dizziness, headache
    - Increased risk of malignancies—lymphomas > carcinoma lung, breast, GI tract, renal cell carcinoma (RCC), prostate, melanoma
    - GI—GI perforation, ulcers, diverticulitis
    - Pulm—dyspnea, pulm embolism, ILD, chronic obstructive pulmonary disease (COPD)

- Drug interactions
  - Methotrexate/disease-modifying anti-rheumatic drug—safe at rheumatologic doses
  - Live vaccines—wait atleadt 3 months after therapy completion
  - Killed vaccines—immunize atleast 2 weeks prior to starting JAK inhibitors - not adequate immune response - repeat in 3 months
  - BAs - increased risk of severe infections/myelosuppression
  - High dose CS—increased risk of severe infections/ myelosuppression
  - Other JAK inhibitors—increased risk of serious adverse effects
  - Triazoles—may increase serum concentration of tofacitinib

3 Regimens in Dermatology

Q. What are the regimens used in leprosy?

A. The usual course for antileprosy therapy is mentioned in the chapter on antileprosy drugs. However, new trial regimens are being tried. The combination of Rifapentine, Moxifloxacin, and Minocycline is believed to be a very potent regimen. The following are the newer regimens of MDT in leprosy:

- Highly intense, daily short course regimens:
  - O + D + C × 6 weeks
  - R + O × 4 weeks
  - R + M × 4 weeks
  - Rb + L × 4 weeks
- Monthly administered regimens:
  - Cl + M with/without O
  - O + M
  - R + O + M

  1 year regimen with monthly ROM and daily C + D

  1 year regimen with initial 4 weeks period of O and 1 year regimen of WHO MB-MDT

  O = Ofloxacin, D = Dapsone, C = Clofazimine, M = Minocycline, R = Rifampicin, Rb = Rifabutin, L = Levofloxacin, Cl = Clarithromycin.

Q. Discuss modified steroid pulse regimens.

A.
- Dexamethasone-azathioprine pulse (DAP): This is used in patients who wish to conceive children since cyclophosphamide can render the patient infertile. Azathioprine does not induce gonadal dysfunction, and also has a lower risk of neoplasia with a steroid sparing effect. In this regimen, azathioprine 50 mg daily orally is given during the first 3 phases of pulse therapy, but no bolus is given during the pulse.
- Dexamethasone methotrexate pulse (DMP): Methotrexate has been used in the past as a steroid sparing agent for pemphigus. It can also be considered in patients who want to conceive. Since it has no apparent effect on the outcome of pregnancies, though sperm motility may be abnormal during treatment. Methotrexate is given 7.5 mg weekly, given orally during the first 3 phases of pulse therapy. No bolus of Methotrexate is given.

- Only dexamethasone pulse therapy (DP): This is often given in patients of systemic sclerosis where 100 mg dexamethasone is given IV on 3 consecutive days every month till clinical inactivity is reached.
- Methylprednisolone pulse therapy: Here, Methylprednisolone IV 1,000 mg replaces dexamethasone.
- Oral mini pulse therapy: Often used for treatment of alopecia areata and totalis, lichen planus, and vitiligo. Here, 5 mg of betamethasone or 60 mg Deflazacort is given in two consecutive doses orally.

Q. What are the modifications which can be made to dexamethasone cyclophosphamide (DC) pulse therapy?

A. Standard DC pulse therapy is discussed in chapter on systemic steroids.

Modifications in DCP:

- Low maintenance oral steroids in between pulses
- To induce rapid remission: six cycles of cyclophosphamide 500 mg at 2 weeks interval; three cycles of cyclophosphamide at 4 weeks interval; six cycles of cyclophosphamide at 3 months interval
- 2 weekly bolus of dexamethasone (100 mg IV – 2 doses)
- Omission of IV pulse dose of cyclophosphamide
- Azathioprine orally with monthly dose of IV dexamethasone
- Methylprednisolone or betamethasone in place of dexamethasone
- MTX 15 mg/week or AZT 100–150 mg/day or WAP (300 mg/week) in place of oral cyclophosphamide
- MMF or cyclosporine
- Oral betamethasone pulse
- Pulse dose with injection human insulin in diabetes patients
- Postponement of pulse due to raised blood sugar and septicemia
- Only cyclophosphamide pulse therapy (IV 500 mg + 50 mg daily)
- Add 1 more pint of IV 500 mg of 5% dextrose on 2nd day
- Intralesional steroid injection and topical potent steroid
- Intravenous immunoglobulin (IVIg) (400 mg/kg) for 5 days/month

Q. What are the other drugs which can be given as pulse therapy?

A. The following drugs can be given as pulse therapy:

- Azithromycin 500 mg on 3 consecutive days in a week for acne
- Isotretinoin 40 mg on 2 consecutive days of a week, for severe acne

- Itraconazole 200 mg bd for 7 days in a month is given for onychomycosis. This pulse is given for 2 consecutive months for fingernail onychomycosis and for 3 consecutive months for toenail onychomycosis
- Fluconazole is given 150–450 mg/week in dermatophytic and candidal infections. A single dose of 400 mg Fluconazole can be given for pityriasis versicolor
- Terbinafine can be given 200 mg bd for 7 days in a week for onychomycosis, to be repeated in two or three pulses
- Levamisole 150 mg on 2 consecutive days of the week in case of Vitiligo and resistant warts
- Rituximab 375 mg/m^2 once a week for 4 weeks in case of pemphigus vulgaris
- Etanercept is given as weekly subcutaneous pulses while infliximab is given on days 0, 15 and 30. Please refer to chapter on Biologicals for further details
- Methotrexate is given as weekly pulses in psoriasis. Please refer to chapter on immunosuppressants
- Topical steroids can be given as weekend therapy for maintaining remission in steroid responsive dermatoses
- Topical mupirocin in the nostrils three times daily for 5 days in a week, repeated each month, for recurrent furunculosis

Q. Discuss other regimens in dermatology.

A.

- Regimens in TB: Refer to the chapter on antitubercular drugs
- Regimens in mycetoma:
  - Welsh regimen: Amikacin is given in a dose of 15 mg/kg/day IM or IV for 3 weeks while cotrimoxazole is given in a dose of 8 mg/kg of sulfamethoxazole and 40 mg/kg of trimethoprim orally for 5 weeks. During the last 2 weeks of this regimen, audiometry and renal function should be done. Up to four such cycles can be given depending on persistence of the lesions, positive cultures, or side effects. If the patient is resistant to amikacin, netilmicin is given in the dose of 300 mg IM.
  - Ramam's regimen: Intensive phase with parenteral penicillin and gentamicin along with oral cotrimoxazole for 5–7 weeks followed by maintenance phase with amoxicillin and cotrimoxazole orally for 2–5 months after healing.
  - Modified Ramam's regimen: Oral amoxicillin is used from the beginning instead of parenteral penicillin.
  - Damle's regimen: In this regimen, rifampicin is added to all the drugs of Welsh's regimen.

- Regimens in psoriasis:
  - Goeckerman's regimen: Crude coal tar 2–5% is applied at night. The patient immerses himself in a bath to which liquor carbon has been added, and then is exposed to UVB or natural sunlight. About 2–3 weeks of this regimen can lead to remission in psoriasis. Irritation because of the tar can occur.
  - Ingram's regimen: 0.5% dithranol in a stiff zinc paste is applied on the lesions and may be covered by dressing. The patient takes a tar bath in the morning and is exposed to sunlight (optional). About 2–3 weeks of this regimen can lead to remission. Discoloration can occur due to anthralin may occur.
  - Stanford regimen: Topical steroids 2–3 times/day, added to the Ingram's regimen.
  - Short contact anthralin therapy (SCAT): 1–2% Anthralin is applied only for 20 mins, especially for palmoplantar psoriasis.
  - Calcipotriol-steroid therapy: Here, potent steroids are applied in the day, and 0.005% calcipotriol is applied at night.

Q. What is the CMC regimen for recurrent furunculosis?

A. The Chlorhexidine, Mupirocin, Clindamycin (CMC) regimen consists of skin disinfection with chlorhexidine for 21 days, nasal mupirocin ointment for 5 days, and oral clindamycin 1,800–2,400 mg for 21 days.

4 Miscellaneous Drugs

COAL TAR

Q. What mechanism is tar believed to have an antiproliferative and anti-inflammatory effect?

A.
- Tar exerts its antiproliferative effect on epidermis through suppression of deoxyribonucleic acid synthesis and reduction of mitotic activity.
- Anti-inflammatory action: Inhibition of chemotaxis of neutrophils.

Q. What are its indications?

A.
- Chronic plaque psoriasis
- Seborrheic dermatitis
- Atopic dermatitis
- Eczematous dermatitis

Q. What is Goeckerman regimen?

A. Coal tar in combination with UVR for psoriasis.

Q. What are the side effects of coal tar?

A.
- Carcinogenesis
- Phototoxicity
- Contact allergy
- Irritation
- Pruritus
- Folliculitis
- Comedones
- Acneiform eruptions
- Keratoses and keratoacanthomas

Q. What are the doses and preparations?

A.
- 1% coal tar lotions
- Coal tar 20% can be compound in creams, ointments, and paste
- Also available as soaks, shampoos, baths, topical emulsions
- It is frequently combined with salicylic acid

Q. What are the major carcinogenic agents in tar?

A. Benzopyrene and anthracene along with pyridines are the carcinogenic agents.

Q. What is the major disadvantage of coal tar?

A. The major disadvantage is poor compliance, foul smell, appearance and capacity to stain clothes and other items.

Q. What is ichthammol?

A. Addition of Sulfuric acid and ammonia to shale oil produces ichthammol.

ANTHRALIN

Q. What is the mechanism of action of this drug?

A. Anthralin inhibits DNA synthesis and anti-Langerhans cell effect.

Q. What are its indications?

A.
- Chronic plaque psoriasis
- In children and adults with extensive alopecia areata
- Alopecia totalis

Q. What are the side effects?

A.
- Irritant contact dermatitis
- Staining of clothes, skin, and nails
- Nephrotoxicity-extensive application causes systemic absorption and causes toxicity

Q. What are the doses and pregnancy status?

A.
- 0.1% or 0.25% cream
- Triethanolamine spray is available to reduce irritation and staining noted with anthralin.
- Pregnancy category: C

Q. What is Ingram's dithranol paste?

A. 0.02–0.08% dithranol, 2% salicylic acid, 24% each zinc oxide and starch and 2.5% hard paraffin. The patient soaks and washes in 90 mL bath to which 120 mL of alcoholic solution of coal tar is added. After drying, small doses of UVB are given, the dosage increasing gradually to suberythemogenic dose. Following the UVB therapy dithranol in Lassar's paste is applied to each plaque, sprinkled with talcum powder and dressed in a gauze suit. This is removed from the following morning.

Q. What is Ingram's regimen?

A. See chapters on regimens in dermatology.

Q. What is short contact anthralin therapy (SCAT)?

A. It consists of the application of anthralin by an applicator for a short period of 20–30 minutes to avoid irritation. The surrounding area is smeared with white soft paraffin prior to application of anthralin. After anthralin 20–30 minutes anthralin is washed with liquid paraffin or other oil.

BASIC FIBROBLASTIC GROWTH FACTOR (B-FGF)

Q. What is B-FGF and its mechanism of action?

A.
- Basic fibroblastic growth factor is a decapeptide.
- B-FGF is a selective growth factor for melanocytes.

Q. What is its indication?

A. Vitiligo

Q. What are the doses and preparations?

A. Decapeptide lotion for once daily application for 6–8 weeks.

Note: It is recommended to be used at bedtime followed by sun exposure for 10–15 minutes the next day.

PHENOLS

Q. What is the mechanism of action?

A. Phenol is an aromatic hydrocarbon derived from coal tar or manufactured from monochlorobenzene, which causes the denaturation of proteins. It has anesthetic properties.

Q. What are its indications?

A.
- Chemical cauterization
- Spot peeling
- Acne scar revision
- Alopecia areata
- Lichen simplex chronicus
- Prurigo nodularis
- Lichen amyloidosis
- Ear lobe repair
- Vitiligo
- Facial rejuvenation

Q. What are the side effects of phenol toxicity and how can they be prevented?

A.
- Phenol is a protoplasmic poison and causes progressive renal failure, cardiac arrhythmia, central nervous depression, respiratory embarrassment and hepatotoxicity

- It can be prevented by intake of plenty of oral fluids pre and post peel
- Alternatively, the patient can be infused 1 pint of Ringer lactate before the procedure and 2 pints during the peel

BRIMONIDINE

Q. What is brimonidine?

A. Brimonidine is a relatively selective alpha 2 adrenergic agonist. It is a vasoconstrictor.

Q. Where is it used in dermatology?

A. In August 2013, the USFDA approved the use of 0.33% brimonidine gel for the treatment of persistent facial erythema of rosacea in adult patients. It is not useful for the treatment of papules and pustules of rosacea.

Q. What is the mechanism of action?

A. The erythema of rosacea may be related to dysregulated cutaneous vasomotor response. This is antagonized by alpha adrenergic receptors whose action is increased by brimonidine. Thus it causes vasoconstriction of the dilated blood vessels.

Q. How is brimonidine applied?

A. A pea sized amount of the drug is applied in a thin layer over the affected areas of the face once daily for up to 1 year.

Q. What are the precautions to be taken?

A. It should be used with caution in patients with cerebral or coronary insufficiency, Raynaud's phenomenon, scleroderma or Sjögren's syndrome. Serious adverse reactions have been reported with accidental ingestion of this gel by children requiring intubation. It has not been properly evaluated in pregnancy or lactation.

Q. What are the drug interactions of brimonidine?

A. Systemic brimonidine can cause hypotension in patients on concomitant beta-blockers. It can cause additive effects with CNS depressants.

Q. What are the side effects of brimonidine?

A. The common side effects are erythema, flushing, burning sensation, contact dermatitis, nasopharyngitis and headache.

Q. What are the other uses of topical brimonidine?

A. It is used for the treatment of ocular hypertension.

BIMATOPROST

Q. What is bimatoprost?

A. Bimatoprost is a synthetic prostaglandin analogue used initially to treat patients with Glaucoma. It was noticed that topical use of bimatoprost had the side effect of stimulating eyelash growth as well as darkening the eyelashes. Hence it was marketed as a 0.03% solution for the treatment of hypotrichosis of the eyelashes.

Q. What is the mechanism of action of bimatoprost?

A. Bimatoprost is a compound derived from fatty acids. It binds to the prostaglandin receptors which are present in the hair follicle. This increases the percentage of anagen hair, and increases the duration of anagen. Bimatoprost also increases the size of the hair papilla. The net result is that the hair becomes longer and thicker. Bimatoprost also stimulates pigment cells.

Q. What are the off label indications of bimatoprost in dermatology?

A.
- Increasing the growth of eyebrows and making them fuller
- Treatment of androgenetic alopecia in both males and females
- Alopecia areata
- Localized stable vitiligo

Q. What are the precautions to be taken?

A.
- Bimatoprost is used for the skin of the upper eyelid margins and not for the lower eyelid. The bottom eyelashes receive the drop from the upper eyelashes while blinking
- The effect of bimatoprost is very gradual and not apparent for at least 2 months. Moreover, the effect is temporary and the eyelashes return to the pretreatment stage after stopping bimatoprost
- Bimatoprost contains benzalkonium chloride as a preservative, which is absorbed by soft contact lenses. These should be removed before application of bimatoprost but may be reinserted 15 minutes later
- Bimatoprost should be used cautiously if there is a history of abnormal intraocular pressure or intraocular inflammation

Q. What are the side effects of bimatoprost?

A. The side effects are relatively minor but include a burning sensation in the eye, redness, increased lacrimation, iris darkening, and discoloration around the eyelids. There is no adequate pregnancy or lactation data.

INGENOL MEBUTATE

Q. What is ingenol mebutate?

A. Ingenol mebutate is an extract from the plant Euphorbia peplus. It induces cell death by primary necrosis. It is available as a gel formulation (0.015%, 0.05%) for use in the treatment of superficial skin cancers including actinic keratoses. In January 2012, the US Food and Drug Administration (FDA) approved ingenol mebutate gel for the treatment of actinic keratoses on the face, scalp, trunk and extremities. Topical ingenol mebutate is currently in phase II trials for eradicating BCC and SCC in situ.

Q. How is ingenol mebutate gel administered?

A. Application of ingenol mebutate gel is not recommended until the skin has completely healed from any previous surgical or drug use. Ingenol mebutate gel is applied to a sun-damaged area. The concentration used and duration of treatment varies according to the site of the keratoses.

- On the face and scalp, ingenol mebutate gel 0.015% is applied once daily for 3 days
- On the trunk and extremities, ingenol mebutate gel 0.05% is applied once daily for 2 days
- The treated area is allowed to dry for 15 minutes after application and should not be washed or touched for 6 hours after treatment. The treated area can be gently washed after that. Excessive sweating should be avoided
- Treated areas become inflamed, often crusted, and then heal over a few days

Q. What is the mechanism of action of ingenol mebutate?

A. The following are the postulated mechanisms of action:

- Causes rapid swelling of mitochondria of dysplastic keratinocytes and cell death by primary necrosis
- On topical application, there is protein kinase C activation, which promotes neutrophilic infiltrate
- Neutrophil infiltrate prevents relapse of tumor by mediating antibody dependant cellular cytotoxicity
- Promotes normal healing as well as restoration of clinical and histologic morphology

Q. What are its drug interactions?

A. As ingenol mebutate is not absorbed through the skin, interactions with oral drugs are unlikely.

Q. What are the adverse effects of its use?

A. Irritations of the application site are very common. This includes redness, scaling, crusting, pain, pruritus, and sometimes infection. Other side effects include eye irritation such as periorbital edema (3%), headache (2%) and nasopharyngitis (running nose, 2%). There is no available data regarding use in pregnancy and children.

NICOTINAMIDE

Q. What is nicotinamide?

A. Nicotinamide/niacinamide/nicotinic acid amide, is the water-soluble, active form of vitamin B3 (nicotinic acid/niacin). Niacin is converted to nicotinamide in vivo, and though both have similar vitamin functions, the pharmacologic and toxic effects of niacin differ completely from nicotinamide. Both are readily absorbed from the GIT.

Q. What is the mechanism of action of nicotinamide?

A. The broad clinical effects of nicotinamide may be explained by its role as:

- An energy precursor in cells
- A modulator of inflammatory cytokines
- Stabilizes leukocytes, inhibits lymphocytic transformation, and the production of antibodies
- An inhibitor of the nuclear enzyme poly adenosine diphosphate-ribose polymerase (PARP), which alters leukocyte chemotaxis
- Topically stabilizes epidermal barrier function by reducing transepidermal water loss
- Sebo-suppressive

Q. What are the dermatological uses of nicotinamide?

A. Oral uses:

- Prophylaxis and treatment of pellagra (primary and secondary)
- Autoimmune bullous diseases (pemphigoid, pemphigus, dermatitis herpetiformis, linear IgA dermatoses). In AIBDs, nicotinamide is administered in oral doses of 500 mg three times daily administered along with oral tetracycline
- Acne vulgaris (recently being used as oral therapy for acne)

Topical uses:

- Acne vulgaris (2–4% gel)
- Rosacea
- Aging skin
- Solar keratoses (additive in sunscreens)

Q. What are the adverse effects due to nicotinamide use?

A. Oral use: Headache and GIT complaints, rarely hepatotoxicity. Very high doses may cause nausea. It does not cause flushing which was associated with niacin use.

LOCAL ANESTHESIA

Q. What is local anesthesia?

A. Local anesthesia is the reversible loss of sensation in a defined area of the body and is achieved by the topical application or injection of agents that block the generation and/or journey of nerve impulses in tissue. Regional anesthesia or field block is essentially local anesthesia but covers a larger area of subcutaneous tissue or larger peripheral nerves. Local anesthesia is used in many dermatological procedures and surgical operations. The aim is to minimize pain and suffering and maximize patient comfort.

Q. Classify local anesthetics.

A. Local anesthetics belong to two classes, amino-amides and amino-esters.

1. Amino-esters:
   - Aminobenzoic acid esters: Procaine chloroprocaine tetracaine benzocaine
   - Benzoic acid esters: Cocaine piperocaine
   - Others: Diathane intracaine
2. Aminoamides:
   - Lignocaine
   - Mepivacaine
   - Bupivacaine
   - Xylocaine
   - Prilocaine
   - Etidocaine
   - Propitocaine
   - Dibucaine

Q. Discuss lignocaine.

A. Lignocaine (lidocaine) is the local anesthetic most frequently used as it is effective, acts rapidly and is relatively free from toxicity and sensitivity. It is the local anesthetic by which all other anesthetics are compared. It is also the only local anesthetic available in many different formulations – spray, patch, ointment, and injection.

Q. What is EMLA?

A. Eutectic (Easily melted) Mixture of Local Anesthetics (EMLA) consists of a 1:1 mixture of 2.5% lignocaine with 2.5% prilocaine in oil in water emulsion. An application time of 1 hour is required for most procedures. The maximum depth of anesthesia achieved is 5 mm. It is particularly useful for numbing areas that require injection, especially in children. EMLA is also used in many dermatological procedures, including curettage, split-skin grafts, and different laser techniques.

Q. What is the role of adrenaline in local anesthesia?

A. Adrenaline (epinephrine) is sometimes added to local anesthetic formulations. It is used to:

- Prolong duration of anesthesia
- Reduce systemic absorption
- Reduce surgical bleeding
- Increase the intensity of the blockade

Epinephrine along with lidocaine is contraindicated for local infiltration of skin flaps and for blocks of acral parts like the digits/toes or penis where it may cause excessive vasoconstriction and ischemia of the tissues. Epinephrine administered in the presence of inhaled anesthetics causes enhanced cardiac irritability and dysrhythmias. Its systemic absorption may accentuate systemic hypertension and is therefore used with caution in patients with hypertension.

Q. What can be the side effects or complications of local anesthesia?

A.
- Allergic reactions (bronchospasm, urticaria, angioedema) – more with amino-esters
- Injection site reactions—pain, infection, nerve damage.
- CNS toxicity—dizziness, drowsiness, visual and auditory symptoms, twitching, tremors, and seizures rarely.
- Cardiovascular toxicity—sinus bradycardia, fall in blood pressure, sinus arrest (most severe with bupivacaine).
- Metallic taste in the mouth

TOPICAL NITROGEN MUSTARD

Q. What is nitrogen mustard?

A. Nitrogen mustard (mechlorethamine) is an alkylating agent. It is an anticancer agent. Nitrogen mustard powder for injection is administered intravenously to treat certain types of cancers, however topical formulations of nitrogen mustard can be prepared to treat cutaneous T-cell lymphomas, namely mycosis fungoides.

Topical preparations of nitrogen mustard are formulated by mixing the injectable powder with either water or an ointment base. The water preparation is unstable and needs to be used immediately, whereas ointment based preparations of nitrogen mustard are stable for at least a few months.

Q. What is the mechanism of action of nitrogen mustard?

A. Nitrogen mustard forms cyclic iminium rings which alkylate DNA and form inter-strand cross links (ICLs). These lesions force the cell to undergo apoptosis via the p53 mechanism.

Q. What are the uses of topical nitrogen mustard?

A. It is classically used in the treatment of the patch/plaque stage of mycosis fungoides. It is also used for the treatment of Langerhans Cell Histiocytosis.

Q. How is nitrogen mustard applied?

A. There are several different regimens. Topical nitrogen mustard (either the water-based preparation or the ointment-based preparation) may be applied daily until lesions resolve completely. This may be followed by a time of maintenance therapy for about 1–2 months.

The following general measures should be carried out when applying topical nitrogen mustard.

- First apply a small amount of nitrogen mustard to a selected test patch (palm-size) on the skin once a day for 7–10 days. If there is no significant irritation, new rash, redness or itching then the patient is advised to start applying nitrogen mustard over all lesions daily.
- It is applied sparingly to the affected areas; the nitrogen mustard is usually absorbed into the skin within the first hour after application.
- Disposable gloves may be worn to apply the preparation or apply directly with your hands and wash thoroughly afterwards.
- Additional moisturising lotions or creams may be applied throughout the day as necessary.
- Avoid application to sensitive areas such as the face and genitalia

Q. What are the side effects of topical nitrogen mustard?

A. The most common side effect of nitrogen mustard is an allergic reaction that usually results in itching, rash, or redness. This is especially a problem in more sensitive areas such as skin folds and occurs whether an aqueous solution or ointment preparation is used. In most cases, a reduction in the frequency of application or decrease in concentration will lessen the side effects and allow continuation with the medication. Darkening of the skin in the area where the nitrogen mustard was applied may also occur; this is reversible once the medication is stopped.

INSECT REPELLENT

Q. What is insect repellent?

A. Insect repellents are agents that are used to protect the body from the bites of insects. Whilst some bites cause only local skin irritation, others can cause serious illnesses and possibly death as the insects act as carriers or vectors of diseases. Mosquito bites are a common problem throughout the world.

Q. Classify insect repellents.

A.

Chemical repellents	*Natural plant-derived repellents*
DEET	Citronella
IR 3535	Soybean oil
MGK-326	Eucalyptus products
MGK-264 picaridin	Neem oil

Q. What makes an ideal insect repellent?

A. The ideal insect repellent should aim to have the following properties:

- Active against a wide variety of biting insects
- Prolonged activity (remain effective for at least 8 hours between applications)
- Nonirritating to the skin and mucous membranes
- Cosmetically appealing (odorless or have a pleasant odor and greaseless)
- No systemic toxicity
- Resistant to abrasion, washing and sweating
- Chemically stable
- Economically viable for widespread use

Q. What is DEET?

A. DEET is N, N-diethyl-3-methylbenzamide. It is a yellow oil and is the most commonly used active ingredient in insect repellents. It is to be applied onto the skin and clothing protects against mosquito bites, tick bites, fleas and chiggers. It is the most broad-spectrum and most effective insect repellent to be developed to date.

Most proprietary formulations are between 5–40%. When used with caution DEET has an excellent safety record.

Q. How do insect repellents work?

A. Mosquitoes use a combination of sight, heat and smell to detect a blood meal. Most insect repellents including DEET work on the principle of creating a vapor barrier that deters the insect from coming into contact with the skin. To the insect, the vapor has an offensive smell and tastes bad.

Q. What are the side effects of insect repellents?

A. Chemical insect repellents have a higher incidence of side effects as compared to natural agents. DEET has been associated with irritation, epidermal reactions, seizures, and cognitive disturbances. An application under clothing and over broken skin is to be avoided, and lower concentrations are to be used in children. The use of insect repellents in infants is not recommended.

INSECTICIDES

Q. What are insecticides?

A. Insecticides are substances designed to kill insects such as lice, mites, ticks, mosquitoes and fleas. They may be topical or systemic agents.

Q. What is an ideal insecticide?

A.
- Proven effectiveness against the target insect
- Capable of killing the eggs (ovicidal) as well as the adult parasites
- Non irritating to the skin and has no systemic toxicity
- Easy to use and inexpensive

Q. Describe some commonly used insecticide treatments.

A.

Insecticide name	*Properties*	*Effective against*	*Toxicity*
Pyrethrum/ pyrethrin/ phenothrin (can be combined with piperonyl butoxide)	• Topical agents • Naturally occurring insecticide found in the chrysanthemum flower • Not Ovicidal	• Head lice • Pubic lice • Body lice	• Can be toxic to humans in high doses • Seek medical advice before using in children under 2 years of age

Continued

Continued

Insecticide name	***Properties***	***Effective against***	***Toxicity***
Synthetic pyrethroids (e.g. permethrin)	• Topical agents • A synthetic form of pyrethrin • Effective against adult lice and has some ovicidal activity	• Head lice • Pubic lice • Body lice • Scabies • Can be sprayed onto clothes, tents, and mosquito nets to act as an insect repellent • Effective against ticks and fleas	• Has rarely been associated with toxic effects at high doses, including eye and skin irritation, tremors, loss of coordination, hyperactivity and paralysis • Seek medical advice before using in children under 2 years of age
Organo-phosphates (e.g. Malathion)	• Topical agents • Ovicidal	• Head lice • Pubic lice • Body lice • Scabies	• Seek medical advice before using in children under 2 years of age • Contains flammable alcohol, so do not expose lotion or wet hair to open flame or electric heal, such as a hair dryer
Benzyl benzoate	• Topical agent • Hydrocarbon	Scabies	Seek medical advice before using in children under 2 years of age
Ivermectin	Oral tablet	Crusted (Norwegian)	Potential neurotoxicity

Q. What is the best treatment for head lice in children less than 2 years of age?

A. Combing wet hair using a regular conditioner and a fine-tooth louse comb is the treatment of choice for head lice in children younger than 2 years of age.

Q. What are the adverse effects of insecticides?

A.
- People who are allergic to chrysanthemums may experience contact allergic dermatitis to pyrethrin or permethrin, although this is rare. As a precaution, these products should be avoided if chrysanthemum or ragweed allergy is present. Patients who are allergic to turpentine should also avoid pyrethrin-based products
- The most frequent side effect of permethrin is itching (likely related to the condition being treated, such as scabies or head lice, but the itch may be heightened after treatment). Oral antihistamines and/or topical corticosteroids can help relieve itchiness
- Permethrin at 5% concentration (a high dose used for treating scabies) can cause a mild burning or stinging sensation, mild itchiness, tingling, numbness, redness, swelling or rash. These preparations also contain a small amount of formaldehyde, which can rarely cause allergy or contact irritant dermatitis
- Rarely malathion may cause skin irritation, rash, redness and allergic reactions
- Benzyl benzoate may cause skin irritation. Apply to a small area of skin, if tingling or pain is experienced, try an alternative product
- Ivermectin may cause a transient exacerbation of itch at the beginning of treatment. Very rarely, Stevens–Johnson syndrome/ toxic epidermal necrolysis or other hypersensitivity reactions have been reported

MINOXIDIL

Q. What is minoxidil?

A. Minoxidil is an antihypertensive vasodilator medication. Unwanted hair growth was an accidental discovery.

Q. What are the indications of minoxidil?

A. USFDA approved:
- Male pattern androgenetic alopecia
- Female pattern androgenetic alopecia

Off-label dermatologic uses:

- Alopecia areata
- Chemotherapy induced alopecia
- Before and after hair transplantation
- Telogen effluvium

Q. What is the mechanism of action of minoxidil?

A. Minoxidil is an ATP sensitive potassium channel opener. This causes stimulation of VEGF and prostaglandins which in turn increases the duration of anagen phase and gradually enlarges vellus hair into mature terminal hair follicles. It also has a local vasodilator action.

Q. What are the side effects of topical minoxidil therapy?

A. The common side effects are:

- Irritant dermatitis
- Allergic dermatitis
- Unwanted hair growth elsewhere
- Itching and burning of the eyes

Q. What is the pregnancy prescribing status of topical minoxidil?

A. Category C

Q. What instructions should be given to the patient who started on minoxidil?

A. The following instructions should be given to the patient:

- 1 mL application twice daily on the scalp
- To expect increased hair fall in the first few months of treatment
- Earliest clinical signs of hair regrowth can be observed 4–5 months after initiating therapy
- On stopping treatment, the pretreatment appearance would return within 3–4 months and stopping treatment after many years of therapy will result in loss of all hair genetically programmed to fall off at that age

Q. How to increase the efficacy of minoxidil?

A. The efficacy of minoxidil can be increased by the concurrent use of a topical retinoid.

Q. What are the commercial preparations of minoxidil?

A. Minoxidil is available as a 2%, 5% and 10% solution and foam.

AMINEXIL

Q. What is aminexil?

A. It is 2,4 diaminopyrimidine oxide.

Q. How does it work?

A. It acts as an antifibrotic agent and prevents collagen formation thus increasing survival of the hair follicle.

Q. What concentration is available?

A. 1–5% solution.

Q. What are the other unapproved agents for treatment of hair loss?

A.
- Progesterone (used topically)
- Cimetidine (used orally 300 mg five times a day)
- Plant extracts like serenoa repens (a type of berry)
- A hair rejuvenation program whose active ingredients contain glycoproteins, hyaluronic acid and amino acids along with nicotinic acid, sodium pantothenate and biotin. It claims to block DHT
- Zinc acetate and zinc sulphate used topically which block DHT production
- Prezatide copper which is an anti-inflammatory superoxide dismutase. It is a wound healing agent but has been used in hair loss
- Copper chloride in cream form can be combined with saw palmetto
- Thymus extract which is an immunomodulating agent

Q. What are the new agents undergoing investigation?

A.
- FK-143 which inhibits both type I and type II 5α reductase
- Turosteride inhibits type II 5α reductase

Q. What are the devices that claim to induce hair growth?

A.
- Electrical biowave helmet
- Electro trichogenesis
- Laser light therapy

GENTIAN VIOLET

Q. What is gentian violet?

A. Gentian violet is a triarylmethane dye. It gets its name because of its color and is not made from gentian or violet flowers. There have been no clinical trials and there is no evidence about the long-term safety and efficacy of gentian violet.

Q. What are the uses of gentian violet in dermatology?

A.
- Fungal infections like oral thrush, vaginal thrush and dermatophyte infections
- Bacterial infections like impetigo (it also has some action against MRSA)

- Oral hairy leukoplakia in HIV positive patients
- To mark the skin for surgeries
- Gram staining

Q. What are the side effects of gentian violet?

A.
- Staining of the clothes and the skin
- Irritation of mucous membranes and oral ulceration
- Necrotic skin reactions when applied around the skin folds
- Permanent staining of the skin when applied over raw areas
- It has a carcinogenic potential but significant data is not available
- Serious side effects are generally absent when gentian violet is used as a topical agent

HONEY

Q. What is honey and what is its use in dermatology?

A. Honey is a saturated or a super saturated solution of sugars. Honey can be used as a second line topical antibacterial agent in the following conditions:

- Leg ulcers
- Pressure ulcers
- Diabetic foot ulcers
- Infected wounds
- Burns

Honey is used when conventional agents fail. Honey dressings promote rapid healing with minimal scarring.

Q. What is the mechanism of action of honey?

A. Honey has a high osmolality and strong interaction with water molecules in the wounds. This causes a lack of free water which inhibits growth of bacteria. Honey is also diluted by wound exudates which leads to generation of hydrogen peroxide which has antibacterial activity. Honey also has some antibacterial phytochemicals which have a direct action on the bacteria. Honey also appears to stimulate lymphocytic and phagocytic activity.

Q. How to prepare honey dressings for wounds?

A.
- Honey should be sterilized and then spread on a dressing rather than directly applying it over the wound
- Occlusive dressing prevent honey from oozing out of the wounds
- The amount of honey and the frequency of dressings depends on the exudation from the wounds
- Abscesses and penetrating wounds require greater amounts of honey to penetrate deeper

HYDROGEN PEROXIDE

Q. What is hydrogen peroxide?

A. Hydrogen peroxide is a bleach and an oxidizing agent that has activity against a wide variety of microorganisms.

Q. What are the uses of hydrogen peroxide in dermatology?

A.
- Low concentrations 1–5% are used to clean wounds, scrapes and other minor injuries although there is little or no evidence that bacterial counts are reduced in wounds
- 1% hydrogen peroxide cream is used in the treatment of acne. Some studies state that is equally effective as benzoyl peroxide
- As a disinfectant of inanimate objects because hydrogen peroxide is active against bacteria, fungi and viruses
- At concentrations up to 10%, it is used in peroxide based hair dyes

Q. What is an advantage of hydrogen peroxide use?

A. There are no known disease causing bacteria or fungi that have developed resistance to hydrogen peroxide.

Q. What are the adverse effects of hydrogen peroxide?

A.
- Irritation and temporary bleaching of the skin and hair are the common side effects
- Concentrated solutions may cause burns and blistering
- Exposure of low concentration hydrogen peroxide to the eyes causes stinging and burning sensation but exposure to concentrations higher than 10% may cause ulceration, perforation, permanent eye injury and blindness
- Ingestion and inhalation of high concentrations of hydrogen peroxide is toxic and can be fatal and at low concentrations there is irritation of the GIT and respiratory tract

DISINFECTANT RUBS

Q. What is a disinfectant rub?

A. Disinfectant rub is a gel or liquid containing antimicrobial agents that reduce the number of microorganisms over the applied surface. They cannot be used if the respective surfaces are visibly soiled. They are easy to use and cause less dryness and irritation than soap and water and are as effective as chemical wash products used in healthcare settings.

Q. What are the commonly used disinfectant rubs in dermatology?

A. The commonly used disinfectant rubs are:

- Ethanol in concentrations 60% or greater
- Chlorhexidine gluconate 2%
- Iodophors like povidone iodine

A combination of these disinfectants is more effective than each used individually.

Q. Discuss ethanol as a disinfectant.

A. Ethanol at a concentration of 60% or greater is effective against:

- Most bacteria including one's that have developed multi-drug resistance (like MRSA)
- Fungi
- Some viruses like influenza virus, HSV, rotavirus and HIV. Hepatitis viruses and enteroviruses require even higher concentrations of ethanol
- Ethanol disinfectants have limited effectiveness against bacterial spores (*Cl. difficile*), protozoan oocysts and certain viruses. It has a short duration of action. To increases its effectiveness and duration of action it is combined with 2% chlorhexidine gluconate in healthcare settings

Q. Discuss povidone iodine.

A. It is a stable chemical complex of polyvinylpyrrolidone (povidone, PVP) and elemental iodine. It has a broad spectrum antiseptic activity. It has been demonstrated that bacteria do not develop resistance to povidone iodine. It is slightly less effective than the combination of chlorhexidine and alcohol however it causes less irritation compared to ethanol. Povidone iodine is contraindicated in patients with hyperthyroidism (overactive thyroid gland) and other diseases of the thyroid, after treatment with radioiodine, and in patients with dermatitis herpetiformis.

Q. What are the uses of disinfectant rubs?

A.

- As a disinfectant of the skin before minor procedures as well as major surgeries
- It is also used to clean the skin surface after a procedure
- Ethanol and chlorhexidine can also be used as hand sanitizers
- Povidone iodine in aqueous solutions has been used in the treatment of ulcers and wounds
- Povidone iodine has been used for treating vaginitis due to mixed infections and also in the prophylaxis of neonatal conjunctivitis

Q. What are the adverse effects of disinfectant rubs?

A.
- Contact dermatitis (irritant as well as allergic)
- Contact eczema
- A brief stinging sensation with ethanol if the skin is cracked
- Povidone iodine can cause staining of clothes and skin

Q. What are the disadvantages of disinfectant rubs?

A.
- Effectiveness is reduced if product is not used according to directions
- Limited effectiveness against some micro-organisms
- Small children should be supervised while using

CANTHARIDINE

Q. What is cantharidine?

A. Cantharidine is a vesicant derived from blister beetle Cantharis vesicatoria. It is also known as Spanish fly.

Q. What is it used for and how does it work?

A. Cantharidine is used in the treatment of viral warts and molluscum contagiosum. It causes a blister to form on the wart or the growth, lifting the wart of the skin. After a few days when the blister dries up, the wart will come off. The action of cantharidin does not go beyond the epidermis basal layer, hence there is no scarring.

Q. How is it used?

A. It is used only topically and applied by doctors because of its potential side effects. Used as follows: The lesion is first shaved or parred. Then Cantharidine (with a substance that creates a colloidal film) is accurately applied to the wart or molluscum. The liquid is then dried and sealed with a nonporous tape for 4–6 hours, after which the tape is removed and the area is washed with soap and water. Blister formation takes place within 24–48 hours, over the next few days the blister dries up and the lesion falls off. Healing is normally complete in 4–7 days. Resistant warts and new molluscum may require repeat treatment.

Q. What are the precautions and side-effects of Cantharidine?

A. *Precautions*: Cantharidine should not be used for warts and molluscum on mucous membranes, eyelids, nostrils, mouth, areas around the anus and the genitals. It should be used with caution in patients with diabetes, peripheral vascular disease and other circulatory problems.

Side-effects: Resulting blister following cantharidin treatment can be painful and discomforting. Occasionally, patients may develop a ring of small satellite warts surrounding the orignal wart after cantharidin treatment. Complications like inflammation of lymph vessels and cellulitis may occur after the treatment of plantar warts with cantharidin.

CAPSAICIN

Q. What is capsaicin and how does it work?

A. Capsaicin is the purified extracted alkaloid from red chilli peppers (capsicums). This is the substance that makes chilli peppers hot. It has been found to relieve pain by reducing substance P, which is found at nerve endings and is involved in transmitting neuralgic and arthritic pain signals to the brain. Pain relief is not instantaneous after application as it is the cumulative depletion of substance P over a period of weeks that brings the full effect.

Q. Where is it used?

A. Capsaicin is used as a topical cream to relieve pain from some arthritic conditions such as osteoarthritis and rheumatoid arthritis and various neuralgic pain like post-herpetic neuralgia, trigeminal neuralgia, atypical facial pain, brachioradial pruritus, nodular prurigo. It is available as a 0.025% or 0.075% strength cream in 45 g tube.

Q. What are the precautions and side effects of capsaicin?

A. *Precautions*: Do not use capsaicin cream on broken or infected skin. Avoid use near eyes or other sensitive areas of the body. Tight bandages should not be applied on top of capsaicin cream.

Side effects: The most common side effect of capsaicin use is a feeling of warmth and stinging, or a sensation of burning after application. This sensation is related to the action of capsaicin on the skin and is to be expected. This sensation usually diminishes after the first few days of application and in mostly disappears with time and continued use.

DIHYDROXYACETONE (DHA)

Q. What is DHA and how does it work?

A. All effective sunless tanners (stainers)contain DHA. It is a colorless 3-carbon sugar that when applied to the skin causes a chemical reaction with amino acids in the surface cells of the skin producing a darkening effect. DHA does not damage skin as it only affects the outermost cells of the epidermis (stratum corneum).

Q. What are the indications of DHA?

A. Clinical uses as camouflage for skin conditions such as vitiligo, spider nevi. It may provide some protection for individuals with certain photosensitivity disorders such as PMLE, erythropoeitic protoporphyria or drug induced photosensitivity.

Q. What are the side-effects and precautions of DHA?

A. *Side effects*: DHA reacts quickly in the stratum corneum minimizing systemic absorption. Contact dermatitis caused by DHA has rarely been reported. Most causes of sensitivity are due to other ingredients such as preservatives in the preparation.

Precautions: The most important thing to remember when using DHA self-tanners is that they do not protect your skin against the sun, an individual is just as susceptible to harmful UV rays, hence it must be stressed that an overall sun protection program is necessary.

Q. How long does the color change last while using DHA?

A. A color change is usually apparent within an hour of application. Maximal darkening may take 8–24 hours to develop. An artificial tan produced by DHA will last until the dead skin cells rub off, usually 5–7 days with a single application. Depending on the area, the same color can be maintained with repeat applications every 1–4 days.

Q. What are the concentrations of DHA available?

A. Concentrations of DHA can range from 2.5 to 10% or more (mostly 3–5%).

ESCHAROTIC AGENTS

Q. What are escharotic agents?

A. Escharotic agents are caustic, corrosive salves, pastes, poultices and plasters that are purported to destroy cancer cells and cure skin cancers.They are called escharotics because they produce a thick black, dry scab called an "eschar" on the skin. The two most common ingredients used in escharotic agents are zinc chloride and bloodroot (contains the alkaloid sanguinarine that is derived from the root of the plant Sanguinaria canadensis).

Q. Who uses escharotic agents?

A. The use of escharotic agents has fallen out of practice in conventional medicine because their efficacy is unproved and their content is unregulated. People still using escharotic agents are those seeking an alternative treatment to conventional therapy, individuals having a fear of surgery or seeking a natural remedy. With the ever-growing use of the internet, people are able to access information about diseases and remedies more readily. Through these sites individuals are able to purchase escharotic agents directly and self-administer at home.

Q. Why is it not advisable to use escharotic agents?

A. In many patients that use escharotic agents the initial outcome is often pleasing, as the tumor appears to die and fall off. However, the harm that escharotic agents can cause is often not immediately apparent. Several cases have been documented in literature where the use of escharotic agents has had detrimental outcomes.

- The tumor appeared initially to disappear but recurred several years later requiring extensive surgery. The patient later developed metastasis (secondary growths).
- Residual tumor found on biopsy although it appeared initially to have gone.
- Severe scarring as a result of the escharotic agent.
- Other dangers include: Non-selectivity of tissue damage—escharotic agents destroy normal tissue as well as skin cancers. Lesions are often undiagnosed; hence many patients self-treating may be treating anything ranging from completely harmless lesions to dangerous melanomas. The manufacture, marketing and distribution of escharotic agents is unregulated, so the strength and purity is unknown. There is lack of scientific evidence for the efficacy of these agents, or their risks and side effects.

EFLORNITHINE

Q. How does eflornithine work?

A. Eflornithine works by blocking the enzyme ornithine decarboxylase (ODC) that stimulates hair growth. Eflornithine HCl cream 13.9% has been shown to slow the rate of hair growth in animal and human studies.

Q. What are the indications of eflornithine?

A. Eflornithine HCl cream is indicated for the reduction of unwanted facial hair in women secondary to: Genetic Hirsutism or hypertrichosis, menopause and the normal aging process, medical condition such as androgen excess disorder and PCOD, adrenal hyperplasia, medications.

Other indication of eflornithine is treatment of african sleeping sickness

Q. How effective is eflornithine?

A. In two double-blind placebo controlled trials, 35% of patients treated with eflornithine cream show significant improvement after 24 weeks of treatment compared with 9% of patients treated with placebo. It appears that the longer eflornithine is used, the better it works. Over time the need for additional hair removal techniques to maintain a hair-free complexion may reduce.

Q. How is eflornithine to be used?

A. A thin layer of eflornithine HCl cream should be massaged well into the affected area of face twice a day. Wait at least 4 hours before washing your face again. Cosmetics and sunscreens can be applied over the top of eflornithine HCl cream once it has been absorbed into the skin and dried. If using in conjunction with other hair removal techniques, eflornithine HCl cream should be applied at least 5 minutes after performing the first technique. If eflornithine HCl cream is stopped, for an extended period of time, hair will begin growing back at the same rate that it used to.

Q. What are the side-effects of eflornithine?

A. Side effects include redness, stinging, burning, tingling, rash, ingrown hairs (pseudofolliculitis barbae), acne. If skin irritation develops, the dose may be reduced to once a day.

SHAMPOO AND SOAPS

Q. What are shampoos?

A. Shampoos are cleansers designed to clean the hair and scalp.

Q. What are the different types of shampoos available.

A. Clarifying shampoos containing heavy duty surfactants, body building shampoos containing protein that increase the volume of hair, moisturizing shampoos for dry flyaway hair, revitalising shampoo for color treated or permed hair, 2 in 1 shampoo with conditioner and baby shampoos with less amount of detergents.

Q. What are the indications of medicated shampoos?

A. Pityriasis sicca, Seborrheic dermatitis, psoriasis, atopic dermatitis.

Q. What are the skin problems faced due to shampoos?

A. Overwashing can cause following problems:

- Irritation of the scalp
- Ph of the skin can change
- The surface oil film i.e., sebum is removed allowing greater loss of water, de-fatted skin may become excessively dry making it more prone to infections
- Irritant contact dermatitis

Q. What are soaps?

A. Soaps are anionic surfactants made from fats and oils mixed with alkali, forming glyceride and sodium salt of fatty acid.

Q. What are the disadvantages of soaps?

A. Irritates the sensitive skin, alkaline skin degrades quickly, soaps form scum when used with hard water thus stoping the surfactant properties, soap leaves deposits of carbonate salts on skin thus irritating the skin, soaps deteriorate on storage.

POTASSIUM PERMANGANATE

Q. What is potassium permanganate ($KMnO_4$)?

A. It is an oxidizing agent with disinfectant, deodorizing and astringent properties.

Q. What is the other name of potassium permanganate?

A. Condy's crystals

Q. What is potassium permanganate used for?

A. It is used for following dermatological conditions like:

- Infected eczema
- Blistering skin conditions
- Room cleansing especially weeping ulcers or abscesses
- Fungal infections such as athlete's foot

Q. What are the precautions taken for the use of potassium permanganate?

A.
- Potassium permanganate crystals and concentrated solutions are caustic and can burn the skin can cause irritation and repeated use may cause burns. If redness or irritation continues notify the doctor.
- Make sure that the crystals or tablets are fully dissolved in water.
- $KMnO_4$ soaks are not suitable for dry skin conditions

TANNING AGENTS

Q. Name a few tanning agents.

A. Stainers (dihydroxy acetone), Bronzers (diase), Tan accelerators (tyrosine and psoralens) , Psoralea (sun beds and sun lamps).

Q. What is the mechanism of action of DHA?

A. DHA is a colorless free carbon sugar that when applied to skin causes a chemical reaction with amino acids in the surface cells of the skin producing a darkening effect DHA does not damage skin as it only affects the outermost cells of epidermis.

Q. What are the indications for DHA containing preparations?

A. Vitiligo and as a camouflage of some skin irregularity such as spider veins, photosensitivity disorders such as polymorphic light eruptions, erythropoietic protoporphyria or drug induced photosensitivity.

Q. What are the precautions taken while using DHA self tanning preparations?

A. Despite the darkening of the skin individual is just as susceptible to harmful UV rays, thus sunscreen use is also necessary.

WET WRAPS

Q. What are wet wraps?

A. Wet wraps are wet bandages wrapped over emollients, topical steroid peels, hot, weeping eczema(atopic dermatitis), erythroderma.

Q. How does wet wrapping work?

A. It works via three different ways:

1. Cooling—by relieving inflammation itching soreness
2. Moisturizing—by enhancing deep absorption of the medication steroid absorption in both superficial and deep places
4. In addition the bandages provide protection from itching and scratching cycle

Q. What are the benefits of wet wrapping?

A. The benefits of wet wraps include:

- Reduced itching and scratching
- Reduced redness and inflammation
- Skin hydration
- Better skin healing process
- Reduced steroid usage
- Improved sleep

Q. What are the side effects of wet wraps?

A. As the steroids are absorbed better under wet wraps the side effects are more, which include burning irritation stinging.

OATMEAL

Q. What is oatmeal?

A. Oatmeal is derived from oat grains that are ground, crushed or rolled.

Q. What is the use of oatmeal in skin care?

A. Oatmeal is used in following dermatologicals conditions:

- Atopic dermatitis
- Contact dermatitis
- Chickenpox
- Dry skin
- Reactions to insect bites
- Reactions to plants such as poison ivy

Q. What are the side effects of oatmeals?

A. Contact allergic dermatitis when used topically. When eaten, some components of oat may cause a reaction in sufferers of Celiac disease, dermatitis herpetiformis.

Q. How does oatmeal help in skin conditions?

A.
- Colloidal oatmeal binds to the skin and provides a protective barrier against irritants
- It holds moisture against the skin due to its fat content allowing it to act as an emollient. It acts as a buffering agent that can help maintain the skin's normal pH
- It has anti-oxidant and anti-inflammatory activity as well as ultraviolet light absorption
- It protect against sun damage and the inflammation of various skin conditions.
- It helps against photoaging
- Oatmeal has also been used as a cleanser and cosmetically as a common ingredient in facial masks

β-BLOCKERS

Q. Discuss the use of beta blockers for the treatment of infantile hemangioma?

A. Beta blockers were introduced for the treatment of hemangioma in 2008 , as a serendipitous discovery when children given propranolol for cardiomyopathy showed improvement in their hemangioma. Propranolol has been used in the proliferative stage of hemangioma, ulcerated hemangioma, stable hemangioma and even regressing hemangioma. The earlier treatment with propranolol started, the shorter is the treatment required.

The mechanism of action is not exactly known but there seem to be early effect due to vasoconstriction, intermediate effects due to blocking of angiogenic signals and long-term effects because of apoptosis of endothelial cells. Propranolol can also have an inhibitory effect on the renin-angiotensin system which can stimulate angiogenesis.

Q. Discuss the pharmacological properties of propranolol?

A. It is a nonselective synthetic beta adrenergic blocking agent. It has got negative chronotropic and ionotropic effects on the heart as well as a vasodilator effect. It is highly lipophilic and has mutliple drug interactions. Its levels are increased by amiodarone, cimetidine and fluoxetine , while they are decreased by rifampicin, phenytoin and phenobarbitone.

Q. What are the contraindications of propranolol?

A. They are:

- Hypotension
- Bronchial asthma
- Heart block
- Bradycardia

Hence a pretreatment ECG is mandatory, especially when the heart rate is below normal for age or if there is a family history of congenital heart conditions or arrhythmias. Propranolol is available as 20 mg/5 mL oral solution and the recommended dose is initially 1 mg/kg/day tid with a max dose of 3 mg/kg/day.

Q. What are the side effects of propranolol therapy?

A.
- Common side effects: Cold extremities, night terrors
- Rare but potentially serious: Hypoglycemia, hypotension and exacerbation of asthma

Note:

- Instead of propranolol, atenolol may be used which has lesser sleep disturbances. Nadolol may be used because it has less side effects.
- Topical beta blockers can be used for small primarily superficial hemangiomas. 0.25% and 0.5% for timolol. It is well tolerated with minimal side effects but absorption can occur through ulcerated areas.

The following are the recently described modalities of treatment for vascular anomalies

Drugs	***Indications***
Oral beta blockers	Proliferative cutaneous, stable and healing airway, ocular, orificial, ulcerated and hepatic hemangioma
Topical beta blockers	Small, superficial hemangioma
Topical rapamycin	Angiofibroma, adjunct for pot wine stains along with laser therapy
Systemic rapamycin	Used in lymphatic malformations, Kasabach-Merritt phenomenon
Systemic sildenafil	Lymphatic malformations
Topical imiquimod	Adjunct for pot wine stains undergoing laser therapy

5 Lasers in Dermatology

Q. What is the full form of LASER?

A. Light amplification by stimulated emission of radiation.

Q. Who is the Father of Laser medicine and surgery?

A. Dr Leon Goldman (Used blue-green argon laser for retinal surgery)

Q. What are different types of Laser/Lasing media?

A.
- Gas: Argon, CO_2, helium, xenon chloride
- Liquid: Rhodamine dye in organic solvent used for pulsed dye laser.
- Solid: Alexandrite, Nd:YAG, Ruby, Erbium:YAG.
- Semiconductor: Diode (E.g., Aluminium gallium arsenide)

Q. What are chromophores?

A. These are absorbing molecules in the skin/body that exhibit characteristic bands of absorption at certain wavelengths. The photon from the laser targets these chromophores resulting in their excited state and eventually causing the desired action.

Q. What are the three primary skin chromophores?

A. Water, hemoglobin and melanin.

Q. Enumerate the wavelengths of commonly used skin lasers.

A.
- Nd:YAG: 1064 nm and 532 nm
- Fractional CO_2: 10,600 nm
- Erbium glass: 1540 nm
- Diode: 808/810 nm
- Excimer: 308 nm
- Alexandrite: 755 nm
- Pulsed dye laser: 585–600 nm

Q. What is thermal relaxation time (TRT)?

A. TRT for a given tissue structure is defined as the time required for the heated tissue to cool halfway toward its initial temperature.

EXCIMER

Q. What is an excimer lamp?

A. UV light device which uses noble gases, i.e., argon, krypton or xenon.

On electrical stimulation and high pressure inside the discharge tube of device 'EX'cited di 'MER' is created which emits UV spectrum between 157 and 351 nm.

Q. Which gas is used in dermatological application of excimer?
A. Xenon at 308 nm is used.

Q. What are advantages of excimer over other phototherapies?
A.
- Lower UV dose exposure
- Shorter course of therapy
- The possibility of being directed at distinct sites of skin

Q. What is the mechanism of action?
A. It acts by:
- Causing T-cell apoptosis
- Decreasing keratinocyte proliferation
- Decreasing proinflammatory, angiogenic, hyperproliferative cytokines

Q. Indications of excimer.
A.
- Vitiligo
- Psoriasis
- Alopecia areata
- Lichen planus
- Atopic dermatitis
- Cutaneous lymphomas

Q. Operative protocols for excimer.
A. **Vitiligo:**
- Start at 150–200 mj/cm^2 OR alternatively use the standard machine dosage chart
- For hands and feet initial dose can be 300–400 mj/cm^2 to start with.
- Standard phototherapy increments of 20/10/0 to be followed, i.e.:
  - 20% if no erythema
  - 10% if erythema <24 hours
  - 0% if persistent erythema
- In the rare case of severe burns, reduce dose by half.

Psoriasis:
- Determine the induration of plaque
- Apply oil before treatment to allow better penetration of light
- For PASI 1 START AT 400 mj/cm^2
- PASI 2 start at 600 mj/cm^2

- PASI 3 start at 900 mj/cm^2
- Increase the dose by 20% every alternate day.

Note: In any case/disorder, If no significant response seen by 10 sittings stop the treatment.

Q-SWITCHED ND:YAG

Q. What is a Q-switch Nd:YAG laser?

A. Q-switched Nd:YAG laser (Neodymium-doped Yttrium Aluminium Garnet) is the gold standard for pigment and tattoo removal in dark skin.

Q. What is the basic pretreatment advice you will give?

A. Due care needs to be taken with regards to the technique and patient selection to avoid complications. Proper sun protection and priming is helpful in minimizing complications and achieving satisfactory outcomes.

Q. Which theory is used as the basis of dermatological laser therapy?

A. Laser therapy of pigmented lesions is based on the theory of selective photothermolysis that was pioneered by Anderson and Parrish.

Q. What is the mechanism of action.

A.

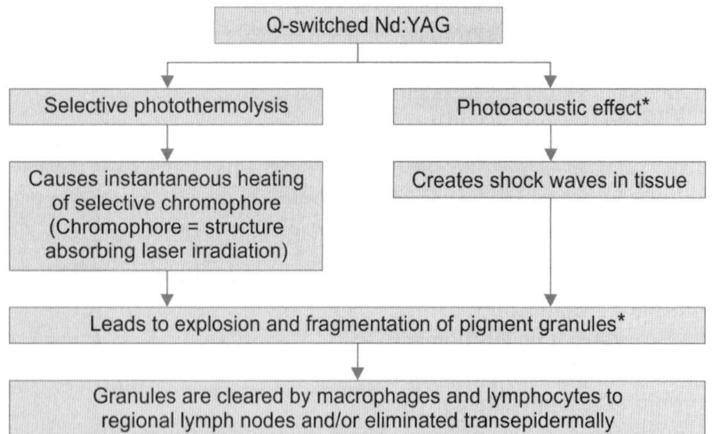

*The brisk whitening of the lesion is due to intracellular steam formation and vacuolization. Whitening is followed by erythema and edema.

Audible popping sound is heard during treatment due to shock wave generation in the treated tissue (Photoacoustic effect).

Q. What is Q-switching?

A. Q-switching is a technique by which a laser can be made to produce extremely high peak power with a shorter pulse duration.

Q. What are the indications?

A.
- Pigmented lesions
  - Lentigines/freckles/CALM
  - Tattoo removal
  - Melasma
- Nevus of Ota/Ito
  - Vascular lesions
  - Nonablative skin rejuvenation/resurfacing

Q. What operative protocols will you follow?

A. Primary step is the selection of appropriate wavelength.

1064 nm:
- Used for dermal lesions, green ink, blue/black ink, carbon peel and laser toning as it has deeper penetration.
- It is poorly absorbed by epidermal melanin and is relatively safer to use.
- Test spots are not mandatory for this wavelength.

532 nm:
- Used for epidermal lesions and red tattoo ink removal.
- This wavelength has very high melanin absorption, has shallow depth of penetration and should be used carefully in darker skin types as the risk of hyper- and hypo-pigmentation is higher.
- Test spots are advisable and low fluences to be used at the beginning.

FRACTIONAL CO_2

Q. What is the difference between ablative and nonablative laser?

A. The basic difference between them is that ablative lasers remove the epidermis while nonablative lasers target the dermis and deeper layers without resulting in epidermal damage. Fractional CO_2 is the Gold standard in ablative lasers.

Q. What is a fractional CO_2 laser?

A. CO_2 laser was invented in 1960 by Chandra Kumar Patel an electrical engineer from Bombay, India. It has an optical cavity which contains active medium containing mixture of CO_2, nitrogen and helium gases. When external electric source enters the optic cavity, the active medium of CO_2 molecules are pumped to high energy vibrational state, they release infrared photons to the wavelength of 10,600 nm and subsequently decay back to the ground state. The reflective mirrors help the photons to re-enter the active medium to stimulate release of more photons.

Q. What does 'fractional' mean?

A. As the term suggests fractional CO_2 works by only ablating the designated 'fraction of skin' allowing for skip areas of normal skin in order to aid in faster re-epithelialization and cover a bigger surface area.

Q. Mechanism of action.

A.

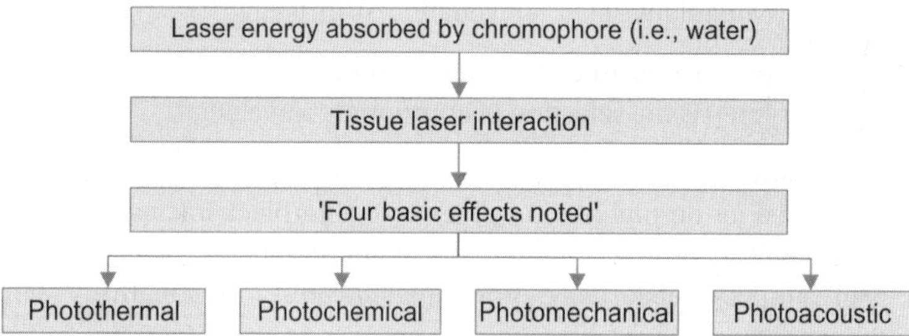

Q. Indications of fractional CO_2 laser.

A.
- Acne scars: Atrophic scars–Skin resurfacing/rejuvenation
- Nonaesthetic: Syringomas, xanthelasma, severe photodamage, verruca plana, DPN, Rhinophyma, sebaceous hyperplasia, pearly penile papules, etc.

Q. Operative protocols for fractional CO_2.

A.
- Usage and operative protocol of CO_2 laser is to be kept at the discretion of senior faculty and individualized for each patient/indication.
- Topical anesthesia (i.e., Eutectic mixture of local anesthetic, Prilocaine 2.5% + Lignocaine 2.5%) to be applied under occlusion for 60 minutes, remove occlusion just before the procedure.

General instructions:
- Ocular protection with opaque glasses for patient and polycarbonate glasses for operator.
- Protection from plume, usage of masks is mandatory by operator and assistant.
- Know about the emergency cut off switch, in case laser beam is emitted even without pressing the foot pad. Point the laser head away from the patient and then press the emergency stop button.
- Wet and dry gauzes to be kept ready to wipe the vaporized lesions if advised by the operator.
- Ice packs to be applied promptly for better tolerance of procedure and reduce postinflammatory changes.

Q. Postoperative care and follow-up.

A. Follow-up the patient on day 7 and day 30, either physically or telephonically.

- Topical antibiotic and sunscreen to be used thrice per day, emphasize on this point.
- Add topical steroid if patient complains of discomfort, excessive irritation, persistent erythema.

DIODE LASER

Q. What are diode lasers?

A. Diode lasers use a single wavelength of light (808 nm) that has a high abruption rate in melanin. Key to successful diode hair removal is the deliverance of high energy into the skin. The energy is selectively absorbed by the melanin of the hair follicle whilst not impacting the surrounding tissue. As the melanin heats up it destroys the root and blood flow to the follicle disabling the hair growth.

Q. What is a triple wavelength diode?

A. A triple wavelength diode uses three different wavelengths in conjunction with each other to get optimum outcome. The wavelengths commonly used are 1064, 810 and 755 nm. Out of these 1064 and 810 nm have potential for deep penetration and hence focus on darker skin tones while 755 can be used to target superficial sensitive structures like eyebrows and upper lips.

Q. What are the alternatives to diode laser for laser hair reduction?

A.
- Long pulse Nd:YAG Laser
- Intense pulsed light (IPL)
- Alexandrite laser

Operative protocols

- General parameters:
  - Stamping mode: Used to target smaller areas like upper lips.
    - Fluence: 8–20 j/cm^2
    - Pulse repetition rate: 1 Hz
  - In motion mode: Used to target larger area like chest, limbs.
    - Fluence: 8–20 j/cm^2
    - Pulse repetition rate: 4–5 Hz
    - Clock: 10–20 seconds
    - Passes: 2–3

6 Chemical Peels

Q. What are chemical peels?

A. A chemical peel refers to the application of one or more chemicals to the skin which 'burn' off damaged cells, resurfacing the skin. The three principal types of chemical peels are alpha-hydroxy acid peels, trichloroacetic acid peels, and the phenol-croton oil peel.

Q. How does a peel work?

A. A peel removes several layers of sun-damaged skin cells, leaving fresh skin which has a more even surface and color. It may stimulate new collagen to be formed improving the skin texture. Peels may result in superficial, moderate depth or deep skin injury.

Q. What are the indications of peels?

A. Chemical peels are most often used on the face, but they are sometimes applied to other sites such as the hands.

A peel may be used to treat damage caused by exposure to the sun (photoaging) including actinic keratoses, to remove pigmentation such as freckles and melasma, to reduce fine lines and wrinkles, and to improve acne.

They are most often used in patients with fair skin, Fitzpatrick skin types I to III. It is wise to wait for 3 to 6 months before repeating a moderate depth peel.

Q. What are contraindications of peels?

A. Patients with Fitzpatrick skin types IV to VI have increased risk of dyspigmentation, hypertrophic, and keloid scarring and chemical peels must be performed cautiously with full patient informed consent.

Q. What is jessner's solution?

A. Resorcinol: 14 g; Salicylic acid: 14 g 85%; lactic acid: 14 g 95%; ethanol: 100 mL.

Q. What are the types of peels?

A. Superficial peels:

- Superficial peels use glycolic acid, salicylic acid and Jessner solution and are well tolerated—the 'lunchtime' peel. They remove thin lesions on the skin surface, reducing pigment and surface dryness.

- The result of the first peel may be disappointing, but after repeated peels, significant improvement is usually evident. A nurse or aesthetician (beauty therapist) may perform superficial peels.

Medium peels:

- Trichloroacetic acid (TCA) is the most common chemical used for a medium depth peel. The results depend on its concentration, usually 20–35%. The treatment is painful and treated areas are swollen, red and crusted for the next week or so.
- It can lead to an impressive improvement in skin texture with a reduction in blotchy pigmentation, freckling and actinic keratoses (dry sunspots). Although fine wrinkles and some acne scars are less obvious, the TCA peel has no effect on deep furrows.

Deep peels:

- Phenol results in deep skin injury. It is rarely used for facial peels nowadays because of the risk of scarring and because of its toxicity. However, it is very effective at improving both surface wrinkles and deep furrows.
- After a phenol peel, the treated skin is pale and smooth but it may be waxy and 'mask-like'.

Q. What are the methods for preparing before peel?

A. A chemical peel is a four-step procedure:

1. Pre-peel preparation
2. Peeling procedure
3. Recovery phase
4. Maintenance phase

Determine whether the peel is required for a focal lesion or for the entire face. Undertake a prepeel classification.

- Fitzpatrick skin phototype: Lighter peels are undertaken in darker skin because of the risk of postinflammatory pigmentation
- Previous experience of skin peels
- A tendency for the skin to develop increased and/or loss of pigmentation at the sites of skin injury

Pre-treatment creams are applied to the face at night for several weeks prior to the peel. By exfoliating the skin and reducing pigmentation themselves, they improve the results seen from chemical peeling. They may also reduce the time needed for healing. The creams usually include one or more of the following:

- Tretinoin
- Alpha hydroxy acid e.g., glycolic or lactic acid

- Hydroquinone for tanned or dark-skinned patients or those with melasma
- Broad-spectrum SPF50+ sunscreen should be used during the day.

Q. What is the procedure method?

A.
- Superficial chemical peels are a minor procedure and no special arrangements are needed. But you may need painkillers, sedation, local anesthetic or even a general anesthetic for deeper peels.
- First, the face is thoroughly washed to remove surface oil. The peeling agent is then applied for several minutes. It stings—how badly and for how long depends on the chemical, its concentration, whether you've had pretreatment with aspirin, and individual factors. A fan can help. The peel is then neutralized, and the burning sensation lessens.
- Individual treatments may include peels with several agents on the same occasion, with the aim of improving results and reducing risks.
- Antibiotics and oral antiviral agents may be recommended after deeper peels

Q. What is the post peel skin care regimen?

A.
- Keep treated areas cool (use a water spray or ice pack).
- Picking should be avoided moisturize—use light preparations after a superficial peel, thicker moisturizers after a deeper peel
- Protect from the sun with sunscreen, especially for the first 6 months
- If advised to do so, tretinoin, glycolic acid and/or hydroquinone at night long-term can be used.

Q. What are the complications of chemical peels?

A Comedones or acne may result from the peel itself or from thick moisturizers used afterwards; ask your dermatologist for treatment.

- Infection due to bacteria, yeast, or virus can be caused by peels
- Scarring may result from infection or picking the scabs, and can be permanent.
- Blotchy pigmentation is most likely in those with darker skin or who had a pigmentation problem before the peel; keep out of the sun and use hydroquinone.

7 Platelet Rich Plasma

Q. What is platelet-rich plasma?

A. Platelet-rich plasma (PRP) is an increased concentration of autologous platelets suspended in a small amount of plasma after centrifugation and used for injection into a wound or a particular skin condition. Platelet-rich plasma is also called autologous platelet gel, plasma rich in growth factors (PRGF), and platelet concentrate (PC).

Blood normally consists of approximately 93% red blood cells (RBC), 1% white blood cells (WBC) and 6% platelets, suspended in plasma. The normal platelet count range is 150,000–350,000/μL of blood. In platelet-rich plasma, the RBC count is lowered to 5 while the platelet count is increased to 94% (three to eight-fold greater than normal).

Q. How is platelet-rich plasma collected?

A. Blood is withdrawn from a patient's arm by syringe.

- The tubes containing withdrawn blood are placed in a centrifuge and spun using a carefully determined protocol.
- The speed and duration of centrifugation are very important to ensure the platelets are not damaged.
- Centrifuging separates the red and white blood cells and platelets and concentrates them at various levels in the tubes.
- Blood plasma that is rich in platelets is drawn off from the appropriate level for therapeutic use.
- An activating agent (e.g., calcium chloride) is added to activate the platelets and release their content prior to use.

Q. Indications for platelet-rich plasma injections.

A.
- Venous and arterial leg ulcers
- Diabetic foot ulcers
- Pressure ulcers (bedsores)
- Skin graft donor sites
- First- and second-degree thermal burns
- Superficial injuries, cuts, abrasions and surgical wounds
- Hair loss – PRP has been shown to reinvigorate dormant hair follicles and stimulate new hair growth in male pattern alopecia

- Post-traumatic scars – PRP combined with centrifuged fat tissue and fractional laser resurfacing improve the cosmetic appearance of scars
- Facial rejuvenation
- PRP injections can treat wrinkles, photodamage and discoloration and is often used in conjunction with other treatments such as facelift, dermal implants, and reconstructive procedures.

Q. Advantages of platelet-rich plasma.

A. As an autologous preparation, PRP is safer to use than allogenic or homologous preparations and is free from concerns over transmissible diseases such as HIV, hepatitis, West Nile fever, and Creutzfeldt-Jakob disease.

Platelet-rich plasma requires no special considerations regarding antibody formation, effectively preventing the risk of graft-versus-host disease and leading to better acceptance by patients.

Q. Role of platelet-rich plasma in wound healing?

A. Platelet-rich plasma effects soft tissue healing via growth factors released after platelet degranulation. These growth factors initiate and enhance physiological processes that contribute to tissue recovery and healing after injury.

Growth-factor molecules associated with platelets include:

- Platelet-derived growth factor (PDGF-AA, PDGF-BB, PDGF-AB)
- Transforming growth factor-beta (TGF-β1, TFG-β2)
- Vascular endothelial growth factor (VEGF)
- Epidermal growth factor (EGF)
- Pro- and anti-inflammatory cytokines [interleukin (IL)-4], IL-8, IL-13, IL-17, tumor necrosis factor-alpha, and interferon-alpha
- Fibroblast growth factor-2 (FGF-2)
- Insulin-like growth factor (IGF)
- Fibrin, fibronectin, vitronectin, thrombin.

These growth factors aid healing by:

- Attracting undifferentiated stem cells into the newly formed matrix and triggering cell division
- Suppressing cytokine release and limiting inflammation
- Attracting macrophages to improve tissue healing and regeneration
- Promoting new capillary growth (new blood vessel formation), and accelerating epithelialization.

Q. Safety, complications and contraindications of platelet-rich plasma.

A. PRP is immunologically neutral and poses no danger of allergy, hypersensitivity or foreign-body reactions.

- Sterile technique must be used at every stage of PRP preparation and application. Sterile technique is especially important if a patient has an underlying medical condition that predisposes to infection.
- The PRP may be injected intralesional or perilesional or mixed with autologous thrombin at a 9:1 ratio, forming a platelet gel and used topically.
- When administered by intradermal injection, a brief period of inflammation at wound sites may be experienced. Nerve trauma is another potential complication.

The following medical conditions are a contraindication for use of PRP:

- Critical thrombocytopenia (low platelet count)
- Hypofibrinogenemia
- Hemodynamic instability (collapse)
- Sepsis (infection)
- Acute and chronic infections
- Chronic liver disease
- Anticoagulation therapy (warfarin, dabigatran, heparin).

8 Intralesional Drugs in Dermatology

INTRODUCTION

The main purpose of intralesional drugs is to achieve a high local therapeutic concentration which persists for a long-time and is not associated with major systemic side effects. Several drugs have been used intralesionally in dermatology, the foremost being corticosteroids but other drugs such as bleomycin, 5-fluorouracil, interferon α, vincristine, methotrexate and antimonials have also been used for various indications.

Q. Discuss intralesional steroids (ILS).

A. Many conditions have been treated with ILS. The main reason is that in these conditions topical steroids cannot penetrate enough due to thickened or impervious epidermal barrier. The classical drug used is injection. Triamcinolone acetonide (10 or 40 mg/mL).

Triamcinolone is preferred for the following reasons:

- Physical characteristics of the molecule: They are small, doesn't crystalline and stay stable for at least 1 week at room temperature and resuspend after being shaken
- Since the particles are small, chances of occlusion or embolism are reduced
- Triamcinolone is the most insoluble of the steroids and it remains at the site of injection for a long time
- Triamcinolone has a long half-life
- The intralesional administration of triamcinolone is relatively painless
- Of the various salts of triamcinolone, acetonide is preferred because it has a longer duration of action and less atrophogenic potential compared to diacetate or hexacetonide

Q. What are the various salts which can be used for intralesional injections?

A. Besides triamcinolone, betamethasone sodium phosphate (6 mg/mL), dexamethasone sodium phosphate (24 mg/mL), dexamethasone (4 mg/mL), prednisolone acetate (50 mg/vial) can also be used. Even hydrocortisone succinate can be used. This is in the form of a solution but the earlier preparations mentioned have to be diluted with sterile water or sodium chloride or dextrose and sodium chloride to make up the strength desired.

Q. What are the indications of intralesional steroids?

A. The following are the common indications:

- Alopecia areata
- Nodulocystic acne
- Keloids
- Hypertrophic scar
- Localized discoid lupus erythematosus
- Localized areas of eczema, e.g., Prurigo nodularis, LSC
- Localized and resistant plaques of psoriasis
- Nail psoriasis
- Hypertrophic lichen planus
- Oral lichen planus
- Nail lichen planus
- Benign lymphocytic infiltrate and lymphocytoma cutis
- Acne (folliculitis) keloidalis nuchae
- Granulomatous cheilitis (part of Melkersson-Rosenthal syndrome)
- Localized sarcoidosis
- Localized lesions of mycosis fungoides
- Myxoid cyst of the fingers
- Pretibial myxedema
- Necrobiosis lipoidica
- Pyoderma gangrenosum

Q. How are intralesional injections given?

A. Intralesional injections are commonly given with a tuberculin or insulin syringe having a nondetachable needle of 30 gauge. This needle helps in precision of dosing. Usually, 0.1 cc is given per cm^2. Another way to give intralesional is by an air-powered gun (Dermojet). The injection can be preceded by optional topical local EMLA application. If required, the solution may be diluted with sterile saline. Xylocaine is not preferred because it stings more. Though the gun is a little less painful, and nonthreatening to children, it can cause disruption of collagen and elastic fibers and should not be used in conditions where tissue destruction is not desired. E.g., Acne, cysts, discoid lupus erythematosus. The air-powered gun has a probably higher risk of introducing infection. It can also cause blindness if injected near the eye or nail dystrophy in the nails. Treatments are repeated every 3–6 weeks with triamcinolone.

Q. What are the side effects of ILS?

A. Immediate:

- Extreme pain at injection site (common with betamethasone)
- Syncopal or vasovagal attack
- Anaphylaxis, especially if lignocaine is used as a diluent
- An extremely rare effect is amaurosis fugax which is transient blindness that occurs after injecting eyebrows in alopecia areata. It is due to embolization in the retinal blood vessels. Though rare, it is extremely alarming.

Early:

- Secondary infections
- Suppression of local tissue healing

Late:

- Atrophy: It is related to the concentration of the steroid injected and the area of the body. Areas like face, genitals, lips, and buccal mucosa are very prone. On these areas it is better to dilute the steroid to make the concentration 5 mg/mL or even 2.5 mg/mL instead of the 10 mg/mL provided.
- Pigmentary changes: Hypo- and hyperpigmentation may occur telangiectasia
- Suppression of the HPA axis: This occurs only with repeated injections over large areas.
- Eye changes—cataract and increased intraocular pressure

Q. Discuss use of ILS in alopecia areata.

A. ILS works best in patients with less than 50% of scalp hair loss, and in those with a shorter duration of hair loss. Patients with extensive AA, rapidly progressive disease and greater than 2 years duration of disease respond poorly. It is seen that patients with a positive hair pull test and exclamation point hairs respond better to ILS because these two signs indicate active inflammation which is best targeted by steroids. The exact mechanism of action of ILS in alopecia areata is uncertain, but immunosuppression is the main mechanism. Steroids suppress the T cell mediated immune attack on the hair follicle (swarm of bees) and change the composition of the local cells from suppressor to effector cells.

Q. Discuss intralesional methotrexate.

A. Methotrexate has been used in the concentration of 12.5–25 mg/mL. It has been used to treat mainly keratoacanthomas. It is recommended that baseline laboratory monitoring like CBC, LFT, BUN and serum creatinine be done. Side effects reported are local pain, erythema, crusting and necrosis while systemically pancytopenia, GI side effects, hepatotoxicity and nephrotoxicity are seen. Concomitant use of probenecid, penicillin and sulfonamides is to be avoided.

Q. Discuss use of intralesional bleomycin.

A. Bleomycins are a group of complex glycopeptides antibiotics which are derived from a *Streptomyces* species. Bleomycin is absorbed by all routes and is mainly detoxified by renal excretion. Intralesional bleomycin has been used for the treatment of recalcitrant warts (especially plantar and periungual) as well as in treatment of BCC, SCC in situ and keratoacanthomas. The drug concentration is 0.5 mg/mL. About three treatments are given at intervals of 7 days between successive injections. The total dose is 1.2 mg (0.4 mg/week). Baseline CBC is recommended. Side effects are pain, erythema, crusting, necrosis, ulceration and flagellate pigmentation while systemically pulmonary toxicity, Raynaud's phenomenon and cutaneous sclerosis. A lot of patients experience pain at the site of injection which is transient. Erythema develops on the day after the injection. An eschar develops 1 week after injection which separates in 2–3 weeks, usually without scarring. Bleomycin inhibits DNA synthesis, and hence works in treatment of warts.

Q. Discuss intralesional 5-Fluorouracil.

A. 5-FU is a pyrimidine antagonist. It inhibits the enzyme thymidilate synthetase, thus disrupting DNA synthesis. Hence it is useful in malignancies. 5-FU is used in the concentration of 50 mg/mL. It can be used in the treatment of keratoacanthomas and basal cell carcinomas, especially those which are recurrent. The side effects are local pain, erythema, necrosis and ulceration, while systemically, pancytopenias can result. 5-FU has also been used in the treatment of keloid, once every 2 weeks, either alone or in conjunction with ILS, pulse-dye laser, and topical imiquimod. 5-FU is found to inhibit fibroblast proliferation also.

Q. Discuss use of interferons intralesionally.

A. IFN-2, 2α and 2β, have been used for treating BCC, SCC, and KA. Intralesional IFN-α and γ have been used to treat BCC. IFNs stimulate macrophages, NK cells, and upregulate MHC antigens. They also induce expression of CD95 receptor, resulting in apoptosis. IFN is usually given in the dose of 3x 106 U injected into the lesion thrice weekly for 2 weeks. Both local and systemic side effects (fever, myalgia etc.,) have been reported.

Q. Discuss use of intralesional rituximab.

A. Rituximab, an anti-CD20 monoclonal antibody has proven activity against B cell lymphomas. It can be used to treat localized primary cutaneous B cell lymphomas in a dose of 10–30 mg/lesion three times weekly for 1 week, and repeated after 4 weeks. The only side effect reported is local pain.

Q. Discuss some other agents used in intralesional therapy.

A. Intralesional mistletoe extract has been used for the treatment of primary cutaneous lymphomas. Interleukin-2 has been used for lymphomas as well as basal cell carcinomas. Aminolevulenic acid, a photodynamic agent, can be used intralesionally for superficial BCC and SCC in situ.

9 Dermatological Drugs in Pregnancy and Lactation

There are three classifications to define pregnancy risk categories of drugs used in pregnancy.

1. The United States Food and Drug Administration (USFDA)
2. The Swedish Catalogue of Approved Drugs (FASS)
3. The Australian Drug Evaluation Committee (ADEC)

We will be only using the USFDA classification throughout this chapter and even elsewhere.

TABLE 1: Percentage of drugs for different classes.

Class	*Definition*	*Clinical studies*	*Animal studies*	*% drugs*
A	Completely safe	No evidence of risk	No evidence of risk	4
B	No evidence of risk to fetus	Limited/not available	No evidence of risk	23
		No evidence of risk	Adverse fetal effects	
C	Risk cannot be ruled out	Not available	Not available	45%
		Not available	Adverse fetal effects	
D	Positive evidence of risk	Shows fetal risks	Adverse fetal effects	22
X	Totally contraindicated	Significant fetal risks	Significant adverse fetal effects	6

TABLE 2: Lactation, the Hale Classification.

Class	*Comment*
L1	Safest
L2	Safer
L3	Moderately Safe
L4	Possibly harmful
L5	Totally contraindicated

TABLE 3: Topical anti-inflammatory drugs in pregnancy.

Name	*USFDA class*	*Lactation class*	*Comment*
Topical steroids	C	L1 (Mild) L2-L3 (Potent)	Usually safe, but avoid potent steroids on nipple area
Topical calcineurin inhibitors	C	L2 but L4 on nipple	Don't use on nipple, since oral absorption is significant
Calcipotriol	C	L3	Use less than 100 g per week, use on <20% body surface area
Anthralin	C	L3	Don't use on nipple, avoid contact with infant's skin
Coal tar	Not available	Not available	Since it is mutagenic, better to avoid in both pregnancy or lactation

TABLE 4: Systemic anti-inflammatory, immunomodulatory and immunosuppressive drugs in pregnancy.

Name	*USFDA*	*Lactation*	*Comments*
Corticosteroids	C	L3	There is a slightly increased risk of cleft palate in first trimester of pregnancy. Lactating mothers should wait for about 4 hours after ingestion to breastfeed. Better to use short courses (<3 weeks) during lactation
Dapsone	C	L4	Neonatal hemolytic anemia and kernicterus recorded in third trimester. Risk of hemolytic anemia exists for breast fed infants. However, it should not be stopped in leprosy patients either in pregnancy or lactation. In other indications, better to stop it in lactation
Hydroxy-chloroquine	C	L2	It is drug of first choice for active lupus in pregnancy. There is slow elimination of HCQS in infant, hence there is a risk of accumulation. Mostly, however, it can be given in lactation

Continued

Continued

Name	USFDA	Lactation	Comments
PUVA	C	L4	Better to avoid in pregnancy. Breastfeeding to be avoided for at least 24 hours after ingestion
Methotrexate	X	L5	Many congenital malformations can occur, including cranial, facial, cardiac, and GI. It can accumulate in the baby's tissues due to immature renal function. Hence totally contraindicated
Mycophenolate	D	L4	Mycophenolate can interfere with hormonal contraception. It can enter breast milk and cause increased frequency of infection and tumors in baby
Azathioprine	D	L3	It interferes with efficacy of IUD contraception can lead to preterm and low birth weight infants. Half the dose is advised 32 weeks gestation to prevent leukopenia in new born. Wait for 4 hours after ingesting it before feeding. Check infant's blood counts periodically
Cyclosporine	C	L3	Risk of prematurity and low birth weights. Can cause maternal hypertension. Infant needs to be monitored for tremors, seizures, hypertension, etc.
Acitretin	X	L5	Should be avoided in lactation due to potential for accumulation in baby
Biologicals	B	L2 (Infliximab) L3 (others)	Higher rate of VATER (Vertebral anomalies, Anal atresia, Tracheoesophageal fistula, Esophageal atresia, Renal abnormalities) in fetus. Live vaccines should be avoided for 6 months in infants with intrauterine exposure to biologicals. Unlikely that high amount of biological are excreted in milk

Continued

Continued

Name	USFDA	Lactation	Comments
Rituximab	C	L2	Preferable to avoid in pregnancy as it can cause hematological problems in neonate. In infants, can cause impaired GI development; avoid in lactation if possible and, if used, monitor blood counts
IVIG	C	L2	Is actually used in infertility, crosses placenta only after 32 weeks and not embryotoxic. No adverse effects in breast fed infants

TABLE 5: Systemic antihistamines in pregnancy and lactation.

Name	USFDA	Lactation	Comments
Chlorpheniramine	B	L3	First line agent in first trimester; transient irritability and drowsiness in infants; no effect on milk production
Diphenhydramine	B	L2	Slight increased risk of cleft palate but overall safe; same as with CPM for lactation
Hydroxyzine	C	L1	Slightly increased risk of congenital malformations; same as with CPM for lactation
Doxepin	C (oral) B (topical)	L5	Can cause hypotonia and weak suckling in infants in third trimester exposure, in lactation can cause sedation and hypotonia in infants
Loratidine	B	L1	Generally safe in pregnancy. Compatible for lactating mothers
Cetrizine	B	L2	Second choice second generation antihistamine in pregnancy. Observe baby for sedation during lactation
Fexofenadine	C	L2	Minimal data, hence use alternatives in pregnancy

TABLE 6: Topical and systemic anti acne (and antirosacea) drugs in pregnancy and lactation.

Name	*USFDA*	*Lactation*	*Comments*
Benzoyl peroxide	C	NA	May be used on limited areas
Clindamycin	B	L2	No known fetal effects and safe in lactation
Erythromycin	B	NA	Presumed safe in both pregnancy and lactation
Azelaic acid	B	L3	No known fetal effects
Metronidazole	B	L3	Compatible topically with pregnancy and lactation
Sulfacetamide	C	NA	No known fetal effects
Tazarotene	X	L3	In lactation, can be used but in limited ares (20%)
Tretinoin adapalene	X	L3	Large studies indicate safety, but most experts do not recommend Can be used in lactation on limited areas
Isotretinoin	X	L5	Isotretinoin embryotoxicity; it accumulates in breast milk and cause toxicity in infants
Spironolactone	D	L2	Feminization of male fetus: possible milk suppression

TABLE 7: Topical anti infective drugs in pregnancy and lactation.

Name	*USFDA*	*Lactation*	*Comments*
Neomycin	C	L2	Local use safe, compatible with breastfeeding
Bacitracin	C	L2	Same as above
Polymyxin	B	L2	Compatible; use with care on nipple area
Mupirocin	B	L1	No known fetal effects, topical antibiotic of choice
Nystatin	A (Vaginal) C (Topical)	L1	Topical antifungal of choice; best studied
Clotrimazole	B	L1	Topical antifungal of choice; best studied

Continued

Continued

Name	USFDA	Lactation	Comments
Terbinafine	B	L2	Low risk in pregnancy; minimal systemic absorption
Ciclopirox	B	L3	Risk minimal; low systemic absorption
Selenium sulfide	C	L3	Local application for limited time; safe in lactation
Trichloro-acetic acid	NA	NA	Safe in pregnancy for condylomas; compatible in lactation
Salicylic acid	C	L3	Use on limited areas for limited time
Podophyllin	X	L3	Maternal fetal death; heart, car and limb defects; uncertain if advisable in lactation
Podofilox	C	L3	Minimal data; uncertain if advisable in lactation
Cantharidin	C	NA	Minimal data; uncertain if advisable in lactation
Imiquimod	C	NA	Minimal data; uncertain if advisable in lactation
Precipitated sulphur	B	NA	Minimal data; likely to be safe
Benzyl benzoate	C	NA	Banned in USA; but probably safe in lactation
GBH	C	L4	Teratogen; avoid in lactation causes seizures, hypersensitivity and liver derangement
Crotamiton	C	NA	Likely safe in both pregnancy and lactation
Permethrin	B	L2	First line therapy in both pregnancy and lactation.
Pyrethrin	C	L2	Second line therapy for lice (first line is occlusive therapy)
Malathion	B	L4	Avoid if possible in lactation, can cause respiratory depression

TABLE 8: Systemic Antiinfectives in Pregnancy and Lactation.

Name	*USFDA*	*Lactation*	*Comments*
Penicillin	B	L1	Antibiotic of choice in both pregnancy and lactation
Cephalo-sporins	B	L1-L2	Older cephalosporins preferred
Erythromycin	B	L2	Can cause maternal hepatotoxicity hence not preferred; can cause heart defects/ pyloric stenosis in fetus/ newborn
Azithromycin	B	L2	Second line macrolide after erythromycin
Clarithromycin	C	L2	Second line macrolide after erythromycin
Clindamycin	B	L2	Risk of colitis and use if all above are ineffective
Sulfonamides	C	L3	Peripartum hyperbilirubinemia, avoid lactation in G6PD deficient infants
Trimethoprim	C	L2	Causes folate depletion in pregnancy; supplement breastfeeding infant with folates
Rifampicin	C	L2	Rx of choice for TB and leprosy, give vitamin K prophylaxis in peripartum period
Tetracyclines	D	L4	Contraindicated due to bone growth defects and teeth discoloration
Quinolones	C	L2	Use only in antibiotic resistance; observe for diarrhea in breastfeeding infants
Griseofulvin	C	L2	Avoid in pregnancy (cases of conjoined twins); minimal data in lactation: best avoid
Keto/ Flu/Itra/ conazole	C	L2	Risk during pregnancy but safe in lactation
Terbinafine	B	L1	Can be given for severe infections
Acyclovir	B	L2	First line therapy for herpes genitalis
Valacyclovir	B	L1	Second line therapy for herpes genitalis
Famciclovir	B	L2	Third line therapy for herpes genitalis

TABLE 9: Miscellaneous Topicals and Systemic Agents in Pregnancy and Lactation.

Name	***USFDA***	***Lactation***	***Comments***
Lignocaine	B	L2	Safe in pregnancy and lactation
Epinephrine	C	L1	Safe in pregnancy and lactation in low doses
Minoxidil	C	L2	Best avoid in pregnancy as cases of newborns with birth defects reported: compatible in lactation
Botulinum toxin	C	L3	Best avoid in pregnancy but compatible in lactation
Hydroquinone	C	L3	Avoid in pregnancy (mutagen) but use in lactation probably safe
Spironolactone	D	L2	Male feminization occurs during pregnancy; possible suppression of milk in lactation
Ivermectin	C	L3	Only if topical permethrin fails, then use
Finasteride	X	NA	Can cause feminization of genitalia of male fetus; not known whether excreted in breast milk

Index

Page numbers followed by *t* refer to table

B

C

D

E

Q

R

S

U

V

W

X

Z